Medical Care of the Liver Transplant Patient, 3E

Medical Care of the Liver Transplant Patient, 3E

Total Pre-, Intra- and Post-Operative Management

Edited by

Paul G. Killenberg, MD
Professor of Medicine
Division of Gastroenterology
Duke University Medical Center
Durham, North Carolina, USA

Pierre-Alain Clavien, MD, PhD
Professor and Chairman
Department of Visceral and Transplantation Surgery
University Hospital Zurich
Zurich, Switzerland

Associate Editors

Alastair Smith, MD
Associate Professor
Medicine – Gastroenterology
Duke University Medical Center
Durham, North Carolina, USA

Beat Müllhaupt, MD
Gastroenterology-Hepatology
University Hospital Zurich
Zurich, Switzerland

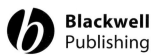

Blackwell
Publishing

Blackwell Publishing, Inc.,
350 Main Street, Malden,
Massachusetts 02148-5020, USA

Blackwell Publishing Ltd,
9600 Garsington Road,
Oxford OX4 2DQ, UK

Blackwell Publishing Asia Pty Ltd,
550 Swanston Street, Carlton,
Victoria 3053, Australia

Second edition published 2001

Third edition published 2006

2   2008

Library of Congress Cataloging-in-Publication Data
Data available

ISBN: 978-1-4051-3032-5

A catalogue record for this title is available from the British Library

Set in Palatino 10/14pt
by SPI Publisher Services, Pondicherry, India
Printed and bound in India by Replika Press Pvt. Ltd

Commissioning Editor: Alison Brown
Development Editor: Mirjana Misina
Production Controller: Kate Charman

For further information on Blackwell Publishing, visit our website:
http://www.blackwellpublishing.com

The publisher's policy is to use permanent paper from mills that operate a sustainable forestry policy, and which has been manufactured from pulp processed using acid-free and elementary chlorine-free practices. Furthermore, the publisher ensures that the text paper and cover board used have met acceptable environmental accreditation standards.

Contents

List of Contributors

Kaushik Agarwal, B Med Sci (Hons), MD, MRCP (UK),
Regional Liver and Transplant Unit,
Freeman Hospital,
Newcastle upon Tyne, UK

Barbara D. Alexander, MD,
Division of Infectious Diseases,
Department of Medicine,
Duke University Medical Center,
Durham, North Carolina

Peter Bauerfeind, MD,
Department of Gastroenterology and
   Hepatology,
University Hospital Zurich,
Zurich, Switzerland

M. Jordi Bruix, MD,
BCLC Group, Liver Unit,
   Hospital Clinic,
University of Barcelona,
Barcelona, Spain

Leo Bühler, MD,
Department of Surgery,
University Hospital Geneva,
Geneva, Switzerland

Martin Burdelski, MD,
Department of Pediatrics,
Children's Medical Center,
University Hospital Hamburg-Eppendorf,
Hamburg, Germany

S. Ravi Chari, MD,
Division of Hepatobiliary Surgery and
   Liver Transplantation,
Vanderbilt University Medical Center,
Nashville, Tennessee

Robyn Lewis Claar, PhD,
Department of Psychiatry,
Harvard Medical School,
Children's Hospital Boston,
Boston, Massachusetts

Pierre-Alain Clavien, MD, PhD, FACS,
Department of Visceral and
   Transplantation Surgery,
University Hospital Zurich,
Zurich, Switzerland

Bradley H. Collins, MD,
Department of Surgery,
Duke University Medical Center,
Durham, North Carolina

ix

Jeffrey T. Cooper, MD,
Department of Surgery,
Tufts-New England MedicalCenter,
Boston, Massachusetts

Dev M. Desai, MD, PhD,
Department of Surgery,
Duke University Medical Center,
Durham, North Carolina

Jean-François Dufour, MD,
Clinical Pharmacology,
University of Bern,
Bern, Switzerland

Richard B. Freeman, MD,
Department of Surgery,
Tufts-New England Medical Center,
Boston, Massachusetts

Judith W. Gentile, RN, MSN, ANP,
Division of Gastroenterology,
Department of Medicine,
Liver Transplant Coordinator,
Duke University Medical Center,
Durham, North Carolina

Kimberly Hanson, MD,
Adult Infectious Diseases and Medical
  Microbiology,
Duke University Medical Center,
Durham, North Carolina

Michael A. Heneghan, MD, MRCPI,
Institute for Liver Studies,
Kings College Hospital,
London, UK

M. David N. Howell, MD, PhD,
Department of Pathology
Duke University Medical Center,
Durham, North Carolina

Julie S. Hudson, RN, MSN,
Liver Transplant Coordinator,
Duke University Medical Center,
Durham, North Carolina

Mark Hudson, MB, FRCP, FRCPE,
Liver Transplant Unit, Freeman Hospital,
Newcastle upon Tyne, UK

Zakiyah Kadry, MD,
Department of Surgery,
The Milton S. Hershey Medical Center,
Hershey, Pennsylvania

Wesley Kasen, MD,
Division of Gastroenterology/Hepatology,
University of Colorado Health Sciences,
Denver, Colorado

Paul G. Killenberg, MD,
Division of Gastroenterology,
Department of Medicine,
Duke University Medical Center,
Durham, North Carolina

Paul C. Kuo, MD, MBA,
Departments of Anesthesiology and
  Surgery,
Duke University Medical Center,
Durham, North Carolina

Juan-Carlos Martinez, MD,
Division of Dermatology,
Department of Medicine,
Duke University Medical Center,
Durham, North Carolina

Richard L. McCann, MD,
Department of Surgery,
Duke University Medical Center,
Durham, North Carolina

Lucas McCormack, MD,
Department of Visceral and
   Transplantation Surgery,
University Hospital Zurich,
Zurich, Switzerland

Andrew J. Muir, MD,
Division of Gastroenterology,
Department of Medicine,
Duke University Medical Center,
Durham, North Carolina

Beat Müllhaupt, MD,
Division of Gastroenterology &
   Hepatology,
University Hospital Zurich,
Zurich, Switzerland

Sarah A. Myers, MD,
Division of Dermatology,
Department of Medicine,
Duke University Medical Center,
Durham, North Carolina

Karli S. Pontillo, CSW,
Clinical Social Worker,
Duke University Medical Center,
Durham, North Carolina

Robert J. Porte, MD, PhD,
Section of Hepatobiliary Surgery and Liver
   Transplantation,
Department of Surgery,
Groningen University Medical Center,
Groningen, The Netherlands

Eberhard L. Renner, MD,
Internal Medicine,
University of Manitoba,
Winnipeg, Canada

Kerri M. Robertson, MD,
Department of Anesthesiology,
General Vascular and Transplant Division,

Duke University Medical Center,
Durham, North Carolina

Don C. Rockey, MD,
Division of Digestive and
   Liver Diseases,
Department of Medicine,
University of Texas,
Southwestern Medical Center
Dallas, Texas

Xavier Rogiers, MD,
Department of Hepatobiliary and
   Transplantation Surgery,
University Hospital Hamburg-Eppendorf,
 Hamburg, Germany

Margarita Sala, MD,
Barcelona Clinic Liver Center Group,
Hospital Clinic,
Barcelona, Spain

Rebecca A. Schroeder, MD,
Department of Anesthesiology and
   Surgery,
Duke University Medical Center,
Durham, North Carolina

Nazia Selzner, MD, PhD,
Division of Hepatology,
Department of Visceral & Transplantation
   Surgery,
University Hospital Zurich,
Zurich, Switzerland

Marcus Selzner, MD,
Department of Visceral and
   Transplantation Surgery,
University Hospital Zurich,
Zurich, Switzerland

**Alastair D. Smith, B Med Biol, MB ChB,
   FRCP (Glasg),**
Division of Gastroenterology,

Duke University Medical Center,
Durham, North Carolina

Stephen R. Smith, MD, MHS,
Division of Nephrology,
Department of Medicine,
Duke University Medical Center,
Durham, North Carolina

Paul Suhocki, MD,
Division of Vascular and Intervention,
Department of Radiology,
Duke University Medical Center,
Durham, North Carolina

David A. Tendler, MD,
Division of Gastroenterology,
Duke University Medical Center,
Department of Medicine,
Durham, North Carolina

James F. Trotter, MD,
Division of Gastroenterology/Hepatology,
University of Colorado Health,

Science Center,
Denver, Colorado

Janet E. Tuttle-Newhall, MD,
Division of Transplant Surgery,
Department of Surgery,
Duke University Medical Center,
Durham, North Carolina

Maria Varela, MD,
Barcelona Clinic Liver Center Group,
Hospital Clinic,
Barcelona, Spain

Mary K. Washington, MD, PhD,
Department of Pathology
Vanderbilt University,
Nashville, Tennessee

Marco Piero Zalunardo, MD,
Institute of Anesthesia,
University Hospital Zurich,
Zurich, Switzerland

Introduction

▼   ▼   ▼   ▼   ▼   ▼   ▼   ▼   ▼

THE PRACTICE of liver transplantation continues to evolve. Recently there has been increased attention on new developments such as the Model of End-stage Liver Disease (MELD) system for stratifying potential recipients, as well as to the issue of retransplantation in the context of limited donor organs and the closely related problem of recurrence of the original liver disease in the liver graft. Although the basic principles of medical care for the liver transplant patient have not changed, the context in which we view these patients has. In this third edition, we have incorporated some of these topical issues and have added new authors from several countries. Our objective remains to provide to both transplant and nontransplant physicians a frame of reference for the management of patients who are contemplating or who have already undergone liver transplantation.

We are grateful to our many colleagues who have agreed to author chapters in this book. We are also grateful to our colleagues at Blackwell Science: Alison Brown, Claire Bonnett, and, most recently, Mirjana Misina whose interest in this project has been so very important.

PGK
P-A C

Management of the Potential Transplant Recipient

Selection and Evaluation of the Recipient (including Retransplantation)

▼　　▼　　▼　　▼　　▼　　▼　　▼　　▼　　▼

Don C. Rockey

■ INTRODUCTION

End-stage liver disease (ESLD; cirrhosis) is a major health problem, causing more than 25,000 deaths each year in the USA. Although therapeutic options for cirrhosis are limited, it has become clear over the last decade that liver transplantation is an effective, and often life-saving, intervention for the cirrhotic patient. Indeed, given the excellent survival currently afforded by liver transplantation, it has become an accepted form of therapy for patients with ESLD. Further, as refinements in surgical technique, intensive care, diagnosis, and immunosuppression continue, survival is likely to improve; this has led to an ever-increasing number of centers performing transplantation. Transplantation carries significant operative risk; the success of liver transplantation is in part due to care in the selection of appropriate transplant recipients. Liver transplantation consumes enormous medical resources and requires that the patient remains on immunosuppressive medication for life. Thus, careful patient selection is critical.

The transplant community is currently faced with a major organ shortage. This has led to extraordinary pressure on organ allocation programs; many patients become seriously ill or die while on waiting lists. Since a successful outcome requires optimal patient selection and timing, the issue of which patients to list for transplant and when to transplant cirrhotic patients has generated great interest as well as considerable controversy. Many issues surround which patients are most appropriate to list for transplantation; in addition, there has been much recent discussion about the subject of timing of transplantation. For example, the transplant community has recently implemented the use of the model for end-stage liver disease (MELD) scoring system in an effort to more objectively allocate organs (see Chapter 6). Nonetheless, in the absence of more definitive guidelines about selection and timing of trans-

Table 1.1 *Steps in Referral of Patients for Transplantation*

1. Establish the presence of significant liver disease.
2. Assess the likelihood that transplantation will prolong survival and/or improve the quality of life.
3. Determine the level of interest on the part of the patient in transplantation.
4. Exclude the presence of severe underlying comorbid processes (infection, HIV, severe cardiopulmonary disease, malignancy).
5. Discuss with the patient the most appropriate transplant center(s).
6. Contact the transplant team.

plant, management of cirrhotic patients has truly become an art and requires more expertise than ever before.

In the context of the view that liver transplantation is potentially life-saving, yet at the same time, a limited resource, this chapter will provide an overview of the currently accepted indications and contraindications for transplantation. In addition, it will highlight controversial areas in patient selection and discuss the optimal timing of referral and timing of transplantation. The steps in referral of patients for liver transplantation are shown in Table 1.1.

■ WHO SHOULD BE CONSIDERED A CANDIDATE FOR LIVER TRANSPLANTATION?

Transplantation in the patient with chronic liver disease has two major purposes: the first is to prolong survival and the second is to improve the quality of life. Simply stated, therefore, transplantation should be considered in any patient with liver disease in whom the procedure would extend life expectancy beyond what the natural history of the underlying liver disease would predict or in whom transplantation is likely to improve quality of life. Having said this, the challenge in transplantation comes in selecting patients most appropriate for transplantation in the context of what is known about the natural history of disease and clinical factors impacting on the quality of life. Assessing these issues is the most critical step in referral of patients for transplantation. From a practical viewpoint, transplantation is indicated in patients who have an estimated expected survival of less than 1 year because of liver disease or an intolerable quality of life because of liver disease.

The survival of most patients with advanced liver disease is poor. Life expectancy for those with cirrhosis can be estimated by the criteria found in the Child–Turcotte–Pugh (CTP) classification system (Table 1.2). Survival of a patient with "Child's C cirrhosis" is on the order of 20–30% at 1 year and less than 5% at 5 years. In contrast, the survival rate after transplantation is 85–90% at 1 year and over 70% at 5 years. By the time the patient has evidence of advanced clinical liver disease (Child's C cirrhosis), the patient may not survive long enough to be evaluated, and ultimately transplanted. Survival can also be estimated using MELd (see chapter 6).

The quality of life of patients with cirrhosis is often poor, typically being adversely affected by fatigue, ascites, encephalopathy, and/or gastrointestinal bleeding. The quality of life after transplantation varies, with many patients reporting good general health, little bodily pain, and acceptable physical functioning [1]. Transplant recipients have reported large gains in those aspects of quality of life most affected by physical health, but smaller improvements in areas affected by psychological functioning [2] (see Chapter 28). Thus, patients' quality of life 1 year after transplantation may be difficult to predict based on pretransplantation variables, making it difficult to assess preoperatively whether transplantation will benefit some patients' quality of life [3,4]. For a variety of reasons, a significant number of patients undergoing transplantation remain unemployed and some patients perceive their health status to be poor [1]. Further, patients typically require lifelong immunosuppression, which is associated with its own set of risks and complications. It is important that both

Table 1.2 *Child–Turcotte–Pugh Classification of the Severity of Cirrhosis*

Clinical and Biochemical Measurements	*CTP Points Scored for Increasing Abnormality*		
	A (1)	*B (2)*	*C (3)*
Encephalopathy (grade)	None	1 and 2	3 and 4
Ascites	None	Slight	Moderate
Bilirubin (mg/dl)	1–2	2–3	>3
Albumin (g/L)	3.5	2.8–3.5	<2.8
Prothrombin time (s>)	1–4	4–6	>6

Child grade	Total score
A	5–6
B	7–8
C	≥10

The point-score system estimates the severity of cirrhosis. A point total of 10 or greater portends an extremely poor short-term prognosis.
Adapted from [49].

Table 1.3 *Indications for Transplantation*

Cholestatic disorders	**Acute fulminant hepatic failure**
Primary biliary cirrhosis[a]	Hepatitis A, B, or C[a]
Primary sclerosing cholangitis	Toxin
Cystic fibrosis	Amanita poisoning
Biliary atresia	Wilson's disease
	Unknown[a]
Chronic parenchymal diseases	
Hepatitis C cirrhosis[a]	**Rare indications**
Hepatitis B cirrhosis	Rare metabolic disorders
Cryptogenic cirrhosis[a]	Polycystic liver disease
Alcohol-related cirrhosis[a]	Budd–Chiari Syndrome
Autoimmune-related cirrhosis	Neoplasm
Hemochromatosis	Amyloidosis
Alpha-1-antitrypsin disease	
Wilson's disease	

[a]Most common.

the primary physician and the transplant team carefully assess the likelihood that transplantation will improve the individual patient's quality of life.

The effectiveness of transplantation is well established for most forms of liver disease. Currently, transplantation is commonly performed in patients with the diseases shown in Table 1.3. Although transplantation is commonly accepted for these indications, there are important considerations specific to some of these disorders that should be kept in mind; these are reviewed in several of the following chapters.

■ CONTRAINDICATIONS TO LIVER TRANSPLANTATION

Currently, there are few absolute contraindications to liver transplantation. Indeed, conditions that were thought to preclude transplantation 15 years ago are no longer considered even relative contraindications for transplantation. In general, the conditions that preclude transplantation (see Table 1.4) are those in which there has been enough experience to determine that the outcome of the patient, if transplanted, is not acceptable. It is important to emphasize that contraindications to transplantation are dynamic and ever-changing, and further, that contraindications to transplantation vary among liver transplant centers, reflecting local expertise. Generally accepted contraindications to transplantation are highlighted below.

Table 1.4 *Contraindications to Transplantation*

Absolute

Uncontrolled infection

Extrahepatic malignancy

Advanced hepatic malignancy

Active substance abuse

Medical noncompliance

Irreversible brain damage

Relative

Very old or young age

Anatomic difficulties

Severe extrahepatic disease

Adverse psychosocial factors

Absolute Contraindications

Uncontrolled Infection

Obligatory immunosuppression after transplantation impairs the natural host defense mechanisms and precludes successful transplantation. Since cirrhotic patients are predisposed to a number of infections prior to transplant, it is imperative that patients be carefully monitored and evaluated for infection. Although active infection precludes transplantation, most infections are ultimately curable. Important active infections in cirrhotics include routine pneumonia and its complications, urinary system infections, bone infections, especially osteomyelitis. Patients with cirrhosis are also predisposed to bacteremia, probably due to inefficient clearing of translocated gut bacteria. This appears to be a particular problem in patients with acute variceal hemorrhage. A number of studies have demonstrated a reduction in the incidence of bacteremia at the time of acute bleeding with the use of intercurrent antibiotics [5]. Thus, transplantation in the setting of acute variceal hemorrhage requires caution.

Special situations include patients with ascites and those with biliary obstructive diseases such as primary sclerosing cholangitis. Again, these conditions do not preclude transplantation, but must be addressed. Patients with ascites are at risk for spontaneous bacterial peritonitis; it is critical to emphasize that this disease may present with subtle clinical symptoms and signs (i.e. the classic triad of abdominal pain, fever, and leukocytosis is actually uncommon). Evidence now suggests that the incidence of spontaneous bacterial peritonitis can be reduced by prophylactic antibiotics; this is now routinely used in cirrhotics with ascites. Patients with biliary obstruction or primary sclerosing cholangitis are at risk for cholangitis or other localized hepatic infectious processes. A high level of suspicion and vigilance are required to detect and manage infection in these patients.

Tuberculosis may complicate liver transplantation and active tuberculosis (especially without ongoing therapy) precludes it. Liver transplantation is a risk factor for development of tuberculosis because of possible activation of latent infection or primary tuberculosis in those receiving immunosuppression post-transplantation [6]. A tuberculin skin test should be performed preoperatively in transplant candidates, and preventive treatment implemented in those with positive results. Radiographic signs of previous granulomatous disease may be important when the tuberculin skin test is negative, unknown, or anergy is present. With a high degree of suspicion and a proactive program, most cases of tuberculosis in transplant recipients can be avoided. Like tuberculosis, reactivation of latent fungal disease has been reported, but fortunately is extremely rare. A high level of suspicion is often required to make a specific diagnosis. For patients with a history of fungal infection, infectious disease consultation is recommended prior to transplantation.

The timing of transplantation in patients with acute infection or treated chronic infection is an important consideration. Transplantation should be delayed until there has been a clear clinical response to antibiotics; the precise timing of transplantation in the setting of infection typically requires coordination between the infectious disease consultant and the transplant team. A final important and practical consideration is that a number of highly resistant organisms are emerging in many hospitals; therefore, it is recommended not only to minimize use of antibiotics preoperatively but also to keep preoperative transplant patients out of the hospital if at all possible.

Malignancy

Immunosuppression impairs innate surveillance mechanisms; therefore, extrahepatic cancers typically exhibit an accelerated course following transplantation. For this reason, it is important to carefully evaluate for malignancy. The presence of hepatobiliary malignancy represents an important challenge in liver transplantation (see Chapter 8). Small hepatic tumors (<2–3 cm) do not appear to adversely impact outcome. In contrast, large or multicentric tumors pose a considerable risk of local spread and distant metastasis. Rare exceptions to this include patients with more benign tumors such as the fibrolamellar variant of hepatocellular carcinoma. Some centers are actively examining aggressive protocols of adjuvant and neoadjuvant therapy in patients with more advanced local malignancy.

Active Substance Abuse

Active substance abuse, including use of ethanol, is generally considered to be a contraindication to transplantation. The reasons for this are many, including the risk of recidivism, noncompliance, and potential injury to the graft and/or other organs (see Chapter 9). It is now common practice for transplant centers to require a period of absolute ethanol abstinence of at least 6 months. One of the most important reasons for this is that a certain proportion of patients who discontinue ethanol consumption will improve to the point where transplantation is not necessary. Additionally, a period of abstinence allows members of the health care team to develop a relationship with the patient and to more readily appreciate the social issues likely to be critical in the individual patient's long-term care. However, it is important to realize that the ''6-month abstinence rule'' is not perfect, and its use alone forces a significant number of patients with a low relapse risk, as assessed by other models such as the High Risk Alcoholism Relapse (HRAR) Scale, to wait for transplantation [7]. It is important for patients with any form of substance abuse to undergo extensive psychiatric evaluation before transplantation is considered.

Medical Noncompliance

As with active substance abuse, medical noncompliance raises many ethical issues in transplantation. Post-transplantation management, in large part due to the requirement for lifelong immunosuppression, is extremely challenging, even in the best of circumstances. Therefore, noncompliant patients generally should not be transplanted. If transplantation is even to be considered in such a patient, extensive psychiatric evaluation and counseling are essential.

Irreversible Brain Injury

Irreversible brain injury is most often an issue in patients with fulminant hepatic failure, and typically occurs as a result of cerebral edema and brain-stem herniation. The presence of irreversible brain injury is suggested by typical neurologic examination findings, computed tomographic abnormalities, or by documented intracerebral pressures greater than 50 mmHg. Management of these issues in the setting of fulminant hepatic failure is typically performed by the transplant center team after the patient has been moved to a transplant center. Irreversible brain injury can occur rapidly in the patient with fulminant hepatic failure, emphasizing the need for careful evaluation at all stages as well as the importance of early referral of patients with this process (see Chapter 13).

The other clinical situation in which the topic of irreversible brain injury becomes an issue is in the patient with chronic liver disease who presents with altered mental status. This is typically due to worsened encephalopathy as a result of medical noncompliance, gastrointestinal bleeding, or infection, to name a few causes. It should be noted, however, that neurological deterioration in patients with chronic liver disease can result also from cerebral edema due to increased intracranial pressure [8]. It is important to differentiate between the two conditions since cerebral edema places the patient at too high a risk for liver transplantation.

Relative Contraindications

Clinical conditions that may adversely affect the outcome of liver transplantation, but do not absolutely proscribe it, are considered relative contraindications (see Table 1.4). The list of relative contraindications varies among centers and is actively evolving. Since this area is rapidly changing, it is best for clinicians caring for patients who may have a relative contraindication to transplantation to have a low threshold for referring them to a transplant center.

Age

Transplantation in either very young or very old patients is difficult; however, age boundaries are not fixed, and are continually being extended. Transplantation can be performed successfully in patients over the age of 60, as well as in children as young as 1 year. Transplantation in the first year of life is associated with low survival rates, and thus should be delayed in this period if possible (see Chapter 31). Further, transplantation has been successfully performed in patients as old as 70, although an age of 65 is generally considered to be the upper limit for transplantation. When questions about age arise, they should be discussed with the transplant center team.

General Medical Conditions

Liver transplantation can be safely performed in patients with minimal degrees of coronary artery disease. Advanced coronary artery disease has been traditionally considered to be an absolute contraindication to transplantation because chronic liver failure increases the surgical risk for coronary artery bypass grafting. However, simultaneous coronary artery bypass grafting and liver transplantation has been successfully performed [9]. Thus, in selected cases, the presence of advanced coronary artery disease may not preclude transplantation.

Pulmonary and renal disease may also pose important problems for the patient undergoing transplantation. In patients with significant chronic pulmonary or renal disease, it is best for the transplant center to evaluate the risk of surgery in the context of the potential benefit of transplantation. It should further be noted that multiorgan transplantation (i.e. liver/kidney, liver/lung), though complicated, is feasible.

Surgical

Anatomic difficulties resulting from previous abdominal trauma and previous abdominal surgeries pose significant potential problems for patients who are otherwise good transplant candidates. These issues are best addressed by individual transplant centers. Portal vein thrombosis also poses added risk for transplantation, but portal vein reconstruction or thrombectomy is often possible. In contrast, extensive mesenteric thrombosis typically precludes transplantation. Transplantation has been performed in cases of congenital anomalies including situs inversus and dextrocardia. Again, expertise varies among centers, requiring referral to a transplant center for assessment as to the feasibility of transplantation.

Human Immunodeficiency Virus

The experience with human immunodeficiency virus (HIV) infection and solid organ transplantation has historically been unfavorable [10]. However, the introduction of highly active antiretroviral therapy (HAART) has substantially changed this position. Patients who had HIV at the time of transplantation typically went on to develop full-blown anti-immunodeficiency syndrome (AIDS); most died due to AIDS-related complications. Many transplant centers have taken the position that the risk of transplantation in patients with HIV infection (even in the absence of AIDS) outweighs the potential benefit. However, recent data suggest that liver transplantation can be performed successfully in carefully selected HIV-infected patients [11,12], typically those controlled on HAART, in whom viral levels are low and CD4 counts are relatively normal. Such patients should be referred to a center with experience and interest in this area – where, if transplanted, they will receive care based on specific protocols. Over the next several years, up to 125 HIV positive liver transplant recipients will be enrolled in a National Institutes of Health (NIH)-funded study (http://spitfire.emmes.com/study/htr/Centers/centers.html) designed to focus on this topic.

■ TIMING OF TRANSPLANTATION

Overview

The timing of transplantation is an important, yet difficult, issue; transplantation should be performed before the patient has experienced complications that endanger life. Thus, timing of transplantation depends on understanding the natural history of the patient's disease, as well as patient-specific factors. Transplantation must be performed early enough so that a satisfactory outcome is probable; outcome is particularly poor in patients who are in an intensive care unit or those with multisystem organ failure at the time of transplantation. However, transplantation should not be performed too early given the shortage of organs, the risk of surgery, and the cost and risks associated with chronic immunosuppression.

Several important variables complicate the timing of transplantation, especially the variability in human physiology and disease; it may be difficult to predict the natural history of disease in specific patients. For example, patients with cholestatic liver diseases (i.e. primary biliary cirrhosis (see Table 1.5) and primary sclerosing cholangitis) typically have a different natural history than those with liver disease that is predicated on hepatocellular injury (i.e. autoimmune hepatitis or hepatitis C virus (HCV)). Thus, transplantation should be timed by combining the best objective prognostic data with subjective assessment of the individual patient.

The Art and Science of Timing Liver Transplantation

Patients who are too well should not be transplanted. Likewise, transplantation of patients who are too sick is associated with poor outcomes. Since the goal of transplantation is to prolong survival, liver transplantation should be performed at the time point when the patient is expected to have greater survival with a liver transplant than without. While there is some art to

Table 1.5 *Calculation of the Mayo Risk Score for Primary Biliary Cirrhosis*

Step 1: Calculate R

$R = 0.871 \times \log_e$ (bilirubin in mg/dl)

$\quad -2.53 \times \log_e$ (albumin in g/dl)

$\quad +0.039 \times$ (age in years)

$\quad +\log_e \times$ (prothrombin time in seconds)

$\quad +0.859$ (if edema is present)

Step 2: To obtain the probability of survival for at least t more years, read $S_0(t)$ from the table and compute $S(t) = [S_0(t)]^{\exp(R-0.57)}$

t (years)	1	2	3	4	5	6	7
$S_0(t)$	0.970	0.941	0.883	0.833	0.774	0.721	0.651

predicting such timing, recent work has provided a more scientific basis for this. Indeed, newer data have led to implementation of the MELD scoring system, which is an objective, data-driven method of organ allocation (see Chapter 6).

In an effort to focus issues related to organ allocation and timing of transplant, the Department of Health and Human Services attempted to more clearly define the relevant principles, policies, and procedures on this subject [13]. It was emphasized that organs should be allocated among transplant candidates based on medical urgency; and that the role of waiting time should be minimized. The Institute of Medicine (IOM) also analyzed waiting times in transplant candidates and concluded that waiting list time did not contribute to an equitable organ allocation system [14]. This report recommended that the use of waiting time as an allocation criterion be abandoned altogether and that a more appropriate system be utilized. Further, it was felt that such an optimal system would allocate organs based on medical need and the natural history of the patient's disease using objective criteria rather than based on waiting times.

Issues with regard to timing and listing criteria for transplantation are less complicated in patients undergoing living donor liver transplantation (LDLT) since the transplant recipient typically identifies a donor, and the transplant is carried out in a controlled fashion (see Chapter 12). However, it is the policy of many centers that patients being considered for LDLT must continue to meet the general criteria for deceased donor (DD) transplantation. That is to say, the patient's predicted survival should be prolonged by transplantation. This is particularly important for LDLT since this procedure puts a healthy donor at risk.

What does the primary provider need to know about timing of transplant? Perhaps the most important caveat is that it is almost never too early to refer a patient for evaluation. If the patient is not ill enough to be considered, the worst outcome is that the patient can be reassured and followed up. On the other hand, if the patient is referred too late, death while awaiting transplantation is a distinct possibility. Thus, from a practical standpoint, a patient who has any evidence of clinically advanced liver disease (i.e. elevated prothrombin time, elevated bilirubin, low albumin, any ascites, hepatic encephalopathy, and/or variceal bleeding) should be immediately considered for transplantation. Indeed, these clinical features identify patients with significant liver disease and should trigger consideration of transplant (see also Table 1.1), unless an obvious and absolute contraindication exists.

In terms of timing of transplantation for specific diseases, the decision to proceed with the transplant must be individualized; it is critical to emphasize that transplantation should be performed when the patient's condition and the natural history of the patient's disease portend a poor short-term survival. The MELD system, while not perfect, is a clear improvement over the previous waiting time-based system and has substantially simplified the process of liver allocation. It is thus important for the clinician to be familiar with MELD.

Retransplantation

An important issue given the large number of patients who have undergone liver transplantation is how to manage those who have graft failure. Currently, retransplantation accounts for approximately 10% of all liver transplants. Further, the number of patients requiring retransplantation is likely to grow as primary transplant recipients survive long enough to develop graft failure from recurrent disease. The limited supply of organs further complicates this issue as does the close relationship that often develops between transplanted patients and their care providers. Current clinical practice and some data suggest that retransplantation is effective in the setting of primary nonfunction [15]. However, data now demonstrate that survival after retransplantation for late-onset graft failure is less than after initial transplantation [16–18].

Perhaps the most controversial issue, with regard to retransplantation, concerns retransplantation for graft failure due to recurrent hepatitis C. Recurrence of HCV is nearly universal after transplantation [19] and appears to adversely affect outcome [20]. Further, despite advances in therapy for HCV, treatment of HCV in the immunosuppressed patient after transplantation is difficult. Indeed, recurrent HCV clearly leads to graft loss, and those who undergo retransplantation for HCV appear to have poorer outcomes than those who undergo retransplantation for other diseases [21–23]. Indeed, the experience of many centers with retransplantation for HCV has been grim. Thus, it has become the policy of some transplant centers to abandon the practice of retransplantation of HCV patients.

An important emerging theme is that retransplantation is somewhat different than primary transplantation, and guidelines (in particular use of MELD) for patients requiring retransplantation may not be the same as for those receiving their first transplant. For example, in studies of retransplanted patients, the 1-year and 5-year survival rates for patients with either CTP scores less than 10 or MELD scores less than or equal to 25 were significantly better than in patients retransplanted who had higher scores. Another study suggested that retransplantation should be performed prior to the development of renal insufficiency [15]. Thus, the message seems to be that retransplantation should be considered early, and the current MELD-based timing methodology may need to be adjusted for retransplantation. Most importantly, the decision to undergo retransplantation is one that should take into account patient-specific as well as center-specific variables.

■ **SUMMARY**

In compliant patients who meet the criteria for clinical severity, and have an understanding of the implications of transplantation (i.e. the requirement for close follow-up, lifelong immunosuppression, etc.), detailed evaluation is indicated. This evaluation includes assessment of medical and surgical risks, psychological evaluation, and continued patient education (see Chapter 2). Following completion of this evaluation by the transplant team, a meeting of the whole team is held to determine the suitability of the patient for transplantation. If it is agreed that transplantation will prolong survival and/or improve quality of life, the patient is listed for transplantation using standard guidelines. For certain diseases the timing of transplantation can be difficult. The objective nature of the MELD system has removed much of the subjective nature of "waiting" from the transplant scenario. Nonetheless, this system is not perfect, and patients will continue to either die while waiting for transplantation or will become too ill to undergo transplantation. Finally, given the growing population of patients already having undergone liver transplantation, the role of retransplantation, particularly for HCV, is under evolution.

■ **ACKNOWLEDGMENTS**

This work was supported by the Burroughs Wellcome Fund.

■ **REFERENCES**

1. Hunt CM, Tart JS, Dowdy E, et al. Effect of orthotopic liver transplantation on employment and health status. Liver Transpl Surg 1996;2:148–153.

2. Bravata DM, Olkin I, Barnato AE, et al. Health-related quality of life after liver transplantation: a meta-analysis. Liver Transpl Surg 1999;5:318–331.

3. Gross CR, Malinchoc M, Kim WR, et al. Quality of life before and after liver transplantation for cholestatic liver disease. Hepatology 1999;29:356–364.

4. Boker KH, Dalley G, Bahr MJ, et al. Long-term outcome of hepatitis C virus infection after liver transplantation. Hepatology 1997;25:203–210.

5. Bernard B, Grange JD, Khac EN, et al. Antibiotic prophylaxis for the prevention of bacterial infections in cirrhotic patients with gastrointestinal bleeding: a meta-analysis. Hepatology 1999;29:1655–1661.

6. Chaparro SV, Montoya JG, Keeffe EB, et al. Risk of tuberculosis in tuberculin skin test-positive liver transplant patients. Clin Infect Dis 1999;29: 207–208.

7. Yates WR, Martin M, LaBrecque D, et al. A model to examine the validity of the 6-month abstinence criterion for liver transplantation. Alcohol Clin Exp Res 1998;22:513–517.

8. Donovan JP, Schafer DF, Shaw BW, Jr, et al. Cerebral oedema and increased intracranial pressure in chronic liver disease. Lancet 1998;351:719–721.

9. Benedetti E, Massad MG, Chami Y, et al. Is the presence of surgically treatable coronary artery disease a contraindication to liver transplantation? Clin Transplant 1999;13:59–61.

10. Bouscarat F, Samuel D, Simon F, et al. An observational study of 11 French liver transplant recipients infected with human immunodeficiency virus type 1. Clin Infect Dis 1994;19:854–859.

11. Ragni MV, Belle SH, Im K, et al. Survival of human immunodeficiency virus-infected liver transplant recipients. J Infect Dis 2003;188:1412–1420.

12. Stock PG, Roland ME, Carlson L, et al. Kidney and liver transplantation in human immunodeficiency virus-infected patients: a pilot safety and efficacy study. Transplantation 2003;76:370–375.

13. Organ Procurement and Transplantation Network – HRSA. Final rule with comment period. Fed Regist 1998;63:16296–16338.

14. Institute of Medicine Analysis of waiting times. In: Committee on Organ Procurement and Transplantation Policy, ed., Organ procurement and transplantation: assessing current policies and the potential impact of the DHHS final rule. Washington, DC: National Academy Press, 1999:57–78.

15. Bilbao I, Figueras J, Grande L, et al. Risk factors for death following liver retransplantation. Transplant Proc 2003;35:1871–1873.

16. Facciuto M, Heidt D, Guarrera J, et al. Retransplantation for late liver graft failure: predictors of mortality. Liver Transpl 2000;6:174–179.

17. Kim WR, Wiesner RH, Poterucha JJ, et al. Hepatic retransplantation in cholestatic liver disease: impact of the interval to retransplantation on survival and resource utilization. Hepatology 1999;30:395–400.

18. Watt KD, Lyden ER, McCashland TM. Poor survival after liver retransplantation: is hepatitis C to blame? Liver Transpl 2003;9:1019–1024.

19. Testa G, Crippin JS, Netto GJ, et al. Liver transplantation for hepatitis C: recurrence and disease progression in 300 patients. Liver Transpl 2000;6:553–561.

20. Russo MW, Galanko J, Beavers K, et al. Patient and graft survival in hepatitis C recipients after adult living donor liver transplantation in the United States. Liver Transpl 2004;10:340–346.

21. Rayaie S, Schiano TD, Thung SN, et al. Results of retransplantation for recurrent hepatitis C. Hepatology 2003;38:1428–1436.

22. Neff GW. Factors that identify survival after liver retransplantation for allograft failure caused by recurrent hepatitis C infection. Liver Transpl 2004;10:1497–1503.

23. Yao FY, Saab S, Bass NM, et al. Prediction of survival after liver retransplantation for late graft failure based on preoperative prognostic scores. Hepatology 2004;39:230–238.

Monitoring the Patient Awaiting Transplantation

▼ ▼ ▼ ▼ ▼ ▼ ▼ ▼ ▼

Beat Müllhaupt

■ INTRODUCTION

Liver transplantation is the only treatment for patients with end-stage liver disease (ESLD). The success of liver transplantation led in most countries to a marked increase of patients on the waiting list, whereas the number of liver transplantations during the same time period increased only slightly. With the growing discrepancy between the numbers of donors and recipients, the median waiting time for liver transplantation has increased dramatically, exceeding in some countries 1–2 years. As a result, the number of patients who die while waiting is increasing and many others die after removal from the list because their clinical deterioration precludes successful transplantation. Accordingly, the management of patients on the waiting list is getting more important with the aim to maintain clinical stability so that liver transplantation can eventually be successfully performed. This is achieved by (1) prophylactic measures to prevent complications of ESLD and (2) early recognition and treatment of complications of advanced liver disease. Most stable patients can be managed as outpatients, with regular controls at the transplant center and in close collaboration with the referring physicians. The frequency of controls is determined by the clinical condition and the current treatment regimen (e.g. treatment for hepatitis C) and by the requirements of the national transplant and allocation organization. In the USA, for example, the frequency of blood controls is determined by the actual model for end-stage liver disease (MELD) score. Since the MELD score is a good predictor of 3 months' mortality on the waiting list, it is useful to see the patients at the intervals outlined in Table 2.1.

The most common complications of advanced liver disease, encountered in patients on the waiting list include refractory ascites, spontaneous bacterial peritonitis (SBP), hepatorenal syndrome (HRS), fluid and electrolyte disturb-

Table 2.1 *Adult Patient Reassessment and Recertification Schedule*

MELD Score	Status Recertification	Laboratory Values no Older Than
≥25	every 7 days	48 h
≤24 but >18	every 1 month	7 days
≤18 but ≥11	every 3 months	14 days
≤10 but >0	every 12 months	30 days

http://www.optn.org/PoliciesandBylaws/policies/docs/policy_8.doc

ances, portal hypertensive bleedings, hepatic encephalopathy (HE), hepato-cellular carcinoma (HCC), malnutrition and progress of other medical diseases. In addition, there are disease-specific aspects such as control of viral hepatitis and prevention of alcohol relapse. In this chapter the different aspects in the care of patients on the waiting list will be reviewed.

Refractory Ascites

The management of ascites and its complication is extensively covered in Chapter 3. Ascites is the most common complication in patients with ESLD. Approximately 50% of patients with compensated cirrhosis will develop ascites over a 10-year period [1]. Development of ascites is associated with 50% mortality after 2 years. The International Ascites Club recently recommended a new grading system for patients with ascites:

Grade 1: ascites can only be detected by ultrasound;
Grade 2: moderate ascites with symmetrical distention of the abdomen;
Grade 3: large or tense ascites with marked abdominal distension [2].

At the onset, ascites (Grade 2) usually can be easily controlled with diuretics and salt restriction (see Chapter 3), but with worsening portal hypertension the development of treatment-refractory or treatment-resistant ascites (Grade 3) is increasing. In this situation aggressive diuretic therapy places the patient at risk of developing renal failure, electrolyte disturbances, volume depletion and HE. Therefore, renal function and electrolytes have to be monitored carefully and any deterioration of renal function should be fully investigated. If ascites can no longer be controlled with diuretics or the use of diuretics is associated with renal insufficiency and electrolyte disturbances, patients can either be treated with large-volume paracentesis and plasma expanders or transjugular intrahepatic portosystemic shunt (TIPS).

In recent years five large randomized controlled trials have compared TIPS to repeated large-volume paracentesis [3–7]. In all studies ascites was better controlled with TIPS compared to large-volume paracentesis. In contrast to large-volume paracentesis, which has no effect on the mechanisms leading to ascites, TIPS is associated with a reduction in portal hypertension that decreases the activity of sodium-retaining mechanisms and improves the renal response to diuretics. Whether TIPS also improves survival is still controversial. In two studies the survival was improved in the TIPS group; however, this could not be confirmed in the other studies. There is also no evidence that TIPS improves the outcome after transplantation. Whether TIPS increases the technical difficulties of transplantation in some patients is controversial but such difficulties are usually uncommon in experienced centers [8,9].

Until recently the major disadvantages of TIPS were (1) the high rate of shunt stenosis (up to 75%), which led to the reappearance of ascites and (2) the development of HE (up to 77%) [10]. However, the recent introduction of polytetrafluoroethylene (PTFE)-covered prostheses improves TIPS patency and decreases the number of clinical relapses and reinterventions without increasing the risk of encephalopathy [11].

Paracentesis with albumin replacement remains the first treatment option for patients with refractory ascites on the waiting list [2]. Paracentesis with plasma volume expansion is safe, less costly and more widely available. Plasma volume expansion with albumin is superior to other plasma expanders (saline, polygeline, dextran-70) for large-volume paracentesis greater than 5 L [12,13]. To reduce the frequency of repeated paracentesis, patients should continue to receive diuretics as tolerated. If the frequency of paracentesis is greater than three times per month, the International Ascites Club recently recommended considering TIPS insertion [2]. In addition, TIPS should be considered for patients who do not tolerate large-volume paracentesis or where large-volume paracentesis is ineffective due to multiple adhesions or loculated ascites (Fig. 2.1).

Although randomized studies are lacking, TIPS should also be considered for patients with treatment-refractory hepatic hydrothorax. This results in resolution of the hepatic hydrothorax in approximately 70% of patients [14].

The peritoneovenous shunt (Le Veen shunt) is rarely used today due to the higher complication rate compared to TIPS or large-volume paracentesis [15]. In addition shunt-related adhesions can make subsequent liver transplantation more difficult. Therefore, the Le Veen shunt should not be considered in patients on the waiting list.

Spontaneous Bacterial Peritonitis

SBP is characterized by infection of the ascitic fluid in the absence of any known intra-abdominal source of infection. The diagnosis is established when there is a positive ascites culture and/or a polymorphonuclear cell

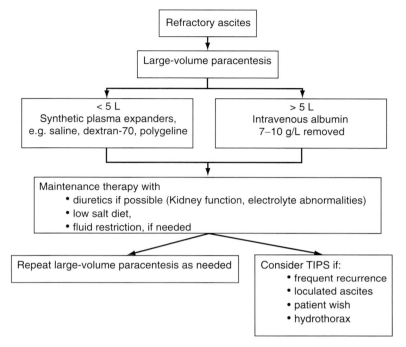

Fig. 2.1 *Treatment options for patients with refractory ascites.*

count (PMC) ≥ 250 cells/mm^3. The prevalence of SBP ranges between 10% and 30% in patients with ascites and is sufficiently common to justify a diagnostic paracentesis in every cirrhotic patient with ascites admitted to the hospital [16]. In addition, a paracentesis should be performed whenever there is clinical evidence for peritonitis (abdominal pain, rebound tenderness), clinical signs of infections (fever, leucocytosis, elevated C-reactive protein (CRP)), development of renal insufficiency, or HE.

In patients with a previous episode of SBP, the 1-year probability for a recurrent SBP ranges between 40% and 70% [17]. In addition, patients who never had SBP but have an increased bilirubin ($>40\,\mu$mol/L) and/or a low total ascitic fluid protein count ($>10\,$g/dl), as well as patients with variceal bleeding, have an increased risk for SBP. In patients with a previous history of SBP, the continuous administration of norfloxacin (400 mg/day) significantly reduced the 1-year probability of SBP from 68% in the placebo group to 20% in the norfloxacin group [18]. Secondary long-term prophylaxis is therefore recommended for all patients with a history of SBP (Table 2.2).

Patients without a history of SBP who have high ascitic fluid protein content ($>10\,$g/dl) have a low risk of infection (0% at 1 year, 3% at 3 years); primary prophylaxis is probably not justified in this patient population. It is unclear whether primary prophylaxis is justified in patients at high risk for SBP such as patients with an ascitic fluid protein content $<10\,$g/L or an

Table 2.2 *Diagnostic Criteria of Hepatorenal Syndrome*

Major criteria

1. Chronic or acute liver disease with advanced hepatic failure and portal hypertension.
2. Low glomerular filtration rate, as indicated by serum creatinine >133 μmol/L (1.5 mg/dl) or 24-h creatinine clearance <40 ml/min.
3. Absence of shock, ongoing bacterial infection, volume depletion, and current or recent treatment with nephrotoxic drugs.
4. No sustained improvement in renal function (decrease in serum creatinine to 1.5 mg/dl or less, or increase in creatinine clearance to 40 ml/min or more) following diuretic withdrawal and expansion of plasma volume with 1.5 L of isotonic saline.
5. No proteinuria (<500 mg/dl) and no ultrasonographic evidence of obstructive uropathy or parenchymal renal disease.

Additional criteria

1. Urine volume <500 ml/day in patients with cirrhosis.
2. Urine sodium <10 mEq/L.
3. Urine osmolality greater than plasma osmolality.
4. Serum sodium concentration <130 mEq/L.

Type of hepatorenal syndrome

Type 1: progressive impairment in renal function as defined by a doubling of initial serum creatinine above 220 μmol/L (2.5 mg/dl) in less than 2 weeks.

Type 2: stable or slowly progressive impairment in renal function not meeting the above criteria.

From [28].

elevated serum bilirubin (>40 μmol/L). In one study, the long-term antibiotic prophylaxis for primary prevention was superior compared to short-term prophylaxis, which was administered only if patients were hospitalized [19]. However, the emergence of infections caused by norfloxacin-resistant bacteria was significantly higher in the continuous long-term prophylaxis group. The benefits of primary prophylaxis in this patient group must therefore be carefully weighed against the selection of norfloxacin-resistant bacteria, but might be justified in selected cases on the waiting list (Table 2.3).

Patients with an upper gastrointestinal bleeding in the presence or absence of ascites are at high risk for severe bacterial infection including SBP. Several studies of gastrointestinal (GI) bleeders with oral or intravenous antibiotics showed a significant reduction of infections including SBP in the antibiotic group [20–25]. No difference was found whether the antibiotic was adminis-

Table 2.3 *Prevention of Complications in Patients on the Waiting List*

Aim	Intervention
I. Prevention of infections	
A. Acute variceal bleeding	First choice: oral norfloxacin 2 × 400 mg for 7 days
	Alternative: oral ciprofloxacin 2 × 500 mg for 7 days
B. Primary prevention of SBP	
1. Ascitic fluid protein high (>10 g/L)	Prophylaxis unnecessary
2. Ascitic fluid protein low (<10 g/L)	Prophylaxis controversial
	Short-term (during hospitalizations) or long-term prophylaxis with daily norfloxacin or trimetoprim-sulfamethoxazole can be considered
C. Secondary prevention of SBP	First choice: norfloxacin 400 mg daily
	Alternative: trimetoprim-sulfamethoxazole daily
II. Prevention of HRS in patients with SBP	Intravenous albumin (1.5 g/kg day 0 and 1 g/kg after 2 days)
III. Prevention of variceal bleeding	
A. Primary prevention of variceal bleeding	First choice: propranolol or nadolol (stepwise increase in dose until 25% reduction in heart rate)
	Alternative: band ligation
B. Secondary prevention of variceal bleeding	First choice: band ligation alone or in combination with propranolol or nadolol
	Alternative especially as bridge to OLT: TIPS

SBP: spontaneous bacterial peritonitis; HRS: hepatorenal syndrome.

tered orally or intravenously. Antibiotic prophylaxis is recommended in all cirrhotic patients with an upper GI bleed irrespective of the presence or absence of ascites. Although several antibiotic regimes are effective, the oral administration of norfloxacin (2 × 400 mg for 7 days) or ciprofloxacin (2 × 500 mg for 7 days) appear to be the first choice (Table 2.3) [25].

Empiric antibiotic treatment should be started when the neutrophil count is >250/mm^3 and SBP is suspected. Currently intravenous treatment with a third-generation cephalosporin (e.g. cefotaxime 2 g every 8–12 h, ceftriaxone 1 g/24 h for 5–7 days) is recommended [16]. Therapy needs to be modified according to the culture results. SBP resolves in approximately 90% of patients. The most important negative predictor of survival is the development of renal insufficiency. The administration of albumin (1.5 g/kg at diagnosis and 1 g/kg at day 3) is able to prevent the development of renal insufficiency and reduces the mortality from 30% to 10% (Table 2.3) [26].

Renal Failure, Fluid, and Electrolyte Disturbances

Patients with ESLD are at increased risk to develop renal failure, either spontaneously (HRS) or due to iatrogenic interventions (diuretics, nephrotoxic drugs). Patients with advanced cirrhosis and ascites are at highest risk. Renal vasoconstriction associated with advanced liver disease leads to severe renal vasoconstriction and functional renal insufficiency [27]. Renal failure occurs in up to 10% of patients with advanced liver disease and even more frequently in patients on the waiting list.

HRS can only be diagnosed after other causes of renal failure have been excluded, including obstruction, volume depletion, glomerulonephritis, acute tubular necrosis, and drug-induced nephrotoxicity [28]. All diuretics should be stopped and a fluid challenge with 1.5 L of isotonic saline should be administered to exclude volume depletion (Table 2.2). From the clinical presentation, two types of HRS can be distinguished:

1. Type I HRS is characterized by rapidly progressive renal failure with an increase in the serum creatinine to more than 220 μmol/L within 14 days and marked oliguria. Type I HRS occurs mostly in patients with type II HRS with a recent precipitating event (severe infection, e.g. SBP, large-volume paracentesis without plasma volume expansion).
2. Patients with type II HRS have refractory ascites with stable or slowly progressive impairment in renal function (Table 2.2).

The prognosis of patients with HRS is poor with a median survival of only 15 days in patients with type I and 150 days in patients with type II [29]. Until recently there was no effective therapy apart from liver transplantation, but fortunately this has changed in recent years. The combination of vasoconstrictor drugs, such as vasopressin analogues, noradrenaline, and the combination of midodrine and octreotide together with plasma volume expansion with albumin (1 g/kg intravenously on day 1, 20–40 daily thereafter) is effective in approximately two-thirds of patients (Fig. 2.2) [10]. It has been shown

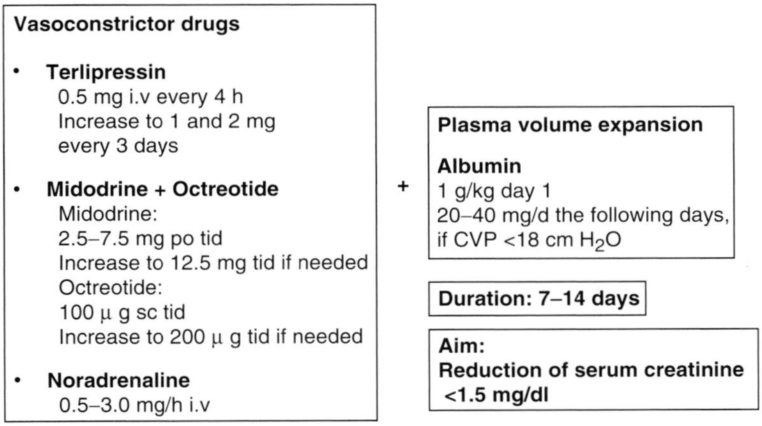

Fig. 2.2 *Therapeutic options for patients with hepatorenal syndrome.*

that the combination of terlipressin and albumin is clearly more effective than terlipressin alone [30]. Surprisingly the recurrence rate is low and responders have a higher rate of survival than nonresponders [30,31]. The response to treatment increases the probability that the patients with HRS survive long enough to undergo transplantation. There is some preliminary evidence that the improvement of renal function reduces post-transplantation morbidity and mortality [32]. There is also evidence that TIPS is effective in patients with HRS [33,34]. For both treatment options the available information is still insufficient; results from randomized controlled trials are lacking.

Hemodialysis has no effect on survival and should not be used routinely. However, as a bridge to transplantation, it might be useful in patients who fail to respond to medical treatment.

Patients with advanced liver disease and portal hypertension have a decreased effective arterial blood volume with activation of the renin–angio-tensin–aldosterone system, the sympathetic nervous system, and increased secretion of antidiuretic hormones (ADHs). The activation of these counter-acting regulatory mechanisms leads to renal vasoconstriction. In this situation renal perfusion is dependent upon prostaglandin-mediated vasodilatation. Nonsteroidal anti-inflammatory drugs (NSAIDs), which inhibit prostaglandin synthesis, may lead to a further decrease in renal blood flow and may precipi-tate acute renal failure [35]. Therefore, NSAIDs should be avoided in patients with ESLD. In addition, all potentially nephrotoxic drugs should be used with caution and overtreatment with diuretics should be avoided. It is generally recommended to stop diuretics if serum creatinine is greater than 1.7 mg/dl (150 μmol/L) and serum urea is greater than 22 mg/dl (8 μmol/L). Several studies have clearly shown that pretransplant renal function significantly impacts on post-transplant survival [36,37].

The most common electrolyte abnormality in patients with advanced liver cirrhosis is dilutional hyponatremia defined as a serum sodium <130 mmol/L. This occurs as a consequence of an impaired free water clearance by the kidney due to a nonosmotic hypersecretion of ADH. Impaired free water clearance occurs several months after the onset of sodium retention and ascites formation and therefore represents a late event in the course of decompensated liver disease. Hyponatremia indicates a poor prognosis and for some authors is an important predictor of survival. It has been proposed to incorporate serum sodium concentration in the MELD score; however, this remains controversial [38]. As long as the serum sodium remains above 125 mmol/L, no specific prophylactic measures are required.

If the serum sodium concentration falls below 125 mmol/L, diuretics should be withheld and an attempt made to expand the effective circulating blood volume by infusion of albumin (100 g/24 h) or red blood cells. This will usually result in a transient drop in the serum sodium concentration, following which the sodium will rise as ADH secretion is turned off by the increased blood volume. Once the serum sodium starts to rise, the colloid infusion can be tapered. Free water restriction should be instituted although there is no data-supported specific threshold for initiating fluid restriction [39].

It is important to remember that attempts to rapidly correct hyponatremia with hypertonic saline can lead to more complications [40]. Transplantation is contraindicated if the serum sodium is below 120 mmol/L due to the risk of developing central pontine myelinolysis.

Portal Hypertensive Bleeding

The management of portal hypertensive bleeding is extensively covered in Chapter 3. In this section only the prophylactic measures will be reviewed. Several studies have been published regarding the result of upper GI endoscopy in patients being evaluated for liver transplantation. Overall 66–85% of these patients had varices and 16–46% presented with large (Grade III to IV) varices [41–43]. Therefore, it is generally accepted that at the time of listing all patients should undergo an upper GI endoscopy. In the rare patients, where no varices are found, endoscopy should be repeated in 2–3 years, and in patients with small varices, who do not undergo some kind of primary prophylaxis, endoscopy should be repeated yearly [44].

Prevention of a First Variceal Bleed (Primary Prophylaxis)

The high mortality rate of a first variceal bleeding episode justifies the development of prophylactic regimes to prevent the development of, and bleeding from, varices. Noncardioselective beta-blockers such as propranolol and nadolol have been the mainstay of primary prevention. In cirrhotics with esophageal varices, both propranolol and nadolol have been shown to reduce the risk of an initial bleeding episode by 40–50%; there was a trend toward reducing mortality [45,46]. It is customary to adjust the dose of beta-blockers until a 25% fall of the heart rate is achieved. About 30% of patients will not respond to beta-blockers with a reduction in hepatic venous pressure gradient (HVPG), despite adequate dosing. These nonresponders can only be detected by invasive measurements of HVPG. Beta-blockers may cause side-effects such as fatigue and impotence that may lead to noncompliance, especially in younger males.

While the side-effects of endoscopic sclerotherapy outweigh its benefit in primary prophylaxes of esophageal variceal hemorrhage [47], endoscopic band ligation has recently been shown to be effective and well tolerated [48]. Thus, in summary, the following scheme is recommended for primary prophylaxis of variceal hemorrhage:

1. Selection of patients with at least medium-sized esophageal varices and/or red color or "red wale signs."
2. Noncardioselective beta-blocker (propranolol or nadolol) dose titrated to reach a reduction of resting heart rate of at least 25%, but not to lower than 50–55/min.
3. In patients with esophageal varices who do not tolerate or have contraindications to beta-blockers, endoscopic band ligation is indicated (Table 2.3).

Secondary Prevention of Variceal Bleeding

About 60% of patients surviving an acute variceal hemorrhage will develop recurrent bleeding within the first year [9,50]. Clinical predictors of early recurrence include severity of the initial hemorrhage, the extent of the underlying liver disease, impaired renal function, and encephalopathy. Endoscopic features include active bleeding at the time of endoscopy, large varices, and stigmata of a recent hemorrhage [51]. There is a strong correlation between the severity of portal hypertension, the survival rate, and the rebleeding risk. The high rebleeding rate with its associated morbidity and mortality justifies the implementation of a secondary prevention program. Different pharmacologic agents have been used for secondary prevention of variceal bleeding, but there is sufficient evidence of efficacy only for noncardioselective beta-blockers [52].

In a meta-analysis of 10 randomized trials comparing propranolol to endoscopic sclerotherapy for secondary prevention, both treatment options were similarly effective [46]. However, sclerotherapy was associated with significantly higher rates of side-effects. Sclerotherapy has also been compared to band ligation in several trials, which were summarized in a recent meta-analysis [53]. Ligation is associated with a lower rebleeding rate (25% versus 30%), fewer complications, lower overall costs and higher rates of survival. In a recent randomized trial the combination of nadolol plus endoscopic banding was more effective for the prevention of variceal rebleeding than endoscopic banding alone [54].

Therefore, endoscopic treatment should be considered in the context of a combined pharmacologic and endoscopic strategy (Table 2.3) [55]. TIPS is currently considered an effective bridge to transplantation by most clinicians. Meta-analysis comparing TIPS with endoscopic treatment found a lower rebleeding rate in patients with TIPS placement [56,57]. However, TIPS was associated with a higher incidence of encephalopathy, and no difference was found regarding the overall survival.

Additionally, the long-term use of TIPS is limited by the frequent shunt occlusion. During the first year, 50–70% of TIPS occlude and as a consequence 20% of the patients develop rebleeding [58]. Regular investigation, usually with Doppler ultrasound and intervention, is often required to avoid shunt occlusion. Misplaced TIPS in the portal vein or vena cava may complicate later liver transplantation [8]. For this reason TIPS placement should be restricted to experienced interventional radiologists.

Hepatic Encephalopathy

Clinically detectable encephalopathy (HE) is found in one-third of patients with ESLD [59]. Usually it presents with changes in mental status as a result of a precipitating event (see below). An important precipitating event is the use of benzodiazepines, prescribed for sleep disturbances. Rarely, patients present with recurrent episodes of HE without an obvious precipitating event. This can either be due to the presence of new spontaneous portosystemic shunts or as the result of severe parenchymal liver disease. Several recent studies describe the presence of subtle changes in mental function in 30–70% of patients that can only be detected by neuropsychological testing in patients who appear otherwise neurologically intact (minimal HE) [60,61].

It is important to remember that the diagnosis of HE is a diagnosis of exclusion. Other etiologies such as intracranial space-occupying lesions, vascular events, other metabolic disorders, and infectious diseases should be excluded. Ammonia levels are widely scattered in patients with liver disease; individual values are a poor predictor of the degree of encephalopathy. In spite of these limitations, ammonia levels are frequently useful when there is uncertainty if mental changes are the result of HE. Changes in ammonia levels should not be considered an indicator of therapeutic benefit; improvement in mental status is the sole therapeutic end point. The severity of HE is most commonly graded according to the West Haven criteria (Table 2.4) [62].

Table 2.4 *West Haven Criteria for Semiquantitavie Grading of Mental State*

Grade 1

    1. Lack of awareness

    2. Euphoria or anxiety

    3. Shortened attention span

Grade 2

    1. Lethargy or apathy

    2. Minimal disorientation for time or place

    3. Subtle personality change

    4. Inappropriate behaviors

    5. Impaired performance of subtraction

Grade 3

    1. Somnolence to semistupor but responsive to verbal stimuli

    2. Confusion

    3. Gross disorientation

Grade 4

    1. Coma (unresponsive to verbal or noxious stimuli)

As soon as deterioration in the mental status is recognized, a search for a precipitating event should be immediately started. Among the factors are:

1. Renal and electrolyte abnormalities, especially uremia and hypokalemia and dehydration.
2. Gastrointestinal bleeding (increases the nitrogen load in the gut).
3. Infection – cultures, especially from ascites to exclude spontaneous bacterial peritonitis are important.
4. Constipation.
5. Use of benzodiazepines, narcotics, or other sedatives (sometimes urinary screening is necessary to exclude their presence).
6. Excessive dietary protein intake.
7. Worsening liver function, e.g. portal vein thrombosis.
8. Noncompliance with medications, especially lactulose or lactilol.

Development of acute HE is associated with a poor prognosis. In a recent study 1- and 3-year survival was only 42% and 23%, respectively [63].

    The mainstay of therapy centers on correcting the precipitating event. Depending on the level of consciousness, intubation has to be considered to prevent aspiration. In these patients a nasogastric tube should be placed and treatment with nonabsorbable disaccharides such as lactulose or lactilol should be started. In cooperative patients this can be given by mouth. The usual starting dose is 20 ml, 3–4 times daily with the aim of achieving 2–4 soft bowel movements per day. Although recent reviews have pointed out the weaknesses of the clinical trials that support the use of the nonabsorbable disaccharides, they are still first-line treatment [64,65].

If patients are not improving after correcting the precipitating cause and administration of lactulose, neomycin 3–6 g/day in divided doses might be added. Alternatively, metronidazole can be used [66]. Classically, low protein diet (minimum 30 g/day) is recommended for patients with encephalopathy. During an acute episode of HE, enteral nutrition is frequently interupted for a few days due to coma or delirium. During this period the patient relies on gluconeogenesis from protein to maintain glucose metabolism in the brain. Gluconeogenesis is one of the most significant sources of endogenous ammonia production and can lead to worsening of the encephalopathy. Therefore, stuporous or comatose patients should be provided with a minimum of 400 calories per day in the form of intravenous glucose to minimize gluconeogenesis.

Once the patient recovers from an intercurrent episode of clinical encephalopathy, a moderate dose of protein (40 g/day) is instituted and is increased up to the maximum tolerated dose within the next few days. It is important to avoid long-term protein restriction to prevent further worsening of the nutritional status. Changes in the diet might help to increase the tolerance for proteins; there is some evidence that vegetable and milk proteins are less encephalogenic in than equal quantities of meat protein [67]. Other therapeutic interventions such as ornithine-aspartate, sodium benzoate, and branched-chain amino acids are less well established [59,68].

■ PORTOPULMONARY HYPERTENSION AND HEPATOPULMONARY SYNDROME

Portopulmonary Hypertension

Portopulmonary hypertension (PPHTN) is defined by:

1. Increased pulmonary arterial pressure (PAP; mean pressure determined by right heart catherization of >25 mmHg at rest and >30 mmHg during exercise)
2. Increased pulmonary vascular resistance (PVR; >240 dyne/s/cm^5).
3. Pulmonary wedge pressure of less than 15 mmHg in patients with portal hypertension [69].

Reports on the incidence of PPHTN vary greatly. In a recent study in patients with cirrhosis and refractory ascites, 16% of the patients fulfilled the criteria for PPHTN [70]; whereas in other studies the incidence was significantly lower [71]. So far no clear relationship between the severity of hepatic dysfunction or the degree of portal hypertension and the severity of pulmonary hypertension has been conclusively established [71]. In addition, little is known about the risk of developing PPHTN while waiting for liver transplantation.

The detection of PPHTN before liver transplantation, however, is crucial because the presence of pulmonary hypertension of any severity increases the perioperative and long-term risk of liver transplantation [72,73]. The most common presenting symptom is progressive dyspnea on excertion; however, patients with even severe PPHTN can be completely asymptomatic.

Echocardiography is the screening method of choice [74,75]. Using a systolic right ventricular pressure (RVsys) of more than 50 mmHg as a cutoff, the sensitivity and specificity to detect moderate to severe PPHNT is 97% and 77%, respectively. Only these patients need to undergo right heart catheterization to fully characterize pulmonary hemodynamics. If moderate to severe PPHNT is confirmed, treatment with pulmonary vasodilators should be instituted with the aim of decreasing PAP to <35–40 mmHg and PVR to <400 dyne/s/cm^5 [76]. Although rare, PPHTN can develop after the initial evaluation for liver transplantation [76,77]. In another study PPHNT was diagnosed in 65% of patients only in the operating room prior to transplantation [73].

These data clearly suggest that regular echocardiographic examinations of liver transplant candidates on the waiting list are mandatory, although the optimal screening frequency remains to be determined. In patients with normal echocardiographic findings at initial evaluation, the echocardiography should be repeated annually and in patients with an RVsys between 35 and 50 mmHg, every 6 months (Table 2.5) [76].

Hepatopulmonary Syndrome

Hepatopulmonary syndrome (HPS) is defined as a triad consisting of:

1. Chronic liver disease.
2. Hypoxemia (PaO$_2$ <70 mmHg or alveolar to arterial oxygen gradient >20 mmHg).
3. Intrapulmonary arteriovenous dilatation or shunts as detected by contrast echocardiography, lung perfusion scanning, or pulmonary angiography [69].

Table 2.5 *Recommended Follow-up Examinations for Patients on the Waiting List*

Complication	Examination	Time Interval
Portopulmonary hypertension	Echocardiography	12 months, if baseline examination normal; 6 months, if RVsys at baseline between 35 and 50 mmHg
Hepatopulmonary syndrome	Pulse oxymetry in standing position	6–12 months: arterial blood gas analysis if $SpO_2 < 97\%$; if $PaO_2 < 70\,mmHg$, perform echocardiography
	Alternative: arterial blood gas standing	6–12 months: if $PaO_2 < 70\,mmHg$, perform echocardiography
Known hepatocellular carcinoma	Abdominal CT or MRI	3 months
	Chest CT	3 months
	Bone scan	3–6 months
Cancer screening:		
Hepatocellular carcinoma	Abdominal ultrasound	3 months
	Alternative: abdominal CT or MRI	6 months
Cholangiocarcinoma	Abdominal ultrasound and CA 19-9	6 months
Colon cancer in primary sclerosing cholangitis patients	Colonoscopy	12 months
Breast cancer in women >40 years	Mammography	12 months
Cervical cancer in women >40 years	Cervical smear	12 months
Prostate cancer in men >45 years	Prostate-specific antigen	12 months

HPS is a serious complication that should be diagnosed before liver transplantation. The reported incidence of HPS in patients with chronic liver diseases is variable (4–32%) and depends on the diagnostic criteria and the tests used to detect intrapulmonary shunts [78,79]. A recent prospective study demonstrated that the survival of patients with HPS is significantly shorter (median survival 11 months) compared to patients without HPS (median survival 41 months) [78].

Medical management has so far been disappointing. Increasingly, liver transplantation has been advocated as the treatment of choice for patients with HPS; normalization of hypoxemia can be expected in approximately 82% within 15 months after liver transplantation. After liver transplantation up to 30% of patients with HPS will die; this is almost twice the death rate experienced by all other transplant recipients [80]. Although the optimal screening methods and interval have not been defined so far, it is probably useful to screen patients every 6–12 months for signs of hypoxemia (Table 2.5). Hypoxemia is the prerequisite for the diagnosis of HPS; therefore, every diagnostic approach should begin with the documentation of hypoxemia at rest. The routine measurement of arterial blood gases has been advocated in all liver transplant candidates [81]. Considering the prevalence of HPS this would lead to a large number of unnecessary arterial blood gas analyses. Therefore, a recent study evaluated the usefulness of pulse oxymetry for the detection of arterial hypoxemia in liver transplant candidates [82]. If arterial blood gas analysis is restricted to patients with an O_2-saturation below 97% only 32% of all patients would need an arterial blood gas analysis. This would still maintain a high sensitivity (96%) and acceptable specificity to identify hypoxemic patients (75%). If hypoxemia is established, the diagnosis of HPS should be confirmed by echocardiography or lung perfusion scanning. For patients with HPS an increase in the MELD score equivalent to a 15% risk of mortality (MELD score = 24) might be requested in the USA (see Chapter 6).

Hepatobiliary Cancer

Hepatocellular carcinoma can complicate all common forms of liver cirrhosis, but occurs most commonly in hepatitis B- or C-induced liver cirrhosis. HCC may be the indication for liver transplantation or may develop on the waiting list. Follow-up of transplant candidates will differ. The management of patients with hepatoma is considered in detail in Chapter 8.

Cholangiocarcinoma (CCA) is a well-recognized complication of primary sclerosing cholangitis (PSC). The reported frequency is as high as 7–36% in patients undergoing liver transplantation. The occurrence of CCA is unpredictable and is often difficult to diagnose. Liver transplantation is only for a selected group of patients with early-stage CCA who undergo preoperative radiation and chemotherapy in the absence of metastases. The issue of how patients with PSC should be screened on the waiting list is still unresolved. However, screening is important, because if the tumor is detected at early stages, where it is still confined in the biliary tree, transplantation still offers the best chances for cure. Currently the best approach probably consists of an ultrasound or magnetic resonance cholangiography and CA 19-9 level every 6 months (Table 2.5). Management of patients with PSC prior to transplantation is discussed in Chapter 10.

Other Cancers

The most common extrahepatic cancer in PSC patients with ulcerative colitis is colon cancer. Patients with ulcerative colitis should undergo yearly colonoscopy while awaiting liver transplantation.

Annual mammography and cervical smear should be obtained yearly in women over 40 years and an annual prostate-specific antigen (PSA) level should be measured in men over 45 years awaiting liver transplantation (Table 2.5).

■ MANAGEMENT OF OTHER MEDICAL DISEASES

Diabetes Mellitus

Patients with established diabetes mellitus will need careful monitoring to ensure that blood sugar is maintained within acceptable limits. There should be a low threshold for instituting insulin-based control since diabetic transplant recipients almost always require insulin in the initial post-transplantation period.

Hypertension

Patients with arterial hypertension will need monitoring to ensure that blood pressure is optimally controlled. If there are any cardiac abnormalities on screening, electrocardiogram (ECG) and echocardiography should be repeated at 6-monthly intervals.

Preventing Further Liver Damage

Patients with ESLD are at increased risk of developing fatal hepatic failure if they develop superimposed acute hepatitis A [83]. Vaccination against hepatitis A and B is much more effective in patients with compensated liver cirrhosis compared to patients with decompensated disease [84]. Therefore, all patients with chronic liver disease should be vaccinated against hepatitis A and B as early as possible in the course of their disease (see Chapter 7).

If possible, potentially hepatotoxic drugs should be avoided, especially medications that increase the risk of GI bleeding or renal insufficiency.

Malnutrition

Malnutrition is common in patients with chronic liver disease awaiting transplantation, and is a risk factor for mortality following liver transplantation [85,86]. Unfortunately, nutritional supplementation has not been proven to affect outcome [87]. However, most of the studies done to date were either poorly controlled or not adequately powered to detect small differences in survival.

In general, the total amount of calories provided should be at least 30–35 kcal/kg/day [88]. Protein restriction should not be considered routine. Adults can receive daily 1–2 g of protein/kg of dry body weight. Patients with ESLD awaiting liver transplant should take daily multivitamin and other supplements as needed. Specific fat-soluble vitamin supplementation should be provided if a deficiency is present.

Temporary Suspension from the Waiting List

Patients may temporarily be inactivated on the waiting list for several reasons and reactivated as soon as the temporary problem is resolved. The most common reasons for temporary suspension are intercurrent infections and variceal bleeding. Such infections should be vigorously treated; management of bleeding and portal hypertension is discussed in Chapter 3.

Disease-specific aspects of the pretransplantation management of patients with viral hepatitis (Chapter 7), hepatoma (Chapter 8), alcoholic liver disease (Chapter 9), autoimmune diseases (Chapter 10), metabolic diseases (Chapter 11), and fulminant hepatic failure (Chapter 13) are covered elsewhere.

■ REFERENCES

1. Fernandez-Esparrach G, Sanchez-Fueyo A, Gines P, et al. A prognostic model for predicting survival in cirrhosis with ascites. J Hepatol 2001;34(1):46–52.

2. Moore KP, Wong F, Gines P, et al. The management of ascites in cirrhosis: report on the consensus conference of the International Ascites Club. Hepatology 2003;38(1):258–266.

3. Rossle M, Ochs A, Gulberg V, et al. A comparison of paracentesis and transjugular intrahepatic portosystemic shunting in patients with ascites. N Engl J Med 2000;342(23):1701–1707.

4. Lebrec D, Giuily N, Hadengue A, et al. Transjugular intrahepatic portosystemic shunts: comparison with paracentesis in patients with cirrhosis and refractory ascites: a randomized trial. French Group of Clinicians and a Group of Biologists. J Hepatol 1996;25(2):135–144.

5. Gines P, Uriz J, Calahorra B, et al. Transjugular intrahepatic portosystemic shunting versus paracentesis plus albumin for refractory ascites in cirrhosis. Gastroenterology 2002;123(6):1839–1847.

6. Sanyal AJ, Genning C, Reddy KR, et al. The North American Study for the Treatment of Refractory Ascites. Gastroenterology 2003;124(3):634–641.

7. Salerno F, Merli M, Riggio O, et al. Randomized controlled study of TIPS versus paracentesis plus albumin in cirrhosis with severe ascites. Hepatology 2004;40(3):629–635.

8. Clavien PA, Selzner M, Tuttle-Newhall JE, et al. Liver transplantation complicated by misplaced TIPS in the portal vein. Ann Surg 1998;227(3):440–445.

9. Somberg KA, Lombardero MS, Lawlor SM, et al. A controlled analysis of the transjugular intrahepatic portosystemic shunt in liver transplant recipients. The National Institute of Diabetes and Digestive and Kidney Diseases (NIDDK) Liver Transplantation Database. Transplantation 1997;63(8):1074–1079.

10. Gines P, Cardenas A, Arroyo V, et al. Management of cirrhosis and ascites. N Engl J Med 2004;350(16):1646–1654.

11. Bureau C, Garcia-Pagan JC, Otal P, et al. Improved clinical outcome using polytetrafluoroethylene-coated stents for TIPS: results of a randomized study. Gastroenterology 2004;126(2):469–475.

12. Gines A, Fernandez-Esparrach G, Monescillo A, et al. Randomized trial comparing albumin, dextran 70, and polygeline in cirrhotic patients with ascites treated by paracentesis. Gastroenterology 1996;111(4):1002–1010.

13. Sola-Vera J, Minana J, Ricart E, et al. Randomized trial comparing albumin and saline in the prevention of paracentesis-induced circulatory dysfunction in cirrhotic patients with ascites. Hepatology 2003;37(5):1147–1153.

14. Siegerstetter V, Deibert P, Ochs A, et al. Treatment of refractory hepatic hydrothorax with transjugular intrahepatic portosystemic shunt: long-term results in 40 patients. Eur J Gastroenterol Hepatol 2001;13(5):529–534.

15. Gines P, Arroyo V, Vargas V, et al. Paracentesis with intravenous infusion of albumin as compared with peritoneovenous shunting in cirrhosis with refractory ascites. N Engl J Med 1991;325(12):829–835.

16. Rimola A, Garcia-Tsao G, Navasa M, et al. Diagnosis, treatment and prophylaxis of spontaneous bacterial peritonitis: a consensus document. International Ascites Club. J Hepatol 2000;32(1):142–153.

17. Tito L, Rimola A, Gines P, et al. Recurrence of spontaneous bacterial peritonitis in cirrhosis: frequency and predictive factors. Hepatology 1988;8(1):27–31.

18. Gines P, Rimola A, Planas R, et al. Norfloxacin prevents spontaneous bacterial peritonitis recurrence in cirrhosis: results of a double-blind, placebo-controlled trial. Hepatology 1990;12(4, Pt 1):716–724.

19. Novella M, Sola R, Soriano G, et al. Continuous versus inpatient prophylaxis of the first episode of spontaneous bacterial peritonitis with norfloxacin. Hepatology 1997;25(3):532–536.

20. Rimola A, Bory F, Teres J, et al. Oral, nonabsorbable antibiotics prevent infection in cirrhotics with gastrointestinal hemorrhage. Hepatology 1985;5(3):463–467.

21. Bleichner G, Boulanger R, Squara P, et al. Frequency of infections in cirrhotic patients presenting with acute gastrointestinal haemorrhage. Br J Surg 1986;73(9):724–726.

22. Soriano G, Guarner C, Tomas A, et al. Norfloxacin prevents bacterial infection in cirrhotics with gastrointestinal hemorrhage. Gastroenterology 1992;103(4):1267–1272.

23. Bernard B, Cadranel JF, Valla D, et al. Prognostic significance of bacterial infection in bleeding cirrhotic patients: a prospective study. Gastroenterology 1995;108(6):1828–1834.

24. Pauwels A, Mostefa-Kara N, Debenes B, et al. Systemic antibiotic prophylaxis after gastrointestinal hemorrhage in cirrhotic patients with a high risk of infection. Hepatology 1996;24(4):802–806.

25. Bernard B, Grange JD, Khac EN, et al. Antibiotic prophylaxis for the prevention of bacterial infections in cirrhotic patients with gastrointestinal bleeding: a meta-analysis. Hepatology 1999;29(6):1655–1661.

26. Sort P, Navasa M, Arroyo V, et al. Effect of intravenous albumin on renal impairment and mortality in patients with cirrhosis and spontaneous bacterial peritonitis. N Engl J Med 1999;341(6):403–409.

27. Schrier RW, Arroyo V, Bernardi M, et al. Peripheral arterial vasodilation hypothesis: a proposal for the initiation of renal sodium and water retention in cirrhosis. Hepatology 1988;8(5):1151–1157.

28. Arroyo V, Gines P, Gerbes AL, et al. Definition and diagnostic criteria of refractory ascites and hepatorenal syndrome in cirrhosis. International Ascites Club. Hepatology 1996;23(1):164–176.

29. Gines A, Escorsell A, Gines P, et al. Incidence, predictive factors, and prognosis of the hepatorenal syndrome in cirrhosis with ascites. Gastroenterology 1993;105(1):229–36.

30. Ortega R, Gines P, Uriz J, et al. Terlipressin therapy with and without albumin for patients with hepatorenal syndrome: results of a prospective, nonrandomized study. Hepatology 2002;36(4, Pt 1):941–948.

31. Moreau R, Durand F, Poynard T, et al. Terlipressin in patients with cirrhosis and type 1 hepatorenal syndrome: a retrospective multicenter study. Gastroenterology 2002;122(4):923–930.

32. Restuccia T, Ortega R, Guevara M, et al. Effects of treatment of hepatorenal syndrome before transplantation on posttransplantation outcome: a case–control study. J Hepatol 2004;40(1):140–146.

33. Guevara M, Gines P, Bandi JC, et al. Transjugular intrahepatic portosystemic shunt in hepatorenal syndrome: effects on renal function and vasoactive systems. Hepatology 1998;28(2):416–422.

34. Brensing KA, Textor J, Perz J, et al. Long-term outcome after transjugular intrahepatic portosystemic stentshunt in non-transplant cirrhotics with hepatorenal syndrome: a phase II study. Gut 2000;47(2):288–295.

35. Boyer TD, Zia P, Reynolds TB. Effect of indomethacin and prostaglandin A1 on renal function and plasma renin activity in alcoholic liver disease. Gastroenterology 1979;77(2):215–222.

36. Gonwa TA, Klintmalm GB, Levy M, et al. Impact of pretransplant renal function on survival after liver transplantation. Transplantation 1995;59(3):361–365.

37. Nair S, Verma S, Thuluvath PJ. Pretransplant renal function predicts survival in patients undergoing orthotopic liver transplantation. Hepatology 2002;35(5):1179–1185.

38. Heuman DM, Abou-Assi SG, Habib A, et al. Persistent ascites and low serum sodium identify patients with cirrhosis and low MELD scores who are at high risk for early death. Hepatology 2004;40(4):802–810.

39. Runyon BA. Management of adult patients with ascites due to cirrhosis. Hepatology 2004;39(3):841–856.

40. Sterns RH. Severe symptomatic hyponatremia: treatment and outcome: a study of 64 cases. Ann Intern Med 1987;107(5):656–664.

41. Rabinovitz M, Yoo YK, Schade RR, et al. Prevalence of endoscopic findings in 510 consecutive individuals with cirrhosis evaluated prospectively. Dig Dis Sci 1990;35(6):705–710.

42. Weller DA, DeGuide JJ, Riegler JL. Utility of endoscopic evaluations in liver transplant candidates. Am J Gastroenterol 1998;93(8):1346–1350.

43. Zaman A, Hapke R, Flora K, et al. Prevalence of upper and lower gastrointestinal tract findings in liver transplant candidates undergoing screening endoscopic evaluation. Am J Gastroenterol 1999;94(4):895–899.

44. Merli M, Nicolini G, Angeloni S, et al. Incidence and natural history of small esophageal varices in cirrhotic patients. J Hepatol 2003;38(3):266–272.

45. Poynard T, Cales P, Pasta L, et al. Beta-adrenergic-antagonist drugs in the prevention of gastrointestinal bleeding in patients with cirrhosis and esophageal varices: an analysis of data and prognostic factors in 589 patients from four randomized clinical trials. Franco-Italian Multicenter Study Group. N Engl J Med 1991;324(22):1532–1538.

46. D'Amico G, Pagliaro L, Bosch J. Pharmacological treatment of portal hypertension: an evidence-based approach. Semin Liver Dis 1999;19:475–505.

47. Teres J, Bosch J, Bordas JM, et al. Propranolol versus sclerotherapy in preventing variceal rebleeding: a randomized controlled trial. Gastroenterology 1993;105(5):1508–1514.

48. Imperiale TF, Chalasani N. A meta-analysis of endoscopic variceal ligation for primary prophylaxis of esophageal variceal bleeding. Hepatology 2001;33(4): 802–807.

49. Bosch J, Garcia-Pagan J. Prevention of variceal bleeding. Lancet 2003;361:952–954.

50. D'Amico G, Pagliaro L, Bosch J. The treatment of portal hypertension: a meta-analytic review. Hepatology 1995;22:332–354.

51. de Franchis R, Primignani M. Why do varices bleed? Gastroenterol Clin North Am 1992;21(1):85–101.

52. Bernard B, Lebrec D, Mathurin P, et al. Beta-adrenergic antagonists in the prevention of gastrointestinal rebleeding in patients with cirrhosis: a meta-analysis. Hepatology 1997;25:63–70.

53. Laine L, Cook D. Endoscopic ligation compared with sclerotherapy for treatment of esophageal variceal bleeding: a meta-analysis. Ann Intern Med 1995;123:280–287.

54. Lo G, Lai K, Cheng J, et al. Endoscopic variceal ligation plus nadolol and sucralfate compared with ligation alone for the prevention of variceal rebleeding: a prospective, randomized trial. Hepatology 2000;32:461–465.

55. Sharara AI, Rockey DC. Gastroesophageal variceal hemorrhage. N Engl J Med 2001;345(9):669–681.

56. Papatheodoridis G, Goulis J, Leandro G, et al. Transjugular intrahepatic portosystemic shunt compared with endoscopic treatment for prevention of variceal rebleeding. Hepatology 1999;30:612–622.

57. Luca A, D'Amico G, LaGalla R, et al. TIPS for prevention of recurrent bleeding in patients with cirrhosis: meta-analysis for randomized clinical trials. Radiology 1999;212:411–421.

58. Casado M, Bosch J, Garcia-Pagan J, et al. Clinical events after transjugular intrahepatic portosystemic shunt: corrolation with hemodynamic findings. Gastroenterology 1998;114:1296–1303.

59. Lizardi-Cervera J, Almeda P, Guevara L, et al. Hepatic encephalopathy: a review. Ann Hepatol 2003;2(3):122–130.

60. Groeneweg M, Quero JC, De Bruijn I, et al. Subclinical hepatic encephalopathy impairs daily functioning. Hepatology 1998;28(1):45–49.

61. Amodio P, Del Piccolo F, Marchetti P, et al. Clinical features and survival of cirrhotic patients with subclinical cognitive alterations detected by the number connection test and computerized psychometric tests. Hepatology 1999;29(6):1662–1667.

62. Atterbury CE, Maddrey WC, Conn HO. Neomycin–sorbitol and lactulose in the treatment of acute portal-systemic encephalopathy: a controlled, double-blind clinical trial. Am J Dig Dis 1978;23(5):398–406.

63. Bustamante J, Rimola A, Ventura PJ, et al. Prognostic significance of hepatic encephalopathy in patients with cirrhosis. J Hepatol 1999;30(5):890–895.

64. Cordoba J, Blei AT. Treatment of hepatic encephalopathy. Am J Gastroenterol 1997;92(9):1429–1439.

65. Butterworth RF. Complications of cirrhosis III: hepatic encephalopathy. J Hepatol 2000;32(suppl 1):171–180.

66. Blei AT. Diagnosis and treatment of hepatic encephalopathy. Baillieres Best Pract Res Clin Gastroenterol 2000;14(6):959–974.

67. Bianchi GP, Marchesini G, Fabbri A, et al. Vegetable versus animal protein diet in cirrhotic patients with chronic encephalopathy: a randomized cross-over comparison. J Intern Med 1993;233(5):385–392.

68. Riordan SM, Williams R. Treatment of hepatic encephalopathy. N Engl J Med 1997;337(7):473–479.

69. Hoeper MM, Krowka MJ, Strassburg CP. Portopulmonary hypertension and hepatopulmonary syndrome. Lancet 2004;363(9419):1461–1468.

70. Benjaminov FS, Prentice M, Sniderman KW, et al. Portopulmonary hypertension in decompensated cirrhosis with refractory ascites. Gut 2003;52(9):1355–1362.

71. Hadengue A, Benhayoun MK, Lebrec D, et al. Pulmonary hypertension complicating portal hypertension: prevalence and relation to splanchnic hemodynamics. Gastroenterology 1991;100(2):520–528.

72. De Wolf AM, Scott VL, Gasior T, et al. Pulmonary hypertension and liver transplantation. Anesthesiology 1993;78(1):213–214.

73. Krowka MJ, Plevak DJ, Findlay JY, et al. Pulmonary hemodynamics and perioperative cardiopulmonary-related mortality in patients with portopulmonary hypertension undergoing liver transplantation. Liver Transpl 2000;6(4):443–450.

74. Torregrosa M, Genesca J, Gonzalez A, et al. Role of Doppler echocardiography in the assessment of portopulmonary hypertension in liver transplantation candidates. Transplantation 2001;71(4):572–574.

75. Kim WR, Krowka MJ, Plevak DJ, et al. Accuracy of doppler echocardiography in the assessment of pulmonary hypertension in liver transplant candidates. Liver Transpl 2000;6(4):453–458.

76. Minder S, Fischler M, Muellhaupt B, et al. Intravenous iloprost bridging to orthotopic liver transplantation in portopulmonary hypertension. Eur Respir J 2004;24(4): 703–707.

77. Colle IO, Moreau R, Godinho E, et al. Diagnosis of portopulmonary hypertension in candidates for liver transplantation: a prospective study. Hepatology 2003;37(2): 401–409.

78. Schenk P, Schoniger-Hekele M, Fuhrmann V, et al. Prognostic significance of the hepatopulmonary syndrome in patients with cirrhosis. Gastroenterology 2003;125(4):1042–1052.

79. Mandell MS. Hepatopulmonary syndrome and portopulmonary hypertension in the model for end-stage liver disease (MELD) era. Liver Transpl 2004;10(10, suppl 2):S54–S58.

80. Arguedas MR, Abrams GA, Krowka MJ, et al. Prospective evaluation of outcomes and predictors of mortality in patients with hepatopulmonary syndrome undergoing liver transplantation. Hepatology 2003;37(1):192–197.

81. O'Brien JD, Ettinger NA. Pulmonary complications of liver transplantation. Clin Chest Med 1996;17(1):99–114.

82. Abrams GA, Sanders MK, Fallon MB. Utility of pulse oximetry in the detection of arterial hypoxemia in liver transplant candidates. Liver Transpl 2002;8(4):391–396.

83. Reiss G, Keeffe EB. Hepatitis vaccination in patients with chronic liver disease. Aliment Pharmacol Ther 2004;19(7):715–727.

84. Arguedas MR, Johnson A, Eloubeidi MA, et al. Immunogenicity of hepatitis A vaccination in decompensated cirrhotic patients. Hepatology 2001;34(1):28–31.

85. Shaw BW, Jr, Wood RP, Gordon RD, et al. Influence of selected patient variables and operative blood loss on six-month survival following liver transplantation. Semin Liver Dis 1985;5(4):385–393.

86. Muller MJ, Loyal S, Schwarze M, et al. Resting energy expenditure and nutritional state in patients with liver cirrhosis before and after liver transplantation. Clin Nutr 1994;13(3):145–152.

87. Le Cornu KA, McKiernan FJ, Kapadia SA, et al. A prospective randomized study of preoperative nutritional supplementation in patients awaiting elective orthotopic liver transplantation. Transplantation 2000;69(7):1364–1369.

88. Aranda-Michel J. Nutrition in hepatic failure and liver transplantation. Curr Gastroenterol Rep 2001;3(4):362–370.

Management of Portal Hypertension and Biliary Problems Prior to Transplantation

▼　　▼　　▼　　▼　　▼　　▼　　▼　　▼　　▼

Nazia Selzer, Janet E. Tuttle-Newhall, and Beat Müllhaupt

E ND-STAGE liver disease (ESLD) results from many etiologies and eventually leads to complications due to portal hypertension. These include bleeding and ascites, hepatic encephalopathy, and eventually, liver failure. Rapid deterioration secondary to portal hypertension in pretransplant patients is not uncommon and can result in death before an organ becomes available. Due to the rapid changes occurring in the fields of vascular radiology, hepatology, and hepatobiliary surgery, there are no clear recommendations easily available regarding the pretransplant therapy for both portal hypertension and biliary complications in patients with ESLD. Transplant programs have established protocols for dealing with these common problems, but typically, these practices are based on the institutional availability of certain therapies or on local experience. This chapter reviews available therapies for portal hypertension and ascites as well as biliary complications in patients with ESLD and the impact of those therapies on potential liver transplantation. In reviewing these manifestations of ESLD, we hope to provide the clinician with a rational plan for caring for these often challenging and complex patients.

■ PORTAL HYPERTENSION

Portal hypertension is a frequent complication in cirrhosis. Pressure rises secondary to increased resistance to increased hepatic portal flow in the cirrhotic liver [1]. It is important to emphasize that contrary to what was traditionally thought, increased hepatic vascular resistance in cirrhosis is due to not only the mechanical consequence of changes in the hepatic architecture but also the active contraction of the vascular smooth muscle cells, myofibroblasts, and other contractile elements within or around hepatic micro-circulation [2,3]. A second contributing factor is an increase in portal flow due to splanchnic vasodilatation and increased splanchnic intravascular volume [4,5]. As a result, venous collaterals form in an attempt to decompress the high pressure in the portal venous system [1]. Despite the formation of these collaterals, which can shunt up to 80% of portal venous flow, the marked increase in splanchnic inflow results in persistently elevated venous pressures. Specific systems of venous collaterals and their anatomic pathways include the gastroesophageal system supplied via the coronary and azygous veins, the splenorenal system via the splenic and retroperitoneal venous systems, the umbilical venous system (which clinically produces the caput medusa), and the hemorrhoidal venous plexus supplied via the inferior mesenteric vein (Fig. 3.1).

■ PREVENTION OF FIRST BLEEDING (PRIMARY PROPHYLAXIS)

The most common and life-threatening disturbance of increased portal venous pressure is upper gastrointestinal bleeding from esophageal varices. The incidence of variceal bleeding in patients with esophageal varices ranges from 20% to 40% at 2 years [6]. Variceal size and the degree of liver dysfunction are the main variables correlated with an increased risk of variceal bleeding. Treatment of the patient with known varices and portal hypertension who has never bled should address two major issues. The first is to prevent the development or the growth of the varices and the second is to prevent variceal hemorrhage in patients with varices that have never bled (primary prophylaxis).

Varices are present in about 50% of patients at the time of the initial diagnosis of cirrhosis. Several studies have demonstrated that the development of varices occurs when the portal pressure gradient (hepatic venous pressure gradient (HVPG)) increases above 10–12 mmHg [7]. A recent large multicenter randomized trial reported that an HVGP > 10 mmHg was accompanied by a faster development of varices, ascites, and death, emphasizing the prognostic value of HVGP measurements [8]. However, repetitive portal pressure measurement is not yet part of standard practice. The procedure requires personnel and equipment that are not available in all centers; the cost effectiveness of this technique has not yet been determined.

It is conceivable that early treatment of compensated cirrhotic patients with portal pressure-reducing agents may prevent the development of varices. Unfortunately, the data are not conclusive. In a recent placebo-controlled study, there was no difference in the development of varices by treating cirrhotics with portal hypertension with timolol, a potent nonselective beta-blocker [9].

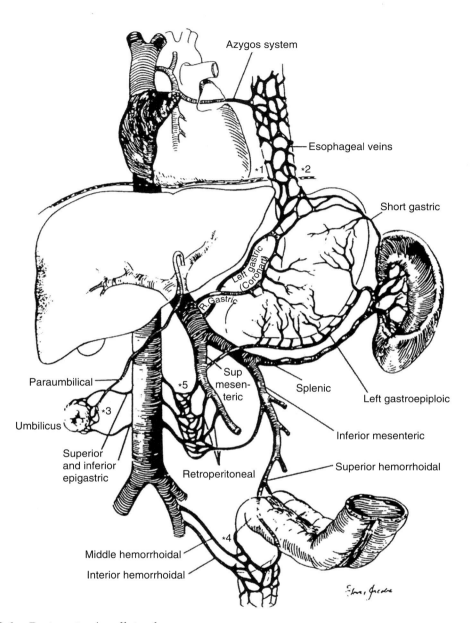

Azygos system

Esophageal veins

*1   *2

Short gastric

Left gastric (Coronary)

R Gastric

Paraumbilical

Sup mesen- teric

Splenic

*5

*3

Left gastroepiploic

Umbilicus

Inferior mesenteric

Superior and inferior epigastric

Retroperitoneal

Superior hemorrhoidal

*4

Middle hemorrhoidal

Interior hemorrhoidal

Fig. 3.1 *Portosystemic collaterals.*

At present, nonselective beta-blockers are the only drugs recommended as monotherapy for the primary prophylaxis of variceal hemorrhage. Beta-blockers not only reduce portal venous flow, but also reduce collateral flow as well. This occurs because of both a decrease in cardiac output from blockade of the beta-1 receptors in the heart and a reduction in splanchnic vascular tone due to blockade of the beta-2 receptors in the splanchnic vessel [10]. Several studies have shown that propranolol and nadolol, both nonselective beta-blockers, are successful in preventing the initial variceal bleeding episode in patients with known portal hypertension. Meta-analysis of these studies concluded that continued propranolol or nadolol prophylaxis reduces the bleeding risk from 25% to 15% over a median of 2 years [11]. This treatment seems to be most beneficial in patients with moderate to large varices (>5 mm) independent of liver dysfunction [12]. In patients with small varices the risk of hemorrhage is small and the treatment does not seem to be cost-effective. Recently, a placebo-controlled trial reported that nadolol prevents the progression of small to large varices [13]. Until these results are confirmed, follow-up endoscopy every year seems to be reasonable in these patients.

Adequate protection against bleeding is achieved if the portal pressure gradient is reduced by 20% or to less than 12 mmHg [14–16]. Unfortunately, portal pressures drop to this level in only 30–40% of patients treated with propranolol [17]. None of the noninvasive methods proposed (Doppler ultrasonography, plethysmography, etc.) are sufficiently precise to predict the portal pressure response. Assessment of HVPG is advised but due to the invasive nature of the measurement and its cost, it is not routinely performed. The most common approach for adjusting the dosage of beta-blockers remains achievement of a 25% reduction in resting heart rate. Therapy with beta-blockers should be maintained indefinitely or until the time of transplantation, as the withdrawal from the treatment is associated with a higher risk of mortality [18].

An approach to increase the proportion of responders to beta-blockers is the addition of a vasodilating drug. The rationale underlying this approach is that some patients who do not respond to propranolol exhibit an increase in portal collateral resistance [19], hindering portal pressure reduction. It has been demonstrated that the addition of isosorbide mononitrate (ISMN) significantly increases the long-term response to beta-blockers [20]. However, it is not yet clear whether this combination has an effect in preventing the first variceal bleeding or rebleeding episode. Indeed, a recent randomized controlled trial comparing nadolol with nadolol plus ISMN demonstrated a significantly lower first bleeding rate in the combination group, but without survival advantage [21–22]. This conclusion has not been confirmed in a large double-blinded multicenter trial [23]. Therefore, combination therapy for primary prophylaxis is currently not recommended [24]. In patients with contraindications to beta-blocker, ISMN alone has no proven efficacy compared with placebo in preventing the first bleeding episode or in affecting survival [25].

About 15–20% of patients cannot be treated with drug therapy because of relative or absolute contraindications [11]. In these patients, endoscopic variceal ligation (EVL) is the only effective alternative for primary prophylaxis. Two recent randomized trails, as well as a meta-analysis of EVL versus propranolol, have shown no difference between the two treatments regarding prevention of hemorrhage or mortality. Therefore, the use of EVL as an alternative in case of contraindications or development of intolerance to beta-blocker therapy is encouraged [26–28].

INITIAL SUPPORT OF THE PATIENT WITH VARICEAL HEMORRHAGE

Variceal bleeding is a medical emergency and its management should be undertaken in an intensive care setting by a team of experienced nurses, hepatologists, endoscopists, and surgeons. The initial therapy is aimed at correcting hypovolemic shock, preventing complications associated with gastrointestinal bleeding, and achieving hemostasis at the bleeding site.

Mortality from an acute variceal bleed can approach 20% within 6 weeks with an immediate mortality from uncontrolled bleeding in up to 8% of cases [29]. This mortality is related not only to the amount of blood lost, but also to the severity of the underlying liver dysfunction. Patients with mild, compensated liver disease have a lower mortality rate compared with patients with severe hepatic dysfunction. The Child–Pugh classification is helpful in stratifying patients into groups by severity of liver dysfunction (Table 3.1) but has been recently replaced by the model for ESLD as a marker of hepatic

Table 3.1 *Child–Pugh Scoring System for Liver Cirrhosis*

Clinical Parameter	Rank	Score
Bilirubin (m/dL)	<2	1
	2–3	2
	>3	3
Albumin (g/dL)	>3.5	1
	2.8–3.5	2
	<3.5	3
Prothrombin ratio (%)	>50	1
	30–50	2
	<30	3
Encephalopathy	Absent	1
	I–II	2
	III	3
Ascites	Absent	1
	Mild	2
	Tense	3

Child's A: 5–6 points; Child's B: 7–9 points; Child's C: >10 points dysfuction and as an allocation tool for liver transplantation in the USA (see Chapter 6) [30,31].

Measures that provide medical support are the most important factors that favorably influence the prognosis of these patients. Peripheral venous catheterization with a large-bore intravenous access for rapid perfusion of blood and fluids is mandatory. The blood bank should be notified of the patient's clinical status and the blood products set up and kept ahead of the patient's needs. Packed red blood cells and clotting factors should be made available when requested. Standard laboratory tests should be done for baseline diagnostic studies including a coagulation profile. Aggressive attempts to replace lost red cell volume should be undertaken. Overtransfusion should be avoided to avoid the rebound increase in portal pressure with a subsequent risk of rebleeding [32]. The placement of a nasogastric tube to empty gastric contents lowers the risk of tracheobronchial aspiration and prepares the stomach for the performance of diagnostic and/or therapeutic upper gastrointestinal endoscopy. In patients with severe hemodynamic alterations and encephalopathy, or patients unable to maintain their airway, orotracheal intubation and mechanical ventilation should be initiated.

Upper gastrointestinal endoscopy should be performed as soon as the patient's clinical status permits. Endoscopy allows specific diagnosis and treatment in 90% of cases. One must never assume that a patient is bleeding from a variceal source without objective confirmation. Patients with cirrhosis can bleed from other causes such as peptic ulcer disease in up to 20% of cases.

In addition, it is important to prevent clinical complications that are frequently seen in portal hypertension patients with gastrointestinal bleeding. This includes the administration of lactulose for the treatment of hepatic encephalopathy and antibiotics (norfloxacin 400 mg/12 h during 5 days) [33] to reduce the incidence of severe bacterial infections produced by microorganism of enteric origin after sclerosis or endoscopic banding.

The currently recommended therapy of variceal bleeding is to resuscitate the patient, start therapy with a somatostatin analog (e.g. Octreotide analog) or a vasopressin analog (e.g. terlipressin), and then to perform an upper gastrointestinal endoscopy [24,34]. Drug therapy may be started upon the patient's transfer to the hospital [35] and maintained up to 5 days to prevent early rebleeding [24]. The rationale for this treatment comes from a number of randomized control trials demonstrating that early administration of medical therapy facilitates endoscopy, improves control of bleeding, and reduces early rebleeding rate [35–36].

The drug of choice for the treatment of variceal bleeding depends on the local resources. These include somatostatin, octreotide, and terlipressin. While terlipressin [34] is the drug of choice in Europe, octreotide is the drug of choice in the USA [35]. In the past, concerns over the potential side-effects of vasopressin have led many clinicians to hold this drug in reserve. In contrast, the safety profiles of somatostatin and octreotide permit clinicians to institute drug therapy in the emergency room as soon as diagnosis of variceal bleeding is suspected. Of note, a recent randomized controlled trial suggested that the use of higher doses (500 µg/h) of somatostatin can result in increased clinical efficacy in the subset of patients with active bleeding at emergency endoscopy [37].

A novel approach is the use of drugs that improve hemostasis. For example, recombinant activated factor VII (rVIIa) has been shown to correct prothrombin time in cirrhotic patients with acute variceal bleeding [38,39]. A recent double-blind trial was unable to show an advantage of this treatment over placebo regarding failure to control bleeding within 24 h or prevention of rebleeding within the first 5 days. However, analysis of the data has demonstrated a benefit of rVIIa in the subgroup of patients with Child's B/C cirrhosis [40]. Further studies need to be performed to verify these findings prior to widespread clinical application.

Endoscopic therapy for variceal hemorrhage has evolved over the past three decades. Two techniques are in common use: endoscopic sclerotherapy (ES) and EVL. Neither procedure reduces portal pressure; however, in the acute setting both can control bleeding. In the acute bleeding patient, either ligation or ES can be used equally depending on the institutional level of expertise. Success rates of 80–90% have been shown in various studies [40], but often more than one session of endoscopy is required and complications may occur.

ES involves injecting sclerosing agents directly into or near the bleeding varix. Complications from this procedure are usually related to the sclerosant, locally or systematically; esophageal perforation can occur but is rare. Ulcerations at the site of the offending varix are common after sclerotherapy. Deep ulcerations may be indicative of a full-thickness injection, and stricture or esophageal perforation may follow. These types of ulcerations are more common in Child's class C patients. Rebleeding from these ulcers can occur in 2–13% of patients [41]. Systemic effects of the sclerosant can include bacteremia, fever, and pulmonary deterioration. The most relevant complication is rebleeding from the initial varices; this is reported in as many as 50% of those patients initially controlled. Varices redevelop in 28–60% of patients following obliteration, with rebleeding in 4–44% of these cases.

Recently, EVL has been advocated instead of sclerotherapy as the therapy of choice for controlling variceal hemorrhage [42]. This treatment is carried out through elastic bands inserted through a device attached to the end of endoscope. Trials comparing the two modalities have shown ligation to be as effective as sclerotherapy in controlling the initial bleeding event with fewer complications. Rebleeding rate and the average number of sessions required to obliterate varices have been reported to be less frequent [43]. However, the performance of EVL may be technically difficult in an esophagus awash in blood, and sclerotherapy might be easier to perform in these situations. Moreover, the major factor influencing survival is the degree of underlying hepatic dysfunction and not the endoscopic modality used to control the bleeding.

If bleeding is not controlled with drug therapy and endoscopy, a Sengstaken–Blakemore or Linton tube should be inserted. The patient's airway should be controlled with an endotracheal tube prior to insertion of the Sengstaken–Blakemore tube to limit the risk of aspiration. Balloon tamponade is effective in 80–90% of patients, but rebleeding occurs in over half of those patients. The physician should plan for a repeat endoscopy after successful balloon tamponade. After unsuccessful endoscopic attempts to control the bleeding, emergency transjugular intrahepatic portosystemic shunt (TIPS) should be considered.

A transvenous, intrahepatic, portosystemic shunt or TIPS is a radiological procedure that involves placement of a metal stent via the internal jugular vein, through the hepatic parenchyma and into the portal vein creating a portosystemic shunt (Fig. 3.2) [44]. The results are a rapid and sustained decrease in portal pressure. The shunt functions physiologically in the same manner as a surgical side-to-side portacaval shunt. A TIPS does not alter the portal vein anatomy, which is an advantage if the patient subsequently undergoes liver transplantation [45]. TIPS has obviated the need for emergent surgical procedures in the majority of patients who fail emergency medical

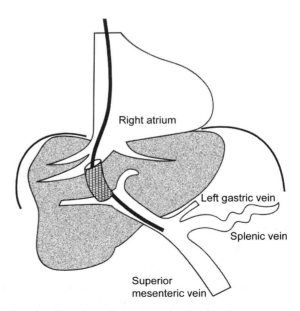

Right atrium

Left gastric vein

Splenic vein

Superior mesenteric vein

Fig. 3.2 *Transjugular intrahepatic portosystemic shunt.*

and endoscopic therapy to control bleeding. Portal pressure can be lowered effectively below 12 mmHg. In addition, the potential to have varices selectively embolized angiographically during the same procedure exists for patients who are actively bleeding [46].

TIPS is quite effective as a salvage hemostatic therapy. The success rate in arresting bleeding is over 90%, but is burdened by a high mortality (38%) [47,48]. In a recent study, Patch et al. [49] identified several factors that independently predicted death following TIPS for acute variceal bleeding. These included the presence of ascites, ventilation problems, serum creatinine, platelet, and white blood cells counts. Some clinicians who routinely treat patients with liver disease have recommended limiting the use of TIPS for emergency control of bleeding to patients who are not ventilated for aspiration, are not septic, have no deteriorating liver and renal function, and are not receiving drugs to support their blood pressure [44]. However, other groups have not found any one of these variables to be predictive of early mortality [48].

Potential candidates for orthotopic liver transplantation (OLT) should have the remainder of their therapy managed with the possibility of transplantation in mind.

Of note, the techniques introduced over the past decades to control active variceal bleeding have resulted in a better prognosis of cirrhotic patients following a first variceal bleeding. Analyzing 28 eligible randomized controlled trails for primary prevention of variceal bleeding between 1960 and 2000, McCormick and O'Keefe [50] reported that the bleeding-related mortality was significantly reduced from 65% to 40% over the past four decades.

PREVENTION OF REBLEEDING

The best modality for the prevention of variceal rebleeding in the patient who is a candidate for transplantation is unknown. Rebleeding rates in untreated patients who have recovered from an episode of variceal hemorrhage range from 55% to 67% at 1 year, with a mortality rate of 20% from each rebleeding episode [51]. Options include medical therapy, intermittent ES or banding, TIPS, certain surgical shunts, or liver transplantation.

Both pharmacological treatment with beta-blockers and endoscopic treatment are accepted as first-line treatment for the prevention of rebleeding. Meta-analysis of studies comparing beta-blocker with placebo consistently demonstrated a benefit for beta-blockers in term of reducing the rebleeding risk and improving survival [11]. Addition of ISMN to beta-blockers decreases the risk of rebleeding from 37–57% to 30–42% [51]. However, ISMN by releasing nitric oxide can cause hypotension and may worsen sodium retention and renal function. Therefore, combination drug therapy in the setting of rebleeding must be done with caution [24].

Some authors have advocated repeated endoscopic therapy for prevention of variceal rebleeding. ES alone reduces the risk of rebleeding to 34–53% [51]. Despite the complete eradication of varices and demonstrable reductions in the rates of rebleeding, repeat ES has not shown to increase survival [33]. It is also accompanied by a greater incidence of complications. ES has been currently replaced by EVL, which is safer and is more effective for prevention of rebleeding (20–43%) [51]. Prophylactic EVL can be performed in all patients including those at high risk for other interventions (i.e. Child's C patients), without adversely affecting hepatic function. Repeat EVL does not affect a patient's candidacy for OLT.

Currently, TIPS is recommended as a bridge to transplantation in patients who have failed other conventional modalities to control rebleeding. The role of TIPS compared with conventional treatment (ES or EVL plus beta-blocker) in the prevention of variceal rebleeding has been investigated in several randomized controlled trials. Meta-analysis of these studies consistently show that TIPS decreases the variceal rebleeding rate (11–22%) compared with endoscopic treatment alone or in combination with propranolol [51]. One-year survival rates in the majority of studies are similar between patients treated with TIPS and those treated with other modalities. Complication of TIPS includes new or worsening hepatic encephalopathy (20–30%) and worsening liver function [52]. Based on these results, it can be concluded that placement of a TIPS decreases the rebleeding rate, while increasing the encephalopathy rate, and has no effect on survival [53]. A cost analysis of TIPS versus endoscopy therapy found that the cost of TIPS was significantly greater at 1 year compared with endoscopy therapy [54] and drug therapy [55].

Maintaining patency of the stent increases the cost of this technique [53]. TIPS stenosis occurs in 18–70% of patients within the first year [52]. Almost uniformly, reintervention is warranted to maintain long-term shunt patency. With close follow-up and frequent Doppler inspections of the shunt to ensure patency (usually every 3 months), early detection of stenosis can be managed with balloon dilatation of the stent or the addition of a new stent. Of note, recently polytetrafluoroethylene-covered stents have demonstrated higher patency with lower rates of dysfunction and encephalopathy [56].

At the time of transplantation, the stent is removed as part of the hepatectomy. Initial improper placement of the stent can significantly compromise the transplant procedure. If the stent is placed into the vena cava, it can be impossible to place a suprahepatic vena caval clamp or, if placed into the portal vein, it can complicate the portal venous anastomosis. It is imperative to have a well-experienced interventional radiologist place these devices to avoid these complications.

■ SURGICAL INTERVENTIONS

In patients who are candidates for OLT but fail nonsurgical therapies, including TIPS, nontransplant surgical interventions may be warranted. Liver transplantation remains the best long-term option for those patients with end-stage hepatic failure who have bleeding varices and nontransplant surgical procedures and must be considered very carefully in this population prior to proceeding. The key in choosing the correct surgical intervention is to balance the degree of hepatic dysfunction against the risk of rebleeding. Shunting procedures may also be appropriate in patients with good hepatic function (therefore, not OLT candidates), who fail medical therapies.

Surgical Shunts

Surgical shunts are categorized into three types: total, selective, and partial. Total shunts involve complete diversion of blood away from the portal circulation and into the systemic circulation. The portacaval shunt is the classic example using either an end-to-side or a side-to-side portal vein to inferior vena caval anastomosis (Fig. 3.3). Due to the complete diversion of blood from the hypertensive portal circulation, these shunts maximally protect against variceal rebleeding. Portacaval shunts are technically straightforward and, historically, have been recommended as the optimal decompression procedure in an emergency setting [57]. Only patients with compensated cirrhosis

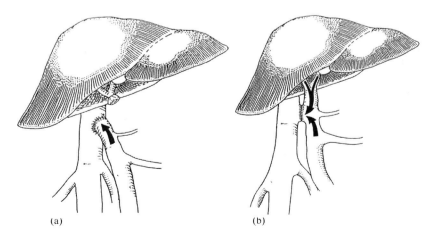

(a) (b)

Fig. 3.3 *(a) End-to-side and (b) side-to-side portacaval shunt.*

(Child's class A and a "good" B) should be considered as candidates for portacaval shunts.

Portacaval shunts should be avoided, if possible, in a candidate for OLT. Although mortality rates for patients undergoing OLT following a portacaval shunt do not differ from those who have not had the procedure, right upper quadrant scarring may substantially complicate the conduct of the transplantation by increasing the operative time and transfusion requirements [58]. This type of shunt is also associated with an increased risk of encephalopathy and accelerated hepatic failure, especially in the patient with limited hepatic reserve. The classic portacaval shunt in the transplant candidate has recently been supplanted by TIPS.

Other options available for total shunts include the mesocaval shunt using a large Dacron interposition graft, 19–22 mm, between the superior mesenteric vein at the root of the small bowel mesentery and the inferior vena cava. This type of shunt is particularly attractive in patients with bleeding varices who have hepatic venous outflow obstruction but require subsequent OLT and in pediatric patients with portal hypertension in whom a distal splenorenal shunt is not feasible secondary to the small size of their venous anatomy. Unlike the portacaval shunt, this type of shunt does not complicate the conduct of the transplant procedure. The shunt itself is easily dealt with during the transplant procedure by interrupting it with heavy sutures or a vascular stapling device. A modification of the classic mesocaval shunt is the partial shunt. Partial shunts preserve portal perfusion to the liver while decreasing portal pressure in order to decrease the risk of variceal bleeding. The most commonly used partial shunt is the superior mesenteric vein to inferior vena cava shunt, using maximum 15-mm Dacron prosthetic graft, an H graft. Due to the smaller size of the prosthetic graft, complete diversion of portal blood flow away from the liver can be avoided. This procedure also avoids the porta hepatis and does not affect any subsequent OLT procedure similar to the classic mesocaval shunt. The advantage to this type of shunt is a lower incidence of encephalopathy but, due to its small size, there is an increased incidence of graft thrombosis.

Selective shunts preserve portal venous flow while selectively decompressing the gastroesophageal varices. The distal splenorenal shunt (Warren shunt) is the most popular shunt currently used in patients who are OLT candidates. This procedure is best offered to patients with recurrent bleeding who are refractory to medical therapy and who have preserved hepatic reserve. In the patient awaiting OLT who is suffering from recurrent variceal bleeding, TIPS is a better bridge to transplantation.

The Warren shunt entails anastomosing the end of the distal splenic vein with the left renal vein and disconnecting the significant venous collaterals such as the coronary and gastroepiploic veins (Fig. 3.4). This results in a

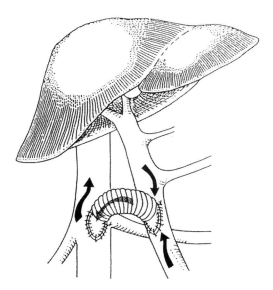

Fig. 3.4 *Distal splenorenal shunt.*

preserved superior mesenteric and portal venous circulation plus a splenor-enal decompressive shunt for the gastric and esophageal varices. This procedure offers the advantages of a lower rate of encephalopathy and decreased incidence of rebleeding especially in those patients with pre-dominantly gastric varices. Unfortunately, this procedure should not be used in patients with preexisting chronic ascites [59]. Patients with adequate or good hepatic function, Child's class A or "good" B patients, can have a reduction in their risk of bleeding to less than 10% and a survival rate reported to be approximately 75% at 5 years. This procedure does not interfere with or increase the risk of subsequent OLT [60]. Unfortunately, in alcoholic cirrhotic patients, the preservation of portal venous flow can be lost over time due to the development of new venous collaterals. This decrease in portal venous flow can lead to an increased incidence of portal vein thrombosis, increasing the rate of variceal rebleeding and potentially complicating an OLT [61]. Some authors have reported better long-term pre-vention of rebleeding in the alcoholic population by using an H-graft, partial mesocaval shunt.

Nonshunting Procedures

Finally, there are several nonshunting therapies available to control recurrent variceal bleeding. These procedures include transesophageal variceal ligation, the Sugiura procedure (or one of its modifications), and the McDermott pro-cedure. A full and comprehensive description and comparison of all these procedures is beyond the scope of this text and they will only be briefly mentioned for completeness. These procedures are usually indicated in patients when a surgical shunt is technically not feasible and in patients that are not candidates for OLT. The modified Sugiura procedure is the most commonly performed nonshunting operation performed at our institution. It is based on the principle of dividing the perforating veins of the esophagogastric varices while preserving the plexus of venous collaterals that connect the coronary vein to the azygous system. The esophagus is devascularized of feeding venous collaterals close to its wall. As stated earlier, the periesophageal veins are preserved. The gastroesophageal junction is likewise devascularized down onto the lesser and greater curves of the stomach. The esophagus is then transected with an EEA stapling device. A splenectomy is added, as is a selective vagotomy and pyloroplasty [62]. Rebleeding rates are low after this type of procedure. One series has reported 76% of their patients free of hemorrhage at 5 years [63]. After this procedure, hepatic function is preserved and subsequently, there is decreased risk of encephalopathy. The most common postoperative complications reported are portal vein thrombosis and esophageal stricture, at 18% and 30%, respectively [63]. In our institutional experience with 15 patients, we have had no episodes of recurrent hemorrhage and only one documented esophageal stricture within a 2-year follow-up period. There are no reports in the literature to date documenting OLT after this procedure.

Recommendation for the Therapy of Portal Hypertension

In conclusion, portal hypertension and subsequent variceal bleeding are major complications of ESLD. As hemorrhage from varices is often massive and life-threatening, aggressive intervention must be used in order to promote patient survival and limit complications. Attention to volume resuscitation, correction of coagulopathies, and early endoscopic evaluation are the cornerstones. Combination of pharmacological therapy with emergency endoscopy is the most promising approach. In most candidates for OLT, the TIPS procedure should be the next step to control bleeding. In patients who have recurrent bleeding despite TIPS, a surgical shunt should be considered. In those patients listed for transplantation, appropriately increasing their status on the waiting list may facilitate OLT, which is definitive therapy. Each patient must be evaluated on an individual basis in order to select the most appropriate operative procedure. Surgeon experience and familiarity must also be a factor in choosing the procedure that should be utilized. Finally, OLT must be considered for patients with rapidly progressive primary liver dysfunction who present with variceal bleeding as a therapy to prevent rebleeding.

Ascites

Ascites in a patient with cirrhosis is often a marker of poor hepatic function and is an indicator of poor long-term survival, with a 2-year survival of only 50% [64]. Many patients are referred for liver transplantation after development of ascites. Therapeutic options for ascites include medical management, surgical options, TIPS, and OLT. The keystones of medical therapy include diuretics, restriction of dietary sodium (2000 mg/day), and serial paracentesis. Fluid restriction is not necessary in most patient with ascites unless serum sodium is below 150 mmol/L [65].

Diuretics must be instituted with care as over aggressive diuretic therapy can reduce intravascular volume and predispose the patient to the hepatorenal syndrome. The usual regimen would be a single morning dose of spironolactone (100 mg) and furosemide (40 mg) [65]. Due to hyperkalemia and the long half-life of spironolactone [66] its use as single-agent therapy is currently recommended only in patients with minimal fluid overload [65]. The dose of both oral diuretics can be increased simultaneously every 3–5 days, if weight loss and natriuresis are inadequate. Maximum doses may be as high as 600 mg/day of spironolactone and 200 mg/day of furosemide. The side-effects of diuretic therapy may include volume depletion, which may precipitate an episode of encephalopathy, or may lead to renal failure. Hyponatremia, hypokalemia or hyperkalemia are not infrequent problems. Care must be taken in using high-dose diuretic therapy in patients with concomitant congestive heart failure, or preexisting renal compromise. Weekly monitoring of electrolytes and changes in the patient's weight must be undertaken when initiating or changing therapy. Encephalopathy, serum sodium less than 125 mmol/L, or serum creatinine greater than 150 μmol/L should lead to cessation of diuretic use.

Paracentesis continues to be an effective means of managing large volume ascites. Two prospective studies have demonstrated that a single 5-L paracentesis can be performed safely without colloid infusion in patients with diuretic-resistant large-volume ascites [67,68]. Larger volumes of fluid can be safely removed with the administration of intravenous albumin. Unfortunately, repeat paracentesis can increase the risk of contaminating the ascitic fluid, leading to peritonitis. Additionally, there is a considerable time investment from both the patient and the physician in using paracentesis as a mode of therapy. Therefore, it is recommended to follow a single large-volume paracentesis by diet and diuretic therapy [65].

Refractory ascites is that which is unresponsive to high-dose diuretics and a sodium-restricted diet. In addition, refractory ascites tends to rapidly recur following paracentesis [69]. Less than 10% of patients with cirrhosis have refractory ascites [70]. Prior to labeling a patient as having medically refractory ascites, an in-hospital trial of dietary management and diuretic therapy should be attempted. Exclusion of nonsteroidal anti-inflammatory drugs is necessary before judging that ascites is refractory to treatment. For patients who fail in-hospital management of their ascites, other options are available. These include serial therapeutic paracentesis, liver transplantation, TIPS, and peritoneovenous shunt.

Serial paracentesis is effective in controlling ascites, even in the subpopulation of patients without any sodium excretion [71]. The development of new paracentesis equipment has significantly improved the speed of paracentesis. The question of colloid replacement following paracentesis remains controversial. Current literature does not support a benefit of colloid replacement for low-volume paracentesis. For larger paracentesis, an albumin infusion of 8–10 g/L of fluid removed should be considered [65].

The peritoneovenous shunt (e.g. LeVeen or Denver) is mentioned for historical interest only. This type of shunt involves placement of a unidirectional valve and catheter system that allows continuous infusion of ascites from the peritoneal cavity into the central circulation. Although this system maintains effective circulating volume and renal perfusion, repeated episodes of infection, poor long-term patency, episodes of disseminated intravascular coagulation, and lack of survival advantage compared with medical therapy limit its use [72].

The placement of TIPS is effective in the majority of patients with refractory ascites. Physiologically, the TIPS mimics a side-to-side portacaval shunt and by reducing sinusoidal hypertension has a positive impact on ascites. Due to increased waiting times for patients listed for OLT, TIPS offers the best long-term solution for both portal hypertension and ascites. TIPS has been compared with sequential paracentesis in several randomized controlled trials [73–76]. A total of 264 patients were included in these studies. All these studies demonstrated that TIPS was effective in reducing the need for repeated paracentesis. There was no advantage in transplant free survival; there was an increased incidence of new or more severe encephalopathy. There was also no improvement in the quality of life in TIPS group. Patients who are on a transplant list and are likely to undergo liver transplantation within a few months are probably better managed by large-volume paracentesis.

In OLT candidates, surgical shunts are rarely used. Historically, a side-to-side portacaval shunt was indicated as definitive therapy for intractable ascites. However, due to the development of better medical and non-surgical options, the use of this particular intervention has fallen out of favor except in the most unusual circumstances. Transplantation is the only effective treatment for the chronic liver disease that predisposes patients to chronic ascites.

BILIARY DISEASE

Biliary Stones in the Patient with End-Stage Liver Disease

Biliary stones, typically pigmented stones, are more common in the cirrhotic than in the noncirrhotic patient. Asymptomatic gallstones should be left untreated as gallstones become symptomatic in the population at a rate of only 1% per year [77,78].

Cholecystectomy should be considered in the pretransplant patient only if symptoms are highly suggestive of biliary colic. In the cirrhotic patient, gallbladder surgery has been reported to be associated with high rates of postoperative morbidity and mortality [79]. The risk of surgery correlates with the degree of liver dysfunction as assessed by Child's classification. Laparoscopic cholecystectomy is feasible in some patients, although the open procedure is sometimes necessary to prevent or control bleeding. These patients are best managed by the surgeons who will be responsible for the transplant procedure.

Management of intrahepatic or common bile duct stones in patients with advanced liver disease is difficult. The therapy for a transplant candidate should focus on prevention of biliary obstruction and subsequent cholangitis. Biliary stricture should be treated by nonoperative means, including endoscopic retrograde cholangiography with stone extraction and sphincterotomy, or transhepatically. The choice of access is based on the location of stones in the biliary tree and the available local expertise. Although it is inefficient in dissolving stones, ursodeoxycholic acid is often used to prevent stone reformation and limit biliary sludging.

CONCLUSION

Portal hypertension, ascites, and progressive biliary diseases are common problems in patients potentially facing hepatic transplantation. Patients with portal hypertension present a challenge to the primary physician from both a medical and social context. Resuscitation and control of hemorrhage are the immediate concerns of initial therapy when a patient presents with bleeding. Once a diagnosis of varices is confirmed, specific, well-thought-out care plans can be initiated. Early recognition of the need for OLT evaluation is paramount. Therapeutic interventions in both the portal hypertensive patient and the patient with progressive biliary disease can have an impact not only on treatment options but also on the outcomes of any further interventions. Early referral to a transplant center can ensure timely evaluation and listing for those patients with progressive liver disease.

■ REFERENCES

1. Benoit JN, Granger DN. Splanchnic hemodynamics in chronic portal hypertension. Semin Liver Dis 1986;6(4):287–298.

2. Rockey DC, Weisiger RA. Endothelin induced contractility of stellate cells from normal and cirrhotic rat liver: implications for regulation of portal pressure and resistance. Hepatology 1996;24(1):233–240.

3. Wiest R, Groszmann RJ. The paradox of nitric oxide in cirrhosis and portal hypertension: too much, not enough. Hepatology 2002;35(2):478–491.

4. Vorobioff J, Bredfeldt JE, Groszmann RJ. Hyperdynamic circulation in portal-hypertensive rat model: a primary factor for maintenance of chronic portal hypertension. Am J Physiol 1983;244(1):G52–G57.

5. Groszmann RJ. Hyperdynamic circulation of liver disease 40 years later: pathophysiology and clinical consequences. Hepatology 1994;20(5):1359–1363.

6. Garcia-Tsao G, Groszmann RJ, Fisher RL, et al. Portal pressure, presence of gastroesophageal varices and variceal bleeding. Hepatology 1985;5(3):419–424.

7. D'Amico G, Pagliaro L, Bosch J. The treatment of portal hypertension: a meta-analytic review. Hepatology 1995;22(1):332–354.

8. Groszmann RJ, Garcia-Tsao G, Makuch RW. Multi-center randomized placebo-controlled trial of non-selective beta-blockers in the prevention of the complications of portal hypertension: final results and identification of predictive factors. Hepatology 2003;38(suppl 1):206A.

9. Merli M, Nicolini G, Angeloni S, et al. Incidence and natural history of small esophageal varices in cirrhotic patients. J Hepatol 2003;38(3):266–272.

10. Conn HO, Grace ND, Bosch J, et al. Propranolol in the prevention of the first hemorrhage from esophagogastric varices: a multicenter, randomized clinical trial. The Boston–New Haven–Barcelona Portal Hypertension Study Group. Hepatology 1991;13(5):902–912.

11. D'Amico G, Pagliaro L, Bosch J. Pharmacological treatment of portal hypertension: an evidence-based approach. Semin Liver Dis 1999;19(4):475–505.

12. Poynard T, Cales P, Pasta L, et al. Beta-adrenergic-antagonist drugs in the prevention of gastrointestinal bleeding in patients with cirrhosis and esophageal varices. An analysis of data and prognostic factors in 589 patients from four randomized clinical trials. Franco-Italian Multicenter Study Group. N Engl J Med 1991;324(22):1532–1538.

13. Merkel C, Marin R, Angeli P, et al. A placebo-controlled clinical trial of nadolol in the prophylaxis of growth of small esophageal varices in cirrhosis. Gastroenterology 2004;127(2):476–484.

14. Groszmann RJ, Bosch J, Grace ND, et al. Hemodynamic events in a prospective randomized trial of propranolol versus placebo in the prevention of a first variceal hemorrhage. Gastroenterology 1990;99(5):1401–1407.

15. Escorsell A, Bordas JM, Castaneda B, et al. Predictive value of the variceal pressure response to continued pharmacological therapy in patients with cirrhosis and portal hypertension. Hepatology 2000;31(5):1061–1067.

16. Bureau C, Peron JM, Alric L, et al. "A La Carte" treatment of portal hypertension: adapting medical therapy to hemodynamic response for the prevention of bleeding. Hepatology 2002;36(6):1361–1366.

17. Feu F, Garcia-Pagan JC, Bosch J, et al. Relation between portal pressure response to pharmacotherapy and risk of recurrent variceal haemorrhage in patients with cirrhosis. Lancet 1995;346(8982):1056–1059.

18. Abraczinskas DR, Ookubo R, Grace ND, et al. Propranolol for the prevention of first esophageal variceal hemorrhage: a lifetime commitment? Hepatology 2001;34(6):1096–1102.

19. Escorsell A, Ferayorni L, Bosch J, et al. The portal pressure response to beta-blockade is greater in cirrhotic patients without varices than in those with varices. Gastroenterology 1997;112(6):2012–2016.

20. Merkel C, Sacerdoti D, Bolognesi M, et al. Hemodynamic evaluation of the addition of isosorbide-5-mononitrate to nadolol in cirrhotic patients with insufficient response to the beta-blocker alone. Hepatology 1997;26(1):34–39.

21. Merkel C, Marin R, Enzo E, et al. Randomised trial of nadolol alone or with isosorbide mononitrate for primary prophylaxis of variceal bleeding in cirrhosis. Gruppo-Triveneto per L'ipertensione portale (GTIP). Lancet 1996;348(9043):1677–1681.

22. Merkel C, Marin R, Sacerdoti D, et al. Long-term results of a clinical trial of nadolol with or without isosorbide mononitrate for primary prophylaxis of variceal bleeding in cirrhosis. Hepatology 2000;31(2):324–329.

23. Garcia-Pagan JC, Morillas R, Banares R, et al. Propranolol plus placebo versus propranolol plus isosorbide-5-mononitrate in the prevention of a first variceal bleed: a double-blind RCT. Hepatology 2003;37(6):1260–1266.

24. de Franchis R. Updating consensus in portal hypertension: report of the Baveno III Consensus Workshop on definitions, methodology and therapeutic strategies in portal hypertension. J Hepatol 2000;33(5):846–852.

25. Garcia-Pagan JC, Villanueva C, Vila MC, et al. Isosorbide mononitrate in the prevention of first variceal bleed in patients who cannot receive beta-blockers. Gastroenterology 2001;121(4):908–914.

26. Lo GH, Chen WC, Chen MH, et al. Endoscopic ligation vs. nadolol in the prevention of first variceal bleeding in patients with cirrhosis. Gastrointest Endosc 2004;59(3):333–338.

27. Schepke M, Goebel C, Nuernberg D. Endoscopic banding ligation versus propranolol for the primary prevention of variceal bleeding in cirrhosis: a randomized controlled multicenter trial. Hepatology 2003;38(suppl 1):218A.

28. Imperiale TF, Chalasani N. A meta-analysis of endoscopic variceal ligation for primary prophylaxis of esophageal variceal bleeding. Hepatology 2001;33(4):802–807.

29. de Franchis R, Primignani M. Natural history of portal hypertension in patients with cirrhosis. Clin Liver Dis 2001;5(3):645–663.

30. Pugh RN, Murray-Lyon IM, Dawson JL, et al. Transection of the oesophagus for bleeding oesophageal varices. Br J Surg 1973;60(8):646–649.

31. McCormick PA, Jenkins SA, McIntyre N, et al. Why portal hypertensive varices bleed and bleed: a hypothesis. Gut 1995;36(1):100–103.

32. Kamath PS, Wiesner RH, Malinchoc M, et al. A model to predict survival in patients with end-stage liver disease. Hepatology 2001;33:464–470.

33. Rimola A, Garcia-Tsao G, Navasa M, et al. Diagnosis, treatment and prophylaxis of spontaneous bacterial peritonitis: a consensus document. International Ascites Club. J Hepatol 2000;32(1):142–153.

34. Levacher S, Letoumelin P, Pateron D, et al. Early administration of terlipressin plus glyceryl trinitrate to control active upper gastrointestinal bleeding in cirrhotic patients. Lancet 1995;346(8979):865–868.

35. Avgerinos A, Nevens F, Raptis S, et al. Early administration of somatostatin and efficacy of sclerotherapy in acute oesophageal variceal bleeds: the European Acute Bleeding Oesophageal Variceal Episodes (ABOVE) randomised trial. Lancet 1997;350(9090):1495–1499.

36. Cales P, Masliah C, Bernard B, et al. Early administration of vapreotide for variceal bleeding in patients with cirrhosis. French Club for the Study of Portal Hypertension. N Engl J Med 2001;344(1):23–28.

37. Moitinho E, Planas R, Banares R, et al. Multicenter randomized controlled trial comparing different schedules of somatostatin in the treatment of acute variceal bleeding. J Hepatol 2001;35(6):712–718.

38. Ejlersen E, Melsen T, Ingerslev J, et al. Recombinant activated factor VII (rFVIIa) acutely normalizes prothrombin time in patients with cirrhosis during bleeding from oesophageal varices. Scand J Gastroenterol 2001;36(10):1081–1085.

39. Bosch J, Thabut D, Bendtsen F, et al. Recombinant factor VIIa for upper gastrointestinal bleeding in patients with cirrhosis: a randomized, double-blind trial. Gastroenterology 2004;127(4):1123–1130.

40. Grace ND. Management of portal hypertension. Gastroenterologist 1993;1(1):39–58.

41. Terblanche J, Kahn D, Bornman PC. Long-term injection sclerotherapy treatment for esophageal varices. A 10-year prospective evaluation. Ann Surg 1989;210(6):725–731.

42. Groszmann RJ, Garcia-Tsao G. Endoscopic variceal banding vs. pharmacological therapy for the prevention of recurrent variceal hemorrhage: what makes the difference? Gastroenterology 2002;123(4):1388–1391.

43. Gimson AE, Ramage JK, Panos MZ, et al. Randomised trial of variceal banding ligation versus injection sclerotherapy for bleeding oesophageal varices. Lancet 1993;342(8868):391–394.

44. Burroughs AK, Patch D. Transjugular intrahepatic portosystemic shunt. Semin Liver Dis 1999;19(4):457–473.

45. Ring EJ, Lake JR, Roberts JP, et al. Using transjugular intrahepatic portosystemic shunts to control variceal bleeding before liver transplantation. Ann Intern Med 1992;116(4):304–309.

46. Rossle M, Haag K, Ochs A, et al. The transjugular intrahepatic portosystemic stent–shunt procedure for variceal bleeding. N Engl J Med 1994;330(3):165–171.

47. Bosch J. Salvage transjugular intrahepatic portosystemic shunt: is it really life-saving? J Hepatol 2001;35(5):658–660.

48. Azoulay D, Castaing D, Majno P, et al. Salvage transjugular intrahepatic portosystemic shunt for uncontrolled variceal bleeding in patients with decompensated cirrhosis. J Hepatol 2001;35(5):590–597.

49. Patch D, Nikolopoulou V, McCormick A, et al. Factors related to early mortality after transjugular intrahepatic portosystemic shunt for failed endoscopic therapy in acute variceal bleeding. J Hepatol 1998;28(3):454–460.

50. McCormick PA, O'Keefe C. Improving prognosis following a first variceal haemorrhage over four decades. Gut 2001;49(5):682–685.

51. Bosch J, Garcia-Pagan JC. Prevention of variceal rebleeding. Lancet 2003;361(9361): 952–954.

52. Boyer TD. Transjugular intrahepatic portosystemic shunt: current status. Gastroenterology 2003;124(6):1700–1710.

53. Burroughs AK, Vangeli M. Transjugular intrahepatic portosystemic shunt versus endoscopic therapy: randomized trials for secondary prophylaxis of variceal bleeding: an updated meta-analysis. Scand J Gastroenterol 2002;37(3):249–252.

54. Meddi P, Merli M, Lionetti R, et al. Cost analysis for the prevention of variceal rebleeding: a comparison between transjugular intrahepatic portosystemic shunt and endoscopic sclerotherapy in a selected group of Italian cirrhotic patients. Hepatology 1999;29(4):1074–1077.

55. Escorsell A, Banares R, Garcia-Pagan JC, et al. TIPS versus drug therapy in preventing variceal rebleeding in advanced cirrhosis: a randomized controlled trial. Hepatology 2002;35(2):385–392.

56. Bureau C, Garcia-Pagan JC, Otal P, et al. Improved clinical outcome using poly-tetrafluoroethylene-coated stents for TIPS: results of a randomized study. Gastro-enterology 2004;126(2):469–475.

57. Orloff MJ, Bell RH, Jr, Orloff MS, et al. Prospective randomized trial of emergency portacaval shunt and emergency medical therapy in unselected cirrhotic patients with bleeding varices (Part 1). Hepatology 1994;20(4):863–872.

58. AbouJaoude MM, Grant DR, Ghent CN, et al. Effect of portasystemic shunts on subsequent transplantation of the liver. Surg Gynecol Obstet 1991;172(3):215–219.

59. Warren WD, Millikan WJ, Jr, Henderson JM, et al. Ten years portal hyper-tensive surgery at Emory. Results and new perspectives. Ann Surg 1982;195(5):530–542.

60. Henderson JM, Gilmore GT, Hooks MA, et al. Selective shunt in the management of variceal bleeding in the era of liver transplantation. Ann Surg 1992;216(3):248–254; discussion 254–255.

61. Sarfeh IJ, Rypins EB. Partial versus total portacaval shunt in alcoholic cirrhosis. Results of a prospective, randomized clinical trial. Ann Surg 1994;219(4):353–361.

62. Sugiura M, Futagawa S. Further evaluation of the Sugiura procedure in the treat-ment of esophageal varices. Arch Surg 1977;112(11):1317–1321.

63. Mariette D, Smadja C, Borgonovo G, et al. The Sugiura procedure: a prospective experience. Surgery 1994;115(3):282–289.

64. D'Amico G, Morabito A, Pagliaro L, et al. Survival and prognostic indicators in compensated and decompensated cirrhosis. Dig Dis Sci 1986;31(5):468–475.

65. Runyon BA. Management of adult patients with ascites due to cirrhosis. Hepatol-ogy 2004;39(3):841–856.

66. Sungaila I, Bartle WR, Walker SE, et al. Spironolactone pharmacokinetics and phar-macodynamics in patients with cirrhotic ascites. Gastroenterology 1992;102(5):1680–1685.

67. Peltekian KM, Wong F, Liu PP, et al. Cardiovascular, renal, and neurohumoral responses to single large-volume paracentesis in patients with cirrhosis and diur-etic-resistant ascites. Am J Gastroenterol 1997;92(3):394–399.

68. Runyon BA. Patient selection is important in studying the impact of large-volume paracentesis on intravascular volume. Am J Gastroenterol 1997;92(3):371–373.

69. Arroyo V, Gines P, Gerbes AL, et al. Definition and diagnostic criteria of refractory ascites and hepatorenal syndrome in cirrhosis. International Ascites Club. Hepatol-ogy 1996;23(1):164–176.

70. Perez-Ayuso RM, Arroyo V, Planas R, et al. Randomized comparative study of efficacy of furosemide versus spironolactone in nonazotemic cirrhosis with ascites.

Relationship between the diuretic response and the activity of the renin–aldosterone system (Part 1). Gastroenterology 1983;84(5):961–968.

71. Runyon BA. Ascites and spontaneous bacterial peritonitis. Philadelphia, PA: WB Saunders, 2002.

72. Gines P, Arroyo V, Vargas V, et al. Paracentesis with intravenous infusion of albumin as compared with peritoneovenous shunting in cirrhosis with refractory ascites. N Engl J Med 1991;325(12):829–835.

73. Lebrec D, Giuily N, Hadengue A, et al. Transjugular intrahepatic portosystemic shunts: comparison with paracentesis in patients with cirrhosis and refractory ascites: a randomized trial. French Group of Clinicians and a Group of Biologists. J Hepatol 1996;25(2):135–144.

74. Rossle M, Ochs A, Gulberg V, et al. A comparison of paracentesis and transjugular intrahepatic portosystemic shunting in patients with ascites. N Engl J Med 2000;342(23):1701–1707.

75. Gines P, Uriz J, Calahorra B, et al. Transjugular intrahepatic portosystemic shunting versus paracentesis plus albumin for refractory ascites in cirrhosis. Gastroenterology 2002;123(6):1839–1847.

76. Sanyal AJ, Genning C, Reddy KR, et al. The North American Study for the treatment of refractory ascites. Gastroenterology 2003;124(3):634–641.

77. Strasberg SM, Clavien PA. Cholecystolithiasis: lithotherapy for the 1990s. Hepatology 1992;16(3):820–839.

78. Aranha GV, Sontag SJ, Greenlee HB. Cholecystectomy in cirrhotic patients: a formidable operation. Am J Surg 1982;143(1):55–60.

Psychosocial Evaluation of the Potential Recipient

▼ ▼ ▼ ▼ ▼ ▼ ▼ ▼ ▼

Robyn Lewis Claar

■ INTRODUCTION

Orthotopic liver transplantation (OLT) is an established and acceptable treatment modality for end-stage liver disease (ESLD) of a variety of etiologies. Unfortunately, many more patients are listed and waiting to undergo OLT than there are donor organs available; in the USA, over 17 000 patients were listed for OLT as of December 2003 [1]. Moreover, short- and long-term survival rates for liver transplant recipients are currently estimated at 79% and 78%, respectively [2]. Therefore, given the scarcity of available livers, as well as the significant mortality risk associated with OLT, potential liver transplant candidates are evaluated carefully to assess medical and psychological comorbidities that might adversely affect post-OLT outcomes.

Pre-OLT psychological evaluation of potential candidates focuses on known psychosocial risk factors that are associated with poor posttransplant outcomes, including active substance abuse, significant psychological distress or impairment, lack of social support, inability to adhere to medical regimens, and lack of readiness for OLT [3]. Certain factors may be considered absolute contraindications to liver transplantation (e.g. continued alcohol use), while other factors may be considered relative contraindications (e.g. mild symptoms of depression). In addition, psychosocial contraindications may vary by transplant center, with certain factors considered to be absolute contraindications at one center but only relative contraindications at another. This chapter focuses on psychosocial risk factors and contraindications to transplantation in the selection process of potential OLT recipients. It is important to note that patients often misconstrue the purpose of psychosocial assessment, believing it to be a means of determining a patient's "social worth" [3]. Thus, it is important to normalize the pretransplant psychological evaluation as an integral component of OLT evaluation. Ultimately, the goal of pretransplant psychological evaluation is to select those patients for OLT who will be able to care for and protect their new organ.

■ SUBSTANCE ABUSE

Alcohol

Many patients referred for consideration of OLT have a history of heavy and sustained alcohol use; alcoholic liver disease (ALD) is the second most common diagnosis in patients undergoing OLT [4]. Although some patients' alcohol use may have been sufficient to cause ESLD, not all patients meet diagnostic criteria for alcohol dependency [5]. It is not uncommon for patients who present for OLT evaluation to report that they consumed large quantities of alcohol yet did not experience clinically significant impairment or distress, a necessary requirement to meet the *Diagnostic and Statistical Manual of Mental Disorders* (4th edition) (DSM-IV) criteria for alcohol dependence [6]. Indeed, some patients claim that they did not experience any impairment from alcohol use until ALD was diagnosed.

Assessment of patients' current alcohol use is crucial to determining whether they are acceptable liver transplant candidates. When conducting clinical interviews, patients are more likely to admit to current alcohol use if questions are phrased with the assumption that they may be drinking. For example, asking "How much alcohol are you drinking?" rather than "Are you drinking alcohol?" typically provides more accurate information. However, because patients may underreport or misrepresent both current and/or past alcohol use, random alcohol screens are useful in providing an objective assessment of whether abstinence has been achieved and is being maintained. Alcohol screens also are warranted when patients provide conflicting reports of their alcohol use to different transplant team members; because conflicting self-reports are highly suspect and concerning, patients' self-reports should be corroborated objectively with random screens.

Current research estimates that between 30% and 50% of patients undergoing OLT for ALD return to some alcohol use 5 years post-OLT [7]. However, it is not surprising that relapse rates are so high, because relatively few patients had been required to participate in a rehabilitation program prior to OLT. Indeed, in a recent literature review, Weinrieb et al. [8] reported that they could find no formal studies of therapeutic interventions for patients with alcoholism who were awaiting or recovering from OLT. Now it is commonplace for liver transplant programs to require participation in a recognized rehabilitation program to minimize the likelihood of relapse. In our program, patients with a history of alcohol abuse are required to complete at least 6 months of abstinence and rehabilitation and to provide written confirmation of participation. This requirement becomes especially important when we consider that 66% of the patients evaluated for transplant at our center in 2004 who had reportedly achieved at least 6 months of abstinence prior to the initial evaluation either were not abstinent by their own admission or relapsed soon after that evaluation. Although vigorous debate continues regarding the utility of a pre-OLT abstinence criteria in predicting post-OLT abstinence, current research suggests that "until further data become available, application of a 6-month rule in most cases provides a safe and prudent means of ensuring that an individual with ALD is an appropriate candidate for liver transplantation" (p. S35) [9]. All patients at our center are informed that abstinence from alcohol is a requirement for continued consideration for OLT, whether or not alcohol was a contributing factor to the development of their ESLD. Lastly, patients are required to sign a behavioral contract (Table 4.1) documenting their understanding of and agreement to maintain abstinence, to seek rehabilitation if indicated, and to undergo random alcohol screens when requested. These random screens can be particularly useful in documenting whether continued alcohol consumption exists; in a recent study by DiMartini et al. [5], blood alcohol levels identified patients who were drinking covertly and were not forthcoming in their psychiatric interviews. Therefore, these researchers encourage inclusion of such screens among routine laboratory testing. Patients are informed at the time of the initial evaluation that a positive alcohol screen and/or failure to undergo a random alcohol screen may result in suspension of evaluation or removal from the waiting list. However, the behavioral contract also stipulates that because setbacks may occur, patients should inform the transplant team about potential relapses when they occur (or ideally prior to their occurrence), rather than waiting for a positive screen, thereby providing access to appropriate rehabilitation treatment and allowing future consideration for OLT.

One aim of the pre-OLT psychological evaluation is to identify those individuals who may be at risk for alcohol relapse when their health improves. For example, some patients have only recently ceased drinking alcohol because of a clinical complication of portal hypertension resulting in a prolonged hospital stay, and thus, are too sick to consume alcohol at the time of their transplant evaluation. However, as their health improves, these patients may be more likely to relapse than those patients who quit drinking alcohol prior to experiencing major medical complications or extended hospitalizations. In addition, because many of these patients have not undergone an alcohol rehabilitation program, the risk of relapse may be high. A recent study identified five significant risk factors for alcohol relapse: (1) living alone, (2) history of suicidal ideation, (3) history of past alcohol-related hospitalization, (4) lack of previous alcohol rehabilitation prior to the pre-OLT evaluation, and (5) failure to accept further alcohol rehabilitation prior to

Table 4.1 *Behavioral Contract*

Duke University Medical Center
Liver Transplant Program

You are being considered for liver transplantation at Duke University Medical Center. The success of the transplant procedure depends on your adherence to a medical program developed by your transplant team. This plan includes the following:

- Attending regular clinic visits
- Taking your medications as prescribed
- Maintaining a healthy weight
- Securing the commitment of family and/or friends to help you care for yourself before and after transplant
- Abstaining from the use of alcohol, tobacco, and drugs not prescribed by your physicians

By signing this contract, I _____ , make a commitment to myself, my family, and the transplant team to take care of myself in the following ways:

_____ 1. I will follow the treatment plan as prescribed by my physicians. I will attend my clinic appointments and take my medications as directed. I will read the pre-transplant educational materials provided by the team and ask questions about any content I don't understand. If I develop a concern or question about any part of the treatment plan or my medications, I will contact my providers if the concern is urgent. If the concern is not urgent, I will raise it at my next scheduled visit.

_____ 2. I understand that alcohol use is prohibited for anyone with liver disease. I commit to not drinking any alcohol—including that found in over-the-counter cold medication—even if alcohol did not cause my liver disease. If alcohol dependence or abuse has been identified as an issue for me, and is a likely part of the cause of my liver disease, I must demonstrate 6 months of abstinence before being considered for listing. I will provide the team with documented evidence of my participation in any recommended treatment programs.

_____ 3. I will not use any substance or drug not prescribed by my physician. If I have used any illegal drugs or substances in the past, I understand that I must demonstrate 6 months of abstinence from illicit drugs before being considered for listing. I will provide the team with documented evidence of my participation in any recommended treatment programs.

_____ 4. I will stop smoking all substances, including marijuana, cigarettes, pipes, and cigars, or using any tobacco products. I must demonstrate 6 months of abstinence from marijuana or any illicit drugs before being considered for listing.

_____ 5. I am willing to have random urine and/or blood tests for evidence of drugs, nicotine, and/or alcohol. I recognize that the transplant team may call me at any time and request that I have this testing at Duke or my local doctor's office. Refusal to comply with this request within 24 hours will be considered a positive test and may result in my removal from the transplant list.

Table 4.1 *Continued*

_____ 6. One drug or alcohol related incident will result in permanent removal from the transplant list.

_____ 7. Failure to keep appointments and/or follow the instructions of the team will also be seen as a lack of commitment on my part. Two serious occurrences may also result in permanent removal from the list at the decision of the team.

_____ 8. I understand that I am responsible for the costs of transplantation. There are likely to be costs to me, as few insurance plans cover all of the expenses in full.

_____ 9. I understand that if I break this contract I may not be eligible for transplantation.
I understand that changing and/or maintaining healthy behaviors is difficult and I may experience setbacks. I commit to seeking immediate assistance to bring any violation of this contract under control. I will be honest in my requests for support in difficult situations. If I feel like I am going to break this contract, I will call a member of the transplant team for assistance.

_____ 10. When I receive a transplant, I understand that these requirements must continue as a lifetime commitment. I understand that failure to comply may result in premature loss of liver function or death.

_____ 11. Other _____

_____

_____

_____

Patient Signature

_____

Date

_____

Witness

_____

Date

OLT [10]. An additional relapse risk factor is past illicit drug use: one longitudinal study demonstrated that a history of illicit drug use at any time prior to OLT was significantly associated with alcohol relapse post transplant [11]. Thus, examination of current and past illicit drug use becomes increasingly important, given that it is a potential risk factor for recidivism/alcohol relapse.

Illicit Drug Use

Many potential transplant candidates have a history of illicit drug use. Continued illicit drug use may undermine both the immediate and long-term success of OLT [12], and so careful assessment is required during the evaluation process prior to recommending that patients be listed for OLT. As with alcohol abuse, patients may attempt to minimize or even rationalize illicit drug use in order to be considered eligible for OLT. For example, some potential OLT recipients will report that continued use of marijuana is for appetite stimulation, when in fact its use is primarily recreational. Almost all centers will insist upon a fixed period of abstinence from illicit drug use prior to evaluation or consideration of listing for OLT, which should be demonstrated by random toxicology screens to verify self-reported abstinence. Rehabilitation also is required for those patients with a past history of significant substance abuse or for those patients who have tested positive for illicit drug use during the evaluation and/or pre-OLT waiting periods. Patients should provide documentation of participation in recommended rehabilitation programs.

Tobacco Use

Smoking increases the peri- and postoperative risk of both myocardial infarction and stroke [12]. Moreover, decreased survival has been documented in transplant patients who smoke [13]. Thus, tobacco cessation is generally recommended but does not constitute an absolute requirement for listing at all liver transplant programs [12]. However, if patients demonstrate equivocal results of pulmonary function testing and/or evidence of important vascular disease, they should be required to abstain from tobacco use prior to OLT listing. All other patients are strongly encouraged to stop smoking. Levenson and Olbrisch [14] note that significant controversies continue to exist among liver transplant programs regarding smoking cessation, despite data that clearly support better outcomes when tobacco abstinence is required. Thus, regardless of whether smoking cessation will be a transplant team medical requirement, all potential OLT patients are advised to quit smoking during their pre-OLT psychosocial evaluations, because smoking is a major cardiovascular risk factor that may affect post-OLT survival. Furthermore, the increased risk of de novo malignant disease among patients transplanted for ALD as opposed to non-ALD is further evidence, if it were needed, that smoking cessation is a vital pre-OLT requirement [15].

As part of the pretransplant psychosocial evaluation, patients are provided with specific behavioral techniques for smoking cessation to cope with their physical addiction to nicotine, including the use of nicotine replacement products. Use of alternative coping mechanisms also may be discussed, as some patients rely on cigarette smoking as a coping method for reducing anxiety. It may be especially difficult for these patients to quit smoking if their anxiety remains untreated. Thus, these patients may benefit from a referral for mental health treatment prior to/in conjunction with addressing their smoking cessation.

■ PSYCHOLOGICAL FUNCTIONING

The pretransplant period can be extremely stressful. Declining health, uncertainty about the possibility of OLT, and inability to continue working and participating in daily activities all may increase the risk of depression and/or anxiety for the transplant candidate. Streisand et al. [16] found that over half of the patients evaluated for OLT at their center reported at least mild levels of depression, and over one-third reported clinically elevated levels of anxiety. Pretransplant psychopathology may predict posttransplant psychological functioning [3]; those patients who experience psychological distress prior to transplantation are likely to experience increased distress after transplantation, which may ultimately impact their recovery from transplantation. Recent research suggests that patients with chronic hepatitis C virus liver disease have a greater incidence of depression and anxiety than patients with other forms of liver disease [17]; thus, these patients in particular should be carefully screened and monitored. Patients who experience depression or anxiety are encouraged—and sometimes required—to seek psychiatric treatment prior to OLT to improve their emotional and physical functioning. While some patients may be resistant at first to pursuing such treatment, we have found that recommendations for treatment are received more positively when framed as a means to improve the patient's success with OLT. Those patients who experience significant psychological distress prior to OLT have increased complications with postsurgical recovery.

In many cases, patients experience psychological distress regarding impending OLT that is not severe enough to limit their ability to care for themselves or their transplanted organ. However, some patients experience psychological distress or impairment that interferes with their health behavior to such an extent that it may prevent them from adhering to medical directives. For example, when patients experience severe symptoms of depression characterized by feelings of worthlessness and/or passive suicidal ideation, they may stop taking prescribed medications. Similarly, a patient who experiences a manic episode characterized by feelings of grandiosity and decreased need for sleep may not engage in necessary personal health care behaviors. These patients should be required to pursue psychiatric services until their functioning is stable enough to be evaluated and satisfactorily listed for OLT. It is important to note that most psychiatric diagnoses are not considered absolute contraindications to OLT, although active schizophrenia is viewed as an absolute contraindication by the over two-thirds of US liver transplant programs [3]. Additional diagnoses that may be seen as absolute contraindications to transplant include untreated psychosis, active suicidal ideation, intractable noncompliance, and significant brain dysfunction (including delirium, dementia, and severe mental retardation) [18,19].

When assessing patients' cognitive functioning and brain dysfunction, it should be remembered that patients with ESLD listed for OLT not uncommonly suffer bouts of hepatic encephalopathy (portosystemic encephalopathy (PSE); Chapters 1 and 2) that affect their global cognitive functioning. Not surprisingly, Streisand et al. [16] found that greater disease severity was associated with poorer cognitive functioning. It is important to assess the onset of cognitive difficulties, because some patients who present for evaluation may have long-standing cognitive limitations that are independent of episodes of PSE. Such patients may benefit from full neuropsychological assessment in order to understand the nature of their deficits as well as to provide them with compensatory strategies with which to undertake the demanding liver transplant regimen. Although a full neuropsychological assessment is both time-consuming and expensive, it is difficult to fully assess and understand the nature of cognitive deficits without such testing. For those patients with significant cognitive limitations, social support and the presence of one or more dedicated caregivers may be crucial to their ability to undergo OLT, as they may be unable to understand the complicated medical regimens without considerable social support. Transplant centers may be cautious in transplanting those patients with significant cognitive limitations; Levenson and Olsbrisch [3] reported that a diagnosis of mental retardation (IQ < 70) is considered a relative contraindication to transplant for 70% of liver transplant centers, and a diagnosis of severe mental retardation (IQ < 50), is viewed as an absolute contraindication to transplant by 46% of centers. Overall, assessing patients' cognitive functioning is important to ensure that patients can understand the pre- and posttransplant medical regimen that is needed for successful outcome to OLT.

Nonadherence

Liver transplant patients must be able and willing to adhere to complex medical regimens both before and after OLT. Note that the term adherence, rather than compliance, is used here as it implies an active partnership between the patient and the medical team in treatment of the medical condition, while the term compliance typically describes a patient's ability to passively follow prescribed medical directives. Lifelong adherence to immunosuppressive therapy post-OLT is crucial for continued success. Patients who do not adhere to medical regimens are at risk for acute and chronic allograft rejection, organ loss, and death [20]. In fact, nonadherence or poor adherence is responsible for as many as 25% of transplant patient deaths after the initial recovery period [21]. In order to predict posttransplant adherence, patients' current adherence behaviors should be closely assessed during the pretransplant psychosocial evaluation. Research demonstrates that one-fifth of transplant patients do not take their medications as prescribed in terms of dosing and timing [20].

When assessing patients' adherence in the pretransplant psychosocial assessment, medication adherence difficulties are normalized (i.e. "Many patients I see have difficulty remembering to take their medications. How have you been doing with that?") so that patients may feel comfortable admitting areas of difficulty. Patients' abilities to afford, remember, and take their medications are assessed. Many OLT patients report that they have difficulty affording current medications and often fail to fill prescriptions or run out of their medications before money is available for a refill. It is critical that these patients meet with a financial coordinator to determine that they will have the necessary financial resources to pay for their expensive posttransplant medications. It is not uncommon for patients to undertake some fund-raising efforts to secure necessary financial resources.

Forgetting to take medications has been cited as the primary barrier to adherence [20]. Patients often report that as the result of episodes of PSE, they cannot recall with certainty whether medications have been taken faithfully. Two common approaches can be used to remedy this situation. First, many patients can enlist assistance from a spouse or other caregiver to remind them to take their medications. In some cases, caregivers will assume responsibility for distributing medications to patients. Second, patients may benefit from using a pill box organizer in which their medications are distributed for each daily dose, usually a week at a time, so that they have a visual reminder and tracking system to facilitate improved adherence.

Many patients may not take their medications because of significant side-effects. In fact, when transplant patients were asked what they most disliked about medications, side-effects was listed as the primary concern [22]. Dissatisfaction with side-effects is often a concern during the pretransplant period also. For example, some patients report that they limit or discontinue certain diuretic medications due to dissatisfaction with their side-effects. These side-effects are likely mild in comparison with some of the side-effects reported for immunosuppressive medications such as seizures, altered mental status, and excessive hair growth [23]. In order to increase the likelihood that patients will adhere to the posttransplant immunosuppressive regimen, they should be asked to demonstrate improved adherence during the pretransplant period, preferably prior to listing for OLT.

Failure to attend clinic appointments may serve as a warning for additional areas of nonadherence and signal that the patient may not be able to adhere to other aspects and demands of the medical regimen. The patient behavioral contract (Table 4.1) includes an item about appointment attendance, and patients are informed that failure to keep appointments is viewed as a serious lack of commitment and adherence to the process. Two occurrences of nonadherence may potentially result in a patient's removal from further evaluation and/or listing.

Social Support

Patients cannot and should not undergo stressful OLT without considerable social support. Depending on the severity of the patient's illness at the time of OLT evaluation, many family members and/or close friends may already have assumed caregiving duties, including overseeing medication and dietary regimens and coordinating the patient's medical appointments. The pre-OLT evaluation includes an assessment of the patient's available social support network as well as designation of primary caregivers. Specifically, the caregiver's relationship with the patient, current functioning, availability, and willingness to provide perioperative care are assessed, as patients will rely heavily upon their caregivers during the perioperative period. Patients also need to identify stable caregivers who can provide reliable transportation and temporarily relocate with them to the transplant center area if they currently reside a significant distance from the transplant center. In addition, the potential caregiver may need to arrange for time away from work and/or for care of other family members in order to assume the transplant caregiving duties. Caregivers' functioning should continue to be assessed throughout the pretransplant period, as caregiving responsibilities have been associated with significant negative impact on caregivers' physical and mental health [24,25].

Some patients may have trouble identifying reliable, stable support. When possible, it is important to meet patients' caregivers in nonemergency settings; sometimes family members or friends only emerge when the patient is in the midst of a life-threatening illness and would not survive without imminent transplantation. Such patterns of support do not bode well. Often these caregivers, although well intentioned, may commit to caring for the patient largely out of a sense of obligation, but may be unable or unwilling to follow through fully with necessary caregiving duties or responsibilities. When caregivers abandon patients after OLT, the complicated task of securing alternate care in structured settings can be faced by the transplant team.

Patients may be asked to continue to bring their caregivers to transplant clinic appointments to assess the caregivers' level of understanding and commitment. Generally, inclusion of caregivers in medical and psychological assessments is viewed as a valuable opportunity to educate and support the family, to monitor family functioning, and to provide referrals for local mental health care as needed [12]. In addition, recommendations can be provided for local support groups to provide family members an opportunity to talk with other transplant patient caregivers and to develop adaptive methods for coping with the stressful transplant process.

Readiness for Transplant

It is important to assess the patient's motivation and readiness for liver transplant. Some patients have only recently learned of the need for liver transplant evaluation and listing and may feel quite overwhelmed and/or unprepared for necessary undertakings. Other patients may be ambivalent about whether they wish to pursue transplantation; in fact, some patients may present for evaluation at the urging of physicians, spouses, or other family members, although they themselves may have ambivalent feelings about pursuing OLT. It can be helpful to speak privately with these patients during the pre-OLT psychological evaluation to determine their personal interest in and commitment to transplantation, because they may be unable to voice their concerns in the presence of individuals who believe that OLT must be pursued at all costs. Certain patients may be in denial regarding the severity of their liver disease, which is viewed as a contraindication to transplant in the majority of liver transplant programs [14]. Alternatively, patients may be uninformed about posttransplant requirements. For example, some patients may be unaware of the lifelong need for immunosuppressive therapy or may think that liver transplantation will completely resolve all remaining health problems. We discuss with patients their knowledge about transplantation and attempt to answer any questions or concerns that they may have. It is important to ensure that patients possess a good understanding of the transplant process; a lack of understanding about transplantation is considered an absolute contraindication to transplant in 15% of liver transplant programs [14]. When assessing readiness for transplantation, patients are reminded of the importance of continued adherence to all medical directives to increase the success of liver transplantation.

■ SUMMARY

Psychosocial evaluation of the potential OLT patient is an important part of pretransplant evaluation in order to determine the patient's suitability for transplantation and the likelihood of successful outcomes. This evaluation should focus primarily on known psychosocial risk factors associated with poor transplant outcomes including substance abuse, psychiatric distress, and medical nonadherence. Patients should be asked to demonstrate their understanding of these risk factors by signing a behavioral contract documenting their commitment to self-care both before and after transplantation. Specifically, they must commit to substance abstinence, medical adherence, and recommendations designed to increase their success with OLT (e.g. rehabilitation to maintain alcohol abstinence or psychotherapy for treatment of depression). The ultimate goal of pretransplant psychosocial evaluation is to assess whether patients are suitable candidates for OLT, and if they are not appropriate candidates at the present time, we strive to provide the resources and support to assist them in becoming better candidates in the future.

■ REFERENCES

1. Scientific Registry of Transplant Recipients. About transplant: fast facts. Available at www.ustransplant.org/facts.html. Accessed September 23, 2004.

2. 2003 Annual Report of the US Organ Procurement and Transplantation Network. Available at http://www.optn.org/AR2003/909b_li.pdf. Accessed May 4, 2004.

3. Levenson JL, Olbrisch ME. Psychosocial screening and candidate selection. In Trzepacz P, DiMartini A, eds., The transplant patient: biological, psychiatric, and ethical issues in organ transplantation. Cambridge: Cambridge University Press, 2000:21–41.

4. Belle SH, Beringer KC, Detre KM. Liver transplantation for alcoholic liver disease in the United States: 1988–1995. Liver Transpl Surg 1997;3:212–219.

5. DiMartini A, Day N, Dew M, et al. Alcohol use following liver transplantation: a comparison of follow-up methods. Psychosomatics 2001;42:55–62.

6. Diagnostic and statistical manual of mental disorders, 4th ed., Washington, DC: American Psychiatric Association, 1994.

7. Lucey MR, Weinrieb RM. Liver transplantation and alcoholics: is the glass half full or half empty? Gut 1999;45:326–327.

8. Weinrieb RM, Van Horn DHA, McLellan AT, et al. Alcoholism treatment after liver transplantation: lessons learned from a clinical trial that failed. Psychosomatics 2001;42:110–116.

9. Lim JK, Keeffe EB. Liver transplantation for alcoholic liver disease: current concepts and length of sobriety. Liver Transpl 2004;10:S31–S38.

10. Karman JF, Sileri P, Kamuda D, et al. Risk factors for failure to meet listing requirements in liver transplant candidates with alcoholic cirrhosis. Transplantation 2001;71:1210–1213.

11. Foster PF, Fabrega F, Sedat K, et al. Prediction of abstinence from ethanol in alcoholic recipients following liver transplantation. Hepatology 1997;25:1469–1477.

12. Olbrisch ME, Benedict SM, Ashe K, et al. Psychological assessment and care of organ transplant patients. J Consult Clin Psychol 2002;70:771–783.

13. Cosio FG, Falkenhain ME, Pesavento TE, et al. Patient survival after renal transplantation: II. The impact of smoking. Clin Transplant 1999;13:336–341.

14. Levenson JL, Olbrisch ME. Psychosocial evaluation of organ transplant candidates: a comparative survey of process, criteria, and outcomes in heart, liver, and kidney transplantation. Psychosomatics 1993;34:314–323.

15. Jain AB, Fung JJ. Alcoholic liver disease and transplantation. Transplant Proc 2003;35:359–360.

16. Streisand RM, Rodrigue JR, Sears SF, et al. A psychometric normative database for pre-liver transplantation evaluations: the Florida cohort 1991–1996. Psychosomatics 1999;40:479–485.

17. Singh N, Gayowski T, Wagener MM, et al. Vulnerability to psychologic distress and depression in patients with end-stage liver disease due to hepatitis C virus. Clin Transplant 1997;11:406–411.

18. Holmes VF. Psychiatric evaluation and care of the liver transplant patient. In Killenberg PG, Clavien PA, eds., Medical care of the liver transplant patient. Malden, MA: Blackwell Science, 2001;92–109.

19. Surman OS. Psychiatric aspects of liver transplantation. Psychosomatics 1994;35:297–307.

20. Laederach-Hofmann K, Bunzel B. Noncompliance in organ transplant recipients: a literature review. Gen Hosp Psychiatry 2000;22:412–424.

21. Bunzel B, Laederach-Hofmann K. Solid organ transplantation: are there predictors for posttransplant noncompliance? A literature overview. Transplantation 2000;5:711–716.

22. Kory L. Nonadherence to immunosuppressive medications: a pilot survey of members of the transplant recipients international organization. Transplant Proc 1999;31:14S–15S.

23. Muir AJ. Pharmacology of immunosuppressive therapy. In Killenberg PG, Clavien PA, eds., Medical care of the liver transplant patient. Malden, MA: Blackwell Science, 2001;361–377.

24. Dew MA, Goycoolea JM, Stukas AA, et al. Temporal profiles of physical health in family members of heart transplant recipients: predictors of health change during caregiving. Health Psychol 1998;17:138–151.

25. Meltzer LJ, Rodrigue JR. Psychological distress in caregivers of liver and lung transplant candidates. J Clin Psychol Med Settings 2001;8:173–180.

Financial Considerations

▼   ▼   ▼   ▼   ▼   ▼   ▼   ▼   ▼

**Paul C. Kuo and
Rebecca A. Schroeder**

I N T H E four decades since orthotopic liver transplantation (OLT) was first performed, it has evolved from an unproven experimental therapy to an accepted state-of-the-art therapy for patients with end-stage liver disease (ESLD) or various metabolic diseases. Correspondingly, the number of transplantations performed in the USA and in Europe has increased dramatically in the past decade. The number of transplantations performed more than doubled from 2201 in 1989 to 4700 in 1999 (USA), and likewise from 2103 in 1990 to 4228 in 1999 (Europe) [1,2]. Currently, the number of transplantations performed is limited by the availability of suitable donor organs, evidenced by the ever-increasing number of patients on the liver transplant waiting list: 2997 patients in 1993 to 14 709 patients in 1999. The average 1-year patient survival rate in the USA for patients undergoing transplantation increased from 81.5% in 1993 to 86.2% in 1997, reported by the United Network for Organ Sharing (UNOS) [1]. In Europe, the data are similar; between 1990 and 1994, 1-year patient survival was 76%. By 2001, this figure had reached 83% [2].

Although liver transplantation has been a success story of modern medicine, it is a particularly resource-intensive medical procedure. OLT remains severely resource-limited in terms of organ availability and cost. It is one of the most expensive surgical procedures and can have a major impact on health system expenditures [3]. Critics of liver transplantation suggest that it is an inappropriate and unacceptable allocation of public resources in a time of limited health care funding. In this modern era, the challenges presented to the liver transplant community are to: (1) determine the relative societal benefits of this therapy, and subsequently, (2) devise strategies that lower societal costs while maintaining or improving clinical outcomes. While only one of the many factors that are relevant, there can be no doubt that the relative economic costs and benefits of OLT must be considered. As a result, the mandates of economics may significantly impact implementation of clinical therapeutic strategies. In this chapter, we introduce the relevant concepts of an economic approach to this analysis and their application to liver transplantation in the adult cadaver and living donor settings.

■ ECONOMIC CONSIDERATIONS

In regard to health care analysis, Evans [4] defines six relevant economic concepts: cost, charge, reimbursement, price, resource use, and expenditures.

Cost: The economic value of both labor and resource inputs required to provide a service or perform a procedure.

Charge: The amount a patient or third-party payer is actually billed by a health care organization.

Reimbursement: The amount a patient or third-party payer actually pays based on billed charges. The amount can be determined retrospectively or prospectively. There is often a shortfall between billed charges and payment.

Price: The amount a third-party payer has determined in advance (i.e. prospectively) that it will pay for a service or procedure.

Resource use: A nonmonetary summary of the labor and resource inputs required to perform a procedure or provide a service (e.g. length of stay, number of laboratory tests).

Expenditures: The total amount of money spent to provide health care to a defined population over a specified period of time.

To date, health care economic analyses are complicated by the use of charges versus costs. True economic costs are not easily observable or measurable. Typically, proxies are used, such as charges, accounting costs, reimbursement payments, or program costs. The appropriateness of the measure depends on the perspective being considered, for example, payer versus societal. Charges, the total amount (including profit) billed to a patient and/or third-party payer, are typically greater than economic costs, the value of resources used to provide medical care. In addition, charges reflect many other parameters besides cost, exhibit regional and interhospital variation, and, generally, can introduce considerable error into calculations. As a result, evaluation of societal benefits of OLT requires a reliable cost assessment method and adequate follow-up information to permit identification of key cost determinants and the performance of cost–outcome analyses of OLT. In this regard, activity-based cost accounting systems have been suggested to provide a more accurate assessment of resource utilization.

A number of methods are available for economic analysis [4]. Each technique is tailored to the particular needs of each analysis type.

Cost-minimization analysis: This technique identifies the least costly technology among one or more alternatives, all of which are assumed to be of equal benefit. Costs are expressed in monetary terms; benefits are not measured.

Cost–outcome or cost-consequences analysis: This method forces the decision makers to identify the best technology among one or more alternatives. Cost (e.g. hospital charges) and outcomes (e.g. reduced incidence of heart failure) are listed in a disaggregated form but not assigned weights or values.

Cost-effectiveness analysis: This technology measures the costs and outcomes of providing a technology, compared with one or more alternatives. Costs are expressed in monetary terms; benefits are expressed in common units for each alternative, including life years gained.

Cost-utility analysis: This technique measures the cost and outcomes of providing a technology, compared with one or more alternatives. Costs are expressed in monetary terms; benefits are expressed in terms of a common scale for each alternative, including quality-adjusted life years (QALY).

Cost–benefit analysis: This technique measures the net financial loss or gain to society of providing a technology. Costs are expressed in monetary terms; benefits are also assigned monetary values.

Health care economic analysis aims to identify cost-effective technologies that can be deployed in an economically efficient health care delivery system. This would be a state of "clinical utilitarianism," as coined by Evans [4].

■ ADULT LIVER TRANSPLANTATION

Liver transplantation has never been, most likely will never be, the subject of a randomized controlled trial, and there remains uncertainty about the magnitude of benefit and cost-effectiveness for specific patient groups. An alternative approach would be the financial analysis of the management of complications in patients while waiting for an organ. Brand et al. [5] hypothesized that an increase in the number of organ grafts would decrease health care costs in patients with liver disease by eliminating the cost of waiting for an organ. The authors examined treatment costs for a consecutive series of liver transplant candidates listed between November 1, 1996 and December 31, 1997. Costs were estimated for inpatient stays, outpatient visits, and posttransplant medications for $2\frac{1}{2}$ years from the date of listing. Of the 58 study patients, 26 (45%) received transplants, 7 of whom died within $2\frac{1}{2}$ years. A total of 11 patients (19%) died while waiting for an organ, and another 21 patients (36%) were still waiting after the conclusion of the study. Pretransplantation costs accounted for 41% of the total cost. Transplanting all 58 candidates without delay through a hypothetical increase in the supply of organs to meet demand would have more than doubled the number of transplants while increasing costs in this cohort by only 37% (from $123 000 to $169 000 per patient). These authors conclude that the savings achieved by transplanting all candidates without delay offset a large portion of the added cost of these additional transplants. However, it remains unknown whether there is a cost savings achieved by utilization of liver transplantation.

As a first step in the process of examining OLT, it is imperative that the "cost" be determined. In the USA, many studies utilize charge data rather than cost data. In an attempt to remedy this issue, Best [1] utilized Medicare reimbursement data for OLT during the period from 1993 to 1999. Average first-year expenditures (base year: 2000) decreased from $201 000 in 1993 to $143 000 in 1998. In a parallel fashion, inpatient costs decreased from $179 000 in 1993 to $120 000 in 1998. Substantive cost reductions during this time were the result of a reduction in total days of hospitalization. The authors caution that generalizability was in question as only 10% of transplants in this country were covered under Medicare. Longworth [6] examined the economics of adult liver transplantation in England and Wales for the diagnoses of alcoholic cirrhosis, primary biliary cirrhosis (PBC), and primary sclerosing cholangitis (PSC). Cost-effectiveness was measured using incremental cost per QALY. The results of a comparison group, representing results in the absence of liver transplantation, were estimated with published prognostic models and observed data from patients waiting for transplantation. The extent of this increase in QALY differs among the groups, with lower cost-efficacy estimates for alcoholic liver disease compared with PBC and PSC. The survival and estimated gain in QALY was positive for all three diagnostic categories. In lieu of formalized prospective randomized trials of OLT, the bulk of the data suggests that OLT is associated with added life expectancy, albeit at great cost.

Multiple attempts have been made for determining the true costs of OLT and their sources. In recognition of the weakness of using charge data, Whiting et al. [7] analyzed activity-based costs at the University of Cincinnati for 53 transplants during the period 1995 to 1996. Professional fees and outpatient medication costs were not included. Actual costs were masked. Multivariate analysis revealed that length of stay, retransplantation, and postoperative dialysis were significantly and independently associated with costs ($r^2 = 0.605$). Length of stay was the strongest predictor of total costs. Subsequently, the authors performed stepwise logistic regression on Length of stay (LS) and found that recipient age, the UNOS status, donor age, and major bacterial or fungal infection were significantly associated; in fact, 50% of the variability of posttransplant costs can be explained by LS alone. Interestingly, allograft rejection was not a factor. The authors discuss the financial strategy of avoidance of complex cases to achieve the best possible outcomes with the lowest possible costs. In a similar fashion, an analysis of cost in the Canadian system was performed by Taylor [8] and encompassed 119 patients who underwent OLT between 1991 and 1992. The cost of pretransplantation, posttransplantation, and transplantation phases was determined. Professional fees were included. Costs were calculated using a standardized technique applied to all services in the Canadian province of Ontario. In many cases, the mean cost was dramatically higher than the median, suggesting a large range of values with extremely skewed data points. The largest single measured cost was inpatient care. The combination of intensive and ward care accounted for 49% of the overall cost. Pretransplant correlates of higher cost included female recipient, alcoholic cirrhosis, recipient age >60 years, and severity of illness. For the transplant phase, severity of illness, additional surgical procedures, and biliary complications were associated with significantly higher costs. Overall, elevated costs were correlated with severity of illness, additional surgical procedures, CMV infection, and biliary complications. In a similar European study, Filipponi et al. [3] examined liver transplant costs in an Italian National Health Services hospital. Their series consisted of a total of 235 adult transplants performed from 1997 to 2000. Staff and diagnostic costs accounted for the largest proportion of liver transplantation costs. Three baseline characteristics significantly impacted costs: portal vein thrombosis, elevated serum creatinine, and fulminant hepatic failure. Finally, the authors link cost-to-outcome ratio to an adequate annual volume of OLT (i.e. >25 per year). However, center-specific characteristics make the relevance of these data difficult to extrapolate as viral hepatitis was the principal diagnosis for 75% of their OLT volume. Additional factors can also play a role. Schnitzler et al. [9] specifically examined the role of preservation time on the economics of OLT. Interestingly, each additional hour of preservation time incurred an additional 1.4% in standardized hospital resource utilization. However, there was no effect on patient survival and retransplantation rates. These studies demonstrate the variability in economic analyses that are center- and disease-dependent.

In the realm of retransplantation, Markmann [10] retrospectively reviewed 1148 consecutive adult liver transplants at UCLA to determine preoperative factors associated with resource utilization. They identified five variables that have independent prognostic value in predicting graft survival: donor age, recipient age, donor sodium and recipient creatinine concentrations, and recipient ventilator requirement before the transplant. Of these, recipient ventilator requirements and elevated creatinine concentration were associated with significant increases in resource utilization. The combination of both these variables correlated with 140% increase in the intensive care unit (ICU) length of stay and 49% increase in hospital charges. In a similar fashion, Azoulay et al. [11]

found that retransplantation was associated with significantly longer hospital and ICU lengths of stay, and higher total hospital charges. Three patient variables in this setting correlated with poor outcomes: age, creatinine concentration, and urgency of retransplantation (with the exception of primary nonfunction). These data allow clinicians to rationally select patients for retransplantation with an aim toward cost control and resource utilization.

Finally, recouping the societal costs of OLT would typically take the form of return to work. Little is known about this, but a study by Loinaz [12] provides a detailed evaluation of employment patterns of 137 patients before and after transplantation at a center in Spain. Only 28% were still working at the time of OLT; after transplant, 56% returned to work at an average of 2.6 months posttransplant. Patients less than 50 years of age and those who worked within 12 months of transplant were significantly more likely to return to work. These results suggest that a return to work is a realistic outcome for many patients following OLT.

■ LIVING DONOR LIVER TRANSPLANTATION

Living donor liver transplantation (LDLT) is an emerging technology for the treatment of ESLD. Theoretically, this would increase the number of patients undergoing transplantation. However, the economic realities of this approach are not fully known as yet. In a center-specific analysis from the University of Colorado, Trotter et al. [13] performed a cost comparison of adult-to-adult right hepatic lobe LDLT with cadaver transplantation (CT) [13]. A total of 24 LDLTs and 43 CTs were performed between August 1997 and April 2000. A majority of recipients were UNOS status 2B. The authors examined all medical costs, including those of rejected donors and follow-up costs for a period of 365 days after surgery. The costs incurred for rejected donors were averaged over the entire population of LDLT recipients. Their costs were presented as an arbitrary cost unit (CU). The source of these cost data is unclear and professional fees were not included. Nevertheless, a number of valid conclusions can be drawn. The cost of pretransplant care encompassing the 90-day period prior to transplantation was almost twofold greater in the LDLT recipients. Mean length of stay was 50% higher in LDLT recipients. The cost of the transplant admission was 24% higher for LDLT. These LDLT recipient costs include all donor evaluations, donor hepatectomy, and donor medical care for one postoperative year. Medical care for LDLT recipients for 1 year after transplant was 4% lower than for CT. Total cost for CT was 21% lower than for LDLT. Interestingly, the cost for evaluation and surgery of successfully evaluated donors was not statistically different from the organ acquisition cost for CT. However, only 10% of donors underwent liver biopsy, endoscopic retrograde cholangiopancreatography (ERCP), or arteriography. When donor costs were further analyzed, evaluation, hepatectomy, and medical care for the first year after donation comprised 13%, 74%, and 7%, respectively, of total costs. Interestingly, the cost of failed donor evaluation was only 6% of total costs. Overall, these authors conclude that LDLT costs are 21% higher than CT, although this difference did not reach statistical significance.

The perceived advantage of LDLT with increased donor numbers and reducing waiting list mortality requires verification. In an attempt to address cost-effectiveness of LDLT, Sagmeister et al. [14] utilized a Markov model to compare outcomes and costs among ESLD patients treated conservatively, or using CT or CT/LDLT. The authors' model utilizes an intent-to-treat decision and models cohorts with ESLD to compare outcomes of the natural history of ESLD and the potential treatment options of CT and LDLT. An annual mortality of 24% is assumed. Again, given the vagaries of center specificity such as differing availability of LDLT and CT organs, revealing results are presented. The natural history of ESLD in the absence of transplantation is associated with a life expectancy of 4 years, with 98% of deaths as the result of liver disease. The combination of CT and LDLT availability increases life expectancy to 12 years, with 52% of patients dying with a natural age- and sex-specific mortality. CT adds 6.2 QALY and accrues an additional €139 000 to society. The availability of both CT and LDLT adds an additional 1.3 QALY with an additional cost of €31 000. Overall, the costs associated with liver transplantation remain high. Mean patient lifetime costs were €191 000 for CT and €222 000 for LDLT. This translates into €22 000 and 23 000 per QALY for CT and LDLT, respectively. Clearly, more analysis of LDLT is required.

■ CONCLUSION

Liver transplantation is a well-accepted standard of care for patients with ESLD. However, the economic realities of the present era necessitate rational utilization of this expensive treatment modality that utilizes the scarce resource of the cadaver donor liver allograft. Economic analysis of the societal benefits of liver transplantation is ongoing. Studies are flawed, but give some inkling of the overall costs generated by transplantation. Identification of appropriate candidates for transplantation will continue to be an issue for debate. Studies have demonstrated that performing transplantation in the sickest patients is cost-ineffective. Evans [4] states that society can no longer underwrite ineffective medical care. Whether liver transplantation will survive under the scrutiny of society and health care economists is presently unclear, but economic mandates will inevitably alter clinical disposition of liver transplantation utilization for the future.

■ **REFERENCES**

1. Best JH, Veenstra DL, Geppert J. Trends in expenditures for Medicare liver transplant recipients. Liver Transpl 2001;7:858–862.

2. Adam R, McMaster P, O'Grady JG, et al. Evolution of liver transplantation in Europe; report of the European Liver Transplant Registry. Liver Transpl 2003;9:1231–1243.

3. Filipponi F, Pisati R, Cavicchini G, et al. Cost and outcome analysis and cost determinants of liver transplantation in a European national health service hospital. Transplantation 2003;75:1731–1736.

4. Evans RW. Liver transplantation in a managed care environment. Liver Transpl Surg 1995;1:61–75.

5. Brand DA, Viola D, Rampersaud P, et al. Waiting for a liver. Hidden costs of the organ shortage. Liver Transpl 2004;10:1001.

6. Longworth L, Young T, Buxton MJ, et al. Midterm cost-effectiveness of the liver transplantation program of England and Wales for three disease groups. Liver Transpl 2003;9:1295–1307.

7. Whiting JF, Martin J, Zavala E, et al. The influence of clinical variables on hospital costs after orthotopic liver transplantation. Surgery 1999;125:217–222.

8. Taylor MC, Greig PD, Detsky AS, et al. Factors associated with the high cost of liver transplantation in adults. Can J Surg 2002;45:425–434.

9. Schnitzler MA, Woodward RS, Brennan DC, et al. The economic impact of preservation time in cadaveric liver transplantation. Am J Transplant 2001;1:360–365.

10. Markmann JF, Markmann JW, Markmann DA, et al. Preoperative factors associated with outcome and their impact on resource use in 1148 consecutive primary liver transplants. Transplantation 2001;72:1113–1122.

11. Azoulay D, Jinhares MM, Huguet E, et al. Decision for retransplantation of the liver: an experience and cost-based analysis. Ann Surg 2002;236:713–721.

12. Loinaz C, Clemares M, Marques E, et al. Labor status of 137 patients with liver transplantation. Transplant Proc 1999;31:2470–2471.

13. Trotter JF, Mackenzie S, Wachs M, et al. Comprehensive cost comparison of adult–adult right hepatic lobe living-donor liver transplantation with cadaveric transplantation. Transplantation 2003;75:473–476.

14. Sagmeister M, Mullhaupt B, Kadry Z, et al. Cost-effectiveness of cadaveric and living-donor liver transplantation. Transplantation 2002;73:616–622.

Donor Organ Distribution

▼ ▼ ▼ ▼ ▼ ▼ ▼ ▼ ▼

**Richard B. Freeman, Jr
and Jeffrey Cooper**

6

THE FUNDAMENTAL problem in modern organ transplantation is the overwhelming disparity between the number of patients potentially treatable with donor organs and the severely limited supply of these grafts. This disparity motivates concerted efforts to improve the number of individuals who consent to have organs removed for donation and is the driving force for organ allocation policy. The scarcity problem is compounded by the increasing variety of conditions for which liver transplantation offers reduction in mortality risk and/or improvement in the quality of life. In addition, as primary caregivers and the public become more aware of the benefits of liver transplantation, more patients with accepted indications for liver transplantation are identified and referred. Consequently, the demand for liver transplantation outweighs the supply of donated organs and there is increasing pressure to deliver organs to those most in need while maintaining acceptable results. The two principles of treating those in need and of achieving good results represent a stewardship conflict for those practicing liver transplantation. This conflict in principles is made most acute in situations where the disparity between donated organs and waiting candidates is widest. The acuity of this conflict can be reduced by increasing organ donation rates on the supply side and by making the liver allocation process more transparent and evidence-based on the demand side. In this chapter, we outline both approaches to alleviating the tension of this stewardship conflict and highlight areas where future efforts are likely to be fruitful.

■ ORGAN DONATION EFFORTS

Organ donation rates vary considerably across the world and within various regions of individual countries (Table 6.1). Recently, researchers have tried to identify underlying reasons for these differences and apply practices from the best performing areas to areas where donation has not been as successful. In Spain, where organ donation rates have been consistently high, the *Organization Nacional Transplantation* has outlined their methodology for maximizing donation [1,2] and has actively disseminated their practices elsewhere [3]. Through the Spanish efforts and refinements by many others, five main imperatives thought to be important for maximizing organ donation have been emphasized. In the USA and elsewhere, these tenets are being applied and there are government-sponsored efforts to continue to identify and implement best practices and techniques [4].

First and foremost, health care authorities must make hospitals accountable for their organ donation efforts. In the USA, the Joint Committee for Accreditation of Hospitals has recently required that hospitals develop and promulgate organ donation polices and procedures and will consider the presence of these policies and procedures as indicators of hospital quality and accreditation [5].

Second, hospitals, and caregivers within, must consistently identify potential organ donors. The Spanish model employs part-time physicians who are compensated for overseeing and implementing organ donation efforts, and who are held accountable for organ donation results within each hospital [6]. This requires a thorough understanding of the few medical contraindications to organ donation and an in-depth appreciation for end-of-life decision making. Consequently, a concerted and persistent education effort is required to inform the bedside caregiving teams of these issues. In addition, the public must be educated regarding the opportunity for donation. Donor registries can be effective in this respect [7].

Third, the process of obtaining consent should be performed only by those experienced and well acquainted with end-of-life decision making, prevailing laws regarding informed consent, presumed consent, donation after cardiac death, and brain death. There is evidence that experienced persons who are culturally similar to potential donor families have a higher likelihood of getting a positive result [8].

Fourth, ongoing accounting through retrospective chart review of the incidence of brain death and/or withdrawal of care in medically suitable patients, the frequency with which these are identified, the frequency that consent is requested for the identified donors and obtained, the frequency with which the consented donors have organs recovered, and the

Table 6.1 *Deceased Donors per Million Population Data*[a]

Area	Deceased Donors per Million Population
Alabama	20.4
Arizona	13.0
Arkansas	12.8
California	15.9
Colorado	18.4
Connecticut	9.1
Florida	21.4
Georgia	16.3
Hawaii	14.5
Illinois	17.0
Indiana	15.0
Iowa	18.1
Kansas	38.7
Kentucky	19.6
Louisiana	21.7
Maryland	11.0
Massachusetts	26.4
Michigan	15.8
Minnesota	29.4
Mississippi	11.9
Missouri	18.6
Nebraska	18.9
New Jersey	12.7
New Mexico	14.0
New York	16.8
North Carolina	16.2
Ohio	18.6
Oklahoma	18.5
Oregon	22.7
Pennsylvania	32.6
South Carolina	18.2
Tennessee	22.0
Texas	17.7
Utah	22.9
Virginia	11.0
Washington	17.8

Table 6.1 *Continued*

Wisconsin	24.6
US total	17.9
Eurotransplant[b]	15.5
France	18.3
Italy	18.5
Spain	33.8
Scandiatransplant[c]	15.0
UK	12.1

[a]US data are the average donors per million per year from 1993 to 2003 based on 2003 census data (provided by UNOS/OPTN). European data are based on deceased donors recovered in 2003 only.
[b]Eurotransplant includes Germany, Belgium, Netherlands, Austria, Luxembourg, and Slovenia.
[c]Scandiatransplant includes Denmark, Norway, Finland, and Sweden.

frequency that organs recovered from consented donors are transplanted must be tracked and compared.

Finally, these data should be given back to the local organ donation organization to inform them as to best practices and performance. Through promotion of these principles and through refinements in their implementation from hospital to hospital, the number of organs retrieved for transplantation can be maximized.

A recent study of organ donor potential in the USA estimated that the organ donor pool is potentially twice as large as the number of actual donors converted (Table 6.2) [9]. In this study, the authors noted that inability to obtain consent for donation is the single largest impediment to realizing the donor potential that exists. They also noted that the vast majority of potential donors reside in the larger hospitals and efforts to increase donation rates should focus on these institutions.

Living Liver Donation

Despite the best efforts of organ donation teams, it is unlikely that deceased donors will ever completely meet the demand for liver transplantation. It is for this reason that living donor liver transplantation has developed. Also, in some areas of the world the only source for transplantable liver tissue is living donors because removal of organs from deceased individuals is not culturally acceptable. Living liver donation was first performed from a parent donating to a child [10]. However, compared with adults, children put a much smaller demand on the deceased donor liver supply, with adults on the waiting list carrying a much larger burden of mortality risk. The pressure of this mortality risk while waiting led families to ask for,

Table 6.2 *Estimates of Total Possible Donors in the USA*

	1997	1998	1999
US donors	5 477	5 801	5 849
Donors in the study	2 763	2 628	2 399
Potential donors in the study	6 843	6 219	5 462
Estimate of national pool	13 565	13 728	13 317

Adapted from Sheehy E, Conrad SL, Brigham LE, Luskin R, Weber P, Eakin M, Schkade L, Hunsicker L. Estimating the number of potential organ donors in the United States. N Engl J Med 2003;349(7):667–674.

and transplant centers to deliver, adult-to-adult living liver transplantation [11,12]. Ethical considerations of informed consent for the donor and questions about whether the donor risk is justified for the recipients' benefit have been raised [13] and continue to surface [14]. Unlike renal transplantation where transplantation of a living donor kidney can be expected to offer results for the recipient that are superior to deceased donor renal transplantation, living donor liver transplantation and graft survival have been reported as equal [15,16] or slightly inferior [17,18] to deceased donor liver transplantation (Fig. 6.1). Cheng et al. [19] published a simulation model to compare the benefit of earlier liver transplantation (offered by a living liver transplantation) for candidates with hepatocellular carcinoma (HCC) with waiting longer for a deceased donor liver and found that earlier transplantation made possible by a living donor achieved better results overall, even when the mortality risk for the living donor was included in the model. Several recent reviews [20–22] of living liver transplantation have been published and a large multicenter trial is under way in the USA [23] to more completely address the risk and benefits to donors and recipients.

The timing of liver transplantation for a recipient who has a willing and able living donor is a critical issue. Candidates waiting for deceased donor organs are subject to the allocation policies under which their transplant center operates (allocation of deceased donor livers is discussed in detail later in the chapter). Theoretically, a transplant candidate with a living donor could receive a transplant at any time in the course of his or her disease; however, the optimal timing for this procedure has not been studied extensively. Some reports have suggested that extremely ill adult candidates have reduced patient and graft survival rates when they are given a living donor graft [24,25] but others have suggested that acutely ill adults [26] and almost all children regardless of the severity of their disease [27,28] can achieve success rates that are comparable with transplantation of deceased donors. The cause for the inferior results in some series has not been well described but has been

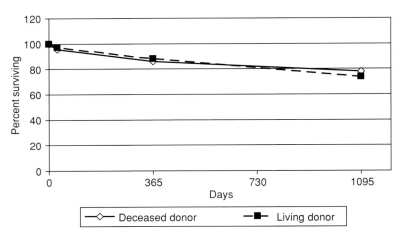

Fig. 6.1 *Patient survival for first adult (>18 years old) recipients of first liver grafts.*

attributed to the "steep learning curve" encountered by centers practicing this technically demanding procedure [29] and/or the need for more than minimal liver mass in the more severely ill recipient [24,30]. The exact place for living donor liver transplantation within the field remains to be determined, but better understanding of liver preservation, injury, and regeneration will help improve results for donors and recipients alike.

Expanded Criteria Donors

The growing disparity between donor supply and recipient need has refocused attention on the use of so-called marginal or expanded criteria for deceased liver donors. This refers to the use of donor livers that possess characteristics that indicate a greater chance of initial poor graft function and decreased graft survival overall. Many of these livers are not procured given the concerns about the increased risk of a poor outcome, although many of these livers may, in fact, be quite useable. In an effort to expand the donor pool, attempts are being made to define exactly what characteristics preclude the use of a particular deceased donor liver.

Much of this work has a counterpart in the field of kidney transplantation, where concerted efforts have been made to maximize use of deceased donor kidneys. In 2001, members of the transplant community met at Crystal City, Virginia, to develop guidelines to maximize the use of deceased donor organs, particularly those recovered from donors over the age of 60, where the discard rate of procured kidneys is almost 50% [31]. It was estimated that the increased utilization of such kidneys could increase the donor pool by 38% [32]. They proposed that a separate list of kidney recipients who are willing to accept older organs be set up in an effort to expedite kidney transplantation for these individuals. Using the data from the Scientific Registry of Transplant Recipients, additional donor risk factors other than age were identified. These included a history of hypertension, stroke as the cause of death, and the preprocurement of creatinine at greater than 1.5 mg/dL. These risk define the extended criteria donor kidney as one whose relative risk of graft failure is 1.7 times greater than that obtained from an ideal kidney donor. One-year graft survival of extended donor kidneys is 82%, versus 89% from standard kidney donors performed during the same time interval [32]. It is hoped that these results will lead to the increased use of older kidneys and decrease the discard rate of such kidneys.

As in the case of kidneys, donor age is known to play a significant role in determining liver graft performance. In a review of the United Network for Organ Sharing (UNOS) database that examined the results of 32 514 deceased donor liver transplants performed in the USA between 1992 and 2000, the relative risk of graft failure was shown to increase 1.3% for every additional year of donor age, beginning at age 31 (Fig. 6.2) [33]. Thus, donor age of between 60 and 69 years is associated with an increased relative risk (75%) of graft failure, and donor age greater than 70 years is associated with 90% increase in graft failure risk when compared with donors 20–40 years of age [33]. Hence, donor age is an important, independent risk factor in determining the rate of graft failure. These factors take on increasing importance considering the increasing average age of the donor population (Fig. 6.2).

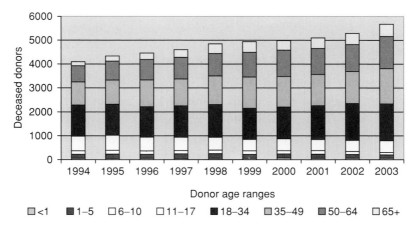

Fig. 6.2 *Distribution of deceased donor ages.*

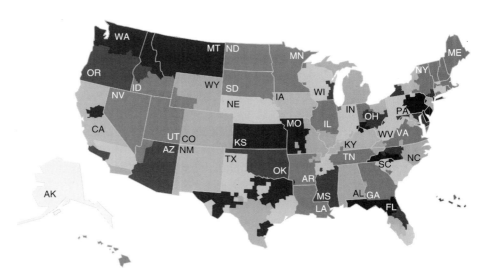

Fig. 6.3 *Donor Service Areas for 56 Organ Procurement Organizations (OPOs) in the USA.*

However, many studies have shown that grafts from elderly donors can be safely used with good results. In particular, Emre et al. [34] demonstrated 1-year graft and patient survival rates of 85% and 91%, respectively, using liver grafts from donors greater than 70 years of age. There seemed to be no significant difference in early graft function between these livers and grafts from younger donors, as evidenced by intraoperative blood product usage, post-operative peak aspartate aminotransferase (AST) and international normalized ratio (INR), as well as by length of postoperative hospital course. Of note, 27 of the 36 elderly donors were "suboptimal," in that they had either a peak alanine aminotransferase (ALT) of greater than 120, high-dose pressor use, a period of profound hypotension, cardiac arrest, or high serum osmolality. No additional screening was used for donors greater than 70; however, no elderly donors with macrosteatosis greater than 30% were used. Average cold ischemic time was 9 h on average. These results are particularly encouraging as the 35 recipients of these grafts included four emergent candidates and 19 were in the previous UNOS status 2 categories at the time of transplantation.

Similarly, Cescon et al. [35] have demonstrated 3-year graft survival of 75% using grafts from donors greater than 80 years of age. Unlike the previously cited study, criteria for donation were stricter for this population, as all donors had to be hemodynamically stable, have normal preprocurement liver function tests, and have less than 30% macrosteatosis. This meant that 50% of possible donors greater than 80 years of age were rejected by this center. Also, unlike the previous study, recipients of these grafts were relatively more stable, with only 2 of 12 recipients falling into the former categories of UNOS status 2A or 1. Of interest, Cescon et al. saw earlier hepatitis C virus (HCV) recurrence in recipients of elderly grafts. This has been confirmed in other studies as well [36]. Thus, livers derived from elderly donors can be safely used, although attention must be paid in ruling out other potential problems in the graft, such as excessive macrosteatosis. In addition, special efforts must be made in limiting cold ischemic times, and such grafts may need to be preferentially placed in more stable recipients and where the cause of liver failure is not HCV.

As previously mentioned, the degree of macrosteatosis is an important variable in determining the utility of a particular liver graft. Multiple studies have shown a relationship between macrosteatosis and primary nonfunction (PNF) [37,38]. Adam et al. [38] reported that 13% of grafts with steatosis greater than 30% had Primary non-function (PNF) versus 2.5% with PNF in those without steatosis. In an Italian study that recorded the results of 860 liver transplants performed between 1990 and 2001, of all donor and recipient variables, only macrovesicular steatosis greater than 15% correlated with decreased patient and graft survival [39]. The relative risk of graft failure and mortality was 1.7 and 1.5, respectively. Such steatotic livers also seem to be particularly sensitive to the deleterious effects of cold ischemia. These authors also found that for each hour of cold ischemic time greater than 10 h, the death rate increased by 15%. They concluded that the combination of donor age greater than 65 and macrosteatosis greater than 30% increased the relative risk of graft failure to 2.5. These effects also seem to be magnified if the recipients were hepatitis C-positive, again emphasizing the potential risk of placing extended donor livers in hepatitis C recipients. These findings have been confirmed in others studies [40]. In contradistinction to macrosteatosis, microsteatosis does not seem to negatively impact early graft function or survival [41].

A third category of so-called expanded criteria cadaveric liver donors includes those who donate after cardiac death (DCD), previously termed "non-heart-beating" donors. Interest has increased because of estimates that the number of donor organs could rise 25% through the expanded use of DCD donors [42]. The Organ Procurement and Transplantation Network (OPTN) data reveal a 4.2% increase in the number of DCD donors in the USA since 1994: 114 liver transplants using DCD donors were performed in 2003 alone. Early results revealed higher rates of PNF and decreased graft survival, in comparison with donors who donated after neurologic death (DND) [43]. This was particularly true of so-called uncontrolled donors, where controlled withdrawal care of care cannot be performed. In one series, the rates of PNF and 1-year graft survival were 17% and 50%, respectively, in livers procured from uncontrolled DCD donors [44]. However, with additional experience, the results of liver transplants performed using controlled DCD livers have gradually improved [45]. Most recently, a single center analysis of 36 liver transplants has been published [46]. The PNF rate was 2/36, and no cases of PNF occurred in the last 30 transplants performed, when a protocol of intravenous prostaglandin E1, vitamin E, and *N*-acetylcysteine via NG tube was initiated. No significant difference in early postoperative function, as measured by INR and bilirubin, was noted in comparison with organs from brain dead donors. However, there was a significantly higher rate of biliary stricture, hepatic artery stenosis, and hepatic abscess formation. There were also a significantly decreased graft and patient survival rates at 1 and 3 years (56% versus 80% 3-year graft survival ($P = 0.002$), and 68% versus 84% 3-year patient survival ($P < 0.01$)). Foley et al. also showed that both graft function and survival worsened with increasing donor age, particularly when the donor was greater than 40 years of age. These results demonstrate that controlled DCD donors can be successfully used to provide liver grafts, albeit with increased postoperative complications and decreased graft and patient survival.

To expand the donor pool even further, procurement of livers from donors infected with either hepatitis B or hepatitis C has become more commonplace. For those donors who have an isolated finding of anti-hepatitis B core antibody (HBcAb), the risk of de novo HBV infection in the recipient has been estimated to be from 25% to 95% [47–49]. However, excellent long-term results have been achieved for HBV-naïve recipients of these grafts in conjunction with the use of chronic lamivudine prophylaxis [50]. Likewise, there is growing evidence supporting the use of HCV-infected livers in HCV-positive recipients. Multiple studies have shown no difference in graft and patient survival for HCV-infected recipients, compared with HCV-positive recipients of uninfected grafts [51–53]. One study from the University of California, Los Angeles (UCLA) showed equivalent graft and patient survival rates, but a significantly shorter time to HCV recurrence, 22.9 months versus 35.7 months, in those HCV-positive recipients who received HCV-positive grafts [52]. In the absence of effective HCV prophylaxis, livers from HCV-positive donors should be reserved for HCV-positive recipients. Livers from donors infected with other pathogens can transmit infection to recipients, but in general, these risks are low and, with the use of effective antimicrobial agents, consequences can be minimized for recipients [54]. Informing recipients of the potential for transmission of donor diseases is paramount.

With time, the pressure to use expanded criteria donors will increase. As seen, there has been a gradual acceptance in using donor livers that previously would have been rejected, either on demographic or on histologic grounds. As the limits to what is acceptable have expanded, there will always be a conflict in using organs with a higher risk of graft failure in a system that funnels organs into the sickest patients, where outcomes, by definition, will not be as good. Ultimately, it will be up to the individual clinician, patient, and family to decide when to use a particular organ. Use of expanded criteria grafts requires that potential recipients be fully informed of the risks associated with these grafts and of risk–benefit calculations in general terms, which makes use of these grafts reasonable. Unfortunately, complete definition of the expanded criteria donor liver is not well established as yet, but with additional research in this area, these decisions will become easier to make.

Deceased Donor Allocation

The tremendous disparity between the number of donor livers available and the number of patients waiting necessitates that there be some method for selecting which of the many waiting candidates should get a donor liver when one becomes available. Despite the increasingly global availability of technology, all resources are, to some degree, limited in their distribution by geography. Deceased or living liver donors occur with differing frequencies in different areas of the world and with differing frequencies within countries as evidenced by the donor data presented earlier in this chapter. In addition, there are ample data documenting that prolonged preservation of liver grafts results in increasing rates of graft failure [55–59]. These preservation time limitations necessitate that some limit be imposed on the distance over which liver grafts are transported from donor sites to recipient centers. Thus, there must be some defined area in which potential recipients are collected for a given donor. These organ distribution units can be defined as the areas in which all potential candidates are culled for a given donor occurring within that area. In the USA, the smallest liver distribution unit is generally defined as the Donor Service Area (DSA) of a given Organ Procurement Organization (OPO) (Fig. 6.3). In other instances, the distribution unit might be a transplant center as in systems where a rotational organ distribution system is employed. Liver distribution units can be sequential as in the US system where, if a donor organ is not accepted within the smallest distribution unit, the organ is offered to a larger distribution unit, the OPTN region (Fig. 6.4). In most cases, liver distribution units are defined more on political, geographic, or organizational grounds rather than by optimal organ preservation limits or by the number of waiting candidates. Indeed, the number of candidates listed in any given OPO appears to be linked to subsequent waiting times for liver transplantation [60].

In almost all cases, each liver distribution unit has more than one waiting liver transplant candidate, so some form of prioritizing these candidates for a donor liver offer must be employed. This prioritization process defines donor organ allocation or, the process by which, from among all of the potential recipients for liver transplant, candidates are ranked in order of preference and selected for that organ offer. This relative selection process, or ranking all individuals from a group of deserving candidates, is extremely important in establishing principles of allocation policy and will be discussed later.

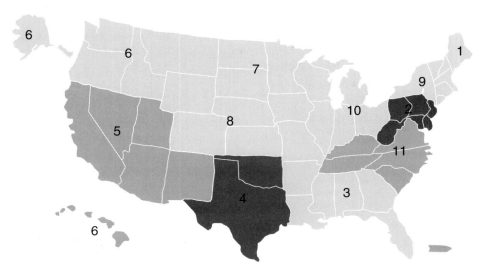

Fig. 6.4 *United Network for Organ Sharing's (UNOS) Organ Procurement and Transportation Network (OPTN) regions in the USA.*

In considering liver allocation, two main ethical principles – individual justice and overall utility – must be accounted for and weighed. Individual justice can be defined as meeting the needs of the individual, whereas medical utility can be defined as achieving the best results with a given therapy for the population under consideration. Allocating organs to candidates based on individual need, by definition, must use individual patient characteristics and rank these to prioritize all waiting candidates. Allocating organs to achieve medical utility might also use individual characteristics but would rank patients in order of likelihood of achieving the best results for the whole.

In order to prioritize candidates according to need, some quantification of need is required; so patients with a higher quantity of need are ranked ahead of those with less need. There are many potential measurements that could be envisioned for this purpose; variables include length of waiting time, potential loss of income, potential loss of support for families, loss of potential to contribute to society, or potential cost to the health care system, etc. One can readily see however, that for many of these and other possible estimates of need, development of objective measurements or end points would be difficult and controversial.

Past liver allocation systems used waiting time as a measure of priority; however, this measure was more often a quantification of lack of need instead of true need, because patients who could wait a long time for a transplant were more likely to survive without a transplant [61]. In this case, candidates with stable or slowly progressing disease could be ranked ahead of those with more severe or rapidly worsening disease; so those who were most likely to progress to death were not necessarily likely to gain high priority in waiting time-driven systems. Progressive liver allocation policy changes in the USA have attempted to focus more on defining individual need by severity of disease. At first, location of care (home, hospital, intensive care unit (ICU)) was used as a surrogate for severity of disease. However, it soon became clear that location of care was more a reflection of physician behavior than an intrinsic characteristic of the patient's disease state. In later allocation policy iterations the Child–Turcotte–Pugh score was used to measure disease severity. This metric was limited by the subjective nature of some of the variables and it imposed categorization of patients into broad classes of patients with a ceiling effect [62].

In 2002, US policymakers chose the model for end-stage liver disease (MELD) [63,64], a mathematical model that defined the risk of death for patients with chronic liver disease using three laboratory values to better prioritize waiting liver transplant candidates with chronic liver disease. In this allocation system, waiting candidates are ranked according to their risk of death using laboratory values only (Fig. 6.5). This continuous system does not categorize patients into broad groups (status designations) and is based

MELD and PELD Scores Used in US Liver Allocation System

MELD = (0.957 × LN(creatinine) + 0.378 × LN(bilirubin) +1.12 × LN(INR) + 0.643) × 10

Values less than 1.0 are rounded to 1.0 to avoid negative MELD scores. Patients on dialysis are assigned a creatinine of 4.0. The MELD score is capped at 40 maximum.

PELD = (0.436 × Age*) – (0.687 × log(albumin)) + (0.480 × log(bilirubin)) + (1.857 × log(INR)) + (0.667 × growth failure†) × 10

* Age <1 year gets 1, Age >1 year gets 0
† growth failure = 1, no growth failure = 0

Values <1.0 are not rounded up so negative PELD scores are possible. The PELD score is not capped.

Fig. 6.5 *Model for end-stage liver disease (MELD) and pediatric end-stage liver disease (PELD) scores used in US liver allocation system.*

solely on variables that are intrinsic to the patient, that are objective, and that are not subject to behavioral biases.

Unique in the development and application of MELD for liver allocation was the prospective validation of this model to make sure that it consistently predicted 3-month mortality risk for waiting liver patients with a variety of disease etiologies [65,66]. These studies documented that for liver transplant candidates, the MELD score was very good, but not perfect, for predicting who would live and who would die. Even though the results consistently showed that the MELD score was highly predictive for most patients, policymakers recognized at the outset that there may be additional factors that could improve the MELD score's applicability to all patients [62]. Recent reports suggest that addition of either hyponatremia [67] or serum sodium [68,69] variables to the MELD equation may improve the model's predictive accuracy, especially for those patients with otherwise low MELD scores. The OPTN database is currently collecting serum sodium values for candidates in the waiting list to prospectively assess this potential improvement. Variation in reagents used for prothrombin time assays can also result in MELD score differences for the same individual [70] and may contribute to imperfections in mortality risk quantification.

Liver transplant clinicians recognize that the risk of death is not the only appropriate measure of need for liver transplantation. Many recent reports document that liver transplantation offers excellent long-term results for patients with hepatocellular cancer (HCC), often better than results achieved with resection [71–75]. However, many patients with HCC present with relatively mild intrinsic liver disease and thus have a relatively low risk of dying in the near term. Prioritizing these patients using mortality risk alone would rank them below the majority of waiting candidates non-malignant conditions. More importantly, the need for liver transplantation for patients with HCC candidates is defined by the risk of progression beyond the favorable early stages of their cancer [76]. Similarly, there are other conditions such as heptopulmonary syndrome, familial amyloidosis, and metabolic liver diseases where mortality risk is not an appropriate definition of need [77]. For these patients, the risk of reaching some end point beyond which the transplant is likely to be of no benefit is a much more accurate measure of need. Unfortunately, models for risk of progression to these end points have not been developed and will require natural history data that have not been systematically collected for these diagnoses. At the present time because there are limited natural history data for the other conditions, the US system employs a regional peer review process to assess centers' requests for patients with conditions where mortality risk is not an applicable prioritization end point.

Defining end points beyond which no benefit accrues to the waiting candidate requires that some definition of benefit be articulated. Recently, Merion et al. [78] compared mortality risk on the waiting list with mortality

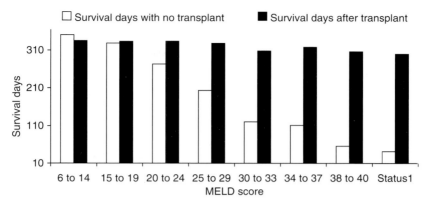

Fig. 6.6 *Comparison of average number of days alive for model for end-stage liver disease (MELD) score ranges.*

risk after transplant and reported the difference in survival. Using this methodology, one can define the benefit of liver transplantation at least for the candidates whose need for transplant can be equated to their mortality risk. In this analysis, candidates with low MELD scores (low mortality risks) had a lower risk of death within the first year without a transplant than if they received a graft at that low score (Fig. 6.6). This indicates that the surgical risk for these candidates is higher than their one-year mortality risk without a transplant. In addition, a benefit in terms of lifetime gained was achieved even for patients with the highest high MELD scores that were selected by centers for transplantation. Assuming that risk models can be developed for other disease end points, one could envision similar estimates of transplant benefit. However, the mortality risk of the liver transplant procedure must always receive some weight against other lesser, nonfatal, end points. Thus, future liver allocation systems may have to consider if there would be circumstances where a candidate with a high risk of attaining a nonfatal end point such as progression to an unfavorable morbidity would receive more priority than a candidate at a higher mortality risk.

The transplant benefit premise allows for additional evidence-based evolution in liver allocation policy. Since the goal of allocation is to rank in order of need the entire group of waiting candidates, patients thought most likely to receive the most benefit in the group at the time of an organ offer should be ranked highest. In addition, the patients with the most to gain can be exposed to higher probabilities of transplant by expanding the distribution units for patients with these characteristics, leaving those who are not likely to benefit for smaller distribution units. Recently, the US organ allocation system has adopted a first step in this approach [79]. After offering to emergent candidates, deceased donor liver will be offered only to those candidates with MELD scores >15 in the DSA followed by candidates with MELD scores >15 in the region. Only after these groups have had the opportunity to receive the organ offer, will the organ be offered to candidates less likely to benefit.

From the above discussion, it is clear that liver distribution and allocation is an evolving process. Today, with computerized data systems, it is essential that data analysis be ongoing to assess the effects of the allocation and distribution systems, to develop and test new policies and methods, and to optimize results. No system will achieve perfection, and codifying policy to make it immutable will not be in the best interest of waiting patients. However, evidenced-based decision making with objective variables and end points makes the process much more transparent and measurable. Liver transplantation depends on the donor resource, whether from deceased or from living donors. If donor procurement ever meets the demand, the need for allocation and distribution policies will be eliminated. This should be the goal of the liver transplant community.

■ REFERENCES

1. Matesanz R, Miranda B, Felipe C, et al. Continuous improvement in organ donation. Transplantation 1996;61:1119–1121.

2. Matesanz R, Miranda B. A decade of continuous improvement in cadaveric organ donation: the Spanish model. J Nephrol 2002;15:22–28.

3. Freeman RB. The Spanish model: world leaders in organ donation. Liver Transpl 2000;6:503–506.

4. Final report of the Organ Donor Break through Collaborative is available at http://www.organdonor.gov/bestpractice.htm.

5. Anon. Joint Commission examines the issue of organ donation. Perspectives 2003;23(12):1–12.

6. Matesanz R, Miranda B, Felipe C. Organ procurement in Spain: the impact of transplant coordination. Clin Transplant 1994;8:281–286.

7. Gabel H. Donor registries throughout Europe and their influence on organ donation. Transplant Proc 2003;35(3):997–998.

8. Callender CO, Bey AS, Miles PV, et al. A national minority organ/tissue transplant education program: the first step in the evolution of a national minority strategy and minority transplant equity in the USA. Transplant Proc 1995;27:1441–1443.

9. Sheehy E, Conrad SL, Brigham LE, et al. Estimating the number of potential organ donors in the United States. N Engl J Med 2003;349:667–674.

10. Strong RW, Lynch SV, Ong TH, et al. Successful liver transplantation from a living donor to her son. N Engl J Med 1990;322:1505–1507.

11. Lo CM, Fan ST, Liu CL, et al. Extending the limit on the size of adult recipient in living donor liver transplantation using extended right lobe graft. Transplantation 1997;63:1524–1528.

12. Yamaoka Y, Washida M, Honda K, et al. Liver transplantation using a right lobe graft from a living related donor. Transplantation 1994;57:1127–1130.

13. Singer PA, Siegler M, Whitington PF, et al. Ethics of liver transplantation with living donors. N Engl J Med 1989;321:620–622.

14. Cronin DC, 2nd, Millis JM, Siegler M. Transplantation of liver grafts from living donors into adults – too much, too soon. N Engl J Med 2001;344:1633–1637.

15. Marcos A, Fisher RA, Ham JM, et al. Liver regeneration and function in donor and recipient after right lobe adult to adult living donor liver transplantation. Transplantation 2000;69:1375–1379.

16. Bak T, Wachs M, Trotter J, et al. Adult-to-adult living donor liver transplantation using right-lobe grafts: results and lessons learned from a single-center experience. Liver Transpl 2001;7:680–686.

17. Garcia-Retortillo M, Forns X, Llovet JM, et al.. Hepatitis C recurrence is more severe after living donor compared to cadaveric liver transplantation. Hepatology 2004;40:699–707.

18. Broelsch CE, Malago M, Testa G, et al. Living donor liver transplantation in adults: outcome in Europe. Liver Transpl 2000;6(suppl 2):S64–S65.

19. Cheng S, Pratt D, Freeman RB, et al. Living-related versus orthotopic liver transplant for small hepatocellular carcinoma: a decision analysis. Transplantation 2001;72:861–868.

20. Trotter JF, Wachs M, Everson GT, et al. Adult-to-adult transplantation of the right hepatic lobe from a living donor. N Engl J Med 2002;346:1074–1082.

21. Gondolesi GE, Varotti G, Florman SS, et al. Biliary complications in 96 consecutive right lobe living donor transplant recipients. Transplantation 2004;77: 1842–1848.

22. Lo CM, Fan ST, Liu CL, et al. Lessons learned from one hundred right lobe living donor liver transplants. Ann Surg 2004;240:151–158.

23. Information about the design, participating centers, and data collection is available at http://www.nih-a2all.org.

24. Goldstein MJ, Salame E, Kapur S, et al. Analysis of failure in living donor liver transplantation: differential outcomes in children and adults. World J Surg 2003;27:356–364.

25. Freeman RB. The impact of the model for end-stage liver disease on recipient selection for adult living liver donation. Liver Transpl 2003;9(10 suppl 2):S54–S59.

26. Miwa S, Hashikura Y, Mita A, et al. Living-related liver transplantation for patients with fulminant and subfulminant hepatic failure. Hepatology 1999;30:1521–1526.

27. Otte JB, Reding R, de Ville de Goyet J, et al. Experience with living related liver transplantation in 63 children. Acta Gastroenterol Belg 1999;62:355–362.

28. Cole CR, Bucuvalas JC, Hornung R, et al. Outcome after pediatric liver transplantation impact of living donor transplantation on cost. J Pediatr 2004;144:729–735.

29. Brown RS, Jr, Russo MW, Lai M, et al. A survey of liver transplantation from living adult donors in the United States. N Engl J Med 2003;348:818–825.

30. Emond JC, Renz JF, Ferrell LD, et al. Functional analysis of grafts from living donors. Implications for the treatment of older recipients. Ann Surg 1996;224:544–552.

31. Rosengard BR, Feng S, Alfrey EJ, et al. Report of the Crystal City meeting to maximize the use of organs recovered from the cadaver donor. Am J Transplant 2002;2:1–10.

32. Metzger RA, Delmonico FL, Feng S, et al. Expanded criteria donors for kidney transplantation. Am J Transplant 2003;3(suppl 4):114–125.

33. Rustgi SD, Marino G, Halpern MT, et al. Impact of donor age on graft survival among liver transplant recipients: analysis of the United Network for Organ Sharing database. Transplant Proc 2002;34:3295–3297.

34. Emre S, Schwartz ME, Altaca G, et al. Safe use of hepatic allografts from donors older than 70 years. Transplantation 1996;62:62–65.

35. Cescon M, Grazi GL, Ercolani G, et al. Long-term survival of recipients of liver grafts from donors older than 80 years: is it achievable? Liver Transpl 2003;9:1174–1180.

36. Machicao VI, Bonatti H, Krishna M, et al. Donor age affects fibrosis progression and graft survival after liver transplantation for hepatitis C. Transplantation 2004;77:84–92.

37. Ploeg RJ, D'Alessandro AM, Knechtle SJ, et al. Risk factors for primary dysfunction after liver transplantation – a multivariate analysis. Transplantation 1993;55: 807–813.

38. Adam R, Bismuth H, Diamond T, et al. Effect of extended cold ischemia with UW solution on graft function after liver transplantation. Lancet 1992;340:1373–1376.

39. Salizzoni M, Franchello A, Zamboni F, et al. Marginal grafts: finding the correct treatment for fatty livers. Transpl Int 2003;16:486–493.

40. Verran D, Kusyk T, Painter D, et al. Clinical experience gained from the use of 120 steatotic donor livers for orthotopic liver transplantation. Liver Transpl 2003;9:500–505.

41. Fishbein TM, Fiel MI, Emre S, et al. Use of livers with microvesicular fat safely expands the donor pool. Transplantation 1997;64:248–251.

42. Van der Werf WJ, D'Alessandro AM, Hoffman RM, et al. Procurement, preservation, and transport of cadaver kidneys. Surg Clin North Am 1998;78:41–54.

43. D'Alessandro AM, Hoffman RM, Knechtle SJ, et al. Successful extrarenal transplantation from non-heart-beating donors. Transplantation 1995;59:977–982.

44. Casavilla A, Ramirez C, Shapiro R, et al. Experience with liver and kidney allografts from non-heart-beating donors. Transplantation 1995;59:197–203.

45. Reich DJ, Munoz SJ, Rothstein KD, et al. Controlled non-heart-beating donor liver transplantation: a successful single center experience, with topic update. Transplantation 2000;70:1159–1166.

46. Cooper JT, Chin LT, Krieger NR, et al. Donation after cardiac death: the University of Wisconsin experience with renal transplantation. Am J Transplant 2004; 4(9): 1490–1494.

47. Wachs M, Amend W, Ascher N, et al. The risk of transmission of hepatitis B from HbsAg(−), HbcAb(+), HBIgM(−) organ donors. Transplantation 1995;59: 230–234.

48. Dodson S, Issa S, Araya V, et al. Infectivity of hepatic allografts with antibodies to hepatitis B virus. Transplantation 1997;64:1582–1584.

49. Dickson R, Everhart J, Lake J, et al. Transmission of hepatitis B by transplantation of livers from donors positive for antibody to hepatitis B core antigen. Gastroenterology 1997;113:1168–1174.

50. Yu AS, Vierling J, Colquhoun SD, et al. Transmission of hepatitis B virus infection from hepatitis B core antibody-positive live allografts is prevented by lamivudine therapy. Liver Transpl 2001;7:513–517.

51. Mulligan D, Goldstein R, Crippin J, et al. Use of anti-hepatitis C virus seropositive organs in liver transplantation. Transplant Proc 1995;27:1204–1205.

52. Ghobrial R, Steadman R, Gornbein J, et al. A 10-year experience of liver transplantation for hepatitis C: analysis of factors determining outcome in over 500 patients. Ann Surg 2001;234:384–394.

53. Velidedeoglu E, Desai N, Campos L, et al. The outcome of liver grafts procured from hepatitis C-positive donors. Transplantation 2002;73:582–587.

54. Angelis MA, Cooper JT, Freeman RB. Impact of donor infection on outcome of orthotopic liver transplantation. Liver Transpl 2003;9:451–462.

55. Totsuka E, Fung JJ, Lee MC, et al. Influence of cold ischemia time and graft transport distance on postoperative outcome in human liver transplantation. Surg Today 2002;32:792–799.

56. Porte RJ, Ploeg RJ, Hansen B, et al. Long-term graft survival after liver transplantation in the UW era: late effects of cold ischemia and primary dysfunction. European Multicentre Study Group. Transpl Int 1998;11(suppl 1):S164–S167.

57. Janny S, Sauvanet A, Farges O, et al. Outcome of liver grafts with more than 10 hours of cold ischemia. Transplant Proc 1997;29:2346–2347.

58. Debroy M, Dykstra DM, Roberts RP, et al. The impact of cold ischemic time and donor age on liver transplant outcome. Am J Transplant 2003;3(suppl 5):451A.

59. Levi DM, Nishida S, Kato T, et al. Reconsidering the impact of cold ischemia time on graft and patient survival after liver transplantation. Am J Transplant 2001;1(suppl 1):209A.

60. Trotter JR, Osgood MF. MELD score of liver transplant recipients according to size of waiting list: impact of organ allocation and patient outcomes. JAMA 2004;291:1871–1874.

61. Freeman RB, Edwards EB. Liver transplant waiting time does not correlate with waiting list mortality: implications for liver allocation policy. Liver Transpl 2000;6:543–552.

62. Freeman RB, Weisner RH, Harper A, et al. The new liver allocation system: moving towards evidence-based transplantation policy. Liver Transpl 2002;8:851–858.

63. Malinchoc M, Kamath PS, Gordon FD, et al. A model to predict poor survival in patients undergoing transjugular intrahepatic portosystemic shunts. Hepatology 2000;31:864–871.

64. Kamath PS, Wiesner RH, Malinchoc M, et al. A model to predict survival in patients with end-stage liver disease. Hepatology 2001;33:464–470.

65. Wiesner RH, McDiarmid SV, Kamath PS, et al. MELD and PELD: application of survival models to liver allocation. Liver Transpl 2001;7:567–580.

66. Wiesner RH, Edwards EB, Freeman RB, et al. Model for end stage liver disease (MELD) and allocation of donor livers. Gastroenterology 2003;124:91–96.

67. Ruf AE, Yantorno SE, Descalzi VI, et al. Addition of serum sodium into the MELD score predicts waiting list mortality better than MELD alone – a single center experience. Am J Transplant 2004;4(suppl 8):438.

68. Biggins SW, Eodriguez HJ, Bacchetti P, et al. Serum sodium predicts mortality in patients listed for liver transplantation. Hepatology 2005;41:32–39.

69. Heuman DM, Abou-Assi SG, Habib A, et al. Persistent ascites and low serum sodium identify patients with cirrhosis and low MELD scores who are at high risk for early death. Hepatology 2004;40:802–810.

70. Trotter JF, Brimhall B, Arjal R, et al. Specific laboratory methodologies achieve higher model for endstage liver disease (MELD) scores for patients listed for liver transplantation. Liver Transpl 2004;10:995–1000.

71. Mazzaferro V, Regalio E, Doci R, et al. Liver transplantation for the treatment of small hepatocellular carcinomas in patients with cirrhosis. N Engl J Med 1996;334:693–699.

72. Llovet JM, Furster J, Bruix J. Intention to treat analysis of surgical treatment for early hepatocellular carcinoma: resection versus transplantation. Hepatology 1999;30: 1434–1440.

73. Figueras J, Jaurrieta E, Valls C, et al. Resection or transplantation for hepatocellular carcinoma in cirrhotic patients: outcomes based on indicated treatment strategy. J Am Coll Surg 2000;190:580–587.

74. Hemming AW, Cattral MS, Reed AI, et al. Liver transplantation for hepatocellular carcinoma. Ann Surg 2001;233:652–659.

75. Wong LL. Current status of liver transplantation for hepatocellular carcinoma. Am J Surg 2002;183:309–316.

76. Freeman RB. Liver allocation for HCC: a moving target. Liver Transpl 2004;10: 49–51.

77. Freeman RB. Mortality risk versus other endpoints: who should come first on the liver transplant waiting list? Liver Transpl 2004;10(5):675–677.

78. Merion RM, Schaubel DE, Dykstra DM, et al. The survival benefit of liver transplantation. Am J Transplant 2005; 5(2): 307–313.

79. A full description of current OPTN policies is available at http://www.optn.org/PoliciesandBylaws/policies/docs/policy_8.doc.

Viral Hepatitis

Paul G. Killenberg

T HE MOST frequent reason for liver transplantation (LT) throughout the world is hepatic damage due to viral hepatitis. The viruses involved in the majority of cases are the hepatotropic, alphabetic viruses A, B (D), C, and E. Hepatitis A, B, D, and E can cause fulminant hepatic failure requiring urgent liver transplantation; hepatitis C infection is rarely identified in this context. Chronic liver disease is not seen following infection with either hepatitis A or hepatitis E; most liver transplants for chronic viral hepatitis are due to hepatitis B virus (HBV) or hepatitis C virus (HCV). This chapter considers the pretransplantation management of chronic HBV and chronic HCV disease. The management of patients with fulminant hepatic failure is discussed in Chapter 13.

Approximately 10% of patients with acute hepatitis B have an unresolved infection resulting in chronic hepatitis and, eventually, in cirrhosis. In contrast, 60–80% of patients infected with hepatitis C exhibit a chronic course. Although only 25% of patients with chronic HCV infection develop cirrhosis and end-stage liver disease (ESLD), HCV-related liver disease is the single most common diagnosis at liver transplantation. Hepatitis D virus (HDV), which requires coinfection by HBV, has a very high rate of chronic infection as well, but is relatively uncommon compared with either hepatitis B or C.

Hepatocellular carcinoma (HCC) occurs in patients with chronic infection by either HBV or HCV; the incidence has been recorded in 1.5–4% of patients per year and increases with the duration of the infection. HCC may occur in patients infected with HBV at any stage of the disease, although HCC is more common in patients with cirrhosis. In contrast, HCC in HCV-infected patients is almost always found in patients with cirrhosis (see Chapter 8) [1].

The progression of chronic HBV or HCV, leading to death from liver failure or HCC, is of concern with respect to the timing of liver transplantation.

In both HBV and HCV, an attempt is made to define a "window" within which the risk of liver transplantation is outweighed by the risk to the patient from progression of disease (see Chapter 6).

The large number of patients with chronic HBV and HCV presents several challenges for liver transplantation. Although the incidence of acute HBV and HCV is falling, the prevalence of chronic liver disease and HCC among those infected is rising [1–3]. The latter trend threatens to further increase the imbalance between the number of potential liver transplant recipients and the number of available donor organs. In addition, liver transplantation for HBV, and particularly for HCV, is relatively inefficient compared with non-viral diseases: in recipients who are infected with HBV or HCV at the time of liver transplantation, the rate of reinfection of the liver graft, potentially leading to a need for subsequent retransplantation, approaches 90% [4,5]. Although there are data suggesting that treatment of HBV and HCV to decrease or eliminate viremia before transplantation may decrease both the rate of reinfection and the rate of damage to the graft, the methods for accomplishing these ends are not established.

Because of the threat of HCC and the potential of damage to the liver graft by reinfection with HBV or HCV, every effort should be made to eradicate the infection prior to transplantation. Indeed, halting further progression of the liver disease may possibly avoid liver transplantation. Although treatment is not always successful in eliminating the virus, there is evidence that even temporary reduction in viremia will decrease the rate of necroinflammatory damage to the liver and reduce the amount and rate of progression of fibrosis [6–8]. Thus, all patients with HBV and HCV infection who exhibit fibrosis beyond the portal tract on liver biopsy should be considered for treatment prior to transplantation. Even if cure of the infection is not accomplished, treatment may buy time until better methods of viral eradication or management of reinfection of the liver graft become available.

■ HEPATITIS B

A decade ago, chronic HBV infection was considered a relative contraindication to liver transplantation except in experimental protocols. Following demonstration that chronic intravenous administration of relatively large amounts of high-titer anti-HBV immunoglobulin (HBIg) immediately pre- and indefinitely posttransplantation would prevent destructive reinfection of the graft in the majority of the liver transplant recipients, liver transplantation became an accepted therapy for HBV-infected patients [9]. Currently, with antiviral treatment before and after liver transplantation, the 1- and 5-year survival of patients transplanted for HBV equals that of patients transplanted for non-HBV disease [10–12].

Present antiviral measures have been directed toward decreasing viral replication and eliminating or decreasing viremia. Data from several observations suggest that the rate of reinfection of the liver graft with HBV is higher in those recipients who are HBeAg+ and HBV-DNA-positive at the time of transplantation [8,13,14]. Lowest risk of reinfection occurs among those with no detectable viremia who are HBeAg-negative or who exhibit anti-HBeAg. Suppression of viral replication also appears to decrease the necroinflammatory changes associated with hepatitis B and to decrease fibrogenesis and in some instances may result in remission of existing fibrosis. There is also a suggestion that the rate of diagnosis of HCC drops (but still remains high) in patients who have eliminated viral replication [14]. Thus, it is generally agreed that treatment directed toward reduction of viremia and viral replication is appropriate for all patients who are awaiting liver transplantation.

The question of timing of antiviral treatment is debated. Some would argue that it is prudent to wait until transplantation is near at hand (3–6 months away), if that can be predicted [14,15]. This argument cites the high cost of treatment with agents such as HBIg and the probability of mutation and escape from oral antiviral agents. By delaying treatment until close to the time of liver transplantation, one hopes to arrive at transplantation at the point of maximal suppression of viral replication and lowest viral titer. The counter-argument is to treat all patients who by clinical course or histopathology appear to have progressive disease and, therefore, will probably become candidates for liver transplantation in the future. This argument points to the occasional patient for whom transplantation is avoided because of resolution of tissue damage and remission of fibrosis prior to development of decompensated cirrhosis. Advocates of the latter approach also point to the growing number of oral antiviral compounds each of which has a different resistance profile; these agents can be used either in tandem or in combination to overcome viral resistance. A final reason to employ methods that appropriately delay the progress toward liver transplantation is that with each decade we have seen the development of new, more effective strategies for eradication of HBV; the observation that fibrosis and even cirrhosis may resolve with resolution of the necroinflammatory activity may permit a larger fraction of patients with chronic HBV liver disease to maintain acceptable liver function and, thus, avoid liver transplantation.

Parenteral Antiviral Treatment for Hepatitis B
Alpha Interferon

Of the antiviral treatments for chronic HBV infection currently in use, daily or thrice-weekly alpha interferon (aIFN) injection is the oldest. It was apparent shortly after introduction of aIFN for the treatment of HBV that only a minority of patients achieved viral eradication; those who benefited most were patients with very low viral titers and high transaminase levels (the latter signifying a robust immunologic reaction to the virus) [8]. Also detracting from its use was the large number of patients who experienced disabling (and at times, life-threatening) side-effects while under treatment. Depression, loss of energy and endurance, serious infection, and profound malaise often led patients to withdraw from therapy. At present, use of aIFN for the treatment of chronic hepatitis B infection should be limited to patients who are categorized in the "A" cohort according to the Childs–Pugh–Turcotte (CPT) scale [8] (see Chapter 1). The risk of side-effects, especially bacteremia and sepsis, precludes use of aIFN in patients who have more severe liver disease.

Hepatitis B Immune Globulin

Hepatitis B immuneoglobulin (HBIg) was the next of the antiviral treatments to be applied to patients with hepatitis B liver disease who were undergoing liver transplantation. Pre- and posttransplantation administration of HBIg led to a dramatic decrease in the rate of posttransplantation hepatitis B. Rates of reinfection dropped three- to fourfold, making it possible for the first time to consider candidates with HBV infection. Recently, combination therapy with HBIg and oral antiviral agents have been shown to be effective. Combination therapy has permitted a reduction in HBIg dose to a scale compatible with intramuscular administration, reducing cost. In addition, some centers have found that they need to continue HBIg for only a brief time after transplantation; viral control is maintained thereafter with oral agents (see Chapter 24) [3,15,16].

Oral Antiviral Agents

Lamivudine, an oral nucleoside analog, was the first oral agent shown to be of benefit in treatment of HBV. It is safe with almost no side-effects at usually effective doses [3,8,14,17]. It reduces the HBV-DNA titer in the great majority of patients within 3–6 months and has resulted in loss of HBeAg and subsequent appearance of anti-HBeAg. Unfortunately, in all but a very few patients, discontinuation of lamivudine results in return of the HBV-DNA and may be attended by a clinical flare of the disease. Thus, its role is suppressive rather than virolytic. Another problem with lamivudine is that after 1 year of treatment, 10–20% of patients develop a mutant strain (YMDD variant) that is resistant to lamivudine; after 5 years of treatment, the viral escape rate approaches 65% [18]. Development of the YMDD mutant results in increased necroinflammatory activity and may lead to decompensation and death in some patients.

Recently, another oral nucleoside analog, adefovir, has been approved by the Food and Drug Administration (FDA) for use in treatment of chronic HBV infection [8,19]. This agent appears to have an efficacy equal to lamivudine, with less viral resistance over time. Adefovir is effective against the YMDD mutant and, thus, has been used in patients experiencing lamivudine failure. Lamivudine appears to be effective against the infrequent emergence of adefovir-resistant strains of HBV, prompting trials of a combination of the two drugs.

About 10% of patients taking adefovir experience a brief flare of aminotransferase activity. This is self-limited and generally tolerated well. Adefovir also may result in an elevation in the serum creatinine in some patients; this side-effect is dose-related and is more frequently seen in doses above the usual 10 mg dose [8,19]. Dose reduction is recommended in patients with a pretreatment creatinine clearance <50 mL/min. Other antiviral agents including entecavir, tenofovir, emtricitabine, and telbivudine are being tested for use in patients with HBV and may become available in the next few years.

An Approach to Management of the Patient with Chronic HBV

Patients with chronic HBV should be considered candidates for an eventual LT if there is continual necroinflammatory disease, or if there is evidence of cirrhosis on biopsy. All patients with HBV should enter a program of regular surveillance for HCC, including imaging of the liver and determination of alpha-1 fetoprotein levels (see Chapter 8)

In addition, the following steps should be followed for all patients infected with HBV:

1. Eliminate alcohol intake. Although it is not clear that socially acceptable levels of alcohol intake are deleterious, higher levels have been associated with more rapid progression of HBV liver disease [20,21].
2. Encourage weight loss and regular exercise. In addition to obvious benefits, reduction of hepatic fat may slow the rate of progression of fibrosis in HBV [14].
3. Vaccinate all susceptible patients against hepatitis A virus (HAV). Coinfection of HBV patients with HAV can result in death or severe decompensation of the baseline liver disease. The rate of immunity induced by vaccination in patients with advanced liver disease varies with the degree of decompensation. The earlier vaccination occurs, therefore, the more likely will there be protection against coinfection [22,23].

The next step is to decide on antiviral treatment. For patients with no evidence of necroinflammatory changes or fibrosis on liver biopsy (true

HBV carriers), a program of regular monitoring of liver tests confirmed by periodic liver biopsy should be undertaken. For patients with evidence of elevation of serum aminotransferases and fibrosis beyond the portal tract on liver biopsy, treatment should be selected depending on the severity of the liver disease. For patients with CPT scores <7 (i.e. compensated liver disease), treatment with either aIFN or oral antivirals is a possibility. Patients should be screened for contraindications to aIFN therapy, particularly preexisting psychiatric problems that may be exacerbated by aIFN therapy and low levels of hemoglobin (>10.5 g/dL), platelets (>70.000/mm^3) or neutrophils (>1000/mm^3). Results, in terms of elimination of HBV-DNA, are better in patients who are HbeAg-negative. The benefit of treatment in HbeAg-positive patients is questionable. HBeAg-negative patients without advanced cirrhosis should be treated for up to 24 months with 6 million units of aIFN three times a week.

In patients with more advanced cirrhosis (CPT score >7), or who have contraindications to aIFN treatment, treatment with an oral antiviral agent such as lamivudine reduces the necroinflammatory changes and thus, delays the progress of fibrosis. Alanine aminotransferase (ALT) should return to normal within 6 months of initiating therapy. A rebound in ALT would suggest development of the YMDD mutant strain and indicate addition of adefovir to the regimen. The benefit of continuation of lamivudine and addition of adefovir or initiation of the original antiviral treatment with a combination of two oral agents is currently under study.

Patients experiencing HBV-DNA suppression on therapy should be followed for development of HCC or for signs of further deterioration of liver function. Although liver transplantation for decompensated liver disease may be avoided by successful DNA suppression, the risk of HCC, though decreased in such patients, continues. Regular imaging and measurement of alpha-1 fetoprotein should continue [1].

■ HEPATITIS C

Approximately one-third of all liver transplants are done for HCV-related disease. In many parts of the world, HCV-related HCC is more common than any other setting for HCC [1]. As discussed above, although 60–80% of patients infected with HCV become chronically infected, only a minority show progressive fibrosis leading to liver failure, HCC, and a need for a liver transplant. Thus, it is important to identify those with the potential for progression to cirrhosis.

Patients with hepatitis C are usually asymptomatic; they also exhibit a variable relationship between active necroinflammatory changes and serum aminotransferase levels. Thus, the patient and the physician can develop a false sense of comfort in the apparent lack of active liver disease and resist opportunities to intervene in the natural history of the disease. In early compensated disease, the only reliable way to stage the degree of fibrosis and estimate the potential for further progression is by liver biopsy.

Early intervention in those patients exhibiting signs of progression (especially extension of fibrosis beyond the portal tract on biopsy) may have advantages in viral eradication [2]. It is estimated that about 1 million random mutations of the HCV-RNA sequence occur each day in HCV patients. Most of the mutations are lethal to the virus and are not replicated in subsequent cycles; however, some are replicated resulting in "quasispecies." The rules of chance support the notion that the longer the duration of the infection, the more quasispecies with relative or absolute resistance to treatment will develop. Thus, early treatment of patients showing the potential for progression is indicated; treatment before the development of cirrhosis also lessens the likelihood of HCC.

Antiviral Treatment of HCV

Chronic HCV can be effectively treated in many patients by a combination of pegylated aIFN and ribavirin. Combination therapy of this type will result in a sustained viral response (SVR), defined as the absence of detectable HCV viremia 6 months after stopping therapy; this occurs in about half of the patients treated [24,25]. Patients achieving an SVR demonstrate cessation of necroinflammatory change, resolution of fibrosis, and a decreased incidence of hepatic failure and HCC. Thus, early treatment in patients evidencing progress of the disease on liver biopsy may prevent the eventual need for liver transplantation [7,26].

The success of state-of-the-art treatment with pegylated aIFN and ribavirin varies according to both viral and host factors. Of the several viral genotypes, genotypes 1 and 4 have the lowest rate of SVR (~35–45%) while genotypes 2 and 3 have the highest (~60–80%). The relative resistance of genotypes 1 and 4 recommends more prolonged treatment (at least 1 year); treatment for genotypes 2 and 3 is usually stopped after 6 months. Among Americans, Blacks are much less likely to reach SVR compared with similarly treated non-Hispanic Caucasians [27].

As noted earlier, treatment with aIFN is frequently an unpleasant experience; side-effects are to be anticipated and can be lessened by pretreatment of appropriate patients with antidepressants, exercise, and support and understanding from the patient's family and doctor. Problems with marrow suppression as noted above in treatment of HBV disease pertain even more to patients with HCV. Use of hematinics to maintain adequate hemoglobin and neutrophil levels is now standard. There is now evidence that the success of treatment depends in part, on the patient's ability to receive most of the prescribed dose of pegylated aIFN and ribavirin [26]. Careful attention to the possibility of side-effects and rapid response to adverse changes, where possible, can insure that the patient has the best chance of achieving an SVR [6].

Treatment is usually with either pegylated aIFN 2a, also known as PEGASUS, at a fixed dose of 180 mcg subcutaneously or a weight-based dose of pegylated aIFN 2b or PEGINTRON, calculated at 1.5 mcg/kg body weight, administered subcutaneously once a week. Ribavirin is given at a dose >10.6 mg/kg body weight. Treatment continues for 12 weeks at which time the HCV-RNA titer is estimated and compared with the titer obtained before starting treatment. Patients who exhibit a reduction in RNA to less than 1% of the starting titer have an 80% chance of being virus-free at the end of treatment and, therefore, are continued on therapy [28]. Patients who do not show a >99% reduction in RNA titer by 12 weeks are generally not continued on therapy since the potential for achieving eventual SVR approaches nil.

Patients who have been treated before with aIFN ± ribavirin may be retreated. Before retreatment, the patient should be screened for previous non-adherence to the prescribed dosage and the reasons for this behavior explored. Preemptive use of antidepressants and hematinic agents should be considered for those who had reduction in doses of ribavirin or aIFN during past trials because of psychiatric problems or marrow suppression. Consideration should also be given to the possibility of reinfection with HCV; the HCV-RNA status of the spouse or sexual partner should be checked. Finally, it has been postulated that patients with high hepatic iron content exhibit relative resistance to aIFN treatment of HCV; serum iron studies and ferritin should be measured [29]. Although it has not been conclusively shown that reduction of iron content via phlebotomy will result in an overall increase in SVR in the general population, it is probably worth doing in those with excessive iron stores.

Properly screened patients failing retreatment should be considered for any new therapy or regimen designed to inhibit fibrogenesis independent of viral eradication. Trials of amantadine as a third agent, or instead of ribavirin have not been successful. Viramidine, an analog of ribavirin, may have less marrow toxicity; studies of the impact of this drug on the rate of SVR are under way [30]. Ribavirin monotherapy does not work.

In HCV infection even more so than with HBV, it is important to follow the three steps noted for pretransplantation patients with HBV. Elimination of all alcohol intake is even more important with respect to decreasing the acceleration of HCV liver disease and the incidence of HCC in HCV cirrhosis [26]. Weight loss and exercise are important at several levels. Finally, vaccination against HAV is imperative. It is very difficult to prevent HAV infection unless one lives the life of a recluse. HAV superinfection in patients with prior HCV infection can result in death in up to 50% of cases [31]. Hepatitis B infection that requires parenteral exposure is more easily prevented by life choices; however, the vaccine is relatively safe and cheap. Patients with HCV should be immunized against both HAV and HBV.

■ SUMMARY

The role of liver transplantation in the treatment of chronic HBV and HCV is one of the most exciting and rapidly developing fields in transplant medicine. With each year new agents are shown to modify the course of the disease, or decrease the impact of reinfection of the liver graft. The possibility of early intervention in the course of the disease and prevention of liver transplantation is one of the most laudable goals in this field.

■ REFERENCES

1. Kaplan ED, Reddy KR. Rising incidence of hepatocellular carcinoma: the role of hepatitis B and C; the impact on transplantation and outcomes. Clin Liver Dis 2003;7:683–714.

2. Davis GI, Albright JE, Cook SF, et al. Projecting the future healthcare burden from hepatitis C in the United States. Liver Transpl 2002;9:331–338.

3. Curry MP. Hepatitis B and hepatitis C viruses in liver transplantation. Transplantation 2004;78:955–963.

4. Roche R, Samuel D. Evolving strategies to prevent HBV recurrence. Liver Transpl 2004;10(suppl 2):S74–S85.

5. Terrault NA. Prophylactic and preemptive therapies for hepatitis C virus-infected patients undergoing liver transplantation. Liver Transpl 2003;9(suppl 3):S95–S100.

6. Berenguer M, Wright TL. Treatment strategies for hepatitis C: intervention prior to liver transplant, pre-emptively or after established disease. Clin Liver Dis 2003;7:631–650.

7. Arenas JI, Vargas HE. Hepatitis C virus antiviral therapy in patients with cirrhosis. 2004;33:549–562.

8. Lai CJ, Terrault NA. Antiviral therapy in patients with chronic hepatitis B and cirrhosis. Gastroenterol Clin North Am 2004;33:620–654.

9. Lerut JP, Donataccio M, Ciccarelli O, et al. Liver transplantation and HBsAg-positive postnecrotic cirrhosis: adequate immunoprophylaxis and delta virus co-infection as the significant determinants of long-term prognosis. J Hepatol 1999;30:706–714.

10. Steinmuller T, Seehofer D, Rayes N, et al. Increasing applicability of liver transplantation for patients with hepatitis B-related liver disease. Hepatology 2002;35:1528–1535.

11. Fagiuali S, Mirant VG, Pompili M, et al. Liver transplantation: the Italian experience. Dig Liver Dis 2002;34:619–620.

12. Roche B, Samuel D. Evolving strategies to prevent HBV recurrence. Liver Transpl 2004;10(suppl 2):S74–S85.

13. Lok AS. Prevention of recurrent hepatitis B post-liver transplantation. Liver Transpl 2002;8(suppl 1):S67–S73.

14. Fontana RJ. Management of patients with decompensated HBV cirrhosis. Semin Liver Dis 2003;23:89–100.

15. Yao FY, Osorio RW, Roberts JP, et al. Liver Transpl Surg 199;5:491–496.

16. Angus PW, McCaughan GW, Gane EF, et al. Combination low-dose hepatitis B immune globulin and lamivudine therapy provides effective prophylaxis against posttransplantation hepatitis B. Liver Transpl 2000;6:429–433.

17. Ben-Ari Z. Experience with lamivudine therapy for hepatitis B virus infection before and after liver transplantation, and review of the literature. J Intern Med 2003;253:544–552.

18. Lok AS, Lai CL, Leung N, et al. Long-term safety of lamivudine treatment in patients with chronic hepatitis B. Gastroenterology 2003;125:1714–1722.

19. Schiff ER, Lai CL, Hadziannis S, et al, on behalf of the Adefovir Dipivoxil Study 435 International Investigators Group. Adefovir dipivoxil therapy for lamivudine-resistant hepatitis B in pre- and post-liver transplantation patients. Hepatology 2003;38:1419–1427.

20. Nalpas B, Berthelot P, Thiers V, et al. Hepatitis B virus multiplication in the absence of usual serological markers. A study of 146 chronic alcoholics. J Hepatol 1985;1:89–97.

21. Donato F, Tagger A, Chiesa R, et al. Hepatitis B and C virus infection, alcohol drinking, and hepatocellular carcinoma: a case–control study in Italy. Brescia HCC Study. Hepatology 1997;26:579–584.

22. Dumot JA, Barnes DS, Younossi Z, et al. Immunogenicity of hepatitis A vaccine in decompensated liver disease. Am J Gastroenterol 1999;94:1601–1604.

23. Smallwood GA, Coloura CT, Martinez E, et al. Can patients awaiting liver transplantation elicit an immune response to the hepatitis A vaccine? Transplant Proc 2002;34:3289–3290.

24. Manns MP, McHutchison JG, Gordon SC, et al. Peginterferon alfa-2b plus ribavirin compared with interferon alfa-2b plus ribavirin for initial treatment of chronic hepatitis C: a randomised trial. Lancet 2001;358:958–965.

25. Fried MW, Shiffman ML, Reddy KR, et al. Peginterferon alfa-2a plus ribavirin for chronic hepatitis C virus infection. N Engl J Med 2002;347:975–982.

26. Davis GL. New approaches and therapeutic modalities for the prevention and treatment of recurrent HCV after liver transplantation. 2003;9(suppl 3):S114–S119.

27. Muir AJ, Bornstein JD, Killenberg PG. Peginterferon alfa-2b and ribavirin for the treatment of chronic hepatitis C in blacks and non-Hispanic whites. N Engl J Med 2004;350:2265–2271.

28. Davis GL, Wong JB, McHutchison JG, et al. Early virologic response to treatment with peginterferon alfa-2b plus ribavirin in patients with chronic hepatitis C. Hepatology 2003;38:645–652.

29. Bacon BR. Hemochromatosis: diagnosis and management. Gastroenterology 2001;120:718–725.

30. Lin CC, Philips L, Xu C, et al. Pharmacokinetics and safety of viramidine, a prodrug of ribavirin, in healthy volunteers. J Clin Pharmacol 2004;44:265–275.

31. Vento S, Garofano T, Renzini C, Cainelli F, et al. Fulminant hepatitis associated with hepatitis A virus superinfection in patients with chronic hepatitis C. New Engl J Med 1998;338:286–290.

Hepatoma

▼ ▼ ▼ ▼ ▼ ▼ ▼ ▼ ▼

**Maria Varela, Margarita Sala,
and M. Jordi Bruix**

■ INTRODUCTION

Hepatocellular carcinoma (HCC) is the most frequent primary malignancy of the liver and its incidence is increasing worldwide. It accounts for as many as 1 million deaths annually, representing the third largest cause of cancer-related death [1–3]. It mostly affects patients with liver cirrhosis [2,4] and currently is the most frequent cause of death for such patients [5–7]. The annual incidence of HCC in cirrhotic patients ranges between 2% and 8% depending on the degree of liver function impairment and some specific characteristics such as advanced age, male sex, increased baseline alpha fetoprotein (AFP), and active viral replication with increased liver cell proliferation [2,4]. Accordingly, the 5-year cumulative incidence ranges between 10% and 20%.

The optimal strategy to decrease HCC-related mortality is to avoid infection with hepatitis B [8] or C viruses or to reduce excessive alcohol intake, but if chronic infection leading to liver damage is already present the only approach to reduce cancer-related death is early detection allowing effective treatment [4,9]. This is the rationale for involving the population at risk, namely cirrhotic patients, in surveillance programs based on ultrasound (US) and AFP determination every 6 months [4,10,11]. The aim is to detect tumors at an early stage (Fig. 8.1) when they may benefit from effective therapy [4,9]. When US leads to suspicious findings, the confirmation of malignancy can be obtained by biopsy or by the fulfillment of noninvasive criteria [4,9].

Patients with HCC diagnosed at an early stage should be considered for curative options (surgical resection, liver transplantation (LT), or percutaneous ablation) (Fig. 8.2) that may reach long-term complete response and hence improved survival [4,10,11]. There are no randomized controlled trials (RCTs) comparing these different options and thus the selection of one of them as the first-line therapeutic approach will depend on the evaluation of

119
▼

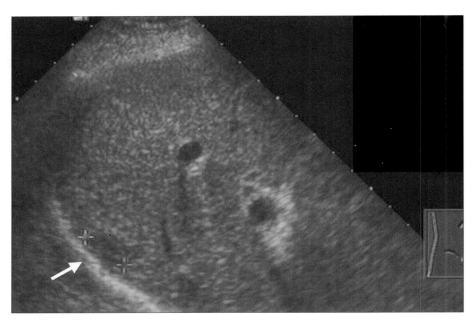

Fig. 8.1 *Small hypoechoic hepatic nodule corresponding to early hepatocellular carcinoma (HCC) diagnosed during surveillance in a cirrhotic patient. Detection at an early stage allows effective treatment to be applied. (Courtesy of Dr L. Bianchi.)*

local resources and human expertise [12]. Unfortunately, early diagnosis is achieved in around 30% of the cases and thus the majority of patients are only considered for palliative approaches [7,13]. Among these, the only therapy that has been proven to increase survival is transarterial chemoembolization [14].

In most units, liver resection is limited to patients with solitary tumors without evidence of vascular invasion or spread outside the liver [15–18]. The best results are obtained in Child–Pugh A individuals without significant portal hypertension and normal bilirubin concentration [15,16]. With this selection criterion there should be almost no postoperative liver failure and associated mortality, and the expected 5-year survival rate may exceed 70%. Unfortunately, even in carefully selected patients, the rate of tumor recurrence is high (50% at 3 years) [15,19–21]. The major predictors of recurrence are the presence of vascular invasion and/or satellites. These characteristics reflect an increased likelihood of dissemination prior to resection, but no doubt some recurrences correspond to metachronic HCC developed in the oncogenic liver [22]. Several options acting against these potential mechanisms have been proposed, including retinoid administration [23], selective localized radiotherapy [24], interferon [25,26], and adoptive immunotherapy [27], but despite encouraging results, none of the options have been incorporated into conventional clinical practice. Patients treated by resection who develop recurrence could be considered for salvage transplantation [28–30], but this has a low

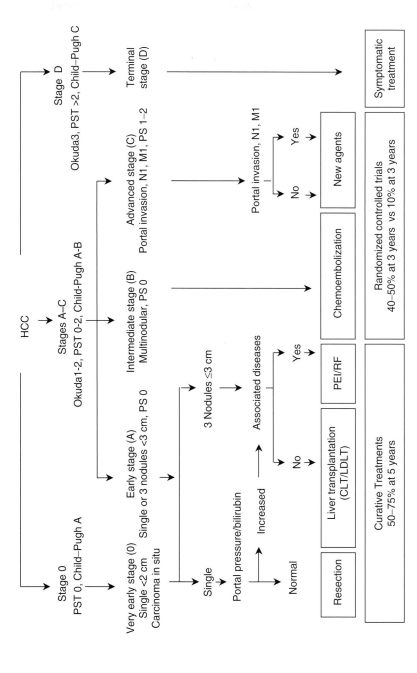

Fig. 8.2 *Barcelona clinic liver cancer (BCLC) staging and treatment strategy for hepatocellular carcinoma (HCC) patients. Patients diagnosed at an early stage (stage A) are considered for options that may provide long-term cure. Patients at intermediate stage (stage B) are considered for transarterial chemoembolization. If patients belong to an advanced stage (stage C) they are considered for research therapeutic trials and if they fit into the end stage (stage D) they just receive symptomatic therapy with avoidance of unnecessary suffering. Stage 0 includes those patients with very early HCC belonging to the so-called carcinoma in situ. This type of tumor is currently very difficult to be diagnosed prior to surgical resection as it lacks characteristic radiological pattern and biopsy is unable to reach confident diagnosis because of very well preserved differentiation degree and architecture. (Reproduced with permission.)*

applicability as most patients will appear as having disseminated disease exceeding enlistment criteria for transplantation [31]. For this reason, in our group we have proposed to offer transplantation to those resected patients in whom pathology evidences a high risk of recurrence (microvascular invasion or satellites) [32].

As mentioned previously, only a minority of the patients (<5%) are adequate for surgical resection due to liver function impairment [32]. Thus, even if diagnosed at an early stage they are better served by LT or percutaneous ablation. The present chapter discusses the issues regarding the selection, enlistment, and follow-up of patients considered for LT, while specific information about the benefits of percutaneous ablation are reported elsewhere [33–36].

Selection of HCC Patients for Liver Transplantation

Patients with advanced nonsurgical HCC were the subjects offered LT at the beginning of the transplant era [37]. The information collected in these pioneering years offered the rationale to limit LT to patients with early HCC. Survival in these patients was not different from non-HCC patients and the recurrence rate was less than 20% at 5 years [38,39]. Simultaneously, it was recognized early on that disease recurrence and death were the rule in patients with macroscopic vascular invasion or extrahepatic spread (lymph nodes or distant metastases) [37,38]. Similarly, it was evidenced that patients transplanted for end-stage cirrhosis who had small "incidental" tumors undetected in the work-up before LT [37] had the same survival as cirrhotics without malignancy and had no HCC recurrence. At that time, incidental HCCs were either minute (Fig. 8.3) and multifocal or solitary < or= 5 cm in size. Tumors larger than this cut-off were already known to have an increased rate of vascular invasion in pathological studies [40,41] and as a result it was proposed that the best candidates for LT would be patients with solitary HCC < or= 5 cm or up to three nodules < or= 3 cm. These were the criteria initially raised by Bismuth et al. [39] and thereafter refined and disseminated by Mazzaferro et al. [42]. Several groups have thereafter confirmed the validity of the criteria nowadays known as "Milano criteria" [43–47], it being well established that patients fitting into these restrictive definitions will achieve survival figures exceeding 70% at 5 years, while the recurrence rate will be less than 25% [45] (Table 8.1). While it is now fully accepted that HCC is an optimal indication for LT and that the best results will be obtained if the Milano criteria are respected, there is a huge controversy as to the extent to which these criteria could be expanded in order to allow more patients to benefit from this life-saving procedure [48,49]. Strict adherence to Milano criteria provides the best results in terms of survival, but it is known that several programs do not exclude patients from the list when

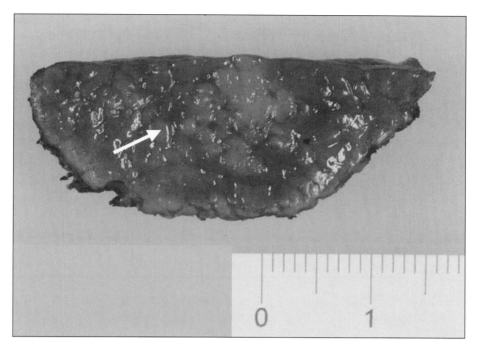

Fig. 8.3 *Small hepatocellular carcinoma (HCC) detected during pathology examin-ation of the explanted liver. Tumor diameter is 10 mm and there is no evidence of vascular invasion or satellites. Tumor margins are ill defined as frequently observed in very early tumor stages. (Courtesy of Dr R. Miquel.)*

follow-up staging while waiting exceeds entry criteria. If the tumor extent is not massive, without vascular invasion and no extrahepatic spread, the results are impaired and only offer a 50% survival at 5 years [38,42,46], but with a higher recurrence rate. This consideration would endorse the potential for an expansion but the critical issue is how to define the new limits [50]. The studies that have proposed an expansion of the limits have been based on the analysis of explanted livers along with assessment of

Table 8.1 *Survival and Recurrence of Patients with Early-Stage HCC Treated with Liver Transplantation*

Author	Year	Number	1-Year Survival Percentage	5-Year Survival Percentage	Recurrence Percentage
Mazzaferro et al.	1996	48	90	75 (4 years)	4 (8%)
Bismuth et al.	1999	45	82	74	5 (11%)
Llovet et al.	1999	79	86	75	3 (4%)
Iwatsuki et al.	2000	344	73	49	83 (24%)
Jonas et al.	2001	120	90	71	20 (17%)
Yao et al.	2001	64	87	73	8 (12%)

outcomes [48,49]. This information is valid but it is obvious that the indication of transplant should be based on radiology and even in experts hands, there will always be a certain degree of understaging [51,52]. This is frequently due to the failure to detect very small additional nodules < 1 cm and/or microscopic vascular invasion [51,53]. Current imaging technology should not miss tumors larger than 15 mm and thus incidental nodules larger than this size should be considered exceptional. The lack of sensitivity of radiology to detect minute additional nodules is critical as the proposed expansion is usually limited to a minor increase in size or to the number of minute additional tumors [48,49] (Table 8.2) that are very unlikely to be detected at staging. Furthermore, if understaging is to be always present, the enlistment of patients

Table 8.2 *Expanded Criteria for Liver Transplantation in Patients with HCC as Proposed by UCSF and Pittsburgh*

Yao et al. (2001)	
Tumor	1 lesion ≤ 6.5 cm
	≤3 lesions, largest ≤4.5 cm and total diameter ≤8 cm
Survival rate	90% at 1 year
	72% at 5 years
Marsh et al. (2000): Modified Pathologic TNM Staging System; patients fitting into stages I, II, and III would be accepted for transplantation	
Stage	Tumor-free survival[a]
I unilobar (any size/no vascular invasion); bilobar (≤2 cm ± microvascular invasion)	190.9 ± 6.9 (177.3–204.6)
II unilobar (>2 cm + microvascular invasion)	127.7 ± 16.7 (95–160.4)
IIIA bilobar (>2 cm)	69.1 ± 10.2 (49.1–89.1)
IIIB bilobar (>2 cm + microvascular invasion)	37.5 ± 10.2 (17.5–57.4)
IVA any lobe, any size, macrovascular invasion	16.4 ± 3.7 (9.1–23.7)
IVB lymph nodes ± metastasis	5.3 ± 1.0 (3.3–7.3)

[a]Tumor-free survival (mean ± SE) in months (95% CI).
Note: Staging is based on the data obtained at pathology and not with imaging techniques.

with more advanced tumor stage as recognized by current imaging techniques will surely translate to transplantation of patients with far more advanced disease and this will no doubt further deteriorate long-term outcome. Accordingly, there is room for expansion, but the data establishing the correlation between staging findings and outcome of patients transplanted with extended indication are nonexistent. Hence, any decision to modify the current definitions has to be put on hold until the availability of studies with well-defined correlation between radiological findings during the waiting time and outcome. Currently, accurate diagnosis and staging requires state-of-the-art dynamic computed tomography (CT) [54] or magnetic resonance imaging (MRI) [51,55] (Fig. 8.4), while Lipiodol injection with delayed CT has no accuracy [56].

A very relevant aspect that has to be taken into account when considering an expansion of criteria is the number of available livers. There is a major shortage of donors and this implies a waiting time between enlisting and transplantation. During this time, the tumor may progress and exceed the criteria used to exclude them from the waiting list. This unfortunate event may affect 25% of the patients with a waiting time of 12 months [15,57].

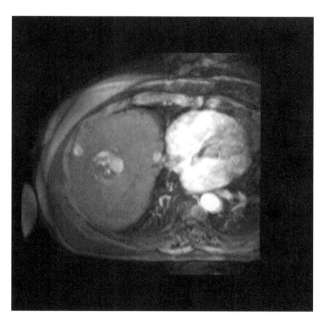

Fig. 8.4 *Hepatic magnetic resonance imaging (MRI) evidences a large HCC in the dome of the liver. Arterial hypervascularization with contrast washout during the venous phase establishes the diagnosis of HCC. Additional hypervascular nodules not detected by ultrasound (US) were also evidenced in the right lobe and excluded the patients from transplantation as this tumor stage exceeds the Milano criteria. (Courtesy of Dr C. Ayuso.)*

This occurs even with the application of treatment upon enlistment and the figures become even higher (50%) if the enlisted patients have more advanced tumors [58].

Some authors have suggested that patients with more advanced disease should be the first to be treated with transarterial chemoembolization and if response to therapy is positive with tumor burden downstaged into the conventional criteria, this would represent a marker of less aggressive disease [59]. Hence, in downstaged patients, transplantation would be successful and potentially could offer long-term survival. This type of "biological" selection is of limited impact. The likelihood of dissemination prior to transplant is not diminished by therapy, the rate of responders is low, the majority of the patients will still progress while waiting, and when the results are expressed according to intention to treat the survival is significantly less than 50% at 5 years [58]. Consequently, it is mandatory that any modification of the enlistment criteria takes into account the impact of the larger number of patients in the waiting list and how this should be handled [60].

Waiting List Management

As mentioned before one of the major unsolved issues in LT is the shortage of donors. This justifies the application of restrictive criteria to select the optimal candidates who will achieve the best possible long-term outcome. Nevertheless, even in countries with a high donation rate such as Spain, there is a continuously growing number of transplant candidates and this creates an expanding waiting list. During the waiting time, the liver disease may progress and impede transplantation [15,57]. There are no homogeneously accepted criteria to prompt exclusion. In most groups, exclusion is based on uncontrolled tumor progression leading to vascular invasion and/or extrahepatic spread. In contrast, in the USA the priority given to patients with HCC is cancelled when the patients exceed the restrictive limits accepted for enlisting [60], and due to the long waiting time in the absence of any priority, this means exclusion.

Waiting time exceeding 6 months is associated with a 25% exclusion rate of the candidates as shown in studies coming from Barcelona and subsequently confirmed in San Francisco [15,57]. This reduces the intention to treat survival to 60% at 2–3 years, a figure clearly below that achieved in the absence of waiting time and dropouts (Fig. 8.5).

There are several strategies aimed at preventing this adverse event. Active health campaigns may increase the number of donations, and active policies within transplant teams may wisely use the so-called marginal livers (advanced age, stetatosis) and those with metabolic disorders (amyloidosis [61], primary hyperoxaluria [62]) or with viral infection without significant liver injury [63]. In addition, highly skilled surgeons may develop the split-liver technique [64].

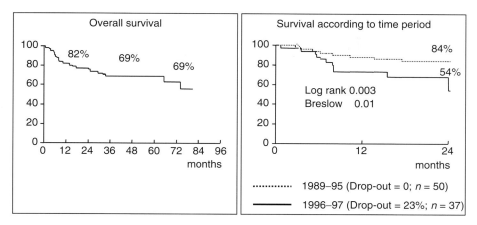

Fig. 8.5 *Survival of patients with hepatocellular carcinoma (HCC) treated by liver transplantation. The left panel represents the overall probability of survival of the whole series of patients. The right panel divides the patients into two periods of time: dotted line represents the period between 1989 and 1995 when the waiting time was reduced and there were no dropouts. Intention to treat survival at 2 years was 84%; continuous line represents the period after 1996 when waiting time expanded and dropouts became a frequent event. The intention to treat survival at 2 years was reduced to less than 60%. (Reproduced with permission.)*

However, the major impact is expected to come from live donation. A simultaneous strategy to impede progression is the application of adjuvant treatment with any of the available options known to be effective: resection, percutaneous ablation, and transarterial chemoembolization. Finally, some groups or countries have established priority policies aiming to transplant those at the highest risk of exclusion due to death or tumor progression.

Treatment upon Enlisting

There are no RCTs comparing any intervention with the best supportive care and thus any suggestion of a therapeutic benefit has to be derived from cohort studies. Unfortunately, most of these investigations merely describe the outcome of those patients that have been finally transplanted and do not offer information about those lost while waiting. The options that are most frequently applied are percutaneous ablation (Fig. 8.6) and chemoembolization. Surgical resection might also be used as a bridge in those patients with moderate surgical risk. Clearly, the decision to treat while waiting has to balance the risk of exclusion with the risk of side-effects related to treatment [65]. Therefore, the usual strategy is to avoid therapy if the expected waiting time is less than 6 months. Systemic chemotherapy has no efficacy and is hampered by severe side-effects [66,67]. Thus, it should not be recommended. Promising results have been reported with percutaneous ablation and chemoembolization [59,68], but

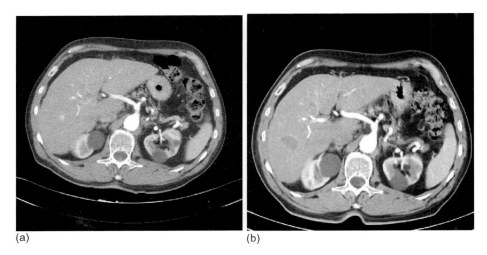

(a)   (b)

Fig. 8.6 *Percutaneous ablation of a small hepatocellular carcinoma (HCC) located in the right lobe of a cirrhotic liver. Patient was enlisted for liver transplantation and due to the long expected waiting time (more than 1 year) it was recommended to treat the HCC by radio frequency. (a) This shows the tumor on baseline conditions. Contrast uptake during the arterial phase indicated viable tumor tissue. (b) This shows the efficacy of treatment: the area occupied by the nodule does not show contrast uptake. The ablated area exceeds the area of the tumor suggesting that a safety rim of surrounding tissue potentially containing satellite foci has also been necrosed. (Courtesy of Dr J. R. Ayuso.)*

there are also studies that do not identify any benefit derived from treatment. Chemoembolization is the approach that has been more widely used. It requires the selective catheterization of the arterial vessels feeding the tumor and after injection of chemotherapy (usually doxorubicin or cisplatin in a Lipiodol emulsion) the artery is obstructed by injection of gelfoam or polivynil alcohol [69]. This combined action results in extensive tumor necrosis that is associated with a reduced tumor growth rate [70,71]. The portal vein should be patent and the liver function should be preserved. Child–Pugh C patients should not receive chemoembolization because of risk of death and Child–Pugh B patients may develop severe decompensation that ultimately may contraindicate transplantation. Chemotherapy administration may also induce side-effects by itself and thus decision to indicate treatment has to carefully balance benefits and risks according to waiting time and tumor profile. Percutaneous ablation has been introduced more recently but it has rapidly shown its advantages and risks [35,72]. The most common techniques to ablate tumors are ethanol injection and radio frequency. Both approaches are highly useful in tumors <2 cm, but radio frequency is more effective beyond this size and in addition it achieves ablation in fewer number of sessions [34,73]. However, side-effects are more frequent and severe with radio frequency as needles are larger and the procedure is done under conscious sedation.

Long-term follow-up and analysis of explanted livers of patients that have received treatment upon enlistment indicate that the rate of complete responses is not as high as reported by radiological examinations based on dynamic CT or MRI [36,74]. However, treatment while waiting does not aim to achieve complete eradication with long-term cure, but rather tumor mass shrinkage with avoidance of progression. It is clear that this might be achieved at least for a given period of time, but it is certain that the efficacy in preventing progression and exclusion will be reduced together with the progressive expansion of the waiting time. Thereby, treatment might be effective when waiting time is kept below 12 months, while in waiting times beyond 24 months, almost any treatment will ultimately fail and not prevent the exclusion of the majority of the patients.

Priority Policies

The establishment of a priority policy is controversial. There is very limited information identifying the parameters that may predict a higher likelihood of progression and thus of exclusion. This impedes the development of an accurate algorithm for clinical decision making. Smaller tumors are less likely to present progressive growth leading to exclusion [57] and tumors that present progression while waiting and exhibit an increased AFP concentration [75] are at higher risk.

A legal mandate forced transplant centers of the USA to develop a priority policy in order to transplant the sickest and avoid time in the waiting list as the major determinant of transplantation. The model for end-stage liver disease (MELD) score [76] was used to establish priority in patients with end-stage disease, but it did not allocate points due to HCC development and thus was useless for HCC patients. To correct this unfair situation, HCC patients were given a fixed number of MELD points according to tumor size and number [77]. The points given initially were excessive as HCC patients had a <90% probability of being transplanted in the first 3 months after enlisting, while the contrary was the case for patients without HCC. The reduction of points partially corrected the lack of equity and in the last modification that was implemented in 2004, it was decided that patients with solitary tumors <2 cm (stage 1) would not get priority because of the low risk of exclusion. Only patients with stage 2 tumors (solitary between 2 and 5 cm, or with up to three nodules less than 3 cm each) would receive priority points [77]. This new proposal is also expected to reduce the number of patients transplanted because of an HCC that ultimately is not confirmed in the explanted liver [77]. Radiological findings may be equivocal in small nodules but hypervascular nodules >2 cm in a cirrhotic liver with a characteristic venous washout on dynamic imaging establish the diagnosis of HCC and avoid the need of a biopsy-proven diagnosis [4]. The continuous analysis of the priority policy results will surely prompt new modifications aiming to obtain optimal results in HCC patients and also ensure that the access to transplant and long-term outcome is homogeneous in all categories of enlisted patients. In this regard, one of the concerns of priority policies upgrading patients with more advanced disease is the potential selection of patients with less favorable profiles and thus with lower probability of long-term survival [60].

Clearly, there is an urgent need to identify the strongest predictors of progression while waiting and it is expected that these will not come from rough assessment of size and number. Better knowledge of the genetic changes and molecular pathways that regulate tumor growth and dissemination should provide the most accurate tools to predict biology and hence allow establishment of a more sensitive selection and priority policy.

Living Donor Liver Transplantation

Living donor liver transplantation (LDLT) is considered an alternative to cadaver liver transplantation (CLT) [78]. In addition to the absence of a relevant waiting time between enlistment and transplantation, it offers the use of an optimal liver with less time between extraction and grafting. In adults, the most common approach is to use the right lobe of the donor. This will have undergone an extensive evaluation to diminish the risk related to major abdominal surgery as much as possible. The assumed death risk for donors is around 0.5% and any program should take this risk into account in order to balance the benefits for the recipient and the risk for the donor, both individually and as a community [79]. Extensive informed consent from the donor and the recipient is of crucial importance. Statistical modeling indicates that LDLT for early HCC offers substantial gains in life expectancy with acceptable cost-effectiveness ratios as compared with conventional CLT when waiting times for transplantation exceed at least 7 months and the outcome after transplant exceeds 70% at 5 years [80].

The outcome after LDLT in patients with HCC does not differ from that of patients receiving a cadaveric liver. A large multicenter study in Japan [81] recruiting 316 patients reinforces this concept and, interestingly, validates the use of the Milano criteria. Thereby, if patients fit into the Milano criteria the survival at 3 years is around 80% (78.7%) and HCC recurrence affects 1.4% of the patients (Fig. 8.7). In contrast, if the Milano definitions are not met, the survival is significantly impaired (60.4% survival at 3 years) and the recurrence rate affects 22.2% of the patients (Fig. 8.7). Despite these encouraging data in Japan, several aspects still need clarification. Some studies have suggested that hepatitis C virus reinfection of the graft might have a more aggressive evolution in LDLT [82]. Others have not found any difference [83,84]. Evolu-

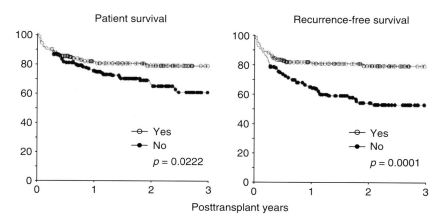

Fig. 8.7 *Survival of hepatocellular carcinoma (HCC) patients treated by live donor liver transplantation in Japan. The probabilities of overall survival and of survival without disease recurrence are divided according to Milano criteria. If these are respected both overall survival and disease-free survival are significantly better that in patients in whom the limits are exceeded. Interestingly, the data reproduce the results of transplantation using cadaveric livers and thus the validity of live donation for this entity is clearly supported. (Reproduced with permission.)*

tion to cirrhosis would be faster and this might counteract the benefits of avoiding exclusion while waiting. Ongoing investigations have to clarify to which extent the more aggressive evolution of viral infection is due to the origin of the graft or merely due to the combination of some immunosuppressive regime combined with a higher rate of biliary complications leading to cholestatic damage. Antiviral treatment and surgical improvements may help to ameliorate these aspects, but until these are fully clarified and solved, live donation should still be seen as a highly promising approach whose full incorporation into conventional clinical practice is not yet achieved.

One of the major controversies raised by live donation is to which extent its indication should be restricted to the criteria used for cadaver livers or, if on the contrary, the criteria could be expanded [81,85,86]. This would allow patients with cancer stage beyond Milano criteria to benefit from transplantation and thus achieve long-term survival that otherwise would be unlikely. Following this reasoning, some groups have established a very liberal policy and proceed to live donation if there is no extrahepatic dissemination or invasion of a major blood vessel. Others, such as the Barcelona group, have proposed a moderate expansion in terms of size and number of tumors [87], in part paralleling the proposals for expansion commented before for cadaveric donation. The major issue here is to balance the risk incurred by the donor (mortality around 0.5%), with the benefit offered to the recipient. It is easy to assume that desperate patients in whom the probability of success is nil should not be allowed to compromise the life of a donor. However, there is no

Table 8.3 *Barcelona Expanded Criteria for Living Donor Liver transplantation in HCC Patients*

Single HCC ≤7 cm

Multinodular HCC: 3 nodules ≤5cm, 5 nodules ≤3 cm

Downstaging: parial response to any treatment lasting
   more than 6 months achieves the cinventional
   criteria of cadaveric liver transplantation

Note. Staging is based on imaging techniques

worldwide minimal life expectancy limit below which live donation should not be offered. Probably, the 50% survival at 5 years frequently proposed as the bottom figure in cadaveric donation [88] should be implemented also in live donation. In keeping with this aim, in Barcelona we have launched a pilot program of live donation with expanded definitions that are reflected in Table 8.3 [87]. The program runs under strict ethical controls and its application is expected to achieve a 5-year survival of 50%. Less than 10% of the HCC patients fit into this indication and the final applicability only involves one-fourth of the potential candidates.

■ CONCLUSION

In summary, LT is an effective therapy for patients diagnosed with HCC at an early stage. Its application is curtailed by the shortage of donors, which prompts a growing waiting time during which the tumor may progress. Antineoplastic treatment may prevent this adverse event, but the best approach would be to increase the number of available livers either through increased cadaver donation or through live donation.

■ REFERENCES

1. Parkin DM, Bray F, Ferlay J, et al. Estimating the world cancer burden: Globocan 2000. Int J Cancer 2001;94(2):153–156.

2. Fattovich G, Stroffolini T, Zagni I, et al. Hepatocellular carcinoma in cirrhosis: incidence and risk factors. Gastroenterology 2004;127(5 suppl 1):S35–S50.

3. Bosch FX, Ribes J, Diaz M, et al. Primary liver cancer: worldwide incidence and trends. Gastroenterology 2004;127(5 suppl 1):S5–S16.

4. Bruix J, Sherman M, Llovet JM, et al. Clinical management of hepatocellular carcinoma: conclusions of the Barcelona-2000 EASL Conference. J Hepatol 2001;35:421–430.

5. Degos F, Christidis C, Ganne-Carrie N, et al. Hepatitis C virus-related cirrhosis: time to occurrence of hepatocellular carcinoma and death. Gut 2000;47(1):131–136.

6. Benvegnu L, Gios M, Boccato S, et al. Natural history of compensated viral cirrhosis: a prospective study on the incidence and hierarchy of major complications. Gut 2004;53(5):744–749.

7. Sangiovanni A, Del Ninno E, Fasani P, et al. Increased survival of cirrhotic patients with a hepatocellular carcinoma detected during surveillance. Gastroenterology 2004;126(4):1005–1014.

8. Chang MH, Chen CJ, Lai MS, et al. Universal hepatitis B vaccination in Taiwan and the incidence of hepatocellular carcinoma in children. N Engl J Med 1997;336(26): 1855–1859.

9. Bolondi L. Screening for hepatocellular carcinoma in cirrhosis. J Hepatol 2003;39(6): 1076–1084.

10. Befeler AS, Di Bisceglie AM. Hepatocellular carcinoma: diagnosis and treatment. Gastroenterology 2002;122(6):1609–1619.

11. Bruix J, Boix L, Sala M, et al. Focus on hepatocellular carcinoma. Cancer Cell 2004; 5(3):215–219.

12. Llovet JM, Burroughs A, Bruix J. Hepatocellular carcinoma. Lancet 2003;362(9399): 1907–1917.

13. Bolondi L, Sofia S, Siringo S, et al. Surveillance programme of cirrhotic patients for early diagnosis and treatment of hepatocellular carcinoma: a cost-effectiveness analysis. Gut 2001;48(2):251–259.

14. Llovet JM, Bruix J. Systematic review of randomized trials for unresectable hepatocellular carcinoma: chemoembolization improves survival. Hepatology 2003; 37(2):429–442.

15. Llovet JM, Fuster J, Bruix J. Intention-to-treat analysis of surgical treatment for early hepatocellular carcinoma: resection versus transplantation. Hepatology 1999;30(6): 1434–1440.

16. Arii S, Yamaoka Y, Futagawa S, et al. Results of surgical and nonsurgical treatment for small-sized hepatocellular carcinomas: a retrospective and nationwide survey in Japan. Hepatology 2000;32(6):1224–1229.

17. Bismuth H, Majno PE. Hepatobiliary surgery. J Hepatol 2000;32(1 suppl):208–224.

18. Song TJ, Ip EW, Fong Y. Hepatocellular carcinoma: current surgical management. Gastroenterology 2004;127(5 suppl 1):S248–S260.

19. Okada S, Shimada K, Yamamoto J, et al. Predictive factors for postoperative recurrence of hepatocellular carcinoma. Gastroenterology 1994;106(6):1618–1624.

20. Shirabe K, Kanematsu T, Matsumata T, et al. Factors linked to early recurrence of small hepatocellular carcinoma after hepatectomy: univariate and multivariate analyses. Hepatology 1991;14(5):802–805.

21. Nagasue N, Uchida M, Makino Y, et al. Incidence and factors associated with intrahepatic recurrence following resection of hepatocellular carcinoma. Gastroenterology 1993;105(2):488–494.

22. Chen YJ, Yeh SH, Chen JT, et al. Chromosomal changes and clonality relationship between primary and recurrent hepatocellular carcinoma. Gastroenterology 2000;119(2):431–440.

23. Muto Y, Moriwaki H, Ninomiya M, et al. Prevention of second primary tumors by an acyclic retinoid, polyprenoic acid, in patients with hepatocellular carcinoma. N Engl J Med 1996;334(24):1561–1567.

24. Lau WY, Leung TW, Ho SK, et al. Adjuvant intra-arterial iodine-131-labelled Lipiodol for resectable hepatocellular carcinoma: a prospective randomised trial. Lancet 1999;353(9155):797–801.

25. Kubo S, Nishiguchi S, Hirohashi K, et al. Effects of long-term postoperative interferon-alpha therapy on intrahepatic recurrence after resection of hepatitis C virus-related hepatocellular carcinoma. A randomized, controlled trial. Ann Intern Med 2001;134(10):963–967.

26. Ikeda K, Arase Y, Saitoh S, et al. Interferon beta prevents recurrence of hepatocellular carcinoma after complete resection or ablation of the primary tumor – a prospective randomized study of hepatitis C virus-related liver cancer. Hepatology 2000;32(2):228–232.

27. Takayama T, Sekine T, Makuuchi M, et al. Adoptive immunotherapy to lower postsurgical recurrence rates of hepatocellular carcinoma: a randomised trial. Lancet 2000;356(9232):802–807.

28. Majno PE, Sarasin FP, Mentha G, et al. Primary liver resection and salvage transplantation or primary liver transplantation in patients with single, small hepatocellular carcinoma and preserved liver function: an outcome-oriented decision analysis. Hepatology 2000;31(4):899–906.

29. Belghiti J, Cortes A, Abdalla EK, et al. Resection prior to liver transplantation for hepatocellular carcinoma. Ann Surg 2003;238(6):885–892.

30. Adam R, Azoulay D, Castaing D, et al. Liver resection as a bridge to transplantation for hepatocellular carcinoma on cirrhosis: a reasonable strategy? Ann Surg 2003;238(4):508–518.

31. Minagawa M, Makuuchi M, Takayama T, et al. Selection criteria for repeat hepatectomy in patients with recurrent hepatocellular carcinoma. Ann Surg 2003;238(5):703–710.

32. Sala M, Fuster J, Llovet JM, et al. High pathological risk of recurrence after surgical resection for hepatocellular carcinoma: an indication for salvage liver transplantation. Liver Transpl 2004;10(10):1294–1300.

33. Livraghi T, Goldberg SN, Lazzaroni S, et al. Small hepatocellular carcinoma: treatment with radio-frequency ablation versus ethanol injection. Radiology 1999;210(3):655–661.

34. Lencioni RA, Allgaier HP, Cioni D, et al. Small hepatocellular carcinoma in cirrhosis: randomized comparison of radio-frequency thermal ablation versus percutaneous ethanol injection. Radiology 2003;228(1):235–240.

35. Gaiani S, Celli N, Cecilioni L, et al. Review article: percutaneous treatment of hepatocellular carcinoma. Aliment Pharmacol Ther 2003;17(suppl 2):103–110.

36. Sala M, Llovet JM, Vilana R, et al. Initial response to percutaneous ablation predicts survival in patients with hepatocellular carcinoma. Hepatology 2004;40(6):1352–1360.

37. Iwatsuki S, Gordon RD, Shaw BW, Jr, et al. Role of liver transplantation in cancer therapy. Ann Surg 1985;202(4):401–407.

38. Bismuth H, Majno PE, Adam R. Liver transplantation for hepatocellular carcinoma. Semin Liver Dis 1999;19(3):311–322.

39. Bismuth H, Chiche L, Adam R, et al. Liver resection versus transplantation for hepatocellular carcinoma in cirrhotic patients. Ann Surg 1993;218(2):145–151.

40. Hsu HC, Wu TT, Wu MZ, et al. Tumor invasiveness and prognosis in resected hepatocellular carcinoma. Clinical and pathogenetic implications. Cancer 1988;61(10):2095–2099.

41. Nakashima T, Kojiro M. Hepatocellular carcinoma. Tokyo: Springer-Verlag, 1987.

42. Mazzaferro V, Regalia E, Doci R, et al. Liver transplantation for the treatment of small hepatocellular carcinomas in patients with cirrhosis. N Engl J Med 1996;334(11):693–699.

43. Llovet JM, Bruix J, Fuster J, et al. Liver transplantation for treatment of small hepatocellular carcinoma: the tumor-node-metastasis classification does not have prognostic power. Hepatology 1998;27(6):1572–1577.

44. Jonas S, Bechstein WO, Steinmuller T, et al. Vascular invasion and histopathologic grading determine outcome after liver transplantation for hepatocellular carcinoma in cirrhosis. Hepatology 2001;33(5):1080–1086.

45. Schwartz M. Liver transplantation for hepatocellular carcinoma. Gastroenterology 2004;127(5 suppl 1):S268–S276.

46. Plessier A, Codes L, Consigny Y, et al. Underestimation of the influence of satellite nodules as a risk factor for post-transplantation recurrence in patients with small hepatocellular carcinoma. Liver Transpl 2004;10(suppl 2):S86–S90.

47. Shetty K, Timmins K, Brensinger C, et al. Liver transplantation for hepatocellular carcinoma validation of present selection criteria in predicting outcome. Liver Transpl 2004;10(7):911–918.

48. Yao FY, Ferrell L, Bass NM, et al. Liver transplantation for hepatocellular carcinoma: expansion of the tumor size limits does not adversely impact survival. Hepatology 2001;33(6):1394–1403.

49. Marsh JW, Dvorchick I. Liver organ allocation for hepatocellular carcinoma: are we sure? Liver Transpl 2003;9:693–696.

50. Bruix J, Fuster J, Llovet JM. Liver transplantation for hepatocellular carcinoma: Foucault pendulum versus evidence-based decision. Liver Transpl 2003;9(7):700–702.

51. Burrel M, Llovet JM, Ayuso C, et al. MRI angiography is superior to helical CT for detection of HCC prior to liver transplantation: an explant correlation. Hepatology 2003;38(4):1034–1042.

52. Krinsky GA, Lee VS, Theise ND, et al. Transplantation for hepatocellular carcinoma and cirrhosis: sensitivity of magnetic resonance imaging. Liver Transpl 2002;8(12):1156–1164.

53. Libbrecht L, Bielen D, Verslype C, et al. Focal lesions in cirrhotic explant livers: pathological evaluation and accuracy of pretransplantation imaging examinations. Liver Transpl 2002;8(9):749–761.

54. Baron RL, Brancatelli G. Computed tomographic imaging of hepatocellular carcinoma. Gastroenterology 2004;27(5 suppl 1):S133–S143.

55. Taouli B, Losada M, Holland A, et al. Magnetic resonance imaging of hepatocellular carcinoma. Gastroenterology 2004;127(5 suppl 1):S144–S152.

56. Bizollon T, Rode A, Bancel B, et al. Diagnostic value and tolerance of Lipiodol-computed tomography for the detection of small hepatocellular carcinoma: correlation with pathologic examination of explanted livers. J Hepatol 1998;28(3):491–496.

57. Yao FY, Bass NM, Nikolai B, et al. Liver transplantation for hepatocellular carcinoma: analysis of survival according to the intention-to-treat principle and dropout from the waiting list. Liver Transpl 2002;8(10):873–883.

58. Roayaie S, Frischer JS, Emre SH, et al. Long-term results with multimodal adjuvant therapy and liver transplantation for the treatment of hepatocellular carcinomas larger than 5 centimeters. Ann Surg 2002;235(4):533–539.

59. Majno PE, Adam R, Bismuth H, et al. Influence of preoperative transarterial Lipiodol chemoembolization on resection and transplantation for hepatocellular carcinoma in patients with cirrhosis. Ann Surg 1997;226(6):688–701.

60. Sala M, Varela M, Bruix J. Selection of candidates with HCC for transplantation in the MELD era. Liver Transpl 2004;10(10 suppl 2):S4–S9.

61. Azoulay D, Samuel D, Castaing D, et al. Domino liver transplants for metabolic disorders: experience with familial amyloidotic polyneuropathy. J Am Coll Surg 1999;189(6):584–593.

62. Donckier V, El Nakadi I, Closset J, et al. Domino hepatic transplantation using the liver from a patient with primary hyperoxaluria. Transplantation 2001;71(9):1346–1348.

63. Vargas HE, Laskus T, Wang LF, et al. Outcome of liver transplantation in hepatitis C virus-infected patients who received hepatitis C virus-infected grafts [see comments]. Gastroenterology 1999;117(1):149–153.

64. Renz JF, Yersiz H, Reichert PR, et al. Split-liver transplantation: a review. Am J Transplant 2003;3(11):1323–1335.

65. Llovet JM, Mas X, Aponte JJ, et al. Cost effectiveness of adjuvant therapy for hepatocellular carcinoma during the waiting list for liver transplantation. Gut 2002; 50(1):123–128.

66. Stone MJ, Klintmalm G, Polter D, et al. Neoadjuvant chemotherapy and orthotopic liver transplantation for hepatocellular carcinoma. Transplantation 1989;48(2):344–347.

67. Stone MJ, Klintmalm GB, Polter D, et al. Neoadjuvant chemotherapy and liver transplantation for hepatocellular carcinoma: a pilot study in 20 patients. Gastroenterology 1993;104(1):196–202.

68. Bolondi L, Piscaglia F, Camaggi V, et al. Review article: liver transplantation for HCC. Treatment options on the waiting list. Aliment Pharmacol Ther 2003;17(suppl 2):145–150.

69. Bruix J, Sala M, Llovet JM. Chemoembolization for hepatocellular carcinoma. Gastroenterology 2004;127(5 suppl 1):S179–S188.

70. GETCH. A comparison of Lipiodol chemoembolization and conservative treatment for unresectable hepatocellular carcinoma. Groupe d'Etude et de Traitement du Carcinome Hepatocellulaire. N Engl J Med 1995;332(19):1256–1261.

71. Llovet JM, Real MI, Montanya X, et al. Arterial embolization, chemoembolization versus symptomatic treatment in patients with unresectable hepatocellular carcinoma: a randomized controlled trial. Lancet 2002;359:1734–1739.

72. Livraghi T, Solbiati L, Meloni MF, et al. Treatment of focal liver tumors with percutaneous radio-frequency ablation: complications encountered in a multicenter study. Radiology 2003;226(2):441–451.

73. Lin SM, Lin CJ, Lin CC, et al. Radiofrequency ablation improves prognosis compared with ethanol injection for hepatocellular carcinoma < or =4 cm. Gastroenterology 2004;127(6):1714–1723.

74. Mazzaferro V, Battiston C, Perrone S, et al. Radiofrequency ablation of small hepatocellular carcinoma in cirrhotic patients awaiting liver transplantation: a prospective study. Ann Surg 2004;240(5):900–909.

75. Llovet JM, Sala M, Fuster J, et al. Predictors of drop-out and survival of patients with hepatocellular carcinoma candidates for liver transplantation. Hepatology 2003;38(suppl 1):763 (A1250).

76. Kamath PS, Wiesner RH, Malinchoc M, et al. A model to predict survival in patients with end-stage liver disease. Hepatology 2001;33(2):464–470.

77. Freeman RB. Liver allocation for HCC: a moving target. Liver Transpl 2004;10(1):49–51.

78. Chen CL, Fan ST, Lee SG, et al. Living-donor liver transplantation: 12 years of experience in Asia. Transplantation 2003;75(3 suppl):S6–S11.

79. Brown RS, Jr, Russo MW, Lai M, et al. A survey of liver transplantation from living adult donors in the United States. N Engl J Med 2003;348(9):818–825.

80. Sarasin FP, Majno PE, Llovet JM, et al. Living donor liver transplantation for early hepatocellular carcinoma: a life-expectancy and cost-effectiveness perspective. Hepatology 2001;33(5):1073–1079.

81. Todo S, Furukawa H. Living donor liver transplantation for adult patients with hepatocellular carcinoma: experience in Japan. Ann Surg 2004;240(3):451–459.

82. Garcia-Retortillo M, Forns X, Llovet JM, et al. Hepatitis C recurrence is more severe after living donor compared to cadaveric liver transplantation. Hepatology 2004;40(3):699–707.

83. Bozorgzadeh A, Jain A, Ryan C, et al. Impact of hepatitis C viral infection in primary cadaveric liver allograft versus primary living-donor allograft in 100 consecutive liver transplant recipients receiving tacrolimus. Transplantation 2004;77(7):1066–1070.

84. Forman LM, Trotter JF, Emond J. Living donor liver transplantation and hepatitis C. Liver Transpl 2004;10(3):347–348.

85. Steinmuller T, Pascher A, Sauer I, et al. Living-donation liver transplantation for hepatocellular carcinoma: time to drop the limitations? Transplant Proc 2002;34(6):2263–2264.

86. Gondolesi GE, Roayaie S, Munoz L, et al. Adult living donor liver transplantation for patients with hepatocellular carcinoma: extending UNOS priority criteria. Ann Surg 2004;239(2):142–149.

87. Bruix J, Llovet JM. Prognostic prediction and treatment strategy in HCC. Hepatology 2002;35(3):519–524.

88. Neuberger J. Developments in liver transplantation. Gut 2004;53(5):759–768.

Alcoholism and Alcoholic Liver Disease

▼   ▼   ▼   ▼   ▼   ▼   ▼   ▼   ▼

Mark Hudson and Kaushik Agarwal

S TARZL ET AL. [1] first reported successful human orthotopic liver transplantation (OLT) in 1968. Since then OLT has become an established and widely accepted treatment for end-stage liver disease (ESLD), with demonstrable excellent outcomes. One-year patient and graft survival rates average 85%; complications such as late graft loss and chronic rejection are uncommon. From April 1, 2003 to March 31, 2004, 491 elective OLTs were performed in the UK: alcoholic liver disease (ALD) was the underlying etiology in 108 (22%) cases. ALD is the commonest cause of ESLD in both Europe and the USA and is responsible for 7.9 deaths/100 000 population in the USA [2]. Moreover, ALD is the second most common indication for liver transplantation (LT), after viral hepatitis [3,4]. Survival rates following OLT for both ALD and non-ALD etiologies are comparable, and the rate of alcohol relapse post-OLT appears acceptably low.

Nevertheless, ALD remains a controversial indication for OLT. A survey of attitudes toward OLT reported that ALD is the least popular indication for listing and organ allocation amongst both the public and family physicians [5]. However, the prevalence and sheer magnitude of alcoholic cirrhosis means that ALD accounts for a substantial and increasing proportion of all OLT undertaken (Fig. 9.1). Concerns about offering liver grafts to patients with ALD arise from the fear that doing so may be "wasting" a liver on a person with "self-inflicted" disease, in whom there is potential for recidivism, abuse, and recurrent liver disease post-OLT. These concerns are particularly marked in the current era where huge disparity exists between the number of patients listed for OLT and the significant shortage of donor organs (see Chapter 6). In spite of the growth of living donor liver transplantation (LDLT: see Chapter 12), 5–15% of listed patients die while waiting, both in

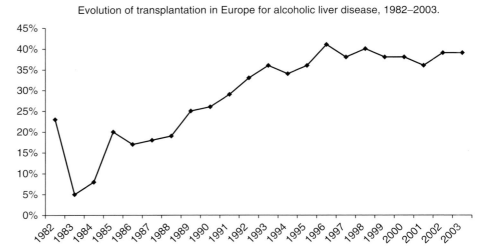

Fig. 9.1 *From May 1968 to December 2003, 8995 liver transplants were performed for alcoholic liver disease (ALD) in Europe. The figure demonstrates the proportion of patients undergoing transplantation for ALD relative to primary biliary cirrhosis (PBC) and virus-related cirrhosis (1982–2003). Adapted from the European Liver Transplant Registry (ELTR), December 2003 (http://www.eltr.org).*

the USA and in Europe [6]. This organ shortage dictates that not all patients who may potentially benefit from OLT will receive a graft. As such the priority that programs should and do give to patients with ALD has been challenged, and this has stimulated much debate. Most centers in Europe and in North America require 6 months' abstinence from alcohol before patients are accepted for OLT listing, and in some cases before evaluation may commence. Some centers demand that patients undergo alcohol rehabilitation, and many centers perform random testing of blood and urine while patients are listed and awaiting OLT. However, few centers follow their own protocols in all instances [7–10]. Overall, evidence suggests that ALD is a very good indication for OLT with similar or better medium-term outcomes after transplantation to most other liver diseases except perhaps cholestatic liver disease [11].

■ ISSUES RELATING TO TRANSPLANTATION FOR ALD

In this review we address the following issues:

1. How can one predict which patient is likely to relapse following OLT and what steps can be taken to prevent such relapse among these patients?

2. Can OLT be justified as effective in patients with ALD compared with those with non-ALD and what criteria should be used to select patients with ALD for liver transplantation?
3. How can one predict who is likely to relapse after transplantation and what steps can be taken to prevent such relapse in these patients?

Classification of the pattern of alcohol consumption and abuse is important in the assessment and management of a potential liver transplant candidate. Heavy consumers may be considered as either abusers or dependent drinkers [12]. Alcohol abuse is distinct from and runs a different course to dependence, there being no evidence that abuse leads to dependence [13,14]. However, there can be a close relationship between alcohol dependence and psychiatric illness (Chapter 4).

There is considerable variation between centers regarding the definition of relapse and recidivism. Some define relapse as any alcohol consumed at all, whereas others define it as consumption of a set amount of alcohol, e.g. 21 units/week for males and 14 units/week for females. In the nontransplant setting, addiction specialists define relapse as >4 units/day or any alcohol consumed daily on 4 or more consecutive days. Return to alcohol consumption of a lesser degree is often referred to as a "slip."

The two principal diagnostic systems for defining alcohol dependence, namely ICD-10 and DSM-IV (Chapter 4), demonstrate reasonably good agreement for classification of alcohol dependence, but poor concordance with respect to abuse or harmful use [15–17]. Moreover, using them to predict which patients will return to excessive drinking is difficult. Recurrence is more likely when patients are truly alcohol-dependent (as defined by DSM-IV or ICD-10) or have coexisting substance misuse [18], have had multiple previous failures at abstinence [19], or have major psychiatric disorders (including depression) [20,21] or posttraumatic stress disorder. Lastly, lack of social support is associated with increased risk of relapse [22]. Risk factors for alcohol relapse after liver transplantation are summarized in a recent review by Neuberger et al. [23], following a workshop on behalf of the European association for studies of the liver (EASL) and the European liver transplant registry (ELTR).

Studies of recidivism following OLT are difficult to compare because of differences both in definition (see above) and in methods of follow-up (from self-reported telephone surveys to intensive counseling with laboratory measures of alcohol-related parameters). Accordingly, reported rates of recidivism vary greatly (9–80%) [24], the majority being between 20% and 30%. Recidivism is considered undesirable because of the potential for recurrent ALD, decreased compliance with immunosuppressive therapy [25], and loss of societal support for transplantation programs with attendant decrease in organ donation rates. Pageaux et al. described 53 patients who underwent transplantation for ALD and compared "relapsers" with those who remained abstinent. They were followed for a mean of 42 (range 1–100) months. Alcohol relapsers had less acute (33% vs. 50%) and chronic (0% vs. 9%) rejection than those who remained abstinent. Furthermore, mean survival (54 months vs. 44 months, $P = 0.004$) was longer and retransplant rates were lower (0% vs. 15%) among those who relapsed than among those who remained abstinent [26], although numbers were small. Other studies support these findings with no adverse effect on graft or patient survival in those who return to moderate drinking [27,28]. Furthermore, Pageaux et al. have followed 128 transplanted patients over a mean of 54 months comparing heavy with occasional drinkers and those who remain abstinent. No difference in survival rates was demonstrated but all episodes of rejection in the heavy drinkers were related to poor compliance with their immunosuppressive therapy. Three deaths were related to heavy alcohol consumption but were independent of recurrent ALD in the graft [29]. In contrast to "recidivism," recurrent ALD has been defined as heavy drinking together with appropriate histological changes. However, very few studies that define the incidence of recurrent ALD exist (see Chapter 24).

The commonest method in use to limit recidivism and thus the potential for recurrent ALD is the "6-month rule" (i.e. requiring abstinence from alcohol for 6 months prior to listing for transplantation). This guideline is standard in the UK, in many European transplant centers [24], and in most US centers. The stated purpose of this guideline is threefold. First, abstinence is said to be associated with a decreased likelihood of recidivism post-LT. However, evidence for this is limited. Bird et al. [9] examined the outcome of transplantation in 24 patients with ALD. Three patients who were drinking heavily prior to LT had laboratory evidence of recurrent alcohol abuse after transplant (although this was denied by all three patients, highlighting the difficulty in obtaining reliable estimates of recidivism). Conversely, only 1 of 21 patients with a record of long-term abstinence returned to alcohol use. Kumar et al. [30] reported recidivism (identified by a telephone survey) amongst 3 of 7 patients (43%) abstinent for less than 6 months compared with 3 of 45 patients (7%) abstinent for longer prior to LT. In contrast, Periera et al. [31] did not find any relationship between duration of abstinence before LT and rates of recidivism. Therefore, evidence that the 6-month rule promotes posttransplant abstinence is somewhat flimsy [32]. Second, the reason for advising at least 6 months of abstinence is to improve the immediate postoperative outcome. Evidence in support of this is again limited [33,34].

Third, the strongest argument for continuing to apply the 6-month rule is to give patients an opportunity to recover spontaneously from advanced liver disease, and thereby avoid transplantation. Many patients present to liver units with very advanced liver disease (as defined by Child–Turcotte–Pugh

(CTP) class [35], high MELD, or Maddrey [36] scores) but improve substantially with prolonged periods of abstinence. The 5-year survival of patients with CTP class C alcoholic cirrhosis and sustained abstinence from alcohol is greater than 50% [37], which compares favorably with liver transplantation. Transplantation can then be considered for patients whose synthetic function does not improve despite abstinence. Unfortunately, this approach does not guide the management of patients who continue to deteriorate to a life-threatening degree within 6 months of stopping drinking or who have the occasional "slip" during this period. In these circumstances, Webb and Neuberger [38] argued recently that death may be the price of proving abstinence. As the length of abstinence prior to transplantation does not reliably predict abstinence afterwards, no justification exists for a fixed arbitrary period of abstinence before transplantation. A degree of flexibility may be required for those sick patients whose condition continues to deteriorate during the 6 months' abstinence period, but who demonstrate clear intent to abstinence and do not have poor prognostic features of alcohol dependence or adverse psychological and psychiatric manifestations. The findings of one study suggest that the number of patients with severe alcoholic cirrhosis to whom LT might be applicable before 6 months of abstinence and rehabilitation has been achieved is very small; and that reassessment at 3 months may help identify those patients whose liver function is not going to recover sufficiently without LT, despite abstinence [39].

No single strategy has been shown to prevent alcohol relapse following transplantation but there is the suggestion that with a multidisciplinary approach the risk can be minimized by continued supportive counseling and good staff–patient relationships. This needs to be supplemented by careful patient selection and treatment of any associated psychiatric conditions [18,32].

Is liver transplantation effective in patients with ALD versus those with non-ALD, and what criteria should be used to select patients with ALD for liver transplantation?

Current evidence supports ALD as an appropriate indication for liver transplantation. Patients with ALD have graft and patient survival outcomes similar to patients who undergo transplantation for non-ALD [11,40]. One- and 5-year patient survival rates for patients with ALD were 82% and 68%, respectively, in the United Network for Organ Sharing (UNOS) database, and 85% and 75%, respectively, in the ELTR database [4,41]. Table 9.1 represents ELTR data on 1-, 5-, and 10-year patient survival rates following LT and is stratified by recipient diagnosis. The outcome among patients with ALD is comparable with that in patients with other diagnoses and superior to those in patients with chronic viral hepatitis at 5 years. Belle et al. [11] revealed that underlying causes of graft dysfunction and loss were similar between patients

Table 9.1 *Patient Survival Post Liver Transplantation*

	1-Year Survival (in Percent)	5-Year Survival (in Percent)	10-Year Survival (in Percent)
Alcoholic liver disease ($n = 8\,890$)	84	72	58
Primary biliary cirrhosis ($n = 3\,353$)	84	78	69
Viral hepatitis ($n = 11\,435$)	82	69	60
Autoimmune hepatitis ($n = 1\,229$)	82	74	66
Hepatocellular carcinoma ($n = 4\,632$)	79	56	43

Adapted from the European Liver Transplant Registry, January 1988 to December 2003 (http://www.eltr.org).

transplanted for ALD and non-ALD, suggesting minimal differences in both graft and patient outcomes overall.

In contrast, outcomes data beyond 5 years are limited. The University of Pittsburgh reported 7-year actuarial patient and graft survival rates of 63% and 59%, respectively, in a cohort of 123 patients with ALD [42]. ELTR data (Table 9.1) demonstrate that survival in ALD patients at 10 years is similar to that in other groups of patients except those undergoing LT for primary biliary cirrhosis (PBC). Interestingly, it appears that survival beyond 5–7 years is worse among patients with ALD because of significant increases in the incidence of cerebrovascular and ischemic heart disease, respiratory failure, and de novo malignancies, particularly of the upper airway (oropharyngeal) and upper gastrointestinal tract [42–44]. This may be the consequence of prolonged exposure to tobacco and alcohol among these patients. These factors should be considered in the routine assessment of patients for ALD.

The minimum criteria necessary for listing for liver transplantation among patients with ALD remain the subject of opinion and debate. However, Lim and Keefe [45] have proposed that in the absence of medical or psychosocial issues that would prevent successful transplantation the following should be adopted: a CTP score ≥ 7; an estimated likelihood to survive 1 year without transplant of <90%; a single episode of spontaneous bacterial peritonitis or the emergence of stage II encephalopathy in the setting of decompensated liver disease. If a patient meets one or more of these criteria and demonstrates no insurmountable impediment to listing for LT then appropriate evaluation should be undertaken (Chapter 1). Some centers incorporate prognostic tools for sobriety and alcoholism acceptance to help guide decision making, e.g. Vaillant's Prognostic Factors for Long-Term Sobriety and the Michigan Alcohol Prognostic Scale [46,47]. Ideally, a psychiatrist or other mental health provider with considerable experience in management of alcohol dependence and concomitant psychiatric diseases should be an integral member of the multidisciplinary team that decides whether or not to list a patient with ALD for liver transplantation.

Particular comorbid issues that may arise in patients with ALD and that require careful consideration during evaluation include cardiomyopathy and neurological disease. Most centers regard cardiomyopathy as a relative contraindication to transplantation, but the limits of left ventricular ejection fraction below which transplantation is contraindicated are not clear and may vary widely, from 20% to 50%. Likewise, ALD may be associated with both central (Wernicke–Korsakoff syndrome, dementia, cerebral atrophy, and hematomas) and peripheral neurological impairment (motor, sensory, and autonomic neuropathy). In a study by Anand et al. [48], 55% of patients with ALD assessed for transplantation had abnormal CT head scans but in only 2 patients did this contribute to decision not to transplant. Peripheral neuropathy does not appear to be associated with a poor outcome; autonomic neuropathy is not uncommon and improves with transplantation. Irreversible brain injury has been discussed in Chapter 1. Nutritional status should always be assessed and optimized aggressively, because malnutrition is associated with adverse outcomes.

In summary, outcomes following LT for appropriately selected patients with ALD are very good, short- and medium-term patient and graft outcomes, being comparable with if not better than those undergoing transplantation for non-ALD. Alcohol relapse rates are acceptably low with little evidence of graft loss related to poor compliance. Abstinence should be recommended for recipients of allografts for ALD but in some it may be possible to return to controlled drinking. However, this remains controversial. Nevertheless, the quality of life after liver transplantation is good even for those who do return to alcohol consumption. Those patients presenting with alcoholic hepatitis pose particular ethical problems. They are very ill, and so the time available for alcohol rehabilitation may be very limited. Anecdotal evidence indicates that 1-year patient survival rates in the UK (~20%) following LT for alcoholic hepatitis are very poor. Therefore, for the time being, alcoholic hepatitis is still not considered a standard indication for liver transplantation.

■ REFERENCES

1. Starzl TE, Groth CG, Brettschneider L, et al. Orthotopic homotransplantation of the human liver. Ann Surg 1968;168(3):392–415.

2. Roizen R, Kerr WC, Fimore KM. Cirrhosis mortality and per capita consumption of distilled spirits, United States, 1949–94; trend analysis. BMJ 1999;319:666–670.

3. Scientific Registry of Transplant Patients. Transplant statistics: center-specific reports. Available at http://www.ustransplant.org/center-adv.html. Accessed December 2004.

4. Adam R, McMaster P, O'Grady JG, et al. Evolution of liver transplantation in Europe: report of the European Liver Transplant Registry. Liver Transpl 2003;9: 1231–1243.

5. Neuberger J, Adams D, Macmaster P, et al. Assessing priorities for allocation of donor liver grafts: survey of public and clinicians. BMJ 1998;317:172–175.

6. McMaster P. Transplantation for alcoholic liver disease in an era of organ shortage. Lancet 2000;355:424–425.

7. Neuberger J. Transplantation for alcoholic liver disease: a perspective from Europe. Liver Transpl Surg 1998;4:S51–S57.

8. Osorio RW, Ascher NL, Avery M, et al. Predicting recidivism after orthotopic liver transplantation for alcoholic liver disease. Hepatology 1994;20:105–110.

9. Bird GL, O'Grady JG, Harvey FA, et al. Liver transplantation in patients with alcoholic cirrhosis: selection criteria and rates of survival and relapse. BMJ 1990;301:15–17.

10. Kumar S, Stauber RE, Gavaler JS, et al. Orthotopic liver transplantation for alcoholic liver disease. Hepatology 1990;11:159–164.

11. Belle SH, Beringer KC, Deire KM. Liver transplantation for alcoholic liver disease in the United States: 1988 to 1995. Liver Transpl Surg 1997;3:212–217.

12. Skinner HA. Spectrum of drinkers and intervention opportunities. Can Med Assoc J 1990;143:1054–1059.

13. Hasin D, Paykin A, Endicott J, et al. The validity of DSM-IV alcohol abuse. J Stud Alcohol 1999;60:746–755.

14. Hasin D, Van Rossem R, McCloud S, et al. Alcohol dependence and abuse diagnoses: validity in community sample heavy drinkers. Alcohol Clin Exp Res 1997;21:213–219.

15. Rounsaville BJ, Bryant K, Babor T, et al. Cross system agreement for substance abuse use disorders: DSM-III-R, DSM-IV and ICD-10. Addiction 1993;88:337–348.

16. Schuckit MA, Hesselbrock V, Tipp J, et al. A comparison of DSM-III-R, DSM-IV and ICD-10 substance use disorders diagnoses in 1922 men and women subjects in the COGA study. Addiction 1994;89:1629–1638.

17. Hasin D, McCloud S, Li Q, et al. Cross-system agreement among demographic subgroups: DSM-III, DSM-III-R, DSM-IV and ICD-10 diagnoses of alcohol use disorders. Drug Alcohol Depend 1996;41:127–135.

18. Beresford TP. Predictive factors for alcoholic relapse in the selection of alcohol-dependent persons for hepatic transplant. Liver Transpl Surg 1997;3:280–291.

19. Gish RG, Lee AH, Keefe EB, et al. Liver transplantation for patients with alcoholism and end stage liver disease. Am J Gastroenterol 1993;88:1337–1342.

20. Merikangas KR, Glernter CS. Comorbidity for alcoholism and depression. Psychiatr Clin North Am 1990;13:613–632.

21. Grant BF, Harford TC. Comorbidity between DSM IV alcohol use disorders and major depression: results of a national survey. Drug Alcohol Depend 1995;39:197–206.

22. Strauss R, Bacon SD. Alcoholism and social stability, a study of occupational integration of 2023 male clinic patients. Q J Stud Alcohol 1951;12:231–260.

23. Neuberger J, Schulz Karl-Heinz, Day CP, et al. Transplantation for alcoholic liver disease. J Hepatol 2002;36:130–137.

24. Neuberger J, Tang H. Relapse after transplantation: European studies. Liver Transpl Surg 1997;3:275–279.

25. Campbell DA, Magee JC, Punch JD, et al. One center's experience with liver transplantation: alcohol relapse over the long term. Liver Transpl Surg 1998;4:S58–S64.

26. Pageaux GP, Michel J, Coste V, et al. Alcoholic cirrhosis is a good indication for liver transplantation even for cases of recidivism. Gut 1999;45:421–426.

27. Belle SH, Beringer KC, Deire KM. Liver transplantation for alcoholic liver disease in the United States: 1988 to 1995. Liver Transpl Surg 1997;3:212–217.

28. Anand AC, Ferraz-Neto BH, Nightingale P, et al. Liver transplantation for alcoholic liver disease: evaluation of a sedation protocol. Hepatology 1997;25:1478–1484.

29. Pageaux GP, Bismuth M, Perney P, et al. Alcohol relapse after liver transplantation for alcoholic liver disease: does it matter? J Hepatol 2003;38:629–634.

30. Kumar S, Stauber RE, Gavaler J, et al. Orthotopic liver transplantation for alcoholic liver disease. Hepatology 1990;11:159–164.

31. Periera SP, Howard LM, Rela M, et al. Quality of life after transplantation for alcoholic liver disease. Liver Transpl 2000;6:62–68.

32. Weinreib RM, Van Horn DHA, McLellan AT, et al. Interpreting the significance of drinking by alcohol-dependent liver transplant patients: fostering candour is the key to recovery. Liver Transpl 2000;6:769–776.

33. Weisner RH, Lombardero M, Lake JR, et al. Liver transplantation for end stage alcoholic disease: an assessment of outcomes. Liver Transpl Surg 1997;3:321–329.

34. Shakil AO, Pinna A, Demetris J, et al. Survival and quality of life after liver transplantation for acute alcoholic hepatitis. Liver Transpl Surg 1997;3:240–244.

35. Child CG, Turcotte JG. Major problems in clinical surgery: the liver and portal hypertension, Vol. 1. Philadelphia, PA: WB Saunders, 1964:49–50.

36. Maddrey WC, Boitnott JK, Bedine MS, et al. Corticosteroid therapy of alcoholic hepatitis. Gastroenterology 1978;75(2):193–199.

37. Powell WJ, Klatskin G. Duration of survival in patients with Laennec's cirrhosis. Influence of alcohol withdrawal and possible effects of recent changes in general management of the disease. Am J Med 1968;44(3):406–420.

38. Webb K, Neuberger J. Transplantation for alcoholic liver disease. BMJ 2004;329: 63–64.

39. Veldt BJ, Laine F, Guillygomarc'h A, et al. Indication of liver transplantation in severe alcoholic liver cirrhosis: quantitative evaluation and optimal timing. J Hepatol 2002;36:93–98.

40. Hoofnagle JH, Kresina T, Fuller RK, et al. Liver transplantation for alcoholic liver disease: executive statement and recommendations. Summary of a National Institute of Health workshop held December 6–7, 1996, Bethesda, Maryland. Liver Transpl Surg 1997;3:347–350.

41. 1997 Annual report of the US Scientific Registry for Organ Transplantation and the Organ Procurement and Transplantation Network. Transplant data, 1988–1997. Bureau of Health Resources and Service Administration, US Dept. of Health and Human Services, Rockville, MD, 1998.

42. Bellamy CO, DiMartini AM, Ruppert K, et al. Liver transplantation for alcoholic liver cirrhosis: long-term follow up and impact of disease recurrence. Transplantation 2001;72:619–626.

43. Duvoux C, Delacroix I, Richardet JP, et al. Increased incidence of oropharyngeal squamous cell carcinoma after liver transplantation for alcoholic cirrhosis. Transplantation 1999;67:418–421.

44. Herrero JI, Lorenzo M, Quiroga J, et al. De novo neoplasia after liver transplantation: an analysis of risk factors and influence on survival. Liver Transpl 2005;11:89–97.

45. Lim JK, Keefe EB. Liver transplantation for alcoholic liver disease: current concepts and length of sobriety. Liver Transpl 2004;10:S31–S38.

46. Vaillant GE. What can long-term follow up teach us about relapse and prevention of relapse and addiction? Br J Addict 1983;83:1147–1157.

47. Lucey MR, Merion RM, Henley KS, et al. Selection for and outcome of liver transplantation in alcoholic liver disease. Gastroenterology 1997;102:1736–1741.

48. Anand AC, Ferraz-Neto BH, Nightingale P, et al. Liver transplantation for alcoholic liver disease: evaluation of a selection protocol. Hepatology 1997;25:1478–1484.

Primary Biliary Cirrhosis, Primary Sclerosing Cholangitis (including Cholangiocarcinoma), and Autoimmune Hepatitis

▼ ▼ ▼ ▼ ▼ ▼ ▼ ▼ ▼

Beat Müllhaupt and Alastair D. Smith

■ INTRODUCTION

Autoimmune forms of liver disease, namely autoimmune hepatitis (AIH), primary biliary cirrhosis (PBC), and primary sclerosing cholangitis (PSC), are relatively uncommon conditions in and of themselves. However, all are incurable, and as a group they are responsible for a not insignificant proportion of liver transplantations (LTs) undertaken both in the USA and in Europe [1,2]. Outcomes following LT are very good, even though recurrent disease may develop in significant numbers of patients given sufficient time. One of the most challenging aspects of management for these patients is the appropriate timing of LT among those with advanced disease: progression may be slow for long periods and episodes of decompensation infrequent, the availability of deceased donor organs is very limited, and symptoms such as fatigue, pruritus, and subtle encephalopathy are extremely disabling but not reflected by the patient's model for end-stage liver disease (MELD) score (Chapter 6). Other important considerations for this group of patients include additional exposure to immunosuppressive therapy prior to LT (AIH), the increased risk of metabolic bone disease and osteoporosis (PBC, PSC, and AIH), and the threat of cholangiocarcinoma (CCA) among patients with PSC. In this chapter we consider each condition in turn, the role that LT plays in management, and the potential strategies for helping patients with end-stage disease (ESLD) reach transplantation in a satisfactory condition.

■ AUTOIMMUNE HEPATITIS

AIH is characterized by progressive fatigue, elevated serum aminotransferase and immunoglobulin G (IgG) concentrations, circulating antinuclear, anti-smooth muscle (type 1), and/or anti-liver kidney microsomal (type 2) antibodies, histological evidence of mononuclear portal tract inflammation in which plasma cells are usually conspicuous, interface hepatitis with varying degrees of periportal and bridging fibrosis, and responsiveness to systemic steroid therapy. A secure diagnosis demands that chronic viral, metabolic, alcoholic, and drug-associated liver injury be excluded by appropriate history taking, corroboration and serologic testing [3]. Like PBC, AIH is more common in women than in men, with a (female:male) gender ratio of at least 3.6:1 [4,5].

AIH has been described in a variety of ethnic and population groups [5–14]. Not only does its prevalence vary, but human leukocyte antigen (HLA) associations also differ. For example, the prevalence of AIH in northern Europe has been estimated at almost 17/100 000 [6], but among native Alaskans it is 2.5 times greater (42.9/100 000) [5]. In northern European and white North American patients AIH is strongly associated with possession of the HLA-A1, -B8, -DR3 (*DRB1*0301*), and -DR4 (*DRB1*0401*) haplotypes [7], whereas in Turkish patients B8 is lacking [8], and among Japanese subjects with AIH the association is almost exclusively with DR4 (DR3 is very uncommon in the Japanese population) [9]. In general, Caucasian patients who possess *DRB1*0301* are younger at diagnosis, less likely to respond to immunosuppressive therapy, more liable to relapse following treatment withdrawal and to require LT than those without *DRB1*0301*. Conversely, patients possessing *DRB1*0401* generally present for diagnosis later in life, respond better to therapy, and have a more benign overall clinical course, with less likelihood of undergoing LT. African American (AA) patients with AIH are younger and demonstrate bridging fibrosis or cirrhosis at diagnosis with greater frequency than Caucasian patients [12,13]. Moreover, they may require larger doses of prednisone to maintain disease remission [12]. Likewise, patients of non-European Caucasoid origin living within the UK were younger and more likely to possess cholestatic biochemical features at diagnosis, and they demonstrated a poorer clinical response to conventional immunosuppressive therapy than Caucasian subjects [14].

As with PBC and PSC the precise etiology of AIH is uncertain, despite knowledge of clear links that exist between AIH and certain HLA types, with respect to both diagnosis and subsequent clinical course. However, the environmental triggers remain elusive. Anecdotal reports have implicated several of the viral hepatitides for the onset of AIH [15]. Molecular mimicry, i.e. homology between viral and body proteins, has been postulated as one potential underlying disease mechanism.

Diagnosis

The greater proportion of patients with AIH present in an insidious fashion, fatigue being the dominant symptom; without intervention, most will progress inexorably thereafter. However, up to 40% of patients may have an acute onset of symptoms [16,17]. Diagnosis requires thorough evaluation (see above) because some other forms of chronic liver disease may exhibit auto-immune features, e.g. Wilson's disease and hepatitis C virus (HCV) liver disease [18]. Liver biopsy is a fundamental requirement not only for diagnostic purposes but also for grading disease severity to help decide whether therapy is necessary and for assessing the fibrosis stage [19,20]. There is poor correlation between serum aminotransferase and IgG concentrations and the extent of histological liver injury and fibrosis. In a small number of patients, disease onset may be very abrupt and pursue a precipitous, fulminant course thereafter [21]. In these circumstances, remission may not be achieved even with potent immunosuppressive agents such as cyclosporine or tacrolimus [20]; therefore, appropriate consideration of and evaluation for LT is vital (Chapter 13). In a small proportion of patients with AIH, clinical, laboratory, pathological, and radiologic features of cholestatic liver disease consistent with either PBC or PSC may be evident, or vice versa [22]. Sometimes, such overlap syndromes coexist from the outset, but on other occasions the diagnoses may be separated from one another by many months. Further consideration of these syndromes is beyond the scope of this chapter.

The clinical features and laboratory parameters that help confirm or refute the diagnosis of AIH have been incorporated into a robust scoring system that has been validated and updated [3]. This should be used whenever there is any uncertainty about the diagnosis, e.g. if the IgG or γ-globulin concentration is normal, or the potential contribution of drug therapy or alcohol is unclear. Moreover, it may be helpful for assessing disease response to drug therapy.

Management

Pharmacologic

Prior to the introduction of prednisone, the 5-year survival rate for patients with AIH was very poor indeed (5–10%) [23,24]. However, this drug and others, notably azathioprine, have improved the outlook significantly for treated patients. More than 80% may anticipate a 20-year life expectancy after diagnosis, and survival is similar to that of sex- and age-matched subjects in the same geographical location who do not have AIH [25]. The following categories of patients with AIH require therapy [20,21]:

1. those whose serum aminotransferase concentrations are greater than 10 times the upper normal limit;
2. those whose serum aminotransferase concentrations are at least five times the upper limit of normal with concomitant elevation of γ-globulin level more than twice the upper limit of normal;
3. those whose liver biopsy demonstrates bridging or multilobular necrosis; and
4. those whose clinical course had an acute mode of onset.

In contrast, it is unclear whether patients who have subclinical disease at diagnosis and/or less aggressive histological abnormalities, i.e. milder disease (such patients were not included in the original studies that established the efficacy of prednisone for severe AIH), should be exposed to the potential risks of immunosuppressive therapy if their outcome in respect of death and requirement for LT is unaffected [26]. Further studies are necessary to answer these questions.

Treatment with prednisone alone, or in combination with azathioprine, offers effective and equally successful remission rates for approximately 80% of patients. The choice of one regimen over the other will depend on physician experience and preference, as well as on patient choice and clinical profile. For example, patients with poorly controlled diabetes mellitus, labile mood, or reduced bone density are more appropriate candidates for therapy with both agents so as to minimize complications of steroid exposure; conversely, patients with AIH who exhibit leukopenia and thrombocytopenia as complications of portal hypertension (PHTN) and hypersplenism, those with thiopurine methyl transferase deficiency, and those who require limited therapy only should be treated with prednisone monotherapy. As many as 13% of patients are intolerant of standard immunosuppressive drug therapy [26], and will require consideration of treatment with agents such as cyclosporine [27] and mycophenolate mofetil [28].

In most cases, symptoms and laboratory parameters improve significantly within 2 weeks of commencing either regimen. Once serum aminotransferase concentrations are within twice the upper limit of the normal range, steroid therapy may be reduced gradually to maintenance levels with the goal of exposing the patient to the lowest daily dose of prednisone such as to maintain disease remission. Histological remission, i.e. resolution of all or virtually all portal and lobular inflammation, lags at least 3 months behind the restoration of aminotransferase and IgG concentrations to normal. Therefore, no attempt at withdrawal of drug therapy during this lag period should be attempted for fear that relapse might be precipitated. Ideally, all patients should undergo liver biopsy after attainment of clinical and laboratory remission to assess the degree to which inflammation and fibrosis have been reduced. However, some patients may be reticent about exposing themselves to potential risks of liver biopsy even though important information may be gained. Patients whose biopsy specimen continues to demonstrate portal and interface hepatitis, despite possessing normal aminotransferase and IgG concentrations, should not be considered for complete withdrawal of drug therapy because this will almost assuredly fail [29,30].

Earlier studies suggested that the overall outcome for patients with cirrhosis at diagnosis was poorer [31]. However, cirrhotic patients can expect to respond as well to glucocorticoid therapy as patients without cirrhosis. Nevertheless, they may experience more drug-related adverse events, probably as a result of increased amounts of unbound serum prednisolone [32,33]. There is growing evidence that clinically important regression of fibrosis may be achieved in response to immunosuppressive therapy [34]. One recent report documented significant hepatic venous pressure gradient reduction in association with regression of fibrosis following successful therapy [35]. Presence of cirrhosis may increase the risk of development of hepatocellular carcinoma (HCC), but compared with patients who have viral ESLD, this appears to be considerably less.

It is estimated that 22% of patients with AIH treated using standard immunosuppressive drug therapy (see above) fail to enter remission, on the basis of either an incomplete response that does not satisfy criteria for remission (13%) or disease progression in the face of satisfactory compliance with drug therapy (9%) [26]. As with those who are intolerant of standard therapy, these groups of patients are eligible for "rescue" therapy using other immunosuppressive therapy, e.g. cyclosporine or tacrolimus. Thus, they, along with patients who demonstrate cirrhosis at diagnosis, are at particular risk of disease progression and need for consideration of LT.

Liver Transplantation

AIH is an excellent indication for LT; 5-year graft and patient survival rates are at least as good as if not better than for any other disease, save for PBC [1,2,36]. Furthermore, one recent study of the United Network for Organ Sharing (UNOS) database revealed that median graft and patient half-lives are 13.4 and 14.8 years, respectively, higher than for any other disease [37]. Although rates of acute and chronic allograft rejection and steroid-resistant rejection are greater among patients transplanted for AIH than for other indications, and the rate of recurrent disease in the transplanted allograft is at least 17% (Chapter 24), it is not clear that these two phenomena are clearly linked to one another, i.e. whether these are cause-and-effect phenomena [38].

Prior to implementation of the MELD scoring system to determine priority for deceased donor organ allocation (February 27, 2002), patients with AIH and manifestations of PHTN who were appropriate LT candidates and had been evaluated and listed (in a timely manner) could anticipate undergoing transplantation after a period of months or years waiting on the list. Symptoms such as fatigue and pruritus, poor quality of life, emergence of ascites and encephalopathy, incomplete response to and complications of standard therapy were important considerations in helping increase a patient's UNOS status for LT. However, since February 2002 none of these factors confers any additional organ allocation priority unless attended by objective evidence of deteriorating liver and renal function, i.e. a rising MELD score. Outside the USA where the MELD scoring system is not used for organ allocation purposes, a patient's priority for LT may be influenced by subjective or some non-MELD factors, e.g. overwhelming fatigue and pruritus, but this latitude is less limited now that was the case 5–10 years ago.

Irrespective of these differences, it is reasonable to target the following groups of patients with AIH for LT evaluation and listing:

1. Those who demonstrate clinical complications of PHTN at or preceding diagnosis.
2. Those whose index liver biopsy reveals cirrhosis even in the absence of complications of PHTN, or in whom subsequent biopsies demonstrate cirrhosis despite laboratory remission [39].
3. Any patient whose clinical, laboratory, and histologic course worsens despite appropriate therapy especially if associated with complications of PHTN, e.g. variceal bleeding.
4. Patients who respond incompletely to standard immunosuppressive therapy (assuming satisfactory treatment compliance), or who relapse promptly as treatment doses are being reduced.

Patients with diabetes mellitus whose blood sugar control has deteriorated or those in whom diabetes mellitus has developed in the face of systemic steroid therapy and who are at increased risk of both hyperlipidemia and ischemic heart disease require detailed assessment. The same holds true for patients with psychiatric illness that may have been precipitated or exacerbated by steroid therapy. The theoretical risk of oncogenesis among patients receiving immunosuppressive therapy for AIH is estimated at 5% with a treatment duration of at least 3.5 years [40]. To this must be added the additional risk of cancer conferred by necessary immunotherapy following LT, especially in the context of an indication known to be associated with greater risk of rejection.

■ PRIMARY BILIARY CIRRHOSIS

PBC is characterized by fatigue and pruritus to varying degrees; cholestatic liver test abnormalities; elevated serum immunoglobulin M (IgM) concentrations; circulating antimitochondrial antibody (AMA); and chronic nonsuppurative inflammation, fibrosis, and eventual destruction of interlobular bile ducts. Disease progression resulting in cirrhosis and eventual liver failure is virtually inevitable, and without consideration of LT, death will follow. In contrast to PSC, PBC is a disease almost exclusively of women, the female:male gender ratio being not less than 9:1 [41,42].

PBC has been described in many different populations and geographic locations, but the reported estimates of incidence and prevailing prevalence rates differ considerably [43–45]. In some areas of both the UK and the USA the prevalence of PBC has been estimated as high as 1 in 4000 persons, making it considerably more common in these locations than, for example, in Africa or South America. Reasons for this variability are unclear, but recent emphasis on case finding may be one explanation, and recognition that the disorder has a wider clinical spectrum than was first appreciated is almost certainly a contributing factor.

In contrast to AIH and other autoimmune disorders, no clear and/or close link between PBC and HLA genotypes exists [41,42]. For example, association with HLA-B8 is stronger among Japanese subjects with PBC than those in the UK and the USA; however, this allele is more prevalent in the Japanese population as a whole and may account for this observed difference. Conversely, there are data to support a familial predisposition to the disease. In comparison with the general population, the prevalence of PBC among first-degree relatives of affected individuals is increased, perhaps by a factor of up to 500. There is debate as to whether the risk is greater for relatives in the same generation or the one that follows.

In common with other autoimmune diseases, a triggering event or insult is believed to be necessary for disease expression [46]. Increased frequency of bacterial (*Escherichia coli*) urinary tract infections among patients with PBC suggests that an infectious agent(s) may be responsible. Moreover, considerable interest and research effort has focused on the potential role of *Chlamydia pneumoniae* as a putative trigger of PBC [47]. However, an open-label pilot study using tetracycline for 3 weeks among 15 patients with PBC who had demonstrated a suboptimal biochemical response to ursodeoxycholic acid (UDCA) revealed no significant improvement (or deterioration) in liver test concentrations [48]. There was no impact on either fatigue or pruritus. The drug was well tolerated.

The role of retroviral infection as the potential trigger for PBC was postulated in 1998 [49], based on the following lines of evidence: identification of virus-like particles in biliary epithelial cells derived from patients with PBC, antiretroviral antibody reactivity among PBC patients with coexisting Sjögren's syndrome, and cloning of a retrovirus from biliary epithelial cells and lymph nodes of patients with PBC [50]. The putative agent referred to as a human betaretrovirus is so named because of the marked similarities it shares with the mouse mammary tumor virus. A recently published study of antiretroviral treatment suggested that combination therapy (lamivudine and zidovudine) was more efficacious than lamivudine alone, resulting in significant liver test and histological improvement for patients [51]. The role of xenobiotics in the development of PBC among certain individuals is possible.

Diagnosis

Unlike AIH, establishing the diagnosis of PBC is usually relatively straightforward, although among patients who lack AMA (at least 5%) careful consideration of other potential causes of cholestatic liver disease may be necessary, e.g. drug-induced liver injury or small duct PSC. The diagnosis of PBC should be considered in any middle-aged female patient who complains of fatigue or pruritus, who is jaundiced, or has other manifestations of portal hypertension, and has clinical evidence of hypercholesterolemia. Likewise, any asymptomatic patient who demonstrates cholestatic liver test abnormalities and/or circulating AMA, especially in the presence of a disorder associated with PBC, e.g. Sjögren's syndrome, autoimmune hypothyroidism, scleroderma, or celiac disease, should probably be considered to have PBC until demonstrated otherwise. Although an uncommon diagnosis among men, it does occur and should not be overlooked [52].

For diagnostic purposes, most workers believe that liver biopsy is unnecessary where clinical and laboratory features point strongly toward PBC and that the procedure should be reserved for patients in whom AMA is lacking, some other diagnostic uncertainty is present, or a possible PBC overlap syndrome with AIH exists [53]. However, sampling error notwithstanding, the histological stage of disease cannot be established clearly without liver biopsy. Since disease stage has been shown to have important implications with respect to therapy [54] and overall outcome [45], it appears logical that patients should undergo liver biopsy at the outset. Follow-up liver biopsy may be necessary among patients who respond poorly or incompletely to drug therapy and therefore the existence of a pretreatment specimen for comparison may be invaluable in this respect also.

Management

Pharmacologic

Only one drug is approved by the US Food and Drug Administration for treatment of PBC, namely UDCA [42,52]. Multicenter, placebo-controlled studies in which daily doses of at least 13–15 mg/kg UDCA were employed demonstrated both symptom and liver test improvement [55–57]; another study revealed an increased duration of liver disease-related survival [58]. Moreover, when results of three of these studies were analyzed together, improved survival rates without requirement for LT were found among those receiving UDCA, although only after the drug had been taken for at least 4 years [59]. Conversely, subsequent meta-analyses have failed to demonstrate benefits from UDCA with respect to complications of liver disease, rates of LT, and overall survival [60,61]. It is claimed that the principal reason for this absence of benefit was the short follow-up period among patients receiving the drug, a fact further highlighted by the outcome of a more recent study [62]. In a further study with follow-up to 12 years, treatment with UDCA did not reduce the risk of LT or death compared with untreated subjects, even though significant improvement in serum bilirubin and alkaline phosphatase concentrations were observed [63]. In contrast, UDCA treatment among patients with stage 1 and 2 disease, but not patients with advanced disease, improved spontaneous survival to that of age- and sex-matched control subjects. The mean treatment duration in the latter study was 8 years [54].

In practical terms it is probably very rare indeed that any patient with PBC is not recommended or offered treatment with UDCA, although one of us (ADS) can recall two individuals who chose not to take the drug when presented with a synopsis of the literature. Furthermore, a few patients will develop unpleasant luminal gastrointestinal side-effects thereby limiting its effectiveness, and for some the drug's cost may be prohibitive. UDCA's effects include increased delivery of bile acids from hepatocyte into biliary cannaliculus, and reduction of damaging intracellular hydrophobic bile acid concentrations. It may also possess immunomodulatory properties [42,52].

Colchicine, prednisolone, azathioprine, cyclosporine, methotrexate, and penicillamine have been tested to varying degrees as potential therapies for PBC. However, all failed to demonstrate clear evidence of benefit when examined in trials of appropriate design or adequate size, or were associated with unacceptable complications, e.g. significant bone density reduction, renal dysfunction, or systemic hypertension [42,52]. Colchicine may offer some benefit in conjunction with UDCA [64]: it is cheap and without important side-effects.

Liver Transplantation

Because PBC is associated with increased rates of liver-related mortality and all cause mortality compared with age- and sex-matched control subjects [45], patients may anticipate the need for LT at some stage. During the early years of LT, PBC was the principal indication in both the USA and Europe. Although it has been overtaken in recent years by hepatitis C virus and alcoholic cirrhosis, LT for PBC continues as one of the top five indications. Furthermore, outcomes for patients with PBC are excellent (Chapter 24).

Whereas the need for and timing of LT among patients with PBC was predicted on the basis of a steadily rising serum bilirubin concentration above 5.9 mg%, and/or the Mayo Clinic model, emergence of the MELD score for estimating 3-month mortality risk and priority for organ allocation has changed this for listed patients in the USA (see earlier). No longer is it possible for patients with overwhelming fatigue, generalized pruritus, severe osteoporosis, or some combination thereof to gain additional priority for LT on the basis of these complications, although such latitude may still exist in other countries. Since PBC may progress very slowly indeed and response to UDCA is variable, the question then arises as to which patients should be evaluated with a view to listing for LT, and at what stage in their disease course? If all patients under 60 with a new diagnosis of PBC were to be evaluated then transplant center teams would find themselves inundated with additional work, and their lists expanded by patients whose likelihood of imminent LT would be remote. Therefore, a balance needs to be struck in giving priority for evaluation to patients whose need is greatest (see below) at the expense of others who may reasonably wait longer:

1. Those who demonstrate clinical complications of PHTN at or preceding diagnosis, or in whom there are concerns about the existence of HCC.
2. Patients whose serum bilirubin concentration is at or close to 5.9 mg% and rising, irrespective of whether they have other clinical complications of PHTN.
3. Those whose index liver biopsy reveals cirrhosis even in the absence of complications of PHTN, or in whom subsequent biopsies demonstrate cirrhosis.
4. Any patient whose clinical, laboratory, and histologic course worsens despite appropriate therapy especially if associated with complications of PHTN, e.g. variceal bleeding.

Patients with autoimmune liver disease in general, and PBC and PSC in particular, may be subject to marked and unheralded clinical decompensation after long periods of disease stability. Such episodes may not be well tolerated and thus permit little time to undertake a given patient's initial LT evaluation, or to update various aspects thereof if several years have elapsed since this was first performed. Furthermore, increasing age, additional comorbid conditions, and minimal functional reserve may render some patients at too high a risk to be transplanted safely. It has been suggested that autoimmune liver disease patients in such circumstances might be appropriate candidates for consideration of live donor LT (Chapter 12).

Specific complications of PBC and their management are well covered in recent review articles and need not be reiterated in detail here [42,52]. However, it is worth emphasizing the importance of proper identification and treatment of vitamin D deficiency and/or osteoporosis among patients with PBC and PSC. The additional impact of the deconditioning accompanying end-stage liver disease, of LT, and of subsequent steroid exposure to these processes should not be underestimated [65], and where possible, should be minimized. It is also worth being aware that recent data have demonstrated that this problem is not confined to patients with cholestatic liver disease [66].

■ PRIMARY SCLEROSING CHOLANGITIS

PSC is a chronic cholestatic liver disease of unknown etiology that is characterized by inflammation, progressive fibrosis, and subsequent obliteration of intra- and/or extrahepatic bile ducts, resulting in cholestasis, biliary fibrosis, and, ultimately, secondary biliary cirrhosis. A recent study from Norway suggests that the incidence is approximately 1.3 and the prevalence 8.5 per 100 000 [67] whereas in Minnesota, USA, the corresponding figures were 1.25 in men and 0.54 in women and 20.9 in men and 6.3 in women per 100 000 population, respectively [68]. PSC occurs predominantly in men (70%) and is characterized by the frequent association with chronic inflammatory bowel disease (IBD; 70–90%), usually ulcerative colitis (UC) [69]. Conversely, only 5–10% of patients with IBD have concomitant PSC.

Natural History

During recent years the number of patients without symptoms at the time of diagnosis has increased from 15–25% to more than 40% [70]. However, progressive liver disease was then observed in 76% of such patients after a mean follow-up of 75 months [71]. Thus, the majority of asymptomatic PSC patients ultimately develop progressive liver disease, just as those with symptoms at diagnosis do. In earlier studies the median survival period for symptomatic patients was estimated at 12 years [70,72,73] whereas results of a more recent study suggest better overall median survival at 18 years [74]. Most but not all patients die from causes related to liver disease, and in a significant proportion

Table 10.1 *Mayo PSC Risk Score*

$$R = 0.03 \times (\text{age in years}) + 0.54 \times \log(\text{bilirubin in mg/dL}) + 0.54 \times \log(\text{AST in IU/L})$$
$$+ 1.24 \times (\text{history of variceal bleeding}) - 0.84 \times (\text{albumin in g/dL})$$

of cases from CCA. Small duct PSC appears to carry a more favorable long-term prognosis than large duct disease [75]; in this study, few patients progressed to large bile duct PSC, and none developed CCA.

Several scoring systems have been developed to assess prognosis for patients with PSC. However, most required patients to undergo biopsy, which clearly limits the utility of any scoring system. The most recent Mayo PSC risk score replaced information from liver biopsy with a history of variceal bleeding (Table 10.1) [76]. This scoring system is better at predicting survival than the Child–Pugh score, especially among patients whose index disease stage was early [77].

Diagnosis

The diagnosis of PSC is based on the constellation of appropriate symptoms, e.g. pruritus, fatigue, jaundice, and features of cholangitis, with cholestatic liver test abnormalities, and characteristic cholangiographic features. The latter include localized or multifocal strictures with intervening segments of normal or dilated bile ducts. Liver biopsy typically reveals evidence of bile obstruction with fibro-obliterative cholangitis, findings that are somewhat nonspecific and must be interpreted carefully alongside clinical and radiological information. Nevertheless, liver biopsy is still performed in a significant proportion of patients to stage disease, and to rule out coexisting liver disease. However, a more recent study questioned the appropriateness of biopsy because the result rarely provided new information that influenced patient management [78]. Liver biopsy remains crucial for the diagnosis of small duct sclerosing cholangitis; this is characterized by typical histological features of PSC in patients whose cholangiogram is normal.

Complications of PSC

Bone Disease

Osteopenia, defined as a T score below −1 is found in almost 50% of PSC patients at the time of referral or diagnosis. Severe osteoporosis (T score below −2.5) occurs in only 10% and is less common than among patients with PBC [79]. However, the severity of bone disease increases with progression of liver disease, such that at the time of transplantation 40% of patients have a bone mineral density below the fracture threshold. One-third of PSC patients develop fractures after LT. Calcium and vitamin D supplementation should be mandatory in these patients [80]. The precise role of bisphosphonates for patients with PSC needs to be determined.

Portal Hypertension

In a large series of 283 patients with PSC, 102 (36%) had esophageal varices, 56% being moderate to large in size. Multivariate analysis revealed that a platelet count of less than 150 000/mL and advanced histological stage were independent predictors for the presence of esophageal varices [81]. Therefore, these patients should be targeted for screening endoscopy. A special complication of PHTN in PSC patients is the development of peristomal varices in patients with an ileostomy. Local treatment is typically not successful and rebleeding episodes are frequent [82]. If ileocolonic surgery is required among patients with PSC, procedures that predispose less to varix formation such as ileoanal, ileorectal, or ileal pouch-anal anastomosis are preferred [83].

Hepatocellular Carcinoma

PSC patients with cirrhosis may develop HCC, although the risk appears to be small. In a recent study only 2% of PSC patients undergoing LT developed an HCC [84].

Cholangiocarcinoma

The risk for CCA is increased in PSC patients, with reported lifetime prevalence rates varying from 5% to 20% [85]. In at least one-third of cases (30–50%) the diagnosis of CCA is established at the same time as the diagnosis of PSC [86]. The prognosis is dismal with a median survival time of 5 months [87]. Confirming the diagnosis of CCA may be very challenging, and possible only when the tumor is at an advanced stage or discovered incidentally at LT. Clinically, CCA should be suspected when a patient shows rapid progression of liver disease with increasing bilirubin concentration and abdominal pain. Endoscopic brushing and biopsies have good specificity, but their sensitivity is usually low. Newer cytological techniques for aneuploidy such as digital image analysis and fluorescence in situ hybridization may increase the diagnostic yield; however, this technology is not yet widely available [88]. Rising serum CA 19-9 and CEA concentrations may support the clinical suspicion of CCA. A combination of tumor markers [(CA 19-9 + (CEA×40)) < 400] has high specificity (100%) and accuracy (85%), but a rather low sensitivity (67%) for CCA [89]. A second study confirmed a reasonably high specificity but even lower sensitivity (33%) [90]. It has been reported that a CA 19-9 value ≥100 IU/L has an 89% sensitivity and 86% specificity for the detection of CCA and is currently used in the Mayo protocol for LT [91]. In this protocol, a CA 19-9 concentration ≥100 IU/L in the presence of a radiographic-appearing malignant stricture without bacterial cholangitis is considered sufficient for the diagnosis of CCA [92]. CCA in PSC patients is usually considered a contraindication to LT because medium-term survival is dismal: only 20–30% of patients achieved 3-year disease-free survival [93]. Conversely, incidental detection of CCA less than 1 cm within the explanted liver has no effect on survival [94]. Recently, an innovative, aggressive treatment protocol using neoadjuvant chemotherapy and radiotherapy has been suggested, in conjunction with staging laparotomy, thereby excluding all patients with extrahepatic disease, followed by LT. An actuarial 82% survival rate at 5 years was reported [92]. Thus, LT might be possible in a highly selected group of PSC patients with CCA.

PSC and Inflammatory Bowel Disease

It is generally accepted that concomitant IBD has no detrimental effect on the natural history and outcome of liver disease for PSC patients following LT. Colectomy does not halt or slow the progression of PSC to cirrhosis, nor does LT protect against exacerbations of IBD [95]. The impact of immunosuppressive therapy on the clinical course of IBD after LT is very heterogeneous, depending largely on the immunosuppressive regimen used, and on the definition of IBD recurrence adopted. The most favorable IBD course has been reported in studies using triple immunosuppression including steroids, whereas the worst outcome has been reported in studies where steroids were routinely withdrawn in the early posttransplant period [95].

Colorectal Cancer

Most studies report an increased risk of colorectal cancer (CRC) among PSC patients with UC, compared with patients with UC alone [85]. In a recent study from Sweden comparing 40 patients with both PSC and UC with 80 age- and sex-matched controls who had UC but not PSC, the absolute cumulative risk of developing colorectal dysplasia and/or cancer was significantly greater in the first group (PSC/UC) [96]. Therefore, it is generally accepted that colonoscopy with multiple biopsies should be performed in all patients with coexisting PSC and IBD, because colitis often runs a quiescent or subclinical course [97]. If UC (or Crohn's colitis) is identified, then these patients should undergo annual colonoscopic assessment beyond LT also because they remain at increased risk of developing CRC (Chapter 24) [98]. Some authors have even recommended 6-monthly colonoscopy during the first 2 years following LT, because most cancers occurred during that period [95].

Management of PSC

Medical Therapy

No specific medical therapy has been found to prevent disease progression or improve long-term survival. Multiple drugs have been evaluated for these purposes, but all have been found wanting. UDCA has been evaluated most extensively: daily doses varying from 10 to 15 mg/kg have some beneficial effects on cholestasis, but no impact on either survival or transplant-free survival has been reported [99]. Higher UDCA doses (15–25 mg/kg) look promising and should be evaluated further [100].

Management of Biliary Strictures

Indications for endoscopic, percutaneous, or surgical treatment of biliary strictures are controversial. Repeated episodes of cholangitis in the presence of a dominant stricture may be managed temporarily by endoscopic and/or percutaneous dilatation and plastic stent or drain placement. In a 12-year prospective trial on the effect of UDCA, 52/106 patients developed a progressive stenosis of major bile ducts. In this study, the combination of UDCA plus endoscopic dilatation of extrahepatic bile duct stenosis improved transplant-free survival over 2 years [101]. Unfortunately, endoscopic manipulation of biliary strictures is often difficult because they are so dense and fibrotic. Currently, we advocate aggressive endoscopic dilatation and stenting of dominant strictures in the potential liver transplant candidate, with repeated brush cytology to assess for CCA.

Management of Infections

Patients with acute cholangitis should be treated with broad-spectrum antimicrobial therapy effective against a range of potential pathogens, e.g. Gram-negative bacilli, enterococci, and *Bacteroides* sp. As described earlier, dominant strictures should be managed aggressively by balloon cholangioplasty. If there is extensive biliary tree involvement resulting in recurrent episodes of cholangitis, long-term antimicrobial prophylaxis with one oral agent (ciprofloxacin, ampicillin, or trimethoprim–sulfamethoxazole) for 3–4 weeks in a rotating fashion may be necessary. Chronic recurrent cholangitis might be difficult to treat and it represents a clear indication for LT, although this in itself has no impact upon the MELD score.

Selection and Timing of Liver Transplantation: Because there is no pharmacological therapy that can prevent disease progression in patients with PSC, LT offers the best prospect of potential cure, improvement in quality of life, and extended survival. Moreover, LT among patients with PSC is associated with excellent 5-year graft and survival rates. The crucial question therefore is what is the optimal time for patients with PSC to undergo LT? This decision is difficult given the variable clinical course and unpredictable risk of development of CCA [102]. Apart from the generally accepted indications, some physicians consider transplantation in PSC patients even in the absence of histologically proven cirrhosis in patients with intractable fatigue, disabling pruritus, severe muscle wasting, chronic or recurrent bacterial cholangitis, and persistent increases in serum bilirubin levels in the absence of CCA. A recent study from the Mayo Clinic demonstrated that posttransplant survival is related to pretransplant Child–Pugh stage [103]. This and the detrimental impact of CCA should alert physicians to refer patients with PSC for consideration of LT compared with other chronic liver diseases.

Survival after OLT

Single-center studies have reported 1-year survival rates of 90–97% and 83–88% at 5 years after LT. A recent disease specific analysis of the UNOS database demonstrated a 5-year survival rate of >80% for patients with PSC [36]. PSC patients usually have higher rates of both acute and chronic allograft rejection and a greater incidence of hepatic artery thrombosis. PSC can recur in the graft and may result in biliary cirrhosis, affecting long-term graft and patient survival (Chapter 24).

■ REFERENCES

1. Scientific Registry of Transplant Recipients. Transplant statistics: center-specific reports. Available at http://www.ustransplant.org/center-adv.html. Accessed December 2004.

2. Adam R, McMaster P, O'Grady JG, et al. Evolution of liver transplantation in Europe: report of the European Liver Transplant Registry. Liver Transpl 2003;9:1231–1243.

3. Alvarez F, Berg PA, Bianchi FB, et al. International Autoimmune Hepatitis Group report: review of criteria for diagnosis of autoimmune hepatitis. J Hepatol 1999;31:929–938.

4. Czaja AJ, Dos Santos RM, Porto M, et al. Immune phenotype of chronic liver disease. Dig Dis Sci 1998;43:2149–2155.

5. Hurlburt KJ, McMahon BJ, Deubner H, et al. Prevalence of autoimmune liver disease in Alaska natives. Am J Gastroenterol 2002;97:2402–2407.

6. Boberg KM, Aadland E, Jahnsen J, et al. Incidence and prevalence of primary biliary cirrhosis, primary sclerosing cholangitis, and autoimmune hepatitis in a Norwegian population. Scand J Gastroenterol 1998;33(1):99–103.

7. Donaldson PT, Doherty DG, Hayllar KM, et al. Susceptibility to autoimmune chronic active hepatitis: human leukocyte antigens DR4 and A1-B8-DR3 are independent risk factors. Hepatology 1999;13:701–706.

8. Kosar Y, Kacar S, Sasmaz N, et al. Type 1 autoimmune hepatitis in Turkish patients: absence of association with HLA-B8. J Clin Gastroenterol 2002;35:185–190.

9. Seki T, Ota M, Furuta S, et al. HLA class II molecules and autoimmune hepatitis susceptibility in Japanese patients. Gastroenterology 1992;103:1041–1047.

10. Pando M, Larriba J, Fernandez GC, et al. Pediatric and adult forms of type 1 autoimmune hepatitis in Argentina: evidence for differential genetic predisposition. Hepatology 1999;30:1374–1380.

11. Gupta R, Agarwal SR, Jain M, et al. Autoimmune hepatitis in the Indian subcontinent: 7 years experience. J Gastroenterol Hepatol 2001;16:1144–1148.

12. Lim KN, Casanova RL, Boyer TD, et al. Autoimmune hepatitis in African Americans: presenting features and response to therapy. Am J Gastroenterol 2001;96:3390–3394.

13. Valdivia EA, Greer J, Cubas IP, et al. Autoimmune hepatitis in the African American population (abstract). Hepatology 2003;34(4):487A.

14. Zolfino T, Heneghan MA, Norris S, et al. Characteristics of autoimmune hepatitis in patients who are not of European Caucasoid ethnic origin. Gut 2002;50:713–717.

15. Manns MP, Strassburg CP. Autoimmune hepatitis. In O'Grady JG, Lake JR, Howdle PR, eds., Comprehensive clinical hepatology. London: Mosby, 2000:3/16.1–3/16.13.

16. Crapper RM, Bhathal PS, Mackay IR, et al. "Acute" autoimmune hepatitis. Digestion 1986;34:216–225.

17. Nikias GA, Batts KP, Czaja AJ. The nature and prognostic implications of autoimmune hepatitis with an acute presentation. J Hepatol 1994;21:866–871.

18. Czaja AJ, Carpenter HA. Histological findings in chronic hepatitis C with autoimmune features. Hepatology 1997;26:459–466.

19. Czaja AJ, Freese DK. Diagnosis and treatment of autoimmune hepatitis (review; 216 references). Hepatology 2002;36:479–497.

20. Heneghan MA, McFarlane IG. Current and novel immunosuppressive therapy for autoimmune hepatitis (review; 50 references). Hepatology 2002;35:7–13.

21. Porta G, Da Costa Gayotto LC, Alvarez F. Anti-liver kidney microsome antibody-positive autoimmune hepatitis presenting as fulminant liver failure. J Pediatr Gastroenterol Nutr 1990;11:138–140.

22. Czaja AJ. Frequency and nature of the variant syndrome of autoimmune liver disease. Hepatology 1998;28:360–365.

23. Cook GC, Mulligan R, Sherlock S. Controlled prospective trial of corticosteroid therapy in chronic active hepatitis. Q J Med 1971;40(158):159–185.

24. Soloway RD, Summerskill WH, Baggenstoss AH, et al. Clinical, biochemical, and histological remission of severe chronic active liver disease: a controlled study of treatments and early prognosis. Gastroenterology 1972;63:820–833.

25. Roberts SK, Therneau TM, Czaja AJ. Prognosis of histological cirrhosis in type 1 autoimmune hepatitis. Gastroenterology 1996;110:848–857.

26. Czaja AJ, Bianchi FB, Carpenter HA, et al. Treatment challenges and investigational opportunities in autoimmune hepatitis. Hepatology 2005;41:207–215.

27. Alvarez F, Ciocca M, Canero-Velasco C, et al. Short-term cyclosporine induces a remission of auto-immune hepatitis in children. J Hepatol 1999;30:222–227.

28. Richardson PD, James PD, Ryder SD. Mycophenolate mofetil for maintenance in autoimmune hepatitis patients resistant to or intolerant of azathioprine. J Hepatol 2000;33:371–375.

29. Czaja AJ, Wolf AM, Baggenstoss AH. Laboratory assessment of severe chronic active liver disease (CALD): correlation of serum aminotransferase and gamma globulin levels with histologic features. Gastroenterology 1981;80:687–692.

30. Czaja AJ, Davis GL, Ludwig J, et al. Complete resolution of inflammatory activity following corticosteroid treatment of HBsAg-negative chronic active hepatitis. Hepatology 1984;4:622–627.

31. Davis GL, Czaja AJ, Ludwig J. Development and prognosis of histologic cirrhosis in corticosteroid-treated hepatitis B surface antigen-negative chronic active hepatitis. Gastroenterology 1984;87:1222–1227.

32. Lewis GP, Jusko WJ, Burke CW, et al. Prednisone side-effects and serum protein levels: a collaborative study. Lancet 1971;2:778–781.

33. Uribe M, Go VLW, Kluge D. Prednisone for chronic active hepatitis: pharmacokinetics and serum binding in patients with chronic active hepatitis and steroid major side effects. J Clin Gastroenterol 1984;6:331–335.

34. Czaja AJ, Carpenter HA. Decreased fibrosis during corticosteroid therapy of auto-immune hepatitis. J Hepatol 2004;40:644–650.

35. Heneghan MA, Ryan JM, Smith AD, et al. Autoimmune hepatitis as a model of physiologic outcome: reversal of fibrosis following therapy is associated with

significant reduction in hepatic venous pressure gradient (abstract). Hepatology 2004;40:181A.

36. Roberts MS, Angus DC, Bryce CL, et al. Survival after liver transplantation in the United States: a disease-specific analysis of the UNOS database. Liver Transpl 2004;10:886–897.

37. Smith AD, Marroquin CE, Edwards EB, et al. What is the anticipated half-life of a liver allograft? (abstract). Gastroenterology 2004;126:A-665.

38. Neuberger J. Transplantation for autoimmune hepatitis (review; 36 references). Semin Liver Dis 2002;4:379–385.

39. Verma S, Gunuwan B, Mendler M, et al. Factors predicting relapse and poor outcome in type 1 autoimmune hepatitis: role of cirrhosis development, patterns of transaminases during remission, and plasma cell activity in the liver biopsy. Am J Gastroenterol 2004;99:1510–1516.

40. Wang KK, Czaja AJ, Beaver SJ, et al. Extrahepatic malignancy following long-term immunosuppressive therapy of severe hepatitis B surface antigen-negative chronic active hepatitis. Hepatology 1989;10:39–43.

41. Neuberger J. Primary biliary cirrhosis. In O'Grady JG, Lake JR, Howdle PR, eds., Comprehensive clinical hepatology. London: Mosby, 2000:3/17.1–3/17.13.

42. Talwalkar, JA, Lindor KD. Primary biliary cirrhosis (review; 140 references). Lancet 2003;362:53–61.

43. Eriksson S, Lindgren S. The prevalence and clinical spectrum of primary biliary cirrhosis in a defined population. Scand J Gastroenterol 1984;19:971–976.

44. Mitchison HC, Lucey MR, Kelly PJ, et al. Symptom development and prognosis in primary biliary cirrhosis: a study in two centers. Gastroenterology 1990;99: 778–784.

45. Prince M, Chetwynd A, Newman W, et al. Survival and symptom progression in a geographically based cohort of patients with primary biliary cirrhosis for up to 28 years. Gastroenterology 2002;123:1044–1051.

46. Parikh-Patel A, Gold EB, Worman H, et al. Risk factors for primary biliary cirrhosis in a cohort of patients from the United States. Hepatology 2001;33:16–21.

47. Abdulkarim AS, Petrovic LM, Kim WR, et al. Primary biliary cirrhosis: an infectious disease caused by *Chlamydia pneumoniae*? (abstract). Gastroenterology 2002;122 (suppl 4):A641.

48. Maddala YK, Jorgensen RA, Angulo P, et al. Open-label pilot study of tetracycline in the treatment of primary biliary cirrhosis. Am J Gastroenterol 2004;99: 566–567.

49. Mason AL, Xu L, Guo L, et al. Detection of retroviral antibodies in primary biliary cirrhosis and other idiopathic biliary disorders. Lancet 198;351:1620–1624.

50. Gershwin ME, Selmi C. Apocolypsal versus apocryphal: the role of retroviruses in primary biliary cirrhosis (editorial; 23 references). Am J Gastroenterol 2004;99: 2356–2358.

51. Mason AL, Farr GH, Xu L, et al. Pilot studies of single and combination antiretroviral therapy in patients with primary biliary cirrhosis. Am J Gastroenterol 2004;99: 2348–2355.

52. Heathcote EJ. Management of primary biliary cirrhosis (review; 105 references). Hepatology 2000;31:1005–1013.

53. Zein CO, Angulo P, Lindor KD. When is liver biopsy needed in the diagnosis of primary biliary cirrhosis? Clin Gastroenterol Hepatol 2003;1:89–95.

54. Corpechot C, Carrat F, Bahr A, et al. The effect of ursodeoxycholic acid therapy on the natural course of primary biliary cirrhosis. Gastroenterology 2005;128:297–303.

55. Lindor KD, Dickson ER, Baldus WP, et al. Ursodeoxycholic acid in the treatment of primary biliary cirrhosis. Gastroenterology 1994;106:1284–1290.

56. Poupon RE, Balkan B, Escwege E, et al. A multicenter controlled trial of ursodiol for the treatment of primary biliary cirrhosis. N Engl J Med 1991;324:1548–1554.

57. Heathcote EJ, Cauch-Dudek K, Walker V, et al. The Canadian multicenter, double-blind, randomized controlled trial of ursodeoxycholic acid in primary biliary cirrhosis. Hepatology 1994;19:1149–1156.

58. Pares A, Caballeria L, Rodes J, et al. Long-term effects of ursodeoxycholic acid in primary biliary cirrhosis: results of a double-blind, controlled multicentric trial: the UDCA–Cooperative Group from the Spanish Association for the Study of the Liver. J Hepatol 2000;32:561–566.

59. Poupon RE, Poupon R, Balkau B. Ursodiol for the long-term treatment of primary biliary cirrhosis. N Engl J Med 1994;330:1342–1347.

60. Poupon RE, Lindor KD, Cauch-Dudek K, et al. Combined analysis of randomized controlled trials of ursodeoxycholic acid in primary biliary cirrhosis. Gastroenterology 1997;113:884–890.

61. Gluud C, Christensen E. Ursodeoxycholic acid for primary biliary cirrhosis. Cochrane Database Syst Rev 2002;1:CD000551.

62. Goulis J, Leandro G, Burroughs AK. Randomised controlled trials of ursodeoxycholic-acid therapy for primary biliary cirrhosis: a meta-analysis. Lancet 1999;354: 1053–1060.

63. Combes B, Luketic VA, Peters MG, et al. Prolonged follow-up of patients in the US multicenter trial of ursodeoxycholic acid for primary biliary cirrhosis. Am J Gastroenterol 2004;99:264–268.

64. Chan CW, Gunsar F, Feudjo M, et al. Long-term ursodeoxycholic acid therapy for primary biliary cirrhosis: a follow-up to 12 years. Aliment Pharmacol Ther 2005;21:217–226.

65. Guichelaar MMJ, Malinchoc M, Sibonga J, et al. Immunosuppressive and post-operative effects of orthotopic liver transplantation on bone metabolism. Liver Transpl 2004;10:638–647.

66. Carey EJ, Balan V, Kremers WK, et al. Osteopenia and osteoporosis in patients with end-stage liver disease caused by hepatitis C and alcoholic liver disease: not just a cholestatic problem. Liver Transpl 2003;9:1166–1173.

67. Boberg KM, Aadland E, Jahnsen J, et al. Incidence and prevalence of primary biliary cirrhosis, primary sclerosing cholangitis, and autoimmune hepatitis in a Norwegian population. Scand J Gastroenterol 1998;33:99–103.

68. Bambha K, Kim WR, Talwalkar J, et al. Incidence, clinical spectrum, and outcomes of primary sclerosing cholangitis in a United States community. Gastroenterology 2003;125:1364–1369.

69. Fausa O, Schrumpf E, Elgjo K. Relationship of inflammatory bowel disease and primary sclerosing cholangitis. Semin Liver Dis 1991;11:31–39.

70. Broome U, Olsson R, Loof L, et al. Natural history and prognostic factors in 305 Swedish patients with primary sclerosing cholangitis. Gut 1996;38:610–615.

71. Porayko MK, Wiesner RH, LaRusso NF, et al. Patients with asymptomatic primary sclerosing cholangitis frequently have progressive disease. Gastroenterology 1990;98:1594–1602.

72. Farrant JM, Hayllar KM, Wilkinson ML, et al. Natural history and prognostic variables in primary sclerosing cholangitis. Gastroenterology 1991;100:1710–1717.

73. Wiesner RH, Grambsch PM, Dickson ER, et al. Primary sclerosing cholangitis: natural history, prognostic factors and survival analysis. Hepatology 1989;10:430–436.

74. Ponsioen CY, Vrouenraets SM, Prawirodirdjo W, et al. Natural history of primary sclerosing cholangitis and prognostic value of cholangiography in a Dutch population. Gut 2002;51:562–566.

75. Björnsson E, Boberg KM, Cullen S, et al. Patients with small duct primary sclerosing cholangitis have a favourable long term prognosis. Gut 2002;51:731–735.

76. Kim WR, Therneau TM, Wiesner RH, et al. A revised natural history model for primary sclerosing cholangitis. Mayo Clin Proc 2000;75:688–694.

77. Kim WR, Poterucha JJ, Wiesner RH, et al. The relative role of the Child–Pugh classification and the Mayo natural history model in the assessment of survival in patients with primary sclerosing cholangitis. Hepatology 1999;29:1643–1648.

78. Burak KW, Angulo P, Lindor KD. Is there a role for liver biopsy in primary sclerosing cholangitis? Am J Gastroenterol 2003;98:1155–1158.

79. Angulo P, Therneau TM, Jorgensen A, et al. Bone disease in patients with primary sclerosing cholangitis: prevalence, severity and prediction of progression. J Hepatol 1998;29:729–735.

80. Leslie WD, Bernstein CN, Leboff MS. AGA technical review on osteoporosis in hepatic disorders. Gastroenterology 2003;125:941–966.

81. Zein CO, Lindor KD, Angulo P. Prevalence and predictors of esophageal varices in patients with primary sclerosing cholangitis. Hepatology 2004;39:204–210.

82. Wiesner RH, LaRusso NF, Dozois RR, et al. Peristomal varices after proctocolectomy in patients with primary sclerosing cholangitis. Gastroenterology 1986;90:316–322.

83. Kartheuser AH, Dozois RR, LaRusso NF, et al. Comparison of surgical treatment of ulcerative colitis associated with primary sclerosing cholangitis: ileal pouch-anal anastomosis versus Brooke ileostomy. Mayo Clin Proc 1996;71:748–756.

84. Harnois DM, Gores GJ, Ludwig J, et al. Are patients with cirrhotic stage primary sclerosing cholangitis at risk for the development of hepatocellular cancer? J Hepatol 1997;27:512–516.

85. Bergquist A, Broome U. Hepatobiliary and extra-hepatic malignancies in primary sclerosing cholangitis. Best Pract Res Clin Gastroenterol 2001;15:643–656.

86. Ahrendt SA, Pitt HA, Nakeeb A, et al. Diagnosis and management of cholangiocarcinoma in primary sclerosing cholangitis. J Gastrointest Surg 1999;3:357–367; discussion 367–368.

87. Rosen CB, Nagorney DM, Wiesner RH, et al. Cholangiocarcinoma complicating primary sclerosing cholangitis. Ann Surg 1991;213:21–25.

88. Kipp BR, Stadheim LM, Halling SA, et al. A comparison of routine cytology and fluorescence in situ hybridization for the detection of malignant bile duct strictures. Am J Gastroenterol 2004;99:1675–1681.

89. Ramage JK, Donaghy A, Farrant JM, et al. Serum tumor markers for the diagnosis of cholangiocarcinoma in primary sclerosing cholangitis. Gastroenterology 1995;108:865–869.

90. Björnsson E, Kilander A, Olsson R. Ca 19-9 and CEA are unreliable markers for cholangiocarcinoma in patients with primary sclerosing cholangitis. Liver 1999;19:501–508.

91. Nichols JC, Gores GJ, LaRusso NF, et al. Diagnostic role of serum CA 19-9 for cholangiocarcinoma in patients with primary sclerosing cholangitis. Mayo Clin Proc 1993;68(9):874–879.

92. Heimbach JK, Haddock MG, Alberts SR, et al. Transplantation for hilar cholangiocarcinoma. Liver Transpl 2004;10(suppl 2):S65–S68.

93. Shimoda M, Farmer DG, Colquhoun SD, et al. Liver transplantation for cholangio-cellular carcinoma: analysis of a single-center experience and review of the literature. Liver Transpl 2001;7:1023–1033.

94. Goss JA, Shackleton CR, Farmer DG, et al. Orthotopic liver transplantation for primary sclerosing cholangitis. A 12-year single center experience. Ann Surg 1997;225:472–481; discussion 481–483.

95. Papatheodoridis GV, Hamilton M, Rolles K, et al. Liver transplantation and inflammatory bowel disease. J Hepatol 1998;28:1070–1076.

96. Broome U, Lofberg R, Veress B, et al. Primary sclerosing cholangitis and ulcerative colitis: evidence for increased neoplastic potential. Hepatology 1995;22:1404–1408.

97. Lundqvist K, Broome U. Differences in colonic disease activity in patients with ulcerative colitis with and without primary sclerosing cholangitis. Dis Colon Rectum 1997;40:451–456.

98. Vera A, Gunson BK, Ussatoff V, et al. Colorectal cancer in patients with inflammatory bowel disease after liver transplantation for primary sclerosing cholangitis. Transplantation 2003;75:1983–1988.

99. Lindor KD. Ursodiol for primary sclerosing cholangitis. Mayo Primary Sclerosing Cholangitis–Ursodeoxycholic Acid Study Group. N Engl J Med 1997;336(10):691–695.

100. Mitchell SA, Bansi DS, Hunt N, et al. A preliminary trial of high-dose ursodeoxycholic acid in primary sclerosing cholangitis. Gastroenterology 2001;121(4):900–907.

101. Stiehl A, Rudolph G, Kloters-Plachky P, et al. Development of dominant bile duct stenoses in patients with primary sclerosing cholangitis treated with ursodeoxycholic acid: outcome after endoscopic treatment. J Hepatol 2002;36(2):151–156.

102. Bjøro K, Schrumpf E. Liver transplantation for primary sclerosing cholangitis (review; 84 references). J Hepatol 2004;40:570–577.

103. Talwalkar JA, Seaberg E, Kim WR, et al. Predicting clinical and economic outcomes after liver transplantation using the Mayo primary sclerosing cholangitis model and Child–Pugh score. National Institutes of Diabetes and Digestive and Kidney Diseases Liver Transplantation Database Group. Liver Transpl 2000;6(6):753–758.

Metabolic Diseases

David A. Tendler

▼ ▼ ▼ ▼ ▼ ▼ ▼ ▼ ▼

S EVERAL METABOLIC diseases may result in progressive liver disease, cirrhosis, and potentially the need for liver transplantation (Table 11.1). In 2002, patients with a primary diagnosis of "metabolic disease," excluding those with nonalcoholic fatty liver disease (NAFLD), accounted for 3.2% of all deceased donor liver transplants, as well as 2.5% of all live donor transplants performed in the USA [1]. Graft and patient survival rates for transplants performed for metabolic disease are excellent, relative to transplantation for other etiologies (Table 11.2). In adults, the metabolic conditions that most often necessitate liver transplantation are NAFLD, idiopathic hereditary hemochromatosis, Wilson's disease (WD), and alpha-1-antitrypsin (AAT) deficiency. In children, liver transplantation may be indicated for correction of inborn errors in metabolism, either because of the development of end-stage liver disease (ESLD) (AAT deficiency, cystic fibrosis, Wilson's disease, glycogen storage diseases (GSDs), tyrosinemia, Byler's syndrome) or to prevent irreversible extrahepatic disease (Crigler–Najjar syndrome, urea cycle disorders, familial hypercholesterolemia, familial amyloidosis). This chapter focuses primarily on the common metabolic liver diseases of adults.

■ NONALCOHOLIC FATTY LIVER DISEASE

NAFLD is a clinico-histopathological entity with histological features that resemble alcohol-induced liver injury, but by definition, occurs in patients with little or no history of alcohol consumption. It encompasses a histological spectrum that ranges from fat accumulation in hepatocytes without significant inflammation or fibrosis (steatosis) to hepatic steatosis with a necroinflammatory component (steatohepatitis) that may or may not have associated fibrosis.

Table 11.1 *Metabolic Disorders that May Be Indications for Liver Transplantation*

Alpha-1-antitrypsin deficiency

Hemochromatosis

Wilson's disease

Nonalcoholic fatty liver disease

Cystic fibrosis

Tyrosinemia

Progressive familial intrahepatic cholestasis (Alagille, Bylers syndrome)

Erythropoietic protoporphyria

Urea cycle enzyme deficiencies

Glycogen storage disease III, IV

Crigler–Najjar syndrome, type 1

Hemophilia A

Homozygous hypercholesterolemia

Protein C deficiency

Galactosemia

Familial amyloidosis

Hereditary oxalosis

Table 11.2 *Kaplan–Meier Survival Rates for Liver Transplants Performed, 1996–2001, for Metabolic Disease [1]*

Years Posttransplant	Graft Survival (%)	Patient Survival (%)
1	84.4	89.9
3	75.8	84.0
5	70.9	79.8

The latter condition is referred to as nonalcoholic steatohepatitis (NASH). The inclusion of NAFLD as a metabolic disease is supported by mounting evidence strongly linking NAFLD to insulin resistance and the metabolic syndrome, also known as "Syndrome X."

Epidemiology

The true prevalence of NAFLD is unknown, but appears to range from 18% to 23%, based on studies of individuals who have undergone evaluation to be liver transplant donors [2], autopsy studies of accident victims [3], as well as a population-based survey of 13 500 adults with abnormal aminotransferase levels, for whom other common causes of liver disease had been excluded [4]. The prevalence clearly increases with increasing body weight, occurring in 60–70% of obese individuals, and 80–90% of morbidly obese patients. Of those patients with NAFLD, approximately 20% will have NASH, which may progress to cirrhosis in 10–20% of patients [5]. The true incidence of cirrhosis attributable to NASH is unknown, and is probably underestimated, as there is generally a loss of steatosis by the time cirrhosis is well established, leaving only nonspecific histological changes. Most patients diagnosed at this stage are labeled as having "cryptogenic" cirrhosis, with NASH suspected based on clinical associations. NASH is now recognized to be a leading cause of "cryptogenic cirrhosis," with components of the metabolic syndrome present in approximately 75% [6,7].

Clinical Associations

Despite the fact that insulin resistance may be subclinical in many patients with NAFLD [8–10], patients will often manifest components of the metabolic syndrome, such as obesity (70–100% prevalence), diabetes mellitus (34–75%), hypertension, or hyperlipidemia/hypertriglyceridemia (20–80%) [11–13]. Additionally, both the risk and the severity of NASH increase exponentially with the presence of each additional component of the metabolic syndrome [14]. The risk of having NAFLD also appears to be increased in patients with polycystic ovarian syndrome (PCOS), another disorder associated with insulin resistance. Other conditions that have been described in association with NAFLD include abetalipoproteinemia, intestinal bypass surgery, rapid weight loss, small bowel bacterial overgrowth, and use of total parenteral nutrition (TPN).

Pathogenesis

The pathogenesis of NAFLD has not been fully elucidated; however, the most widely supported theory implicates insulin resistance as the key mechanism leading to hepatic steatosis, and perhaps also to steatohepatitis. Others have proposed that a "second hit," or additional oxidative injury, is required to manifest the necroinflammatory component of steatohepatitis.

Diagnosis

Criteria proposed for the diagnosis of NASH include:

1. Exclusion of other forms of chronic liver disease, such as hepatitis B, hepatitis C, autoimmune hepatitis, and Wilson's disease. It should be

noted, however, that it is possible for patients with other forms of chronic liver disease to have concomitant metabolic steatohepatitis.

2. Absence of significant alcohol consumption (generally regarded as fewer than 40 g of ethanol per week).

3. Histological findings including macrovesicular steatosis; lobular inflammation, generally with neutrophils; and evidence of liver cell injury, such as balloon degeneration. Mallory bodies and/or fibrosis may be variably present.

Natural History

A major limitation to the understanding of the natural history of NAFLD is a lack of prospective data. Notwithstanding, the risk of progression from NASH to cirrhosis appears to be proportional to the stage of disease at the time of initial liver biopsy. One study of 132 patients followed for a mean of 18 years found that cirrhosis developed in 26% of patients with balloon degeneration on initial biopsy, compared with only 4% of those who had only steatosis present [5].

Mortality risk may also be increased in patients with NASH. One study of 30 patients showed a 5-year survival of 67% and a 10-year survival of 59% [15]. Although overall mortality was similar to age- and sex-matched controls, liver-related mortality was increased. Again, there appears to be an association with the stage of disease at diagnosis, as patients with balloon degeneration and fibrosis and/or Mallory hyaline on initial biopsy had a liver-related mortality of 13% over an 18-year follow-up [5]. Therefore, liver biopsy appears to be an important prognostic tool for establishing the risk of cirrhosis and liver-related mortality. It is important to remember that comorbidities associated with obesity and diabetes, such as cardiovascular disease, frequently contribute to mortality in patients with NASH.

Hepatocellular carcinoma (HCC) may also be a late complication of NASH-induced cirrhosis. A recent study documented histological features of NASH in patients with cryptogenic cirrhosis and HCC [16].

Finally, the natural history of NASH may be altered by successful treatment, as histological improvements, including fibrosis, have been documented following interventions such as weight loss or the use of insulin-sensitizing pharmacotherapy [17–19].

Issues in Management

As insulin resistance is accountable for most, if not all, cases of NAFLD, several measures that improve insulin sensitivity have been shown to be effective avenues for treatment. Antioxidant therapies, such as vitamin E [20] and betaine [21], that target the inflammatory component of NASH may also benefit.

Interventions that have been demonstrated to improve insulin sensitivity, and often, liver histology, include exercise [22], weight reduction [23,24], and the use of insulin-sensitizing medications, such as metformin [25] and thiazolidinediones [17–19]. Exercise has a powerful effect on insulin sensitivity. Obese type 2 diabetics increased their sensitivity to insulin twofold by engaging in low-intensity bicycle riding [26]. Weight loss achieved with orlistat [27] or following gastric bypass surgery [28] has also been shown to yield histological improvements. Numerous pilot studies have shown similar histological improvements in NASH patients treated with insulin-sensitizing medications. Metformin, troglitazone, and pioglitazone have all resulted in significant improvements in aminotransferase levels, as well as steatosis grades, and in some cases levels of inflammation and fibrosis. Two studies of patients with steatohepatitis reported marked improvements in both aminotransferase levels and steatosis grades following short-term therapy with troglitazone and pioglitazone, respectively [18,19], while another study utilizing rosiglitazone for 48 weeks also demonstrated significant improvements in necroinflammatory and fibrosis scores [17].

Larger prospective trials are currently under way and will help establish whether pharmacological therapy is a safe and effective option for these patients. Currently the use of these agents for patients with NAFLD would be considered off-label, and should be reserved for patients with significant histological changes who do not have well-established cirrhosis, and with careful monitoring of blood glucose and liver function studies.

Cirrhotic patients with diabetes present a particular challenge. The use of oral hypoglycemic agents is generally discouraged in patients with established cirrhosis. In addition to the potential for idiosyncratic hepatotoxicity, there is also a hypothetical risk of inducing hypoglycemia, particularly with the use of long-acting sulfonylurea medications, due to impaired hepatic gluconeogenesis and glycogenolysis. Cirrhotic patients may also be at increased risk for the development of metformin-induced lactic acidosis. In this setting, insulin administration is preferable.

Pretransplant Considerations

Because of the prevalence of obesity and diabetes in this population, careful screening of patients with NASH-related cirrhosis for cardiovascular disease should be an important part of pretransplant evaluation. Although generally obtained routinely for most patients undergoing transplant evaluation, patients with NASH-related cirrhosis who warrant transplant consideration should undergo 12-lead electrocardiography to evaluate for evidence of ischemic heart disease, left ventricular hypertrophy, or arrhythmia. Chest radiographs should also be standard to exclude evidence of pulmonary edema or cardiomegaly. More aggressive testing to rule out ischemic heart disease with exercise stress testing, dobutamine stress echocardiography, and cardiac catheterization is also justified. In patients with diabetes mellitus, adequate blood sugar control should be demonstrated, as control of hyperglycemia posttransplant can be quite difficult due to the effect of glucocorticoids. Additionally, the exclusion of significant end-organ disease is paramount. Cardiac catheterization should be obtained in all diabetics, as significant coronary artery disease is a contraindication to transplantation, due to the risk of immunosuppressant-accelerated atherosclerosis. Similarly, patients with a history of cerebrovascular disease are precluded from transplantation. Finally, it is important to obtain a 24-h urine collection for protein and creatinine to look for evidence of diabetic nephropathy.

Impact of NAFLD on Organ Utilization

The presence of significant hepatic macrovesicular steatosis is associated with primary graft nonfunction [29]. As such, most centers do not transplant livers with more than 30% fat. Given that NAFLD is present in approximately 20% of potential donors, fatty liver disease has a significant impact on the availability of transplantable organs. Factors that account for the prevalence of hepatic steatosis in potential donors include the prevalence of NAFLD in the general population and the use of intravenous dextrose in critically ill patients prior to declaration of brain death.

The reason for the suboptimal performance of transplanted steatotic livers is not entirely clear. It has been demonstrated that there is diminished mitochondrial ATP synthesis during cold preservation of fatty livers [30]. Additionally, compared with controls, steatotic animal livers transplanted after cold storage had significant reperfusion injury with significantly lower graft survival, presumably due to the generation of free radical species [31].

Prognosis following Transplantation

Several studies have demonstrated that NAFLD recurs in the majority of patients posttransplantation. One study of 30 patients diagnosed pretransplantation with either NASH or cryptogenic cirrhosis with phenotypic evidence of NASH found the 5-year recurrence of NAFLD to be 100%, compared with a 25% incidence in controls [32]. Several patients developed steatohepatitis and fibrosis, although no increases in graft failure, chronic rejection, or mortality were observed. The time to development of steatosis correlated with the cumulative steroid dose. In contrast, a retrospective study of 71 patients who were transplanted for cryptogenic cirrhosis found that NASH recurred in eight patients and cryptogenic cirrhosis in four, one of whom required retransplantation [33]. Rejection had occurred in 24%. The 5-year cumulative incidence of graft failure was 7%. It is not known how many of these patients had cryptogenic cirrhosis resulting from other forms of liver disease.

■ HEMOCHROMATOSIS

Idiopathic hereditary hemochromatosis is an autosomal recessive disorder that is manifested by excessive intestinal iron absorption, inappropriate for total body iron levels and erythropoietic needs. It is generally caused by a mutation in the hemochromatosis (HFE) gene, located on chromosome 6 [34]. Several mutations that can potentially result in phenotypic hemochromatosis have now been described. Chronic hepatic iron deposition can eventually lead to cirrhosis and HCC, as well as cardiac (cardiomyopathy, arrhythmia), endocrinological (diabetes, thyroid disease, hypogonadism), and joint disease.

Epidemiology

Hemochromatosis is the most common inherited metabolic disorder, occurring principally among persons of northern European descent. Genetic homozygosity is present in approximately 1 per 200 American Caucasians, with approximately 10–14% of Caucasians being heterozygote carriers. It is now recognized that neither phenotypic nor clinical expression of the disease occurs in all homozygotes. Abnormal transferrin saturations consistent with homozygosity have been found in 0.5–3.7 per 1000 individuals screened in population-based studies. One such study showed no clinical signs of the disease in half of the homozygotes, and ferritin levels remained normal in one-quarter over 4 years [35]. Furthermore, it has been shown that phenotypic hemochromatosis can occur in adults without a known HFE gene mutation [34].

Pathophysiology

Hemochromatosis is characterized by excessive iron absorption and deposition in various tissues. The exact mechanism by which the HFE gene regulates iron homeostasis is not known. HFE appears to interact with the transferrin receptor, leading to a diminished affinity of the transferrin receptor for transferrin and, thus, iron storage overload [34]. Three missense mutations of the HFE gene have been described to date. The C282Y mutation is the main mutation responsible for most patients with clinically apparent hemochromatosis, found in 80–90% of affected individuals. Two additional point mutations, the H63D and S65C mutations, are associated with milder forms of the disease.

Clinical Features

The manifestation of symptoms depends on the timing of diagnosis, with the majority of patients who are diagnosed during laboratory screening being asymptomatic. Symptoms are generally not apparent before age 40 and may include fatigue, arthralgias, cutaneous hyperpigmentation, and loss of libido. Men are three times as likely as women to manifest symptoms and have twice the incidence of cirrhosis and diabetes [36]. This is probably explained by chronic iron losses secondary to menstruation. Potential signs of the disease include [37]:

- Serum aminotransferase abnormalities, present in 75%.
- Hepatomegaly, reported in up to 95% of patients.
- Cutaneous hyperpigmentation, seen in approximately 70–90% of patients.
- Splenomegaly.
- Hypothyroidism.
- Cardiac disease, occurring in approximately one-third of patients, including dilated cardiomyopathy and supraventricular arrhythmias.
- Hypogonadism, including amenorrhea, loss of libido, impotence (45% incidence).
- Diabetes mellitus, seen in 30–60% of patients.
- Arthropathy, present in approximately 45% of patients, and infrequently improving with phlebotomy.
- Partial loss of body hair, present in 62%.
- Cutaneous atrophy, most often on the anterior surface of the leg.
- HCC, with at least a 20-fold increase in risk compared with the general population [38].
- Increased risk of certain infections with siderophoric (iron-loving) bacteria, such as *Vibrio vulnificus*, *Yersinia enterocolitic*, and *Listeria* sp. Avoidance of seafood has been advocated for this reason [39].

Diagnostic Evaluation

Measurement of transferrin saturation has been shown to be the screening modality with the highest predictive value. There is no uniform recommendation regarding the level of transferrin saturation at which to initiate a full evaluation; however, a value greater than 45% is generally seen in most patients with hemochromatosis. A value of 60% or more will identify nearly all homozygotes, irrespective of iron loading. A value of 50% or more will identify nearly all homozygotes, irrespective of iron loading or sex [40]. It has been advocated that a level of 60% for men and 50% for women be used as a practical threshold. Ferritin levels are useful for prognosticating extent of disease, as increasing ferritin levels correlate with increased iron deposition in tissue. Values less than 500 ng/mL usually signify precirrhotic disease, whereas values greater than 1000 ng/mL often signify cirrhosis [41].

With the advent of clinically available genetic testing for HFE gene mutations, confirmation of the diagnosis is generally much easier. In patients with elevated transferring saturations, HFE gene mutation analysis can confirm the diagnosis.

Given the ease with which the diagnosis can now be made noninvasively, the decision to pursue liver biopsy should now be based on the need to exclude cirrhosis, which is the main risk factor for HCC. Risk factors for more advanced fibrosis include age >40, abnormal aminotransferase levels, ferritin >1000 ng/mL, and history of significant alcohol consumption. Liver biopsy should be considered in these individuals.

Issues in Management

Patients with homozygosity for hemochromatosis with biochemical and/or histological evidence of iron overload are candidates for phlebotomy. Most experts advocate weekly phlebotomy of 500 mL of blood, which removes 200–250 mg of iron. Phlebotomy schedules can be altered based on tolerance. Generally accepted end points for termination of weekly phlebotomy include the development of iron deficiency anemia and/or the normalization of iron stores. Laboratory values consistent with the accomplishment of successful therapeutic phlebotomy include hemoglobin level <12 g/dL, mean cell volume (MCV) in the low 80s, transferrin saturation <20%, and ferritin level less than 50 ng/mL. Following successful therapeutic phlebotomy, maintenance phlebotomy is typically needed every 2–4 months in order to maintain normal iron stores. Patients should be advised to moderate their intake of iron-rich foods, as well as vitamin C supplementation. Excessive amounts of vitamin C can increase the release and absorption of free iron. It is also important to counsel patients regarding alcohol consumption. One study demonstrated an increased risk for development of cirrhosis in patients who consumed more than 40 g of ethanol per day. The risk was ninefold in those who consumed 60 g or more of ethanol per day [42]. It is also worth noting that red wines have relatively high concentrations of iron.

Special attention needs to be given to patients with cirrhosis, given the significantly increased risk for the development of HCC. It has been estimated to occur in up to 30% of cirrhotics and accounts for one-third of hemochromatosis-related deaths, irrespective of phlebotomy success. The risk of developing HCC in patients with hemochromatosis is significantly increased in patients with a history of excessive alcohol consumption (48% vs. 25%) and tobacco use (50% vs. 18%), compared with hemochromatosis patients without HCC [43]. The existence of occult primary liver cancer is a well-described problem. One study of 37 patients transplanted for hemochromatosis found liver cancer in ten patients, which was unsuspected in seven prior to transplantation [44]. Regular screening with serum alpha fetoprotein (AFP) levels and either ultrasound or CT scan should be performed every 6–12 months in cirrhotic patients with hemochromatosis.

Liver Transplantation for Hemochromatosis

Several studies have demonstrated that patients with hemochromatosis have a relatively worse prognosis following liver transplantation, compared with those who are transplanted for other etiologies. This is most often due to an increased risk for infections, cardiac complications, and recurrence of HCC. Of nine patients transplanted for hemochromatosis in one study [45], three developed congestive heart failure and four cardiac arrythmias, postoperatively. This was despite having no detectable preexisting heart disease after standard cardiac testing. The 25-month actuarial survival was 53%, compared with 89% age- and sex-matched transplant recipient controls. Another study of 22 patients transplanted for hemochromatosis also demonstrated comparatively poor outcomes with survival at 1, 3, and 5 years of 72%, 62%, and 55%, respectively, with most patients dying from recurrent HCC [46]. However, 13 patients had other risk factors for liver disease. Finally, a study of 37 patients transplanted with severe iron overload demonstrated a 5-year survival of 40%, compared with an overall survival rate of 62% [47]. More than half of the deaths in the 1st year were attributed to sepsis, whereas half of the late deaths were due to cardiac complications.

Although iron reaccumulation is not invariable [46], posttransplant biopsies have revealed hepatic iron accumulation in many patients. Therefore careful monitoring and initiation of treatment is paramount.

Impact of HFE Heterozygosity on Liver Transplantation

Heterozygotes for the C282Y mutation that undergo transplantation for ESLD from other causes do not appear to be at increased risk for the development of ESLD [48]. Likewise, it does not appear that HFE heterozygosity for the C282Y mutation in transplanted livers adversely affects survival. Of 141 donor livers, in one study [48], 24 heterozygotes were detected (17%). Survival did not differ between recipients of heterozygous and normal livers. The development of phenotypic hemochromatosis has been reported in one case of an HFE heterozygote recipient who received a heterozygote donor liver [49]. Additionally, it has been shown that increased iron stores may be slow to mobilize in recipients of iron-loaded grafts, which could theoretically compromise graft function [46].

■ WILSON'S DISEASE

WD, also known as hepatolenticular degeneration, is a rare autosomal recessive disorder of copper transport, occurring in approximately 1 in 30 000 individuals [50]. Because of impairment in biliary excretion, copper accumulates in the liver, and if untreated, results in cirrhosis. Hematological, neurological, and renal disease may ensue. Liver disease is generally apparent between the ages of 8 and 16; however, neurological symptoms are uncommon prior to age 12. Most patients present with clinical symptoms between the ages of 5 and 35, although patients as old as age 62 presenting have been reported.

Pathophysiology

WD is caused by a defect in a gene on chromosome 13 that encodes for a copper-transporting ATPase in the liver. As a result of a mutation in the WD gene, there is a failure to adequately transport copper from the liver to bile, which is the major mechanism for copper excretion and a failure to incorporate copper into hepatic apoceruloplasmin [51]. As copper accumulates in hepatocytes, the ability of metallothionein to bind and distribute copper in hepatocytes is exceeded and copper is eventually deposited in lysosomes. Hepatocellular necrosis ensues, likely due to free radical injury, and copper is released into the blood stream. Cirrhosis is typical at this point. Copper then deposits in extrahepatic tissue, such as the cornea, basal ganglia, proximal renal tubules, joints, and red blood cells [52].

Clinical Features

Patients typically present with abnormal liver function testing and/or neuropsychiatric symptoms. In general, hepatic symptoms tend to present early, particularly in adolescents, whereas neuropsychiatric symptoms tend to present later [53]. The most frequent presenting symptoms, according to a study of 283 patients with WD, in order of frequency, are jaundice, dysarthria, clumsiness, tremor, drooling, gait disturbance, malaise, and arthralgias [53]. Fifty-eight patients had neurological symptoms alone, 28 patients had only hepatic symptoms, and 26 patients had hepatic symptoms followed by neurological symptoms. Approximately one-quarter of patients will have evidence of hemolysis as well. By the time neurological symptoms are present, Kayser–Fleisher (KF) corneal rings are usually present.

■ LIVER DISEASE

The spectrum of hepatic disease can be quite variable, with a number of possible manifestations, ranging from asymptomatic elevations in liver function tests to fulminant hepatic failure. The spectrum includes:

- asymptomatic hepatomegaly;
- asymptomatic elevations in aminotransferase or bilirubin levels;
- acute hepatitis with a transient illness resembling viral or autoimmune hepatitis;
- chronic hepatitis, approximately 40% of individuals with WD will present with signs of chronic hepatitis or cirrhosis;
- portal hypertension presenting as isolated splenomegaly and/or thrombocytopenia, representing unapparent cirrhosis;
- fulminant hepatic failure, usually seen in children and young adults.

Hepatocellular necrosis is accompanied by release of copper into the bloodstream, resulting in a hemolytic anemia and possible renal failure. Jaundice is usually apparent.

Liver biopsy findings can be variable as well. Findings may include hepatic steatosis or steatohepatitis that resembles alcoholic liver disease or NAFLD, portal inflammation and fibrosis that may resemble autoimmune or viral hepatitis, and cirrhosis. The histological findings are often nonspecific. Additionally, copper staining has suboptimal sensitivity and may be negative.

■ NEUROPSYCHIATRIC DISEASE

Present in approximately 35% of patients with WD, neuropsychiatric symptoms often signify the presence of cirrhosis. In addition to the common presenting symptoms listed above, patients may experience subtle changes in behavior, concentration, or coordination. In children, this may be manifested by a deterioration in school work. Dysphagia may occur secondary to a pseudobulbar palsy. Migraine headaches, insomnia, depression, anxiety, mania, and emotional lability are possible presenting symptoms. Patients may also present with symptoms that mimic Parkinson's disease, with bradykinesia, rigidity, tremor, speech and gait disturbances, and facial dystonia [51].

Diagnostic Evaluation

The diagnosis of WD may be difficult, as individual diagnostic or physical abnormalities are typically nonspecific. The combination of clinical, biochemical, and histological abnormalities compatible with WD is necessary for diagnosis.

1. Laboratory testing. Abnormalities may include:
   - Abnormal liver function tests.
   - Low serum ceruloplasmin. By itself, a low ceruloplasmin has a very poor predictive value for WD, with one study of 17 patients with

ceruloplasmin levels <20 mg/dL demonstrating a positive predictive value of 6% [54]. Conversely, patients may have WD and normal ceruloplasmin levels, as was found in 12 of 55 patients diagnosed with WD in another study [55].

- Low serum copper. This is usually proportional to low ceruloplasmin levels, as the serum copper consists of both ceruloplasmin-bound copper and non-ceruloplasmin-bound (free) copper. Free copper levels are generally elevated, and may be calculated by subtracting ceruloplasmin-bound copper (ceruloplasmin × 3.15) from total copper levels (in mcg/dL).
- Elevated urinary copper excretion. Levels greater than 100 mcg in a 24-h urine collection are suggestive of WD.
- Low uric acid levels may signify renal tubular disease, such as Fanconi's syndrome.
- Low alkaline phosphatase levels have been described in patients with more acute disease activity, usually in conjunction with hemolytic anemia (Shaver 86).

2. Slit-lamp examination for KF rings. KF rings are caused by copper deposition in Descemet's membrane of the cornea. They are present in more than 90% of patients with neurological symptoms and 50–60% of patients with isolated hepatic disease [55].
3. Liver biopsy. In addition to the histological abnormalities described above, the hepatic copper concentration can be calculated. Values greater than 250 mcg/g of dry weight are suggestive of WD.
4. Genetic testing. Useful for first-degree relatives of WD patients with a specific mutation.

Recommendations

A low ceruloplasmin in the setting of KF rings is generally diagnostic for WD, warranting initiation of therapy and familial screening. Patients with a low ceruloplasmin and no KF rings should have 24-h urine copper measurements. If abnormalities in either liver function testing or 24-h urine copper levels are found, liver biopsy with hepatic copper concentration measurements should be pursued. Similarly, liver biopsy should be performed in patients with abnormal liver function testing who have KF rings, but normal ceruloplasmin levels, present.

Issues in Management

The goals of therapy include the initial removal of accumulated copper from body tissue, followed by the prevention of reaccumulation of copper. Therapy is lifelong. Medical options for patients with compensated liver disease include D-penicillamine, trientine, and zinc. Recommendations pertaining to the selection of these agents have evolved. Traditionally, copper chelation with D-penicillamine was considered first-line treatment; however one-third of patients do not tolerate side-effects. Trientine, another copper chelator, has been demonstrated to be effective first-line therapy, and is generally better tolerated than D-penicillamine. It may also be a better option in patients with neuropsychiatric manifestations. Zinc appears to be an effective treatment option. It works by promoting metallothionein production in enterocytes, which leads to increased copper binding and fecal excretion [56]. Although its use is often delegated to postchelator phase maintenance treatment, successful first-line use has been demonstrated in many patients. It is also prudent to advise patients to avoid copper-rich foods, such as shellfish, mushrooms, liver, nuts, chocolate, and broccoli.

Patients with fulminant hepatic failure should be immediately evaluated for liver transplantation (see Chapter 13). The diagnosis of WD in this group of patients can be challenging. The following characteristics are typical for patients initially presenting with fulminant hepatic failure [57]:

1. Coomb's negative hemolytic anemia
2. Coagulopathy, unresponsive to parenteral vitamin K
3. Rapidly developing renal failure
4. Relatively modest aminotransferase elevations (usually <1000 IU/L)
5. Normal or subnormal serum alkaline phosphatase (often <40 IU/L)
6. Ratio of alkaline phosphatase: total bilirubin is often <2
7. Female to male ratio of 2:1

Patients with hemolytic anemia, hemoglobinurea, and renal failure have a poor prognosis. Fresh frozen plasma exchange may stabilize patients by lowering serum copper levels and reducing hemolysis [58]. One encouraging study in nine patients with hepatic decompensation demonstrated recovery in liver function in all nine patients utilizing combination therapy with trientine and zinc for 4 months, followed by a transition to zinc monotherapy [59].

Liver Transplantation for Wilson's Disease

Indications for liver transplantation include fulminant hepatic failure, decompensated cirrhosis that has not responded to chelation therapy, and, in some circumstances, severe neuropsychiatric symptoms unresponsive to therapy. Liver transplantation for WD is generally associated with excellent long-term, disease-free survival [60–63]. One year posttransplant survival has been reported to range from 79% to 100%, with the majority of deaths occurring in the immediate posttransplant period [63–69]. Long-term survival is generally the rule in patients that survive the first 3 months posttransplant. Normalization of liver function and KF rings are typical.

Liver transplantation for patients with intractable neuropsychiatric symptoms, but preserved liver function, is controversial. Improvements in neuropsychiatric symptoms, ranging from modest to dramatic, have been reported posttransplantation, most of which were performed in patients with coexisting hepatic failure [66,69,70]. Significant improvements have been documented with respect to motor dysfunction, cognitive impairment, and magnetic resonance imaging abnormalities. Because significant neurological improvements are not always appreciated, liver transplantation for patients with preserved hepatic function is currently considered experimental.

■ ALPHA-1-ANTITRYPSIN DEFICIENCY

AAT deficiency is an autosomal recessive disorder, occurring in 1 in 2000 to 1 in 7000 persons [71], generally of European descent. Hepatic disease, although less prevalent than pulmonary disease, develops in approximately 10–15% of affected children and adults and can result in chronic liver disease and cirrhosis, both in children and in adults. It is the most common indication for pediatric liver transplantation, although it is a rare cause of ESLD in adults. It also appears to be an independent risk factor for the development of HCC, even in the absence of cirrhosis [72].

Pathophysiology

In contrast to pulmonary AAT disease, which is caused by proteolytic destruction of elastin by elastase, hepatic disease appears to result from intrahepatocyte accumulation of AAT molecules [73]. Only some AAT genotypes appear to confer a risk for the development of liver disease. The Z, M, and S alleles have been shown to result in AAT accumulation in hepatocytes with resultant disease [74]. Because only some homozygotes develop liver disease, it has been proposed that an additional defect is required, such as decreased degradation of the AAT molecules within the endoplasmic reticulum [73]. This results in increased AAT accumulation in hepatocytes. The mechanism by which intrahepatocyte AAT accumulation leads to hepatocellular injury is not well understood. Putative mechanisms include hepatocyte ballooning and damage with the release of lysosomal enzymes, and increased susceptibility to other insults, such as viral infection or toxin.

Clinical Features

The clinical manifestations of liver involvement from AAT deficiency can be quite variable, including asymptomatic liver enzyme elevations, hepatomegaly, cholestasis, and cirrhosis with manifestations of portal hypertension. The largest natural history study of 127 Pi homozygous children demonstrated cholestatic liver disease in 11%, and liver disease without jaundice in an additional 6% [75]. The remaining 87% of children with AAT remained clinically healthy. Of those with liver damage, one-fifth developed cirrhosis by age seven. In the remaining children with neonatal cholestasis bilirubin levels normalized, generally, by 6 months of age. Early liver enzyme abnormalities generally abate with age. While more than half of young children had elevated liver enzymes, by age 18 only 12% of surviving children had abnormal liver enzyme levels and all were clinically healthy. Males appear to be twice as likely as females to develop chronic liver disease [75].

Adult-onset liver disease, including the development of cirrhosis or HCC, can occur in homozygous individuals without antecedent childhood liver disease. Most patients who present later in life with liver disease are nonsmokers, as smokers tend to die earlier from emphysema, before liver disease becomes apparent. Cirrhosis was found to be the main cause of death in 12 of 17 nonsmokers with AAT (mean age of death, 73 years), in contrast to only 2 of 23 smokers (mean age of death, 56 years) [76]. More than two-thirds of adults with AAT liver disease present after age 60 [77]. The stage of liver disease is generally advanced at the time of diagnosis, with 42% of patients surviving less than 2 years [77]. In a study of 246 adults with Pi homozygosity, 12% were found to have cirrhosis, with one-quarter having HCC [72]. Adults over age 50 with AAT have a 25% risk for the development of cirrhosis and/or HCC [71]. The risk for development of HCC is substantially greater in men than in women, with an odds ratio of 8 [72]. Primary liver cancer has been found in 25–38% of cirrhotics with AAT deficiency.

Heterozygosity for Pi may also confer a risk for the development of liver disease. Of 599 adult liver transplant recipients, 50 were found to be heterozygous carriers, with a significantly greater percentage found in patients with cryptogenic cirrhosis (27%), compared with other liver diseases [78].

Diagnosis and Management Issues

The diagnosis of PI*ZZ AAT deficiency is made by phenotype analysis with isoelectric focusing. While AAT protein levels are useful for screening homozygotes, levels are often normal or only slightly depressed in heterozygote individuals. Additionally, AAT protein levels are considered acute-phase reactants, and may transiently increase during periods of systemic inflammation, confounding its predictive value [73]. As phenotyping is considered to be the gold standard, liver biopsy is not mandatory for establishing the diagnosis, but may be useful for disease staging. It should be noted that periodic acid–Schiff (PAS) inclusions, while present in homozygous AAT deficiency, are often not detectable in heterozygotes (47–65%) or neonates [79,80].

It is recommended that individuals with AAT deficiency and chronic liver disease be vaccinated against hepatitis A and hepatitis B. Because individuals with AAT deficiency often present as adults with advanced liver disease, it is recommended that first-degree relatives of patients with AAT deficiency undergo testing.

Liver Transplantation for Alpha-1-Antitrypsin Deficiency

Liver transplantation is indicated for patients with ESLD secondary to AAT. Transplantation of a phenotypically normal donor liver results in the correction of the disease, with normal production and secretion of AAT. Prognosis following liver transplantation is excellent. Of 97 children with hepatic AAT, 26 developed ESLD, with 24 children undergoing liver transplantation. Two patients died following transplantation [81]. Another review reported a 100% survival after a median follow-up of 40 months [82] among 25 children transplanted for AAT liver disease. A 73% 1-year survival was reported in an analysis of 22 adults transplanted with AAT deficiency, the majority being heterozygotes who presented with cirrhosis and portal hypertension [83]. When evaluating adults with AAT for liver transplantation, careful assessment of pulmonary function is important. Concomitant obstructive pulmonary disease, precluding liver transplantation, was noted in 10 of 19 adults (53%) with AAT [77].

■ GLYCOGEN STORAGE DISEASE

Because it is the body's principal carbohydrate store, glycogen plays a key role in maintaining effective blood glucose homeostasis during periods of fasting and in times of stress. Several enzyme defects that result in impaired glycogen degradation, inadequate maintenance of appropriate blood glucose concentrations, and abnormal accumulation of hepatic glycogen exist [84]. The most clinically important of these are types I, III, and IV, respectively. As a group, GSDs are rare (1/100 000 live births) but they may be associated with complications of liver disease and other body systems such that consideration of orthotopic liver transplantation (OLT) becomes necessary.

Most late teenage and young adult patients with type I and, to a lesser extent, type III GSD have developed hepatic adenomata by virtue of negotiating the challenging demands of early years. In many instances, these are either multiple or large. Although the reported progression of benign lesions to HCC is very low, there may be sufficient concern in some circumstances to justify OLT, e.g. where the number of lesions is too great for all to be biopsied or a large solitary lesion exists that is not amenable to resection. Not only does OLT remove the risk of cancer development but it also corrects the inherited metabolic defect such as concomitant manifestations, namely hyperuricemia, hypertriglyceridemia, lactic academia, and their potential complications, e.g. recurrent pancreatitis. Hepatocyte transplantation may be a realistic alternative to OLT among patients with type I GSD in whom compliance with dietary demands may be difficult or impossible; furthermore, hepatic adenomata may regress following correction of the metabolic defect and restoration of normal blood glucose concentrations. This has been described in at least one instance 9 months after the procedure. The patient, a 47-year-old woman, was eating a normal diet and could fast for up to 7 h without developing hypoglycemia; tacrolimus was her only immunosuppressive therapy [85].

In contrast to patients with type I GSD, those with type III GSD may develop hepatic fibrosis and progression to ESLD. Although, the overall risk of this appears low (10–20%), consideration of OLT may be necessary. OLT offers the only hope of sustained progress and cure for patients with type IV GSD. In general, they present during the first year of life and their clinical course typically comprises failure to thrive, hepatosplenomegaly, evidence of liver dysfunction, and muscular hypotonia [84].

■ **REFERENCES**

1. Annual report of the U.S. Scientific Registry of Transplant Recipients and the Organ Procurement and Transplantation Network: transplant data 1993–2002. Rockville, MD, and Richmond, VA, HHS/HRSA/OSP/DOT and UNOS, 2002.

2. Marcos A, Fisher RA, Ham JM, et al. Selection and outcome of living donors for adult to adult right lobe transplantation. Transplantation 2000;15:2410–2415.

3. Wanless IR, Lentz JS. Fatty liver hepatitis (steatohepatitis) and obesity: an autopsy study with analysis of risk factors. Hepatology 1990;12:1106–1110.

4. Clark JM, Brancati FL, Diehl AM. The prevalence and etiology of elevated amino-transferase levels in the United States. Am J Gastroenterol 2003;98:960–967.

5. Matteoni CA, Younossi ZM, Gramlich T, et al. Nonalcoholic fatty liver disease: a spectrum of clinical pathological severity. Gastroenterology 1999;116:1413.

6. Caldwell SH, Oelsner DH, Iezzoni JC, et al. Cryptogenic cirrhosis: clinical characterization and risk factors for underlying disease. Hepatology 1999;29:664.

7. Bugianesi E, Leone N, Vanni E, et al. Expanding the natural history of nonalcoholic steatohepatitis: from cryptogenic cirrhosis to hepatocellular carcinoma. Gastroenterology 2002;123:134–140.

8. Chitturi S, Abeygunasekera S, Farrell GC, et al. NASH and insulin resistance: insulin hypersecretion and specific association with the insulin resistance syndrome. Hepatology 2002;35:373–379.

9. Marchesini G, Bugianesi E, Forlani G. Nonalcoholic fatty liver, steatohepatitis, and the metabolic syndrome. Hepatology 2003;37:917–923.

10. Marchesini G, Brizi M, Bianchi G, et al. Nonalcoholic fatty liver disease. A feature of the metabolic syndrome. Diabetes 2001;50:1844–1850.

11. Ludwig J, Viggiano TR, McGill DB, et al. Nonalcoholic steatohepatitis: Mayo Clinic experiences with a hitherto unnamed disease. Mayo Clin Proc 1980;55:434–438.

12. Powell EE, Cooksley WG, Hanson R, et al. The natural history of nonalcoholic steatohepatitis: a follow-up study of forty-two patients for up to 21 years. Hepatology 1990;11:74–80.

13. Diehl AM, Goodman Z, Ishak KG. Alcohol-like liver disease in nonalcoholics. A clinical and histological comparison with alcohol-induced liver injury. Gastroenterology 1988;95:1056–1062.

14. Marceau P, Biron S, Hould FS, et al. Liver pathology and the metabolic syndrome X in severe obesity. J Clin Endocrinol Metab 1999;84:1513–1517.

15. Propst A, Propst T, Judmaier G, et al. Prognosis in nonalcoholic steatohepatitis (letter). Gastroenterology 1995;108:1607.

16. Bugianesi E, Leone N, Vanni E, et al. Expanding the natural history of nonalcoholic steatohepatitis: from cryptogenic cirrhosis to hepatocellular carcinoma. Gastroenterology 2002;123:134–140.

17. Neuschwander-Tetri BA, Brunt EM, Wehmeier KR, et al. Improved nonalcoholic steatohepatitis after 48 weeks of treatment with the PPAR-gamma ligand rosiglitazone. Hepatology 2003;38:1008–1017.

18. Caldwell SH, Hespenheide EE, Redick JA, et al. A pilot study of a thiazolidinedione, troglitazone, in nonalcoholic steatohepatitis. Am J Gastroenterol 2001;96:519.

19. Promrat K, Lutchman G, Uwaifo GI, et al. A pilot study of pioglitazone treatment for nonalcoholic steatohepatitis. Hepatology 2004;39:188–196.

20. Lavine JE. Vitamin E treatment of nonalcoholic steatohepatitis in children: a pilot study. J Pediatr 2000;136:734–738.

21. Abdelmalek MF, Angulo P, Jorgensen RA, et al. Betaine, a promising new agent for patients with nonalcoholic steatohepatitis: results of a pilot study. Am J Gastroenterol 2001;96:2711–2717.

22. Ueno T. Therapeutic effects of restricted diet and exercise in obese patients with fatty liver. J Hepatol 1997;27:103–107.

23. Palmer M, Schaffner F. Effect of weight reduction on hepatic abnormalities in overweight patients. Gastroenterology 1999;116:1413–1419.

24. Eriksson S, Eriksson KF, Bondesson L. Nonalcoholic steatohepatitis in obesity: a reversible condition. Acta Med Scand 1986;220:83–88.

25. Uygun A, Kadayifci A, Isik AT, et al. Metformin in the treatment of patients with non-alcoholic steatohepatitis. Aliment Pharmacol Ther 2004;19:537–544.

26. Usui K, Yamanouchi K, Asai K, et al. The effect of low intensity bicycle exercise on the insulin-induced glucose uptake in obese patients with type 2 diabetes. Diabetes Res Clin Pract 1998;41:57–61.

27. Harrison SA, Ramrakhiani S, Brunt EM, et al. Orlistat in the treatment of NASH: a case series. Am J Gastroenterol 2003;98:926–930.

28. Silverman EM, Sapala JA, Appleman HD. Regression of hepatic steatosis in morbidly obese persons after gastric bypass. Am J Clin Pathol 1995;104:23–31.

29. Burke A, Lucey MR. Non-alcoholic fatty liver disease, non-alcoholic steatohepatitis and orthotopic liver transplantation. Am J Transplant 2004;4:686–693.

30. Fukumori T, Ohkohchi N, Tsukamoto S, et al. Why is fatty liver unsuitable for transplantation? Deterioration of mitochondrial ATP synthesis and sinusoidal structure during cold preservation of a liver with steatosis. Transplant Proc 1997;29:412–415.

31. Gao W, Connor HD, Lemasters JJ, et al. Primary nonfunction of fatty livers produced by alcohol is associated with a new, antioxidant-insensitive free radical species. Transplantation 1995;15:674–679.

32. Contos MJ, Cales W, Sterling RK, et al. Development of nonalcoholic fatty liver disease after orthotopic liver transplantation for cryptogenic cirrhosis. Liver Transpl 2001;7:363–373.

33. Sanjeevi A, Lyden E, Sunderman B, et al. Outcomes of liver transplantation for cryptogenic cirrhosis: a single-center study of 71 patients. Transplant Proc 2003;35:2977–2980.

34. Pietrangelo A. Hereditary hemochromatosis – a new look at an old disease. N Engl J Med 2004;350:2383–2397.

35. Olynyk JK, Cullen DJ, Aquilia S, et al. A population-based study of the clinical expression of the hemochromatosis gene. N Engl J Med 1999;341:718–724.

36. Moirand R, Adams PC, Bicheler V, et al. Clinical features of genetic hemochromatosis in women compared with men. Ann Intern Med 1997;127:105–110.

37. Niederau C, Strohmeyer G, Stremmel W. Epidemiology, clinical spectrum, and prognosis of hemochromatosis. Adv Exp Med Biol 1994;356:293–302.

38. Elmberg M, Hultcrantz R, Ekbom A, et al. Cancer risk in patients with hereditary hemochromatosis and in their first-degree relatives. Gastroenterology 2003;125: 1733–1741.

39. Andrews NC. Disorders of iron metabolism. N Engl J Med 1999;341:1986–1995.

40. Edwards CQ, Kushner JP. Screening for hemochromatosis. N Engl J Med 1993;328: 1616–1620.

41. Guyader D, Jacquelinet C, Moirand R, et al. Noninvasive prediction of fibrosis in C282Y homozygous hemochromatosis. Gastroenterology 1998;115:929–936.

42. Fletcher LM, Dixon JL, Purdie DM, et al. Excess alcohol greatly increases the prevalence of cirrhosis in hereditary hemochromatosis. Gastroenterology 2002;122:281–289.

43. Deugnier YM, Guyader D, Crantock L, et al. Primary liver cancer in genetic hemo-chromatosis: a clinical, pathological, and pathogenetic study of 54 cases. Gastro-enterology 1993;104:228–234.

44. Kowdley KV, Hassanein T, Kaur S. Primary liver cancer and survival in patients undergoing liver transplantation for hemochromatosis. Liver Transpl Surg 1995;1: 237–241.

45. Farrell FJ, Nguyen M, Woodley S, et al. Outcome of liver transplantation in patients with hemochromatosis. Hepatology 1994;20:404–410.

46. Crawford DH, Fletcher LM, Hubscher SG, et al. Patient and graft survival after liver transplantation for hereditary hemochromatosis: implications for pathogenesis. Hepatology 2004;39:1655–1662.

47. Tung BY, Farrell FJ, McCashland TM, et al. Long-term follow-up after liver trans-plantation in patients with hepatic iron overload. Liver Transpl Surg 1999;5: 369–374.

48. Alanen KW, Chakrabarti S, Rawlins JJ. Prevalence of the C282Y mutation of the hemochromatosis gene in liver transplant recipients and donors. Hepatology 1999;30:665–669.

49. Wigg AJ, Harley H, Casey G. Heterozygous recipient and donor HFE mutations associated with a hereditary haemochromatosis phenotype after liver transplant-ation. Gut 2003;52:433–435.

50. Frydman M. Genetic aspects of Wilson's disease. J Gastroenterol Hepatol 1990;5: 483–490.

51. Loudianos G, Gitlin JD. Wilson's disease. Semin Liver Dis 2000;20:353–364.

52. Cuthbert JA. Wilson's disease. Update of a systemic disorder with protean mani-festations. Gastroenterol Clin North Am 1998;27:655–681.

53. Saito T. Presenting symptoms and natural history of Wilson disease. Eur J Pediatr 1987;146:261–265.

54. Cauza E, Maier-Dobersberger T, Polii C, et al. Screening for Wilson's disease in patients with liver diseases by serum ceruloplasmin. J Hepatol 1997;27:358–362.

55. Steindl P, Ferenci P, Dienes HP, et al. Wilson's disease in patient presenting with liver disease – a diagnostic challenge. Gastroenterology 1997;113:212–218.

56. Hill GM, Brewer GJ, Prasad AS, et al. Treatment of Wilson's disease with zinc. I. Oral zinc therapy regimens. Hepatology 1987;7:522–528.

57. Roberts EA, Schilsky ML. A practice guideline on Wilson disease. Hepatology 2003;37:1475–1492.

58. Kiss JE, Berman D, Van Thiel D. Effective removal of copper by plasma exchange in fulminant Wilson's disease. Transfusion 1998;38:327–331.

59. Askari FK, Greenson J, Dick RD, et al. Treatment of Wilson's disease with zinc. XVIII. Initial treatment of the hepatic decompensation presentation with trientine and zinc. J Lab Clin Med 2003;142:385–390.

60. Podgaetz E, Chan C. Liver transplantation for Wilson's disease: our experience with review of the literature. Ann Hepatol 2003;2:131–134.

61. Asonuma K, Inomata Y, Kasahara M, et al. Living related liver transplantation from heterozygote genetic carriers to children with Wilson's disease. Pediatr Transplant 1999;3:201–205.

62. Wang XH, Cheng F, Zhang F. Copper metabolism after living related liver transplantation for Wilson's disease. World J Gastroenterol 2003;9:2836–2838.

63. Emre S, Atillasoy EO, Ozdemir S, et al. Orthotopic liver transplantation for Wilson's disease: a single-center experience. Transplantation 2001;15:1232–1236.

64. Bellary S, Hassanein T, Van Thiel DH. Liver transplantation for Wilson's disease. J Hepatol 1995;24:373–381.

65. Nyckowski P, Dudek K, Skwarek A, et al. Results of liver transplantation according to indications for orthotopic liver transplantation. Transplant Proc 2003;35:2265–2267.

66. Schumacher G, Platz KP, Mueller AR. Liver transplantation: treatment of choice for hepatic and neurological manifestation of Wilson's disease. Clin Transplant 1997:11:217–224.

67. Schilsky ML, Scheinberg IH, Sternlieb I. Liver transplantation for Wilson's disease: indications and outcome. Hepatology 1994;19:583–587.

68. Sutcliffe RP, Maguire DD, Muiesan P, et al. Liver transplantation for Wilson's disease: long-term results and quality-of-life assessment. Transplantation 2003;75:1003–1006.

69. Geissler I, Heinemann K, Rohm S, et al. Liver transplantation for hepatic and neurological Wilson's disease. Transplant Proc 2003;35:1445–1446.

70. Stracciari A, Tempestini A, Borghi A, et al. Effect of liver transplantation on neurological manifestations in Wilson disease. Arch Neurol 2000;57:384–386.

71. Anonymous. Alpha 1-antitrypsin deficiency: memorandum from a WHO meeting. Bull World Health Organ 1997;75:397–415.

72. Larsson C. Natural history and life expectancy in severe alpha1-antitrypsin deficiency, Pi Z. Acta Med Scand 1978;204:345–351.

73. American Thoracic Society/European Respiratory Society Statement: standards for the diagnosis and management of individuals with AAT deficiency III. Liver and other diseases. Am J Respir Crit Care Med 2003;168:856–866.

74. Birrer P, McElvaney NG, Chang-Stroman LM, et al. Alpha 1-antitrypsin deficiency and liver disease. J Inherit Metab Dis 1991;14:512–525.

75. Sveger T. Liver disease in alpha 1-antitrypsin deficiency detected by screening of 200,000 infants. N Engl J Med 1976;294:1316–1321.

76. Eriksson S, Carlson J, Velez R. Risk of cirrhosis and primary liver cancer in alpha 1-antitrypsin deficiency. N Engl J Med 1986;314:736–739.

77. Rakela J, Goldschmiedt M, Ludgwig J. Late manifestations of chronic liver disease in adults with alpha-1-antitrypsin deficiency. Dig Dis Sci 1987;32:1358–1362.

78. Graziadei IW, Joseph JJ, Wiesner RH, et al. Increased risk of chronic liver failure in adults with heterozygous alpha 1-antitrypsin deficiency. Hepatology 1998;28:1058–1063.

79. Hultcrantz R, Mengarelli S. Ultrastructural liver pathology in patients with minimal liver disease and alpha 1-antitrypsin deficiency: a comparison between heterozygous and homozygous patients. Hepatology 1984;4:937–945.

80. Clausen PP, Lindskov J, Gad I, et al. The diagnostic value of alpha 1-antitrypsin globules in liver cells as a morphological marker of alpha 1-antitrypsin deficiency. Liver 1984;4:353–359.

81. Francavilla R, Castellaneta SP, Hadzic N, et al. Prognosis of alpha-1-antitrypsin deficiency-related liver disease in the era of paediatric liver transplantation. J Hepatol 2000;32:986–992.

82. Prachalias AA, Kalife M, Francavilla R, et al. Liver transplantation for alpha-1-antitrypsin deficiency in children. Transpl Int 2000;13:207–210.

83. Vennarecci G, Gunson BK, Ismail T, et al. Transplantation for end-stage liver disease related to alpha 1 antitrypsin. Transplantation 1996;61:1488–1495.

84. Quist RG, Baker AJ, Dhawan A, Bass NM. Metabolic diseases of the liver. In: O'Grady JG, Lake JR, Howdle PD, eds. Comprehensive clinical hepatology, 1st edition. London: Mosby, 2000;3/22.1–22.19.

85. Murace M, Gerunda G, Neri D, et al. Hepatocyte transplantation as a treatment for glycogen storage disease 1a. Lancet 2002;359: 317–318.

Living Donor Liver Transplantation

▼ ▼ ▼ ▼ ▼ ▼ ▼ ▼ ▼

James F. Trotter and Wesley Kasen

■ **HISTORY OF LIVING DONOR LIVER TRANSPLANTATION**

The first successful living donor liver transplantation (LDLT) was reported in 1989 with the transplantation of a left hepatic lobe from a 29-year-old woman to her infant son. Following the success of this initial procedure, LDLT became the predominant means of transplantation in Asia where cultural beliefs largely preclude deceased donor (DD) transplantation. In the USA, the widespread application of LDLT occurred much later. Until 1997, fewer than 100 LDLTs were performed each year in the USA, largely from adult (parental) donors to pediatric recipients. Subsequently, there was a rapid growth in the number of adult-to-adult LDLTs. Between 1997 and 2003, the number of cases (percentage of all liver transplantations) increased nearly fourfold, from 86 (2.1%) to 321 (5.6%). The number of LDLTs in 2004 was 323 or 5.2% of all liver transplantations, as depicted in Fig. 12.1. There are two primary reasons for the increased number of LDLTs in adult patients during this time. First, the technical success of the procedure increased measurably with the use of the right hepatic lobe graft, compared with the smaller left hepatic lobe graft. In 1994, the first right hepatic lobe LDLT was reported in Japan, and the first series was documented shortly thereafter. The first adult-to-adult right hepatic lobe LDLT was performed in the USA in 1997. The initial results of right hepatic lobe LDLT were superior to the smaller left hepatic lobe and helped lead to widespread application of the procedure. Second, a critical shortage of DD livers developed during the 1990s when the number of patients listed for transplantation increased nearly 10-fold from 1676 patients in 1991 to 13,999 in 1999, while the number of DD livers available for transplantation increased by only 52% from 2953 to 4478. As a result, the number of patients dying on the transplant list increased more than fourfold from 435 to 1753 over the same period. Therefore, in the 1990s the relative availability of DD livers

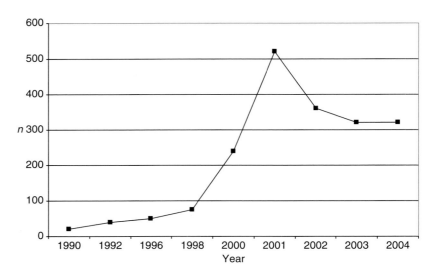

Fig. 12.1 *Number of living donor liver transplantations (LDLTs) versus year.*

decreased due to the growing disparity between the number of patients listed for transplantation compared with a stable donor pool. As a result, the waiting time for transplantation increased and the number of patients dying on the list increased. Consequently, selected transplantation centers began to offer LDLT as a means to expand their donor pool to decrease waiting list mortality by reducing the time to transplantation.

■ SELECTION OF RECIPIENTS

National standards for the selection of recipients (and donors) for LDLT have recently been published by several regulatory bodies. The United Network for Organ Sharing (UNOS) Ad Hoc Committee on Living Donation, the Advisory Committee on Transplantation for the Secretary of Health and Human Services, and the New York State Health Department have each formulated specific recommendations regarding the appropriate selection, evaluation, and perioperative management of donors and recipients. Some of these documents have specified the composition of the evaluation team, the technical experience of the surgeon, and the staffing requirements for nurses, physicians, and trainees during the operative and perioperative periods. In accordance with these guidelines, most transplant centers use a stepwise approach to recipient selection, as shown in Fig. 12.2.

The first step toward consideration of LDLT for the recipient is evaluation and listing for DD transplantation. In general, each LDLT recipient should meet UNOS criteria for listing, since a DD graft may be required if the living donor

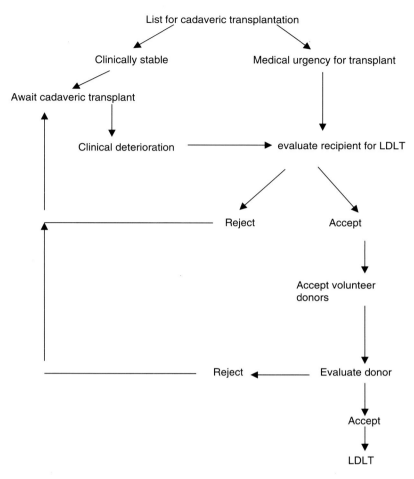

Fig. 12.2 *Evaluation protocol for recipients and donors.*

graft fails. The appropriate selection of recipients for LDLT requires recognition of the potential advantages and disadvantages of both DD and LDLT. Perhaps the greatest advantage of LDLT is a reduction in waiting time. Once a potential living donor is evaluated and found suitable, the transplantation can be scheduled within hours to weeks. For the recipient, a reduction in waiting time may allow transplantation to occur prior to the development of further complications of end-stage liver disease (ESLD) that could lead to death or medical deterioration, thereby compromising the success of the procedure.

Another advantage of LDLT is that the operation is a scheduled procedure, compared with DD transplantation, which occurs with only short-term notice. The scheduled nature of LDLT may allow for treatment and medical stabilization of the recipient so that he/she may be in the best possible medical condition at the time of surgery. Finally, organs from living donors experience very short cold-ischemia time (the time between harvesting of the donor liver and implantation in the recipient), usually less than 1 h. However, cold-ischemia time for DD liver transplantation is between 6 and 10 h in over 50% of patients. Reduction of cold-ischemia time may be beneficial, as prolonged cold-ischemia time has been associated with increased complications and graft dysfunction.

There are also potential disadvantages of LDLT, most notable of which is the risk of complications to the donor. In addition, the graft survival rates in LDLT are significantly less than with DD transplantation. The rate of graft loss in adult LDLT recipients is significantly higher compared with adult DD recipients (hazard ratio 1.66, 95% CI = 1.30–2.11). In addition, several centers have documented a higher incidence of biliary complications in LDLT recipients. As a result, LDLT recipients may require more frequent postoperative procedures (percutaneous cholangiography, endoscopic retrograde cholangiography, and/or reoperation) to treat biliary complications compared with DD recipients. Finally, the right hepatic lobe graft may not provide sufficient hepatic function for patients with severely decompensated liver disease.

The consideration of specific recipients for LDLT must take into account the recognized advantages and disadvantages of the procedure. In general, to be considered "medically eligible" for LDLT, the patient must have an urgent need for an expedited transplantation. One means to objectively measure a patient's requirement for transplantation is the Model for Endstage Liver Disease (MELD) score, which is an objective assessment of the patient's 90-day mortality based on creatinine, bilirubin, and INR. The MELD score is currently the basis by which patients are prioritized for transplantation. The higher the MELD score, the higher the 90-day mortality and the higher the priority for transplantation. There is a significant increase in mortality at MELD scores above 18, as shown in Fig. 12.3. Patients with a MELD score

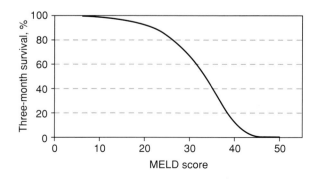

Fig. 12.3 *Three-month survival versus model for end-stage liver disease (MELD) score.*

>18 have a 90-day mortality (>10%), which is approximately equal to the 1-year mortality after LDLT. Therefore, patients with an MELD score higher than 18 may be deemed medically sick to be considered for surgery. While the MELD score provides an objective measure of severity-of-illness in most patients with liver disease, some patients may have life-threatening complications despite a low MELD score. These selected patients may benefit from an expedited transplantation with a living donor, because they have virtually no chance for DD transplantation due to their low MELD score. In our experience, a disproportionate number of patients with cholestatic liver disease are severely ill without a corresponding high MELD score and therefore may be more likely to undergo LDLT compared with patients with noncholestatic liver disease.

Special consideration must be given to patients with severely decompensated liver disease. Patients with chronic liver disease requiring continuous treatment in the intensive care unit have poor outcomes after LDLT. In this group of patients, Testa et al. reported a 57% mortality following LDLT, compared with only an 18% mortality when a DD liver was used. In addition, patients with decompensated liver disease require a larger graft compared with patients who are less sick. Child's A recipients may do well with very small grafts (graft-to-recipient body weight ratio (GRBW) of 0.6%). However, recipients with more advanced liver failure (Child's B and C) had significantly poorer graft survival when the GRBW was less than 0.85% compared with greater than 0.85% (33% vs. 74% graft survival). Therefore, patients with severely decompensated chronic liver disease may not be able to undergo successful LDLT, especially if the size of the donor graft is small.

There is controversy regarding the routine evaluation of patients with clinically stable cirrhosis, i.e. patients with cirrhosis and low MELD score without any complications of liver disease. At some transplant centers these patients are not routinely evaluated for LDLT, because the risks to the donor are considered too great to outweigh the potential benefits to the recipient. However, other transplant teams support LDLT in these stable patients, since transplantation prior to the development of clinical decompensation may give the patient the best chance for a favorable outcome. Therefore, the selection of these patients is based on the experience and judgment of the transplant team.

Once a patient has been deemed "medically eligible" for LDLT, the transplant team must determine if the patient is "surgically suitable" to undergo the surgical procedure. Patients with one or more problems that could jeopardize the success of the procedure may be rejected for further consideration for LDLT. Common problems that may exclude a patient from LDLT include one or more of the following chronic medical conditions: renal failure, coronary artery disease, pulmonary hypertension, hypercoaguable state, extensive mesenteric venous thrombosis, morbid obesity, and/or advanced age. In our

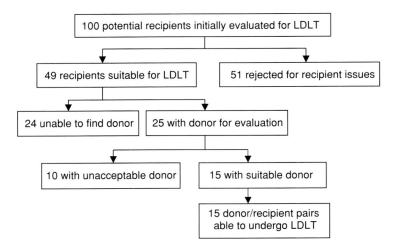

Fig. 12.4 *Outcomes of 100 patients evaluated for living donor liver transplantation (LDLT).*

experience, approximately half of the patients who are found "medically eligible" for LDLT based on the severity of their liver disease are not "surgically suitable" due to underlying major medical or surgical conditions (see Fig. 12.4). The selection of specific patients for LDLT is based on the skill, experience, and judgment of the transplant team. With greater experience, select patients with complex medical problems may be considered for LDLT.

■ DONOR SELECTION

Once a patient has been accepted as a candidate for LDLT, he/she may accept potential donors for evaluation. To be considered for evaluation, the donor must have the following characteristics:

- be between the age of 18 and 55 years,
- have a blood type identical/compatible with that of the recipient,
- not have significant medical conditions,
- not have previous significant abdominal surgeries and must demonstrate a long-term, significant relationship with the recipient.

The donor must also be able to yield a graft of sufficient size for the recipient. At our center, we generally require that the donor's body weight be at least 70% of the recipient, because we have found that smaller donors are unable to provide a right hepatic lobe of sufficient size for the recipient. Other centers may use more objective measures to determine requirement for graft size.

Approximately half of the patients found "medically eligible" and "surgically suitable" for LDLT are unable to identify a potential donor for evaluation. The reasons that a patient may not have a potential donor for evaluation include one or more of the following: estrangement from their family or friends, no family or friends between 18 and 55 year of age, or the presence of an obvious significant medical problem in the potential donor such as morbid obesity or coronary artery disease. One of the most common reasons for rejection of potential donors in the USA is obesity. Obese individuals are more likely to have hepatic steatosis, which is associated with increased operative complications and poor graft function following transplantation. In addition, the prevalence of medical conditions (diabetes, hypertension), which could increase perioperative complications, is higher in obese patients. Therefore, in areas of the country where the incidence of obesity is highest (southeast and north-central USA), the number of suitable donors may be smaller than in western states where obesity is less common. As a result, transplantation programs in regions where obesity is more prevalent may not be able to perform as many LDLTs due to a reduction in the number of suitable donors.

Once a potential donor is identified, he/she is evaluated in a systematic fashion designed to reject unsuitable donors as early as possible in the evaluation process (Table 12.1). The initial phase of donor evaluation is performed by a registered nurse, typically by telephone. Basic data such as age, sex, height, weight, relationship to the recipient, blood type, current medications, medical, psychiatric, and surgical histories are obtained to determine if further evaluation is warranted. The potential donor is then presented to the transplant team to determine if formal evaluation is reasonable, and further evaluation proceeds in a stepwise fashion, including tests shown in Table 12.1. Any potential problems encountered during the second phase of evaluation are further investigated during the third phase, which may include tests such as

Table 12.1 *Living Donor Liver Transplantation Evaluation*

Phase I

Recipient

A. MELD $\geq$ 18 or life-threatening complications

B. Financial clearance for LDLT

C. Absence of significant contraindication:

   1. Morbid obesity (recipient weight >130% ideal body weight)

   2. Severe medical problem compromising outcome (pulmonary hypertension, previous coronary artery bypass graft, etc.)

D. Psychosocially stable

E. Age <65 years

Table 12.1 *Continued*

Donor

A. Age >18 and $\geq$ 55

B. Identical or compatible blood type with recipient

C. Absence of previous significant abdominal surgery

D. Absence of major medical problems (diabetes, severe or uncontrolled hypertension, hepatic, cardiac, renal or pulmonary disease)

E. Demonstrable, significant, long-term relationship with recipient

F. Normal liver function tests, serum electrolytes, complete blood count with differential cell count, negative hepatitis B surface antigen, hepatitis B core antibody and hepatitis C antibody

Phase II

A. Complete medical history and physical examination of potential donor laboratories:

   1. Serum ferritin, iron, transferrin, ceruloplasmin

   2. Alpha-1-antitrypsin level and phenotype

   3. Rapid plasmin reagin (RPR)

   4. Cytomegalovirus antibody (IgG), Epstein–Barr virus antibody (IgG)

   5. Antinuclear antibody

   6. Human immunodeficiency antibody (HIV)

   7. Toxicology/substance abuse screen

   8. Urinalysis

   9. Blood oxygen saturation

B. Chest radiograph

C. Electrocardiogram

D. Formal surgical evaluation of donor

E. Anesthesia preoperative evaluation

F. Magnetic resonance imaging of the liver, biliary system, and hepatic vasculature

Phase III

Other tests or consultations to clarify any potential problems uncovered during evaluation:

endoscopic retrograde cholangiopancreatography, hepatic angiogram, liver biopsy, echocardiogram, stress echocardiogram, etc. (some centers routinely obtain these tests as part of the donor evaluation)

endoscopic retrograde cholangiopancreatography (ERCP), hepatic angiography, liver biopsy, echocardiography, or stress echocardiography; however, these tests are not routinely performed. Approximately half the potential donors who go through formal evaluation are ultimately accepted as donors (see Fig. 12.4).

While nondirected donation (or "Good Samaritan" donation) may be acceptable for renal transplantation, most LDLT centers do not evaluate individuals who present themselves as nondirected or "Good Samaritan" donors. These nondirected donors are excluded from liver donation, because the risk of the donor surgery is up to ten times higher than with kidney donation. Therefore, each potential donor must demonstrate a long-term, significant relationship with the recipient. Psychosocial assessment is an important aspect of donor evaluation that should be performed by a social worker familiar with liver transplantation. Selected donors may require evaluation by a psychiatrist. In psychosocial evaluation any underlying psychological or psychiatric problems should be identified along with the donor's motivation for donation. In addition, the social impact of the surgery on the donor and his or her family should be fully investigated. The donor must also be given the opportunity to withdraw consent for the procedure at any point up to the time of the operation. The privacy of this decision must be protected so that the donor may make this decision without undue coercion from the recipient. Therefore, when a donor is disqualified for donation because of withdrawal of consent, the precise reason for rejection of the donors is not disclosed to the recipient.

■ SURGICAL TECHNIQUE

The most important determinant of donor and recipient outcome is the skill and experience of the surgical team. LDLT should be performed only by surgeons with extensive experience in hepatobiliary and liver transplantation surgery. Surgical technique continues to evolve for LDLT. The details of the surgical technique are beyond the scope of this discussion. However, the general features of the operation are as follows. The recipient undergoes complete removal of the diseased liver through a standard right subcostal incision, while the donor hepatecomy is performed in an adjacent operating room. The right lobectomy represents approximately 60% of the donor's liver volume. A cholecystectomy is performed and the right hepatic artery, right portal vein, and right hepatic vein are isolated and removed with the right lobe from the donor. The right hepatic lobe is then implanted into the recipient with the following anastomoses: donor's right hepatic vein to recipient's right hepatic vein remnant with a caval extension, donor's right portal vein to recipient's portal vein, and donor's right hepatic artery to recipient's hepatic artery. Depending on the donor's and the recipient's anatomy, either choledochocholedochostomy or the Roux-en-Y drainage procedure is performed to connect the biliary system.

Both the remnant liver in the donor and the right lobe graft in the recipient regenerate after surgery. In one study, the volume of the liver graft increased by 87%, from a mean of $862\,cm^3$ at the time of operation to a mean of $1614\,cm^3$ 7 days after the procedure. This correlates to 94% of its final regenerated volume after 1 week. In the same series, the donor's liver remnant doubled in size 1 week after hepatectomy.

■ RECIPIENT OUTCOMES

DD transplantation is the preferred means of liver transplantation in patients with this option, because a living donor is not placed at risk and recipient outcomes are superior compared with LDLT. There is no difference in the unadjusted patient and graft survival rates for LDLT compared with DD transplantation. However, because LDLT recipients are, in general, ideal candidates for transplantation, the risk-adjusted survival rates for LDLT recipients are significantly lower than with DD transplantation. Table 12.2 shows that LDLT recipients are younger, thinner, and less sick at the time of transplantation. In addition, the average MELD score in LDLT patients is 14 compared with 22 for DD recipients. Compared with DD transplantation, the risk-adjusted graft survival is also lower following LDLT. Living donor recipients have a 59% higher relative risk for graft failure than those receiving DD livers.

The spectrum of complications after LDLT is similar to conventional transplantation. However, some problems are more frequent in the LDLT recipients. The most common problem specific to the recipient of an LDLT is biliary complications, i.e. bile leak and biliary stricture, which are two- to threefold more common compared with DD transplantation. At our center, the incidence of biliary problems following DD transplantation is 15% compared with 44% in LDLT patients (see Fig. 12.5). Bile leak after surgery is common because thousands of biliary radicles are transected and exposed on the cut surface of the right hepatic lobe. In our experience, the postoperative biliary leaks are often self-limited and do not require interventions such are cholangiography and/or reoperation. Moreover, as surgical technique continues to improve, so should the rate of complications with LDLT.

Table 12.2 *Characteristics of Living Donor and Deceased Donor recipients*

	Living Donor Recipients (%)	Deceased Donor Recipients (%)
Age >65	7.8	8.4
Body mass index >31 kg/m²	11.6	21.3
MELD score >30	1.3	12.5
Hospitalized in ICU	10.0	13.7
Previous transplant	2.5	9.5

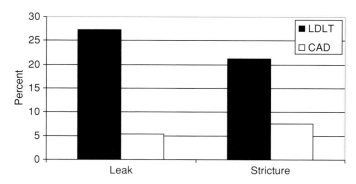

Fig. 12.5 *Biliary complications in living donor and deceased donor recipients.*

The outcomes of LDLT patients infected with hepatitis C are controversial. Some centers have shown that hepatitis C recurs earlier and is more severe in LDLT patients compared with cadveric patients. However, other data suggest that there is no difference in outcome. There are inherent problems in assessing the results in hepatitis C-infected LDLT recipients including small numbers of recipients to evaluate, limited follow-up relative to the natural history of hepatitis C, differences in patient selection between centers, and differences in severity-of-illness at transplant between LDLT and DD recipients. However, at our center, we are cautious in the selection of HCV-infected recipients for LDLT. In our opinion, patients selected for LDLT should have a well-defined medical urgency to warrant LDLT, because recurrent HCV following transplantation may lead to early loss of the graft.

■ DONOR OUTCOMES

There is also a small, but measurable, risk of complication in the donor related to the donor hepatectomy. However, the exact risk to the donor is not known because of the absence of a national database to track such outcomes. Donor complications have been assessed primarily through single-center reports and surveys that may underestimate the severity and prevalence of complications. The most important complication is donor death. Although the exact risk is unknown, the estimated risk of donor death is between 1/100 and 1/500. In addition, nonfatal complications are reported in 10–20% of donors, the most common of which is biliary problems. The most common biliary complication is a bile leak from the cut surface of the liver followed by biliary strictures. Other complications that may be seen in the donor, which are common with all major abdominal surgeries, include blood transfusion, wound infection, small bowel obstruction, and incisional hernia. However, the full spectrum and incidence of complications will likely increase as the duration of follow-up in living donors increases over time. The incidence and severity of complications in donors must be considered as the greatest disadvantage of this procedure and must be considered in the selection of recipients for this procedure. The National Institutes of Health have recently initiated a multicenter prospective trial that will prospectively measure donor (and recipient) outcomes in a large cohort of patients. As discussed later, the results of this study, which will be concluded in several years, will likely provide the most comprehensive picture of donor problems related to this procedure.

The impact of hepatectomy on donor quality of life, one of the most important outcomes of LDLT, has been assessed in several studies. These reports are single-center outcomes in relatively small numbers of patients (fewer than 100). In general, donors have been able to return to their predonation employment about 10 weeks after surgery. Almost all donors have been happy with their decision to donate. However, most donors experience mild ongoing abdominal discomfort related to the surgery. A comprehensive evaluation of the effects of the donor hepatectomy on donor quality of life awaits a prospective study in a larger number of patients (see discussion later).

■ THE FUTURE OF LDLT

During the rapid phase of growth of LDLT after 1997, some surgeons at large LDLT programs projected that up to 50% of all transplants would be performed using living donors and that this procedure could significantly reduce the growing shortage of donor organs in the USA. However, the rapid phase of growth of LDLT has not been sustained. Currently, living donors account for close to 5% of all liver transplants, not 50%. In fact, the number of LDLTs in the USA decreased from its peak of 518 in 2001 to 361 in 2002 and 321 in 2003. The reasons for the decrease in the number of LDLTs are complex and not entirely clear. One reason is related to concern over donor safety. Following the well-publicized death of a living liver donor in 2001, some surgeons may have simply decided that the risk to the donor outweighed any potential benefit for the recipient and therefore decided not to perform the procedure. Another possible explanation is that the initial rise in LDLTs performed between 1997 and 2001 could reflect a "backlog effect," i.e. programs with large numbers of patients listed for transplantation offered the procedure to all potential candidates shortly after the procedure was recognized as a treatment option. Thereafter, the number of cases decreased because most patients listed for transplantation are not candidates for LDLT.

Perhaps the most important reason for the reduction in LDLTs is that only a small fraction of patients listed for transplantation are able to undergo the procedure. LDLT will likely remain an important, but limited, treatment option for selected patients with ESLD. Perhaps the best candidates for the procedure will be patients who are otherwise ideal candidates for surgery with a clear medical urgency for transplantation. Over time, we have found that two types of patients are ideally suited for this procedure: patients with cholestatic liver disease with rapid decompensation and patients with small hepatocellular carcinoma. The role of LDLT in the field of transplantation will largely be determined by prospective assessment of outcomes of donors and recipients of this procedure. These results are likely to be drawn from an ongoing study funded through the National Institutes of Health. The adult-to-adult LDLT (A2ALL) study is a prospective analysis of LDLT that began enrollment in 2004 and will objectively assess the impact of this procedure on donors and recipients including patient and graft survival, quality-of-life outcomes, and surgical complications. The results of this study will be available in several years and will likely provide a rational basis for the application of LDLT. Until that time, clinicians should continue to use their clinical judgment and maintain a generally cautious approach toward this innovative surgical procedure.

■ REFERENCES

1. Trotter JF, Wachs M, Everson GT, et al. Adult-to-adult right hepatic lobe living donor liver transplantation. New Engl J Med 2002;346:1074–1082.

2. Trotter JF. The selection of donors for adult-to-adult living donor liver transplantation. Liver Transpl 2003;9:S2–S7.

3. Ghobrial RM, Busuttil RW. Future of adult living donor liver transplantation. Liver Transpl 2003;9:S73–S79.

Fulminant Hepatic Failure

▼ ▼ ▼ ▼ ▼ ▼ ▼ ▼ ▼

Michael A. Heneghan

■ INTRODUCTION

Fulminant hepatic failure (FHF) describes a pattern of clinical symptoms associated with abrupt arrest of normal hepatic function [1]. The defining state is the presence of hepatic encephalopathy with coagulopathy and jaundice. In many cases, the clinical picture is complicated by cerebral edema, renal impairment, sepsis, and multiorgan failure.

Liver transplantation (LT) is an important treatment option in the management of severe liver failure and constitutes approximately 10% of liver allograft usage in both the USA and Europe. However, the process of selecting appropriate candidates for transplantation rather than relying on intensive care management remains problematic. Prior to reaching a decision in favor of surgery, physicians must be able to identify patients whose prognosis is otherwise poor without operative intervention.

In this chapter we review the clinical and laboratory characteristics that are associated with a poor prognosis in acute liver failure and that accordingly serve as a basis for selecting patients for transplantation. We also consider etiological and management issues including the steps to be taken by physicians prior to the transplant center referral. The minutiae of the critical care of such patients are beyond the scope of this chapter and only key concepts are discussed in detail. The paradigm should, however, be early discussion referral and transfer of patients to the transplant center because the key to successful management and outcome of acute liver failure is the maintenance of other organ function such that the option of transplantation is preserved.

■ DEFINITIONS

The first effort to define FHF was by Trey and Davidson [2] (as part of a surveillance study of liver damage after halothane anesthesia in the USA), who described it as "a potentially reversible condition, the consequence of severe liver injury, with the onset of hepatic encephalopathy within eight weeks of the first symptoms and in the absence of pre-existing liver disease." Within this group of patients are those that present unwell without any symptoms referable to the liver and accordingly it causes difficulty in defining the onset of illness. This definition primarily served to differentiate between patients with true acute deterioration in hepatic failure and those with decompensation or exacerbation of chronic liver disease.

Other definitions have categorized patients into two, and, more recently, into three groups of liver failure [3,4]. These are based on the timing between the development of jaundice and the onset of hepatic encephalopathy. All definitions serve to subdivide patients into prognostic categories.

FHF as defined by Bernau et al. [3] is the development of hepatic encephalopathy within 2 weeks of the onset of jaundice, whereas subfulminant hepatic failure is characterized by the development of hepatic encephalopathy between 2 and 12 weeks after the onset of jaundice. Time considerations have become clear as important indicators of likely progress, and paradoxically groups of patients with the most rapid onset of encephalopathy are those with the best chance of spontaneous recovery. To account for this, an umbrella term of "acute liver failure" has been proposed within which three categories exist [4]. Hyperacute liver failure is used to describe those patients who develop encephalopathy within 7 days of the onset of jaundice. Acute liver failure includes those with a jaundice-to-encephalopathy time of 8 to 28, whereas subacute liver failure is suggested to describe patients with a jaundice-to-encephalopathy time of 5 to 12 weeks. The majority of patients in the hyperacute liver failure group have acetaminophen poisoning but other common causes include acute hepatitis A and B virus infections. The majority of patients within the acute liver failure group have viral hepatitis, whereas the bulk of patients in the subacute liver failure group have non-A, non-B (seronegative) hepatitis. Table 13.1 summarizes the characteristics of patients presenting with each of the three categories of acute liver failure.

For the purpose of this discussion, all patients without preexisting liver disease and who present with jaundice, encephalopathy, and coagulopathy will be termed a fulminant hepatic failure.

■ CAUSES OF FULMINANT HEPATIC FAILURE

The list of potential causes of FHF is long (Table 13.2). Although considerable differences existed in the past pertaining to the etiology of hepatic failure

Table 13.1 *Characteristics of Subgroups and Etiology of Liver Failure in Patients with Acute Liver Failure Classified According to O'Grady et al. (1993)*

	Hyperacute Liver Failure	Acute Liver Failure	Subacute Liver Failure
Encephalopathy	Yes	Yes	Yes
Duration of jaundice (days)	0–7	8–28	29–84
Cerebral edema	Common	Common	Rare
Prothrombin time	Prolonged	Prolonged	Least prolonged
Bilirubin	Least raised	Raised as subacute	Raised as acute
Prognosis	Moderate	Poor	Poor
Acetaminophen	Common	Never	Never
Hepatitis A	Common	Common	Rare
Hepatitis B	Common	Common	Rare
NANB hepatitis	Rare	Common	Common
Idiosyncratic drug reaction	Common	Common	Rare

based on geographical location [3–12], these differences have become less pronounced. In a report from a workshop in the mid-1990s, viral hepatitis accounted for 62% of all causes of acute liver failure in the USA, with hepatitis B being the most common agent [1]. In contrast, a recent publication from the US Acute Liver Failure Study Group involving 17 centers identified acetaminophen toxicity as the most common apparent cause of FHF (39% of cases), with idiosyncratic drug reactions accounting for a further 13% [11]. In contrast to a decade earlier, viral hepatitis A and B combined were implicated in only 12% of cases, whereas 17% of cases of FHF were of indeterminate cause. Hepatitis A virus as a cause of fulminant or subfulminant hepatic failure varies from 13% in the UK to 50% in France and 90% in India [10]. Indeed, in the UK, acetaminophen hepatotoxicity accounted for approximately 70% of all FHF in the 1980s and 1990s [4,5]. However, legislation restricting analgesic pack sizes introduced in September 1998 has changed the pattern of deaths by suicidal overdose with acetaminophen, salicylates, and ibuprofen [12]. Concurrently, the numbers of patients admitted to liver units, listed for LT, and undergoing transplantation for acetaminophen hepatotoxicity have all fallen [12]. Suicidal deaths from acetaminophen and salicylates were reduced by 22% in the year after the change in legislation, and this reduction persisted in the next 2 years. Liver unit admissions and liver transplants for acetaminophen hepatotoxicity were reduced by around 30% in the 4 years after the legislation. Numbers of acetaminophen and salicylate tablets consumed in nonfatal overdoses were reduced in the 3 years after the legislation. Large overdoses were reduced by 20% (9–29%) for acetaminophen and by 39% (14–57%) for salicylates in the

Table 13.2 *Etiology of Acute Liver Failure*

Etiology	Frequency
Viral hepatitis	
A/B, B with D superinfection	Common in developed world
C	Rare
E	Common in endemic areas especially in pregnant women
NANB	Common cause of acute and subacute liver failure
Herpesviruses 1, 2, and 6	Rare except in immunocompromise
Varicella-zoster	Rare except in immunocompromise
CMV/EBV/adenovirus	Rare except in immunocompromise
Hemorrhagic fever viruses	Rare
Drugs	
Acetaminophen	Common
Isoniazid, ketoconazole, tetracycline, cocaine, phenytoin, valproate, carba mazepine, halothane, nonsteroidal anti-inflammatory agents	Relatively common
Herbal remedies	
Germander/chaparal/Jin bu huan	Increasingly common
Others	
Veno-occlusive disease/Budd–Chiari	Common
Wilson's disease	Rare
Pregnancy-related liver disease	Rare
Acute fatty liver/HELLP/liver rupture	
Circulatory failure/ischemic hepatitis	Rare if less than 50 years old
Amanita phalloides	Rare
Malignancy/leukemia	Rare
Heatstroke	Rare

second and third years after the legislation. Ibuprofen overdoses increased after the legislation, but with little or no effect on deaths [12].

Currently, there are over 200 formulations containing acetaminophen in the USA. With increasing acetaminophen use, higher rates of morbidity and mortality have been seen in patients with accidental overdose than in patients who attempted suicide, even though the latter group had ingested more acetaminophen [11,13]. This is accounted for by higher frequency of chronic alcohol abuse, starvation, or by concomitant ingestion of other enzyme-inducing drugs such as phenytoin, carbamazepine, primidone, phenobarbital, rifampicin, and isoniazid [13,14]. Hepatitis C virus rarely causes acute hepatitis in the developed world [7,15] but has been reported in as many as 50% of patients with acute liver failure in some series from Japan and Taiwan [6,8]. In contrast, hepatitis E virus as a cause of FHF is common in subtropical areas, especially in pregnant women, where it is associated with high mortality.

■ MANAGEMENT OF FULMINANT HEPATIC FAILURE

Severe FHF once established follows a predictable course. For this reason, it is appropriate to consider in advance treatment options in such patients. The principles of management of FHF include:

1. Recognition of the tempo of liver failure with attention to the rapidity of onset of encephalopathy from the appearance of jaundice.
2. Establishment of likely etiology (history, physical examination, laboratory studies, radiology).
3. Institution of antidotes where appropriate.
4. Early discussion with the transplant center.
5. Anticipation and prevention of complications of FHF or aggressive treatment (acidosis, renal failure, sepsis, cerebral edema, circulatory failure) where established.
6. Institution of organ support (ventilatory, renal replacement therapy (RRT), inotropes, bioartificial liver/extracorporeal liver assist device (ELAD)).
7. Early consideration of transplantation (orthotopic auxiliary, living donor).

■ MAKING THE DIAGNOSIS

There is no substitute for a detailed clinical history from the patient, a close relative, or a friend. This should include history of recent surgery, prescribed drug intake, transfusions, extent of alcohol intake, recreational drug ingestions (e.g. amphetamines, cocaine), family history, travel history, sexual practice, and exposure to jaundice. Issues such as the premorbid personality should be also discussed as some patients may not be appropriate transplant candidates based on a history of severe psychiatric disease or multiple previous suicidal attempts. In one recent series, over 25% of potential candidates fulfilling transplant criteria for FHF were denied based on past psychiatric history alone [16].

Treatment of FHF for the most part follows general supportive care guidelines, but notable exceptions occur especially in patients whose disease results from specific hepatotoxic insults. The use of antidotes is pertinent in patients with acetaminophen or carbon tetrachloride (CCl$_4$) poisoning in whom even late administration of N-acetylcysteine (NAC) is potentially life-saving [17].

In patients who have consumed the wild death cap mushroom *Amanita phalloides*, penicillin and silibinin may prevent death [18]. Such patients present with marked muscarinic symptoms followed by a period of wellness and subsequent FHF. Transplantation may be the only option if diagnosis and treatment is delayed beyond 12 h of ingestion. The use of NAC may be potentially useful in other cases of fulminant hepatic liver failure, where its benefit arises not from donation of sulfur groups but rather from its antioxidant effects, which prevent the inflammatory response initiated by oxidative damage, and by improvement in microcirculatory blood flow through restoration of normal vascular responsiveness to endothelial-derived relaxing factor. This concept has been the source of recent dispute [19,20].

Syndromes causing FHF that merit further attention include FHF occurring in the context of pregnancy. Liver dysfunction, especially prolongation of the prothrombin time (PT), should trigger expeditious delivery in all cases irrespective of etiology (hypertension-related liver disease, HELLP syndrome, acute fatty liver of pregnancy) [21]. A trial of labor per vaginum can be attempted in selected cases that have no evidence of encephalopathy. In general, the paradigm of management should be parenteral steroid administration to aid maturation of the fetal lung followed by early delivery. Severe unrecognized liver disease may be present and delay in delivery can result in catastrophic consequences including hepatic infarction, subcapsular hematoma, liver rupture, and death. Successful LT has been carried out for FHF occurring in this setting.

In any patient who presents with a marked transaminitis and coagulopathy, it is important also to consider whether or not patients might be presenting with FHF of unusual cause. In some situations such as an acute presentation of Wilson's disease, prognosis without LT is dismal and a high index of suspicion should be present among young adults with FHF of unknown cause with Coomb's negative hemolytic anemia [22]. Although Kayser–Fleischer rings representing copper deposition in Descemet's membrane of the cornea are associated with the condition, they are not pathognomonic and absence thereof should not preclude diagnosis and transplantation. Other useful clues to the diagnosis may be the presence of an elevated serum bilirubin concentration that is out of proportion compared with other hepatic enzymes, a low normal alkaline phosphatase, moderate transaminitis, and a low uric acid level (resulting from a renal tubular defect from copper accumulation).

In contrast to acute presentation of Wilson's disease where LT is appropriate, patients who demonstrate an unusual presentation of other disease processes need to be carefully excluded from transplantation. This includes etiologies such as infiltrative liver disease from acute leukemia, lymphoma, breast carcinoma, melanoma, or oat cell tumors of the lung [23]. Other etiologies that preclude transplantation include ischemic/hypoxic hepatitis and liver failure occurring in the setting of severe sepsis [24].

■ PROGNOSIS WITHOUT LIVER TRANSPLANTATION

In considering further management of these patients, particularly those with grade III or IV coma, specific factors need to be examined in relation to listing for transplantation. Several criteria have been defined, but the commonest in use (King's College Hospital (KCH) and Clichy criteria) are outlined in Tables 13.3 and 13.4, respectively [3,5]. Both sets of criteria offer specificity of 90% in

Table 13.3 *Criteria Adapted for Identifying Patients Who Are Considered for Transplantation in King's College Hospital, London (King's criteria), see O'Grady et al. (1989) [5]*

Acetaminophen

pH <7.30 (irrespective of encephalopathy grade after volume resuscitation)

or

PT >100 s (INR >6.5) + serum creatinine >300 μmol/L

if in grade III or IV coma

Nonacetaminophen

PT >100 s (INR >6.5) (irrespective of encephalopathy grade)

or

Any three of the following (irrespective of encephalopathy grade):

1. Etiology (NANB/indeterminate hepatitis/halothane/drug reaction)

2. Age <10 or >40 years.

3. Jaundice-to-encephalopathy interval >7 days.

4. PT >50 s (INR >3.5)

5. Serum bilirubin >300 μmol/L

Wilson's disease

Encephalopathy alone in patient with FHF

Budd–Chiari syndrome

Encephalopathy and renal failure in patient with FHF

Table 13.4 *Clichy Criteria for Listing for Orthotopic Liver Transplantation Proposed by Bernau et al. (1986) [3]*

Age <30 years	Confusion or coma + factor V level <20%
Age >30 years	Confusion or coma + factor V level <30%

predicting mortality from FHF. Other authors have suggested that LT should be tentatively offered to all patients who have grade III or IV encephalopathy, but the decision to proceed to transplant should be deferred until an organ is identified for that patient [25]. An alternative proposal suggests performing volumetric computed tomography (CT) among patients in whom doubt exists and transplanting all patients whose liver volume is less than 700 ml; repeating CT examinations and observation of patients with a volume between 700 and 900 ml; and not transplanting patients whose liver volume is greater than 900 ml [25]. The latter two concepts have not been subjected to rigorous prospective evaluation.

The difficulty with most currently applied criteria is that they fail to predict those patients who do not need LT. Blood lactate levels may reflect both hepatic dysfunction and the degree of tissue oxygenation in patients with FHF [26]. Threshold values that best identified individuals likely to die without transplantation were derived from a retrospective initial sample of 103 patients with acetaminophen-induced FHF and applied to a prospective validation sample of 107 patients. Predictive value and speed of identification were compared with those of KCH criteria. In the initial sample, median lactate concentration was significantly higher in nonsurviving patients than in survivors both in the early samples (8.5 vs. 1.4 mmol/L, $P < 0.0001$) and after fluid resuscitation (5.5 vs. 1.3 mmol/L, $P < 0.0001$). A threshold value of 3.5 mmol/L applied to the validation sample early after admission had sensitivity of 67%, specificity of 95%, positive likelihood ratio of 13, and negative likelihood ratio of 0.35. Combined early and postresuscitation lactate concentrations had similar predictive ability to KCH criteria but identified nonsurviving patients earlier in the clinical course. Addition of postresuscitation lactate concentration to KCH criteria increased sensitivity from 76% to 91% and lowered negative likelihood ratio from 0.25 to 0.10. Therefore, arterial blood lactate measurement rapidly and accurately identifies patients who will die from acetaminophen-induced FHF and its use could improve the speed and accuracy of selection of appropriate candidates for transplantation.

■ MANAGEMENT ISSUES

Given the general lack of treatments of certain efficacy, except in those cases in which an antidote can be administered, the most fitting place for management of the patient with FHF is the intensive care unit (ICU). Although criteria for admission to intensive care facilities differ from center to center, any patient with altered mental status in conjunction with a prolongation in PT should be managed in this setting on the basis that further deterioration is likely and may occur precipitously, and that the development of complications may be pre-empted by early recognition of other organ system dysfunction. The issues of greatest import in the management of patients with FHF are discussed further.

General Considerations

All patients should have a urinary catheter inserted, cardiac monitoring insti-tuted, and a triple lumen central venous catheter inserted. The most appropriate routes of venous access are the internal jugular and femoral vein approaches. In patients with severe coagulopathy, the subclavian vein should be avoided. In most instances, an arterial line for hemodynamic monitoring and blood sam-pling should be inserted and Swan–Ganz pulmonary artery pressure monitoring should be undertaken in any patient in whom arterial hypotension exists and/or urine output is poor. Intubation and ventilation should be considered early in any patient with grade III or IV encephalopathy. Despite profound coagulopa-thy, bleeding is rarely a problem in patients with FHF and fresh frozen plasma should only be given if active bleeding occurs. The foremost difficulty in treating coagulopathy is that it disallows interpretation of the PT as a prognostic indicator especially in patients with acetaminophen-induced FHF. In contrast, platelet infusions are appropriate in the setting of thrombocytopenia and severe coagulopathy for all procedures.

Intracranial Hypertension

Cerebral edema leading to intracranial hypertension occurs in between 50% and 80% of patients with severe FHF (grade III or IV coma) in whom it is a leading cause of death. Customary measures include placement of the patient in a quiet area with the head elevated at 10–20° above the horizontal. In general, sedation of any kind should be avoided in the early stages of coma. Assisted ventilation should be undertaken in all patients with grade III or IV coma. Gagging, fevers, seizures, arterial hypertension, agitation, head turning, and endotracheal suction are all associated with elevations in intracranial pressure (ICP) and should be avoided. Although paralysis may be needed if patients are particularly difficult to ventilate or if severe hypoxia exists, para-lyzing agents should be avoided as seizure activity may be masked.

Invasive monitoring of cerebral pressure using the Camino fiber-optic catheter tip system is used most commonly used in patients with FHF, and if aggressive correction of coagulopathy and thrombocytopenia is carried out prior to insertion of the extradural monitor, its use is associated with few complications. In most centers including our own, it is inserted in patients who have developed pupillary abnormalities or in patients with grade III/IV coma who are to undergo transplantation. When used in conjunction with jugular venous bulb oxygen saturation measurement, it allows accurate assessment of cerebral perfusion and oxygenation.

The goals of management should be to maintain cerebral perfusion pressure (CPP) greater than 40 mmHg and mean arterial pressure >60 mmHg. In many centers, a CPP of less than 40 mmHg for 2 successive hours is a contraindication to transplantation, although frequent successes have been reported in patients with CPP below this level for longer periods of time. Surges in ICP above 20 mmHg for greater than 5 min or pupillary changes should be treated with mannitol given as a bolus over 30 min (0.5–1.0 g/kg, 20% solution) [27]. A recent novel approach to the management of elevated ICP in FHF is the establishment of moderate hypothermia (in keeping with the principles of neurosurgical management of cerebral trauma victims); however, these promising observations need confirmation prospectively [28].

Close attention should also be paid to serum electrolytes such as magnesium, calcium, and sodium. In a recent randomized controlled trial, the effect of induced hypernatremia to maintain serum sodium concentrations of 145–155 mmol/L using 30% hypertonic saline was examined [29]. In patients randomized to hypertonic saline, norepinephrine dose requirement was less and ICP decreased significantly relative to baseline over the first 24 h. Moreover, the incidence of intracranial hypertension, defined as a sustained increase in ICP to a level of 25 mmHg or greater, was significantly higher in the control group. The objectives of therapy in all cases are to avoid cerebral herniation and the occurrence of fixed dilated pupils on examination.

Circulatory Disturbance

Patients with FHF typically have poor oral intake prior to hospitalization and are dehydrated and hemoconcentrated. Paradoxically, vasodilatation and capillary leak may also be present as a result of Gram-negative sepsis and cytokine release from liver necrosis. Additionally, increased muscle tone and a stress response results in release of epinephrine [27]. The clinical situation is usually one of volume depletion and hypotension in a patient with warm peripheries and tachycardia. The principles of management relate to volume resuscitation with colloid while avoiding high arterial pressure associated with the development of cerebral edema. A pulmonary capillary wedge pressure of 12–14 mmHg is desirable.

The hypotension observed in FHF is frequently seen in association with a reduction in systemic vascular resistance and a hyperdynamic circulation. If pulmonary artery pressures remain low, vascular filling is required and if it persists despite this, fungal or bacterial sepsis should be suspected and treated prophylactically. If arterial hypotension persists and urine output is low, norepinephrine may be required to restore arterial pressure. Prostacyclin, a microcirculatory vasodilator, causes a fall in systemic vascular resistance but mean arterial pressure is maintained by virtue of significant increases in cardiac output. Prostacyclin use results also in an increase in both oxygen delivery and oxygen consumption, suggesting a marked tissue oxygen debt exists in patients with FHF. NAC also results in improving cardiac output and oxygen delivery in FHF [19].

Metabolic and Renal Disturbance

Hypoglycemia occurs early in the clinical course of FHF and results from impaired gluconeogenesis, an inability to mobilize glycogen stores, and an increase in circulating insulin. Blood glucose levels should be monitored every 4–6 h in patients with FHF and the blood sugar concentration maintained using 10% and 20% dextrose solutions. Patients with FHF should also be fed via the enteral route if possible: nasogastric feeding is appropriate in ventilated patients. Hypophosphatemia and hypomagnesemia are seen in those who maintain urine output.

Metabolic acidosis is a frequent finding in FHF. Although originally attributed to liver dysfunction and impaired lactate metabolism, it has been established that much of the acidosis is related to the presence of tissue hypoxia and increased peripheral lactate production. RRT may be appropriate in this situation even prior to the development of renal failure.

Renal failure (urine output <300 ml/24 h) occurs in up to 70% of severe acetaminophen-induced FHF and 30% of FHF from other causes [5,27], with sepsis, hypovolemia, and reduced intravascular filling important contributory factors in its development. Initial management should consist of aggressive volume loading and if oliguria persists "renal dose" dopamine can be instituted. If no effect occurs, intravenous furosemide infusion may be tried. However, it is unlikely that any of these approaches will be successful in the anuric patient, and this should prompt early consideration of RRT.

RRT of some form should be instituted if acidosis, fluid overload, hyperkalemia, or a rising creatinine develops. Access should be achieved via a double-lumen catheter. Continuous venovenous hemodiafiltration (CVVHD) or high-volume hemofiltration are the most appropriate forms of RRT. Intermittent hemodialysis should be avoided, as significant hypotension frequently accompanies hemodialysis and critical falls in CPP is detrimental in these cases [27]. An important concept in the management of FHF is the observation that acute liver failure and septic shock share many clinical features, including hyperdynamic cardiovascular collapse. Adrenal insufficiency may result in a similar cardiovascular syndrome. In septic shock, adrenal insufficiency, defined using the short synacthen test (SST), is associated with hemodynamic instability and poor outcome. Abnormal SSTs have been reported in 62% of patients with FHF [30]. Those who required norepinephrine for blood pressure support had a significantly lower cortisol increment following synacthen compared with patients who did not. Moreover, increment and peak cortisol concentrations following SST were lower in patients who required ventilation for the management of encephalopathy. In addition, increment was significantly lower in those who fulfilled liver transplant criteria or who died compared with those who survived.

Sepsis

Severe immunocompromise typically accompanies FHF, and prevention of infection is a major goal in the management of such patients. Daily blood cultures should be drawn in all cases. In prospective studies, typical markers of infection such as fever and leukocytosis are frequently absent in these patients even in the presence of positive blood cultures [31]. In the same study in whom 80% of all patients had an organism identified, a further 10% had suspected infection without positive cultures. The commonest sites of infection in patients with FHF are chest, urinary tract, sites of cannulae, and intravenous lines. Infection occurs early in the clinical course but also accounts for approximately 25% of late deaths in patients with FHF [31]. The commonest organisms identified are *Staphylococcus aureus* and *Escherichia coli*, whereas *Pseudomonas aeruginosa* is commonly isolated from culture after prolonged intensive care stay.

Fungal sepsis may be identified in up to one-third of patients with FHF [32]. *Candida albicans* is the commonest organism identified and invariably occurs concomitantly with bacterial infection [32]. Change in clinical status should result in collection of culture materials from all body fluids and close attention to antimicrobial cover. The use of prophylactic antibiotics is controversial and their institution should probably be deferred until clinically indicated. However, a recent study of 227 consecutive patients with stage I–II encephalopathy prospectively enrolled in the US Acute Liver Failure Study Group examined the role of infection as a factor in progression of encephalopathy [33]. On multivariate analysis, acquisition of infection during stage I–II encephalopathy was a predictive factor for worsening encephalopathy in patients with acetaminophen-induced FHF. In patients who progressed to deep encephalopathy, the first confirmed infection preceded progression in 15/19 acetaminophen patients and in 12/23 nonacetaminophen patients. In patients who did not demonstrate positive microbiologic cultures, a higher number of components of the systemic inflammatory response syndrome (SIRS) at admission was associated with more frequent worsening of encephalopathy. The use of prophylactic antibiotics in these patients and the mechanisms by which infection triggers hepatic encephalopathy clearly requires further investigation. If prophylaxis is to be administered, ceftazidime with dicloxacillin is probably the most appropriate antibiotic cover [34], although gut decontamination has not been found to add extra benefit to treatment regimens [34].

■ ORTHOTOPIC, AUXILIARY, AND LIVING-RELATED TRANSPLANTATION IN FHF

Apart from the conventional techniques of orthotopic liver transplant procedures utilized for treatment of FHF, some novel approaches to liver replacement therapy have occurred as a result of organ shortage. These include auxiliary LT whereby a lobe of liver from the patient with FHF is removed and replaced with a cadaveric lobe [35]. Following transplantation, immunosuppression is instituted in a similar fashion as for a conventional liver transplant recipient. Over subsequent months, the native liver regenerates and when normal liver function has recovered, immunosuppression is withdrawn to facilitate regeneration of the native liver and atrophy of the transplanted lobe. The goal of this type of surgery is to enable the transplant recipient to have a life free of immunosuppression.

An alternative approach has been living donor LT of either the complete right or the left hepatic lobes in adult patients, and left lateral segments (segments 2 and 3 of the left hepatic lobe) in children [36,37]. In general, 1-year patient survival for patients transplanted for FHF is approximately 65% irrespective of the type of liver graft utilized. A recent review of the United Network for Organ Sharing (UNOS) liver transplant database from 1990 to 2002 identified 15% of transplant recipients with FHF having a drug implicated as the etiology of their acute liver failure at the time of liver transplant during the study period [38]. One-year patient and graft survival for the entire cohort was 77% and 71%, respectively. These results reflect the severity of the disease process pretransplant. Where median waiting times for organs are short, actuarial 1-year survival can approach 95% [39]. These survival data reiterate the value of early referral and transfer.

■ STEPS IN REFERRAL PRIOR TO TRANSFER

Criteria to define which patients with FHF should be transferred from nontransplant to transplant centers are unclear, but the keys to survival are early contact, frequent discussion with the transplant center, early initiation of intensive care management, and early transfer if appropriate. With this in mind, all patients with encephalopathy of any grade, acidosis, prolonged PT, rising creatinine, and rising bilirubin should be discussed with the transplant center. Indeed, the absence of encephalopathy should not discourage contact. A further issue to clarify at an early point in discussions is the preferred transplant center of the patient's insurance carrier, as this will avoid reduplication of effort. Referral should not be delayed while a diagnosis is being sought, the label of FHF being sufficient to warrant discussion regarding transfer to the transplant center.

Although delay may exist on the part of the transplant center, it is usually in the context of arranging accommodation, and communication should continue by frequent phone contact. In the interval between referral and transfer, key pieces of data can be obtained such as blood group, HIV status, hepatitis serology, acetaminophen levels, ultrasound examination of the liver, and past medical and psychiatric history. In contrast to patients with chronic liver disease, the need for urgent clarification on these issues is vital. Table 13.5 summarizes the appropriate steps in referral. Contraindication to transplantation does not preclude transfer. Undeniably, greater resources can be made available to FHF patients in a transplant center than in smaller hospitals where management of this complex metabolic disturbance is not commonplace.

◼ ROLE OF ARTIFICIAL LIVER SUPPORT

In the same way that RRT is life-saving among patients with acute renal failure, it is certain that a proportion of patients could recover fully from the syndrome of FHF if supported through the period of extreme organ dysfunction and physiological stress. This could alter the role or need for LT for this disease, allowing regeneration of the damaged liver and recovery of hepatocyte function. With this goal in mind, several systems that show considerable promise including the bioartificial liver (BAL) and the ELAD exist [40–43]. The HepatAssist liver support system is an extracorporeal porcine hepatocyte-based BAL [42]. In a prospective, randomized, controlled, multicenter trial in patients with severe acute liver failure, a total of 171 patients were enrolled. Although there was no statistically significant difference in survival at 30 days between BAL-treated versus control patients for the complete patient cohort, subgroup analysis identified the group of patients with fulminant or sub-FHF as being more likely to benefit from therapy [42]. The molecular adsorbent recirculating system (MARS) is an emerging option for patients with liver failure, which encompasses a cell-free, albumin dialysis device that enables

Table 13.5 *Steps in Referral of Patients to a Liver Transplant Center*

Step I   Determine the following:

    A. The presence of fulminant to hepatic failure.

    B. Detailed history.

    C. Laboratory studies (HIV test, ABO blood group, syphilis, acetaminophen level, etc.).

    D. Radiographic investigation (chest films and liver ultrasound).

    E. Orders for daily blood cultures.

Step II

    A. Discuss possibility of liver transplantation with patient and family.

    B. Identify social support network.

Step III

    A. Contact the patient's insurance carrier.

    B. Identify the preferred transplant center.

Step IV

    A. Contact the transplant team.

    B. Inform transplant team of patient's clinical status.

Step V

    A. Determine means of transportation with the transplant team (air/ground).

    B. Provide transplant team with contact names and numbers (medical/family).

Step VI

    A. Inform the patient and family of the travel arrangements.

    B. Assemble records (history/laboratory data/X-rays) for transfer.

    C. Designate physician family member to travel with patient.

Step VII

    A. Designate physician and nurse to travel with patient.

    B. Assemble adequate resuscitation equipment, fluids, and drugs for transfer.

    C. Anticipate potential complications during transfer.

    D. Inform transplant center of departure and anticipated arrival time.

the removal of albumin-bound substances. The proponents of albumin dialysis postulate that substances such as bilirubin and bile acids, metabolites of aromatic amino acids, fatty acids, and cytokines that may be responsible for some of the systemic manifestations of FHF and might offer either a bridge to transplant or an alternative treatment choice. Despite positive results from nonrandomized trials and case reports, a recent meta-analysis suggests that MARS treatment does not appear to reduce mortality for patients either with FHF or in patients with acute-on-chronic liver failure compared with standard medical treatment [43]. The goal, however, will be to provide a device with longer-term capabilities.

■ REFERENCES

1. Hoofnagle JH, Carithers RL, Jr, Shapiro C, et al. Fulminant hepatic failure: summary of a workshop. Hepatology 1995;21:240–252.

2. Trey C, Davidson LS. The management of fulminant hepatic failure. In Popper H, Schaffner F, eds., Progress in liver failure. New York: Grune and Stratton, 1970:282–298.

3. Bernau J, Rueff B, Benhamou JP, et al. Fulminant and subfulminant liver failure: definitions and causes. Semin Liver Dis 1986;6:97–106.

4. O'Grady JG, Schalm S, Williams R. Acute liver failure: redefining the syndromes. Lancet 1993;342:373–375.

5. O'Grady JG, Alexander GJM, Hayllar KM, et al. Early indicators of prognosis in fulminant hepatic failure. Gastroenterology 1989;97:439–445.

6. Chu C, Sheen I, Liaw Y. The role of hepatitis C virus in fulminant hepatic failure in an area with endemic hepatitis A and B. Gastroenterology 1994;107:189–195.

7. Sallie R, Silva E, Purdy M, et al. Hepatitis C and E in fulminant hepatic failure: a polymerase chain reaction and serological study. J Hepatol 1994;20:580–588.

8. Yoshiba M, Sekiyama K, Inoue K, et al. Contributions of hepatitis C virus to non-A non-B fulminant hepatitis in Japan. Hepatology 1994;19:829–835.

9. Benhamou JP. Fulminant and subfulminant hepatic failure; definitions and causes. In Williams R, Hughes RD, eds., Acute liver failure: improved understanding and better therapy. London: Mitre Press, 1991:6–10.

10. Acharya SK, Dasarthy S, Kumer TL, et al. Fulminant hepatitis in a tropical population: clinical course, cause and early predictors of outcome. Hepatology 1996;23:1448–1455.

11. Ostapowicz G, Fontana RJ, Schiodt FV, et al. Results of a prospective study of acute liver failure at 17 tertiary care centers in the United States. Ann Intern Med 2002;137:947–954.

12. Hawton K, Simkin S, Deeks J, et al. UK legislation on analgesic packs: before and after study of long term effect on poisonings. BMJ 2004;329:1076–1080.

13. Schiødt FV, Rochling FA, Casey DL, et al. Acetaminophen toxicity in an urban county hospital. N Engl J Med 1997;337:1112–1117.

14. Whitcomb DC, Block GD. Association of acetaminophen toxicity with fasting and ethanol use. JAMA 1994;272:1845–1850.

15. Wright TL, Hsu H, Donegan E, et al. Hepatitis C virus not found in fulminant non-A non-B hepatitis. Ann Intern Med 1991;115:111–112.

16. Bernal W, Wendon J, Rela M, et al. Use and outcome of liver transplantation in acetaminophen-induced acute liver failure. Hepatology 1998;27:1050–1055.

17. Harrison PM, Keays R, Bray GP, et al. Improved outcome of paracetamol-induced fulminant hepatic failure by late administration of acetylcysteine. Lancet 1990;335:1572–1573.

18. Klein AS, Hart J, Brems JJ, et al. Amanita poisoning: treatment and the role of liver transplantation. Am J Med 1989;86:187–193.

19. Harrison PM, Wendon JA, Gimson AES, et al. Improvement by acetylcysteine of hemodynamics and oxygen transport in fulminant hepatic failure. N Engl J Med 1991;324:1852–1857.

20. Walsh TS, Hopton P, Philips BJ, et al. The effect of N-acetylcysteine on oxygen transport and uptake in patients with fulminant hepatic failure. Hepatology 1998;27:1332–1340.

21. Heneghan MA. Pregnancy and the liver. In O'Grady JG, Lake JR, Howdle PD, eds., Comprehensive clinical hepatology. London: Mosby, 2000:28.1–28.14.

22. Berman DH, Leventhal RI, Gavaler JS, et al. Clinical differentiation of fulminant Wilsonian hepatitis from other causes of hepatic failure. Gastroenterology 1991;100:1129–1134.

23. Rowbotham D, Wendon J, Williams R. Acute liver failure secondary to hepatic infiltration: a single centre experience of 18 cases. Gut 1998;42:576–580.

24. Henrion J, Minette P, Colin L, et al. Hypoxic hepatitis caused by acute exacerbation of chronic respiratory failure: a case-controlled, hemodynamic study of 17 consecutive cases. Hepatology 1999;29:427–433.

25. Van Thiel DH. When should a decision to proceed with transplantation actually be made in cases with fulminant or subfulminant hepatic failure: at admission to hospital or when a donor organ is made available? J Hepatol 1993;17:1–2.

26. Bernal W, Donaldson N, Wyncoll D, et al. Blood lactate as an early predictor of outcome in paracetamol-induced acute liver failure: a cohort study. Lancet 2002;359:558–563.

27. Ellis A, Wendon J. Circulatory, respiratory, cerebral and renal derangements in acute liver failure: pathophysiology and management. Semin Liv Dis 1996;16:379–388.

28. Jalan R, Damink SW, Deutz NE, et al. Moderate hypothermia for uncontrolled intracranial hypertension in acute liver failure. Lancet 1999;354:1164–1168.

29. Murphy N, Auzinger G, Bernal W, et al. The effect of hypertonic sodium chloride on intracranial pressure in patients with acute liver failure. Hepatology 2004;39: 464–470.

30. Harry R, Auzinger G, Wendon J. The clinical importance of adrenal insufficiency in acute hepatic dysfunction. Hepatology 2002;36:395–402.

31. Rolando N, Harvey F, Brahm J, et al. Prospective study of bacterial infection in acute liver failure: an analysis of fifty patients. Hepatology 1990;11:49–53.

32. Rolando N, Harvey F, Brahm J, et al. Fungal infection: a common, unrecognised complication of acute liver failure. J Hepatol 1991;12:1–9.

33. Vaquero J, Polson J, Chung C, et al. Infection and the progression of hepatic encephalopathy in acute liver failure. Gastroenterology 2003;125:755–764.

34. Rolando N, Wade JJ, Stangou A, et al. Prospective study comparing the efficacy of prophylactic parenteral antimicrobials, with or without enteral decontamination, in patients with acute liver failure. Liver Transpl Surg 1996;2:8–13.

35. van Hoek B, de Boer J, Boudjema K, et al. Auxiliary versus orthotopic liver transplantation for acute liver failure. EURALT Study Group. European Auxiliary Liver Transplant Registry. J Hepatol 1999;30:699–705.

36. Marcos A, Fisher RA, Ham JM, et al. Right lobe living donor transplantation. Transplantation 1999;68:798–803.

37. Miwa S, Hashikura Y, Mita A, et al. Living-related liver transplantation for patients with fulminant and subfulminant hepatic failure. Hepatology 1999;30: 1521–1526.

38. Russo MW, Galanko JA, Shrestha R, et al. Liver transplantation for acute liver failure from drug induced liver injury in the United States. Liver Transpl 2004;10:1018–1023.

39. Ascher NL, Lake JR, Emond JC, et al. Liver transplantation for fulminant hepatic failure. Arch Surg 1993;128:677–682.

40. Detry O, Arkadouopoulos N, Ting P, et al. Clinical use of a bioartificial liver in the treatment of acetaminophen-induced fulminant hepatic failure. Ann Surg 1999;65:934–938.

41. Ellis AJ, Hughes RD, Wendon JA, et al. Pilot-controlled trial of the extracorporeal liver assist device in acute liver failure. Hepatology 1996;24:1446–1451.

42. Demetriou AA, Brown RS, Jr, Busuttil RW, et al. Prospective, randomized, multi-center, controlled trial of a bioartificial liver in treating acute liver failure. Ann Surg 2004;239:660–667.

43. Khuroo MS, Khuroo MS, Farahat KL. Molecular adsorbent recirculating system for acute and acute-on-chronic liver failure: a meta-analysis. Liver Transpl 2004;10: 1099–1010.

Management in the Perioperative Period

The Transplant Operation

Lucas McCormack, Marcus Selzner, and Pierre-Alain Clavien

■ THE DONOR LIVER

Immediate function of a transplanted liver is essential. Unlike in kidney, pancreas, or, to some extent, heart transplantation, there is no effective artificial support for a hepatic patient in the event of graft failure. Without rapid restoration of hepatic function, death from bleeding or cerebral edema generally ensues within 72 h. However, improvements in knowledge of liver physiopathology and the adoption of a new methodology in intensive care unit management have led to progressive improvements in the treatment of patients with liver failure after liver transplantation (LT) [1]. Recovery after LT, indeed, presents a variety of patterns of evolution ranging from early and complete function of the graft to complete absence of liver function, which can lead to patient death when retransplantation is not performed. Although less frequent than for other organs, such as the kidney, primary graft nonfunction (PNF), defined as non-life-sustaining function of the liver graft, leads to death or retransplantation within 7 days [2,3]. Delayed graft function (DGF) defined as impaired liver function responding to support therapy [4] still occurs in some recipients.

One of the known causes of PNF or DGF is poor organ quality at the time of LT, which can depend on the condition of the donor, cold-ischemia time, and the organ preservation method [4]. The development of perfusion preservation solutions has reduced liver damage related to the harvest/storage procedure. The Euro-Collins solution has been replaced by better preservation solutions such as the histidine–tryptofan–ketoglutarate solution (HTK), University of Wisconsin, or Celsior solutions [5,6] with these newer solutions. Cold storage of the liver explant can be extended up to 12–24 h, allowing for better organ allocation and recipient preparation [3].

Donor Selection

Determining the quality of the donor liver in a heart-beating cadaver remains imprecise; careful attention to the circumstances of the donor's death and the function and morphological characteristics of the organ prior to harvest is critical [7]. The ideal donor can be described as 50 years old or younger; without hepatobiliary disease; with hemodynamic and respiratory stability (systolic blood pressure >100 mmHg and central venous pressure >5 cm H_2O); with acceptable PO_2 and hemoglobin level; without severe abdominal trauma, systemic infection, hypernatremia, or cancer; with diuresis >50 mL/h and normal creatinine; and with low requirement of inotropic drugs. However, this ideal donor is far from the norm and many potential donors are older than 60 years, hemodynamically unstable, and have been treated in the intensive care unit for more than 5 days [8]. In the University Hospital of Zurich more than two-thirds of the cadaveric liver grafts are from marginal donors.

The increase in number of liver transplant candidates and the dramatic rise in waiting list mortality have led to the adoption of a more aggressive approach to organ recruitment, introducing a greater potential risk for postoperative graft dysfunction. Although there is a large body of evidence to show that older donors and fatty livers significantly increase the incidence of PNF or initial poor function of the hepatic allograft, the present donor shortage has encouraged the use of marginal livers and grafts from elderly donors [9]. Abnormal liver test function, long stay in the intensive care unit, hemodynamic instability (prolonged hypoxia or hypotension), donor age over 65 years old, and steatosis are no longer absolute contraindications for organ retrieval [8,9]. Moreover, the progressive expansion of liver-splitting techniques has introduced additional new variables relative to longer harvesting times and parenchymal handling that may influence postoperative graft recovery.

No single parameter defines the acceptability of a donor for organ harvest, donor livers are usually discarded when there is a combination of factors that predicts poor function [9]. The decision to accept or reject a donor liver also must take into consideration the severity of the recipient disease and the urgency of the donor organ. Personal inspection of the liver and histological examination of a liver biopsy performed by an experienced transplant surgeon and pathologist can be very helpful in reaching a decision.

Matching Donor and Recipient

Only donor and recipient ABO types are usually matched according to the standard rules. An additional issue is that of size compatibility. Smaller organs are easily adapted to a large recipient but the opposite is not true. Size reduction of an adult liver or the use of segments was initially implemented only to overcome the need for size-matched grafts in pediatric recipients. Usually segments 2 and 3 or the left hemiliver are used, allowing up to 1/10 weight mismatch between the donor and the recipient weight. The remaining liver was discarded and this procedure led to a shift in donor organs from adults to children. Therefore, living-related LT was introduced as a logical extension of reduced-size and segmental LT [10].

As a next step, split LT was implemented [11,12]. This technique allows a whole liver to be divided into two allografts and therefore the total number of grafts to be increased. However, the incidence of vascular and biliary complications, as well as PNF rates, was higher than after whole organ transplantation. The reason is that splitting of the liver is a time-consuming procedure usually associated with a longer cold-ischemia time and with the risk of some rewarming. Thus, selection of high-quality organs and low-risk recipients is mandatory. Although this procedure could dramatically shorten the waiting list for transplantation, it can be performed in only a small proportion of "optimal" livers (15–20%). Splitting the liver in situ and carefully transecting the bile duct for the left liver or the left lateral segment close to the parenchyma without damaging the vasculature of the right bile duct usually help to reduce cold-ischemia time and prevent biliary complications [13]. Liver transplantation of two adults using a split-liver graft has been also performed [11]. A small recipient must be selected for the left hemiliver since only grafts with more than 1% of the liver volume/recipient body weight ratio or more than 40% of the native liver volume are considered sufficient. The transplanting of less than 1% can be dangerous and could render an elective patient a highly urgent retransplantation. Therefore, such a procedure must be considered very carefully and carried out only in centers with experience in major liver surgery as well as segmental graft LT. The right hemiliver of a living-related adult donor has been also increasingly used over the past few years [14]. This offers an optimal graft with controlled ischemia times, but this strategy is associated with significant risk for the living donor [15].

The Procurement

The procurement of the liver should be performed by an experienced surgeon, with particular care taken to optimize organ viability of the heart-beating cadaver. Cardiovascular and respiratory instability is suggested by the necessity for vasopressor support, poor blood gas values, or other adverse findings familiar to intensive care physicians. If such donors are unstable or if the heart stops beating before the patient has been transferred to the operating room, the kidney might be the only suitable organ for transplantation. However, most brain death donors can be maintained and improved with conventional intensive therapy and then an attempt can be made to coordinate the needs of surgeons who perform transplantation to allow multiple cadaveric organ procurement. Adequate management of the donor prior to and during the harvesting is very important to achieve immediate hepatic function after LT. The surgeon must be aware of common problems of resuscitation including excessive use of vasopressor drugs, prolonged acidosis, hypoperfusion from hypovolemia, persistent anemia, and uncorrected hypernatremia.

A flexible procedure for multiple cadaveric organ procurement should allow excision of various organ combinations without jeopardy to any of the individual grafts. The guiding principle is to avoid warm ischemia of any potential graft. This is achieved by carefully timed and controlled infusion of cold solutions into anatomic regions, the limits of which are defined by preliminary meticulous surgical dissection.

Removal of thoracoabdominal organs must be coordinated with the abdominal team. The organ procurement is generally performed through a midline incision from jugular notch to pubis including median sternotomy. The long incision provides good exposure for removal of the heart, lungs, kidneys, pancreas, small bowel, and the liver. The liver is inspected to be sure that its color and texture are normal. Anomalies are looked for, of which arteries to the left liver from the left gastric artery or to the right liver from the superior mesenteric artery are the most frequent. Failure to complete the arterial revascularization of the graft due to unrecognized aberrant arterial supply is poorly tolerated after cold storage, leading to PNF or acute biliary problems in the recipient.

Complete mobilization of the liver is not required as for a liver resection since a part of the diaphragm in contact with the liver is also resected. The retroperitoneal space is entered by incising the peritoneal reflection of the ascending colon, cecum, and distal part of the small intestine. The distal part of the cava and aorta are dissected free and encircled. The inferior mesenteric vein is ligated and a cannula is placed up to the main portal vein. The left triangular ligament of the liver may be incised and the upper part of the abdominal aorta is encircled just above the origin of the celiac axis (Fig. 14.1). Additional cannulas are placed in the distal part of the aorta and the inferior vena cava. The clamped aortic and portal cannulas are attached to an air-free infusion system through which chilled preservation infusion can later be infused. The clamped vena cava cannula is attached to tubing that leads to a bleeding bag on the floor. When all the teams involved in the harvesting are ready to proceed with the procurement, the aorta is cross-clamped (Fig. 14.1). The cannulas of the portal vein and inferior aorta containing the chilled preservation solution are immediately open to perfuse intraabdominal organs. The effluent is drained out through the inferior vena cava cannula to the bag on the floor. The right atrium is also opened as an extra precaution against overdistention of the liver. Anesthesiologist support is stopped. Topical ice

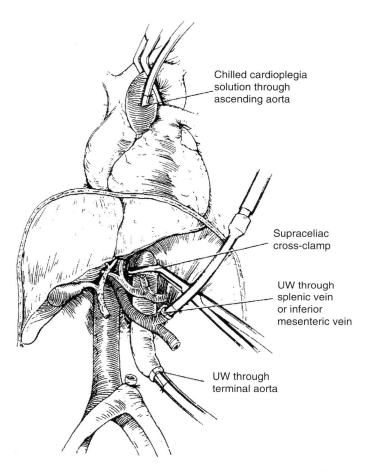

Chilled cardioplegia
solution through
ascending aorta

Supraceliac
cross-clamp

UW through
splenic vein
or inferior
mesenteric vein

UW through
terminal aorta

Fig. 14.1 *Schema of the donor procedure showing the placement of the cannulas for perfusion during multiorganic procurement.*

slush is rapidly applied on the abdominal organs. The gallbladder is incised and bile washed out in order to prevent autolysis of the mucosa of the biliary tract. Hepatic extirpation is performed after removal of heart and lungs and before pancreas and kidneys harvesting.

The hepatogastric ligament is divided. Care must be taken to prevent hepatic artery injury or portal vein transection when simultaneous pancreas harvesting is performed. The vena cava is transected below and above the liver with the surrounding cuff of the diaphragm. Particular care should be taken to prevent caval injury during cardiac retrieval. Finally, a portion of the aorta including the celiac axis and the initial part of the superior mesenteric artery is resected en block to complete the removal of the washed-out liver. Both iliac arteries and veins are harvested systematically in case that vascular reconstruction is required.

■ THE RECIPIENT OPERATION

Few surgical procedures require the same fastidious attention to technical details that is necessary in LT. Technical errors translate directly into poor liver function or infectious or biliary complications. Thus, transplantation should be performed only by surgeons proficient in the procedure. In addition, the operative environment should include experienced nursing and ancillary support. Intraoperative management by a knowledgeable anesthesiologist with experience in LT is critical for a successful result. The procedure presents the challenge of maintaining homeostatic temperature, circulation (including oxygen-carrying capacity and coagulation competence), gluconeogenesis, and electrolyte concentration while establishing adequate anesthesia and muscle paralysis with agents not requiring hepatic function for degradation. In the last decade, improvements in perioperative care during LT have permitted avoidance of venovenous bypass (VVB) during the operation in many centers. In cases of LT using the standard technique with resection of the retrohepatic vena cava, the anesthesiologist should maintain an adequate preload during cava occlusion and correct metabolic abnormalities after release of the congested portal circulation. In cases of LT with preservation of the native vena cava, the hemodynamic consequences of the cross-clamping of the inferior vena cava can be avoided. The most important factor predictive of postoperative success is the stability of the patient during the operation and his or her delivery to the intensive care unit normothermic with adequate circulatory competence.

From the surgical point of view, a successful organ engraftment begins with a controlled recipient hepatectomy. This can be a formidable task in individuals with severe portal hypertension and extensive collateral formation or in patients with multiple previous operations. Particular surgical challenges include patients who have undergone a previous liver resection for hepatocellular carcinoma, prior biliary repairs for biliary tract injuries, portosystemic shunts, or prior liver retransplantation. In general, extirpation follows control of the proximal and distal vessels and lysis of all ligamentous attachments. A specific technical concern includes retaining maximal length of all vessels. The length of the bile duct depends of the planned biliary reconstruction: choledochocholedochostomy vs. choledochojejunostomy. Care to prevent injury to the right adrenal gland during caval dissection is important for preventing bleeding.

For many years, VVB was used to prevent congestion and minimize the release of lactate and other by-products of gut hypoperfusion into the portal circulation. In addition, it improved venous return to the heart during implantation and thus improved hemodynamic stability during the period of caval occlusion. However, several disadvantages related to the use of VVB have been reported: longer operative time, transient hypothermia, cannula and incision-related morbidity, hemodilution, and increment of cost [16]. Many centers employ this technique selectively in some patients without portal hypertension or those with hemodynamic instability during intraoperative trial of portal vein and venacaval clamping.

The classic surgical technique for LT requires resection en block of the retrohepatic vena cava with the recipient's liver and cross-clamping of the cava and the portal veins (Figs 14.2 and 14.3). The "piggyback technique" in which the native vena cava is preserved was originally described using transient cross-clamping of the vena cava in conjunction with VVB. The main advantages over the standard technique are to avoid retrocaval dissection, thereby reducing the risk of bleeding and facilitating caval anastomosis in large-for-small size grafts. To avoid the need of VVB, a modification of this technique permitted the preservation of the caval flow by performing a cavocaval anastomosis or using the middle and left hepatic vein cuff with partial vena cava clamping at its anterior face (Figs 14.4 and 14.5) [17]. Caval preservation has gained acceptance in many centers due to its many advantages, including reduced warm ischemia time, improved intraoperative stability, preservation of renal perfusion pressure, and improved postoperative renal function. In addition, splanchnic venous drainage can be maintained through a transient portacaval anastomosis offering several advantages [17,18] including a decrease in the volume of the native liver, which can facilitate difficult hepa-

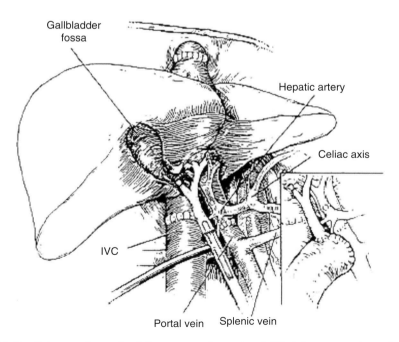

Fig. 14.2 *Schema of standard liver transplantation (LT). The two main techniques for biliary reconstruction are shown: end-to-end cholecocholedochostomy (CC) without T tube and end-to-side Roux-en-Y (RY) hepatojejunostomy.*

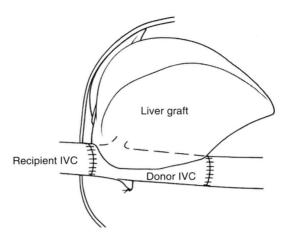

Fig. 14.3 *Liver transplantation using the standard technique with resection of the retrohepatic vena cava. IVC: inferior vena cava.*

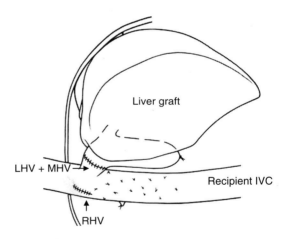

Fig. 14.4 *Liver transplantation with preservation of the recipient inferior vena cava: anastomosis using the middle and left hepatic vein. LHV: left hepatic vein; MHV: middle hepatic vein; RHV: right hepatic vein; IVC: inferior vena cava.*

tectomies. The reduction in portal vein pressure may reduce bleeding, and by avoiding mesenteric congestion, a portacaval shunt promotes hemodynamic stability. This is particularly useful in patients with metabolic disease or fulminant hepatic failure who lack adequate portosystemic collateral in the splachnic area. Nowadays, with all these techniques available, the surgical team can select the optimal technique for each particular patient.

The implantation technique in the classical operation begins with the supra-hepatic caval anastomosis, followed by the infrahepatic caval anastomosis (Figs 14.2 and 14.3). If the cava was preserved, the donor cava can be anasto-mosed either side-to-side or end-to-side with the recipient vena cava (Figs 14.4

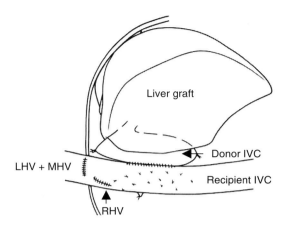

Fig. 14.5 *Liver transplantation with preservation of the recipient inferior vena cava: side-to-side cavocaval anastomosis. LHV: left hepatic vein; MHV: middle hepatic vein; RHV: right hepatic vein; IVC: inferior vena cava.*

and 14.5). When present, the temporary portacaval shunt is taken down. The operation then proceeds to the portal anastomosis as soon as possible to reduce warm-ischemia time of the new liver. Before reperfusion, the liver must be washed out of the hyperkalemic and adenosine-rich Wisconsin preservation solution. Starzl et al. [19] describe flushing the liver via the portal vein with lactated Ringer's solution and then allowing the liver to be reperfused with blood without venting of the vena cava. Others had advocated a 200–300 cc blood flush through the portal vein, with venacaval venting after all venous connections are established but with the suprahepatic cava temporally occluded [20,21]. Both techniques attempt to reduce the release of potassium in the circulation and to ameliorate the postreperfusion syndrome [22]. The hepatic artery anastomosis is the final vascular step in the procedure. Some groups advocate simultaneous arterial and venous reperfusion, arguing that it decreases reperfusion injury and late biliary strictures [23].

The biliary tract reconstruction can be carried out according to two main techniques (Fig. 14.2). The duct-to-duct anastomosis with a cholecocholedochostomy (CC) has become the most widely employed technique of biliary reconstruction and can be performed end-to-end or side-to-side depending on the anatomic situation or the surgeon preference [24]. The Roux-en-Y (RY) hepatojejunostomy is used mostly in some special situations as listed in Table 14.1.

The CC has several advantages over RY: easier to perform, faster, avoids an additional jejunal anastomosis, preserves Oddi's sphincter function, results in more physiological biliary reconstruction, and provides an easy access for subsequent biliary manipulation using endoscopic transpapillary approach.

Table 14.1 *Indications for Roux-en-Y hepatojejunostomy*

- Retransplantation
- Insufficient length of the bile duct
- Small-size pediatric recipient
- Severe mismatch in donor and recipient common bile duct size
- Disease of the extrahepatic bile ducts
    - Primary or secondary sclerosing cholangitis
    - Biliary atresia
    - Bile duct injury
    - Cholangiocarcinoma

Surgical dictum has been to drain biliary anastomosis. The traditional CC over a T tube allows the evaluation of the bile flow and bile quality (color and viscosity) in the immediate posttransplant period. This approach has three additional theoretical advantages as well as a number of disadvantages. First, the tube has the potential to divert the bile and control a biliary fistula when there is a leak in the CC. Second, the drain has the potential to stent the CC and prevent strictures at the anastomotic site. Finally, the T tube provides access for visualization of the biliary tree [25].

Although the T tube may prevent a biliary fistula, its placement may be associated with a leak at the T tube insertion site in the immediate postoperative period or at the time of removal, dislodgment, or cholangitis from partial obstruction [26]. A 2001 randomized trial of CC with or without T tube after LT showed a higher complication rate in the first group (33% vs. 15%); 60% of the complications were related to the presence of the T tube [27]. Bile leakage and cholangitis occurred more frequently in the T tube group (10% vs. 2% and 28% vs. 0%, respectively); the occurrence of early and late strictures did not differ between the two groups [27]. The advantage of being able to visualize the biliary tree must be weighed against the complication rate related to the T tube and the performance of unnecessary cholangiograms. T tube cholangiography tends to become a routine procedure, with occasional cholangitis despite the use of prophylactic antibiotics [27,28]. Access to the biliary tract with a T tube is no longer a justification for its use given the existence of safe and effective procedures for biliary exploration (percutaneous or endoscopic).

A 1999 trial compared end-to-end and side-to-side CC after LT without T tube and showed that the type of biliary anastomosis is of little relevance to the incidence of biliary tract complications [24]. Nowadays, in most of the centers, when it is feasible, the standard procedure for biliary reconstruction is the direct end-to-end CC without stenting to avoid T tube-related biliary complications.

The intraoperative mortality rate is currently very low. Most intraoperative deaths occur in high-risk patients such as those with fulminant liver failure. Blood loss and requirement for transfusion have also decreased significantly with better selection of patients and increased experience with the procedure. Although the blood requirement can still be very high in cases with previous biliary surgery, retransplantation, or previous liver resection, most of the patients receive less than 5 units of packed red blood cells.

■ IMMEDIATE POSTOPERATIVE MANAGEMENT

Postoperative intensive care unit management is similar to that following any major procedure. Ventilatory support and volume replacement are standard. Isolation is not required beyond standard universal precautions. No sedation is given until extubation. For unclear reasons, postoperative pain is usually mild; any discomfort should alert one to possible complications. Monitoring of serum liver test values is critical; increasing abnormalities or failure of liver test values suggest PNF or technical complications such as hepatic artery thrombosis, acute Budd–Chiari syndrome, or portal vein thrombosis. Examination of portal vein and hepatic artery flow by Doppler ultrasound is routinely indicated within the first 24 h after LT or in case of suspicion of any vascular complication. When the evaluation with ultrasound is unclear an urgent angiogram must be done to exclude hepatic artery thrombosis. Early diagnosis with immediate surgery is the only factor separating a return to normal liver function from graft necrosis and death.

Drain management and perioperative antibiotic prophylaxis are not different in this operation from that in any other major abdominal procedure. Closed suction drains should be used and removed early after the threat of postoperative hemorrhage and bile leak is over. One day of antibiotic prophylaxis is appropriate with an agent with adequate skin and biliary organism. Prophylaxis of infection with *Pneumocystic carini*, toxoplasmosis, cytomegalovirus, and Candida may be done according to each center's protocol. Patients with chronic hepatitis B virus infection require special treatment with gamma globulin. Two- or three-drug immunosuppression therapy is started depending on the decision of a multidisciplinary team. Patients are discharged when they are familiar with their medication. Those patients whose homes are more than 2 h from the transplant center must stay in the vicinity of the transplant center for an additional 2–4 weeks. Close monitoring of hepatic function, immunosuppression level, and medical compliance is continued weekly for 4 weeks and then once every 3 weeks until corticoid therapy is completely stopped. After 2–3 months of outpatient control, the patient's care is remanded to their referring physician for long-term follow-up. It is important to establish open lines of communication between the community physician and the transplant center to ensure early diagnosis and referral of postoperative complication and rejection.

■ **REFERENCES**

1. Azoulay D, Samuel D, Adam R, et al. Paul Brousse liver transplantation: the first 1,500 cases. Clin Transpl 2000;14:273–280.

2. Ploeg RJ, D'Alessandro AM, Knechtle SJ, et al. Risk factors for primary dysfunction after liver transplantation – a multivariate analysis. Transplantation 1993;55(4):807–813.

3. Cavallari A, Cillo U, Nardo B, et al. A multicenter pilot prospective study comparing Celsior and University of Wisconsin preserving solutions for use in liver transplantation. Liver Transpl 2003;9(8):814–821.

4. Avolio AW, Agnes S, Chirico AS, et al. Primary dysfunction after liver transplantation: donor or recipient fault? Transplant Proc 1999;31(1–2):434–436.

5. Janssen H, Janssen PH, Broelsch CE. UW is superior to Celsior and HTK in the protection of human liver endothelial cells against preservation injury. Liver Transpl 2004;10(12):1514–1523.

6. Nardo B, Beltempo P, Bertelli R, et al. Comparison of Celsior and University of Wisconsin solutions in cold preservation of liver from octogenarian donors. Transplant Proc 2004;36(3):523–524.

7. Loinaz C, Gonzalez E. Marginal donors in liver transplantation. Hepatogastroenterology 2000;47(31):256–263.

8. Rull R, Vidal O, Momblan D, et al. Evaluation of potential liver donors: limits imposed by donor variables in liver transplantation. Liver Transpl 2003;9(4):389–393.

9. Verran D, Kusyk T, Painter D, et al. Clinical experience gained from the use of 120 steatotic donor livers for orthotopic liver transplantation. Liver Transpl 2003;9(5):500–505.

10. de Santibanes E, McCormack L, Mattera J, et al. Partial left lateral segment transplant from a living donor. Liver Transpl 2000;6(1):108–112.

11. Azoulay D, Castaing D, Adam R, et al. Split-liver transplantation for two adult recipients: feasibility and long-term outcomes. Ann Surg 2001;233(4):565–574.

12. Azoulay D, Marin-Hargreaves G, Castaing D, et al. Ex situ splitting of the liver: the versatile Paul Brousse technique. Arch Surg 2001;136(8):956–961.

13. Yersiz H, Renz JF, Farmer DG, et al. One hundred in situ split-liver transplantations: a single-center experience. Ann Surg 2003;238(4):496–505; discussion 506–507.

14. Tanaka K, Kiuchi T, Kaihara S. Living related liver donor transplantation: techniques and caution. Surg Clin North Am 2004;84(2):481–493.

15. Miller CM, Gondolesi GE, Florman S, et al. One hundred nine living donor liver transplants in adults and children: a single-center experience. Ann Surg 2001;234(3):301–311; discussion 311–312.

16. Chari RS, Gan TJ, Robertson KM, et al. Venovenous bypass in adult orthotopic liver transplantation: routine or selective use? J Am Coll Surg 1998;186(6):683–690.

17. Belghiti J, Ettorre GM, Durand F, et al. Feasibility and limits of caval-flow preservation during liver transplantation. Liver Transpl 2001;7(11):983–987.

18. Figueras J, Llado L, Ramos E, et al. Temporary portocaval shunt during liver transplantation with vena cava preservation. Results of a prospective randomized study. Liver Transpl 2001;7(10):904–911.

19. Starzl TE, Groth CG, Brettschneider L, et al. Orthotopic homotransplantation of the human liver. Ann Surg 1968;168(3):392–415.

20. Fukuzawa K, Schwartz ME, Acarli K, et al. Flushing with autologous blood improves intraoperative hemodynamic stability and early graft function in clinical hepatic transplantation. J Am Coll Surg 1994;178(6):541–547.

21. Brems JJ, Takiff H, McHutchison J, et al. Systemic versus nonsystemic reperfusion of the transplanted liver. Transplantation 1993;55(3):527–529.

22. Millis JM, Melinek J, Csete M, et al. Randomized controlled trial to evaluate flush and reperfusion techniques in liver transplantation. Transplantation 1997;63(3):397–403.

23. Post S, Palma P, Gonzalez AP, et al. Timing of arterialization in liver transplantation. Ann Surg 1994;220(5):691–698.

24. Davidson BR, Rai R, Kurzawinski TR, et al. Prospective randomized trial of end-to-end versus side-to-side biliary reconstruction after orthotopic liver transplantation. Br J Surg 1999;86(4):447–452.

25. Ascher NL. Advances in biliary reconstruction after liver transplantation. Liver Transpl Surg 1996;2(3):238–239.

26. Rolles K, Dawson K, Novell R, et al. Biliary anastomosis after liver transplantation does not benefit from T tube splintage. Transplantation 1994;57(3):402–404.

27. Scatton O, Meunier B, Cherqui D, et al. Randomized trial of choledochocholedochostomy with or without a T tube in orthotopic liver transplantation. Ann Surg 2001;233(3):432–437.

28. Ben-Ari Z, Neville L, Davidson B, et al. Infection rates with and without T-tube splintage of common bile duct anastomosis in liver transplantation. Transpl Int 1998;11(2):123–126.

The Difficult Surgical Patient

▼ ▼ ▼ ▼ ▼ ▼ ▼ ▼ ▼

**Robert J. Porte,
Lucas McCormack,
and Pierre-Alain Clavien**

■ INTRODUCTION

Patients who are considered as a candidate for liver transplantation may vary widely in their medical condition as well as their previous medical and surgical history. With growing success rates of liver transplantation a widening of the acceptance criteria for this procedure has been observed. Nowadays, more and more complex patients with concomitant medical disorders and /or previous history are accepted for liver transplantation. Although the surgical technique of liver transplantation has emerged from an experimental therapy to a more standardized and relatively safe procedure, great differences exist in the complexity of the operation among different patients. Various medical conditions and anatomical abnormalities may make the procedure of liver transplantation technically more challenging and demanding than in the "average" case. Anatomical abnormalities associated with additional surgical difficulties include pre-existing thrombosis or stenosis of one or more of the hepatic vessels (i.e. portal vein thrombosis and Budd-Chiari Syndrome). In addition, previous surgical operations in the upper abdomen may not only have resulted in a distorted anatomy, but will also have led to the formation of intra-abdominal adhesions and scar formation, making a liver transplant procedure technically more complex, especially in the presence of portal hypertension and many venous collaterals. These conditions not only affect the technical aspects of the procedure, but are also associated with higher intraoperative blood loss and transfusion requirement [1,2]. Moreover, postoperative morbidity and mortality rates are higher in these difficult surgical patients [1,3].

■ PREEXISTING THROMBOTIC CONDITIONS

Mesenteric Vein or Portal Vein Thrombosis

Adequate inflow of both portal and arterial blood is essential for successful liver transplantation. About 70–80% of the normal blood flow to the liver is provided by the portal vein and the splanchnic venous circulation. Thrombosis of the portal vein may develop gradually in patients with liver cirrhosis [4,5]. Although the etiology of this is unclear, it is believed to be related to decreased or reversed portal vein flow secondary to increased intrahepatic resistance. Thrombosis of the portal vein may be clinically subtle, but usually results in the development of abundant venous collaterals and ascites. In patients with a preexisting thrombosis of the portal vein and/or of its tributaries, it may be difficult to reconstitute adequate portal venous inflow to the graft during liver transplantation [4,5]. In most cases of portal vein thrombosis, only the main stem of the portal vein is occluded and the confluence of the portal vein and splenic vein remains patent. In this situation, blood flow through the splenic vein is usually reversed and blood from the mesenteric veins is shunted to the systemic circulation via the splenic vein and its collaterals to the left renal vein and/or the paraesophageal venous plexus. In general, portal vein thrombosis in patients undergoing liver transplantation is associated with higher than average costs [6].

Various surgical techniques have been described to deal with portal or mesenteric vein thrombosis in liver transplantation (Table 15.1). The first option in this situation is an eversion thrombectomy of the portal vein in

Table 15.1 *Surgical Alternatives for Portal Vein Reconstruction in Patients with Portal or Mesenteric Vein Thrombosis*

Thrombosis limited to the main stem of the portal vein
- Eversion thrombectomy
- Venous extension graft to the confluence of splenic and mesenteric vein
- Venous jump graft to the superior mesenteric vein

Extensive thrombosis of the portal and mesenteric venous system
- Portacaval hemitransposition
- Arterialization of the portal vein
- Anastomis of donor portal vein with the recipient left renal vein
- Combined liver and small bowel transplantation

order to remove all thrombus mass in its lumen [2,7]. A regular end-to-end anastomosis between the portal vein of the recipient can then be performed in most cases. The endothelium of the surgically recanalized portal vein is mostly absent or at least severely injured and it is generally advised to provide anticoagulation postoperatively for 3 months to avoid rethrombosis of the portal vein. When thrombectomy of the portal vein is technically not possible due to long-standing thrombosis and calcification or fibrosis of the portal vein lumen, creation of a "venous jump graft" to the superior mesenteric vein is indicated (Fig. 15.1) [2,5,8]. A segment of the iliac vein, obtained during organ procurement from the donor, can be used to extend the portal vein of the allograft. This "jump graft" can be positioned prepancreatic in a nonanatomical position and subsequently anastomosed with the superior mesenteric vein using an end-to-side technique. When portal vein thrombosis is present and technical problems during the portal anastomosis can be expected, it is advisable to first reconstruct the hepatic artery and reperfuse the liver graft on the arterial circulation.

In rare cases, thrombosis of the splanchnic venous circulation is more extended and includes the portal vein, splenic vein as well as the superior mesenteric vein, and many of its tributaries [7]. In such patients only multiple friable venous collaterals may be present without any suitable vessel for anastomosis with the portal vein of the donor liver. Four alternative surgical procedures have been described to deal with this situation:

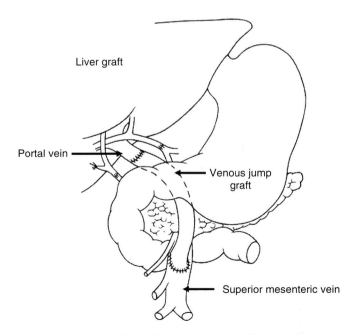

Fig. 15.1 *Venous jump graft from the portal vein to the superior mesenteric vein.*

1. portacaval hemitransposition,
2. arterialization of the portal vein,
3. portal anastomosis with the left renal vein, or
4. a combined liver–small bowel transplant.

Portacaval hemitransposition refers to a direct connection between the infra-hepatic inferior vena cava (IVC) of the recipient and the portal vein of the donor liver (Fig. 15.2) [9–11]. The donor suprahepatic IVC is subsequently anastomosed in a "classical" end-to-end fashion with the IVC of the recipient. The anastomosis between the recipient infrahepatic IVC and the donor portal vein can be either end-to-end or end-to-side. Several groups have reported good short- and long-term outcome in these patients [7,9–11]. Anticoagulation is generally advised in these patients for 3 months. Arterialization of the portal vein can be an acceptable alternative [12,13]. This technique does not seem to have an effect on transplant function. However, the number of successful cases of portal vein arterialization reported in the literature is low, long-term follow up is lacking, and some centers have reported unfavorable results after portal vein arterialization in liver transplantation [14]. The third alternative is a direct anastomosis between the donor portal vein and the left renal vein of the recipient. This technique can be a good alternative in patients with portal vein thrombosis and a previous distal splenorenal shunt [15]. Combined liver

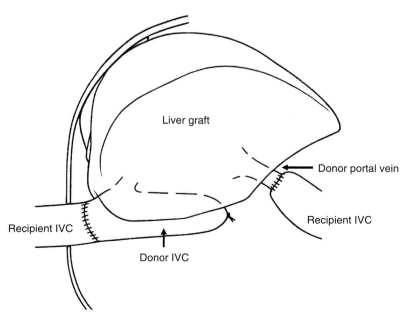

Fig. 15.2 *Portacaval hemitransposition with end-to-end anastomosis between recipient inferior vena cava (IVC) and donor portal vein.*

and small bowel transplantation is indicated in selected patients with concomitant anatomical or functional intestinal failure and dependency on parenteral nutrition. The addition of a small bowel transplant increases the risk of postoperative morbidity and is associated with a lower long-term survival [16]. Main complications after small bowel transplantation are related to infectious conditions due to the direct contact between the small bowel transplant and its nonsterile contents.

Complete absence of the portal vein is a very rare congenital malformation that can be coincidentally found in liver transplant candidates [17]. These patients usually have a large congenital portosystemic shunt, but no portal hypertension and venous collaterals. Although the superior mesenteric in these patients is usually of adequate quality and diameter for direct anastomosis with the donor portal vein, the procedure may be complicated because of formation of massive edema of the viscera during cross-clamping of the superior mesenteric vein [17].

Despite many potential technical difficulties that can be encountered during liver transplantation in patients with extensive portal or splanchnic venous thrombosis, these conditions are no longer considered an absolute contraindication for liver transplantation [2,5]. The best surgical approach may change from patient to patient and is dependent on the anatomical situation as well as on the personal preferences and experience of the surgeon. Studies comparing the various surgical techniques are lacking and most likely will never become available given the low incidence of these conditions.

Hepatic Artery Thrombosis

Adequate arterial inflow to the grafted liver is of paramount importance to avoid ischemic injury of the bile ducts and subsequent biliary complications (see Chapter 21). In the presence of preexisting thrombosis of the hepatic artery, alternative sites should be used for arterial anastomosis with the allograft. The alternative options for hepatic artery anastomosis are summarized in Table 15.2. Most frequently an anastomosis with the abdominal aorta will be made, either directly (if the arterial vasculature of the donor liver is of ad-

Table 15.2 *Surgical Alternatives for Hepatic Artery Reconstruction in Patients with Thrombosis or Severe Stenosis of the Native Hepatic Artery and Celiac Trunk*

Iliac artery conduit to the infrarenal aorta

Indirect anastomosis with the supraceliac aorta via an iliac artery conduit

Direct anastomosis with the supraceliac aorta

Anastomosis with the splenic artery

equate length) or after extension with a donor iliac artery interposition graft [8,18]. Anastomosis with the abdominal aorta can be made below either the origin of the renal arteries (infrarenal) or the cranial from the celiac trunk (supraceliac) (Figs 15.3 and 15.4). Advantage of the anastomosis with the infrarenal aorta is that the liver can first be reperfused on the portal vein, as subsequent cross-clamping of the infrarenal aorta will not lead to a reduction of the portal vein flow. This is in contrast with the situation where the hepatic artery is anastomosed with the supraceliac aorta, at which level cross-clamping of the aorta for constructing the anastomosis will lead to an important reduction in portal vein flow. When the allograft has already been reperfused on the portal vein, cross-clamping of the supraceliac aorta and subsequent reduction of the portal vein flow will lead to additional warm-ischemic injury of the liver as well as the risk of portal vein thrombosis at the site of the anastomosis. On the other hand, a much shorter segment of iliac artery conduit is needed when the anastomosis is made with the supraceliac aorta, compared with the infrarenal aorta. This may facilitate long-term patency of this conduit and the hepatic artery of the graft [18]. Despite acceptable long-term patient survival in these patients, the patency of arterial conduits after liver transplantation is lower than that of direct anastomosis with the native hepatic artery [8,18].

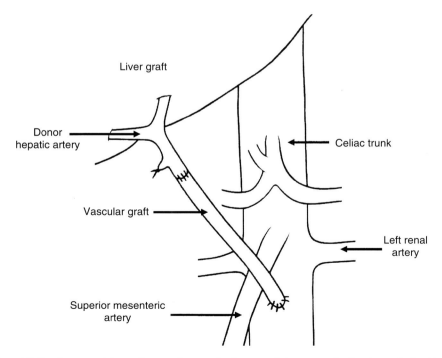

Fig. 15.3 *Interposition of vascular graft for arterial revascularization of the liver graft (infrarenal anastomosis).*

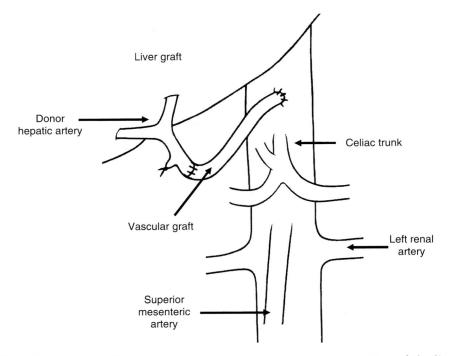

Fig. 15.4 *Interposition of vascular graft for arterial revascularization of the liver graft (supraceliac anastomosis).*

The third alternative for hepatic artery anastomosis is an end-to-end anastomosis with the splenic artery [19]. When using this technique, the recipient splenic artery is dissected free from its origin alongside the pancreas. After obtaining adequate length, the splenic artery is subsequently ligated distally and transsected. The splenic artery is then flipped ventral and toward the right side to facilitate an end-to-end anastomosis with the donor common hepatic artery or celiac trunk. Disadvantage of this technique is that it leads to a 25–40% reduction of blood flow through the portal vein, somewhat increasing the risk of postoperative portal vein thrombosis.

Budd–Chiari Syndrome

Budd–Chiari syndrome is defined as an obstruction of venous drainage of the liver due to various causes, leading to progressive liver damage and portal hypertension [20]. Occlusion may occur at the level of the hepatic veins or the IVC at any point between the entrance of the hepatic veins and the right atrium. Normally, the liver drains into three major hepatic veins and a variable amount of smaller caudate veins that enter directly into the IVC. Pretransplantation occlusion of the hepatic venous drainage, as in Budd–Chiari syndrome, is uncommon and is invariably associated with ascites. In about one-third of the patients no etiological factor can be identified, whereas hematological disorders are identified as the cause of venous occlusion in about 40%. The use of oral contraceptives as well as intra- or extrahepatic tumors has been reported in 10–15% of the patients [20]. Patients with Budd–Chiari syndrome may become a candidate for liver transplantation when liver insufficiency develops or ascites becomes irretractable [21–23]. The typical anatomical abnormalities underlying Budd–Chiari syndrome make liver transplantation in these patients technically more demanding and risky [22]. Much depends on the level of venous occlusion, and adequate preoperative imaging studies of the vascular anatomy are of paramount importance in these patients. Complete anatomical visualization can obtained by venocavography or magnetic resonance imaging (MRI) or computed tomography (CT) scanning, using two-dimensional reconstructions. When the occlusion is predominantly situated at the level of the hepatic veins, leaving the IVC unaffected, liver transplantation can usually be performed in a standard fashion. Based on local and personal preference, this can be either the "classical" technique with two end-to-end anastomoses between the recipient suprahepatic and infrahepatic IVC and the donor IVC, or the "piggyback" technique with an end-to-side or side-to-side anastomosis between the recipient and donor IVC [24] (see also Chapter 14). The surgical procedure may become technically more difficult when the suprahepatic IVC is occluded. To ensure adequate venous drainage of the liver allograft a direct end-to-end anastomosis is required between the donor IVC and the right atrium of the recipient. Adequate exposure is of great importance for this procedure and the diaphragm and pericardium may need to be opened alongside the IVC. In most cases this can be achieved through the abdominal approach, and thoracotomy is rarely necessary. Dissection of the IVC, however, may be difficult and time-consuming due to secondary scarring and perivascular inflammation. In addition, massive hypertrophy of the caudate lobe is found in most patients with Budd–Chiari syndrome and this may seriously hinder surgical access to the IVC [23]. Venovenous bypass may be helpful in these patients to decompress the IVC and to reduce congestion of the liver by decreasing portal blood flow through the liver. This may also reduce blood loss in these technically difficult cases. Some patients with Budd–Chiari syndrome may have had previous decompressive surgery, such as portacaval or mesocaval shunt operations [22]. This will present an additional risk factor in these patients, as outlined later. In addition, concomitant thrombosis of the portal vein has found in up to 83% of the patients undergoing liver transplantation for Budd–Chiari syndrome, further increasing the technical challenges in these patients [20–22,25].

Postoperatively, systemic anticoagulation therapy is indicated, especially in patients with an underlying primary hypercoagulability that has led to hepatic outflow obstruction. Early series have shown a high incidence of recurrent obstruction of the hepatic veins in patients who were not treated with long-term anticoagulant therapy [21,22]. Most centers have adopted a protocol with immediate postoperative administration of heparin (either unfractioned or low-molecular-weight heparin) with subsequent conversion to long-term treatment with warfarin. In patients with an underlying myeloproliferative disorder, long-term therapy directed toward this disease should be continued. Anticoagulant therapy is not indicated in patients with obstructing lesions of the IVC or hepatic veins, such as venous webs, which will be completely removed during transplantation and replacement of the IVC. Reported 3-year survival rates after liver transplantation in patients with Budd–Chiari syndrome range from 45% to 88% [20–23,25]. Long-term survival may be influenced by progression of the underlying hematological disorder [23].

Previous Upper Abdominal Surgery

It is well known that previous abdominal operations can make liver transplantation a surgically more difficult procedure due to the intra-abdominal formation of adhesions and fibrosis. In patients with portal hypertension, multiple venous collaterals may develop in the adhesive scar tissue, resulting in excessive blood loss and difficult dissection of the native liver. Most challenging situations can occur in patients with a history of previous hepatobiliary surgery or portosystemic shunt procedure.

Previous Hepatobiliary Surgery

Surgical operations in the liver hilum and/or on the liver itself lead to perihepatic adhesions and scar formation, which makes it more difficult to mobilize the native liver during a transplant procedure. This is particularly relevant after surgery of the hepatoduodenal ligament, such as cholecystectomy and portoenterostomy in children with biliary atresia [26]. Dissection of the hepatoduodenal ligament can be challenging in these children. In addition, scarring of the liver hilum leads to a higher incidence of portal vein fibrosis and subsequent thrombosis in these children. This contributes to portal hypertension and the formation of venous collaterals and neovascularization in the adhesive scar tissue. It is well recognized that blood loss is higher in children with a previous portoenterostomy. However, overall mortality and morbidity are not different for liver transplantation for biliary atresia or other indications in children, such as metabolic disorders [26].

Similar problems of adhesion and perihepatic fibrous scar formation can be encountered in patients who had a previous partial liver resection, for example for a hepatocellular carcinoma. With growing experience and refinements in surgical technique and anesthesiological management, previous hepatobiliary surgery is certainly no longer an absolute obstacle for liver transplantation and in experienced centers long-term outcome is not different from patients without previous surgery in the right upper quadrant of the abdomen.

Portosystemic Shunt Procedure

Portosystemic shunt procedures, such as a splenorenal shunt or a mesocaval shunt, may be indicated in patients with complications of portal hypertension but still relative preserved liver function [27,28]. Although these procedures are nowadays less frequently performed due to the availability of percutaneous transjugular intrahepatic portosystemic shunts (TIPSS) and better medical management of these patients, a shunt procedure may have been previously performed in a transplant candidate. Apart from the intra-abdominal adhesions due to these surgical procedures, these shunts also reduce portal blood flow to the liver. This may, at least theoretically, increase the risk of portal vein thrombosis after liver transplantation. To avoid future problems with the portal vein anastomosis during liver transplantation, an end-to-side or side-to-side portacaval shunt should best be avoided in patients with chronic liver disease. Types of portosystemic shunts that have the least impact on a possible future liver transplant are the distal splenorenal shunt and a well-positioned TIPSS [27,28]. Given the early occlusion rate and the need for constant surveillance, it is generally advised that TIPSS should be reserved for patients with Child C classification of cirrhosis, whereas a distal splenorenal shunt is a safe, durable, and effective treatment in patients with acceptable operative risk and still good liver function [27]. In case of TIPSS it is important that the proximal and distal ends of the metal shunt do not extend too far inside the portal vein and suprahepatic IVC, because this may seriously hamper adequate mobilization and anastomosis of these vascular structures during a future liver transplant procedure [29].

Extreme Hepatomegaly

Some liver diseases, such as polycystic liver disease or large liver tumors, may be associated with extreme hepatomegaly. The presence of an extremely large liver or a large liver tumor makes it technically more difficult to mobilize the native liver, dissect the IVC, and perform the hepatectomy.

Liver transplantation may be indicated in selected patients with polycystic liver disease and disabling or life-threatening secondary complications [30,31]. Rarely, polycystic liver disease results in liver insufficiency, but progressive compression of hilar strictures, such as the portal vein or bile duct, may lead to massive ascites or jaundice. In most cases, this can be managed with a conservative medical or endoscopic management. In selected patients with areas of relatively spared normal tissue in the polycystic liver, partial liver resection may result in (partial) relief of the symptoms and complaints [32]. When complications become life-threatening or when they have a significant impact on the patient's quality of life, liver transplantation can become a therapeutic option [31,33,34]. In these patients, the size of the liver may have become extraordinary and the liver may almost completely fill up the entire abdominal cavity. Liver transplantation in these patients can be technically demanding due to the difficult exposure and dissection of the hilar vascular structures as well as the IVC. Many patients have associated polycystic kidney disease, also affecting renal function. This further hampers the management of these patients. Combined liver and kidney transplantation may, therefore, become the best treatment option in selected patients with polycystic liver and kidney disease.

Extremely large liver size can also be encountered in patients with very large, rare tumors, such as hemangioendothelioma. Liver transplantation may be indicated in selected patients with hepatic hemangioendothelioma [35,36]. These patients normally have a normal liver function and usually do not have coagulation abnormalities, thereby reducing the risk of major bleeding. Once the native liver has been removed, liver transplantation in these patients usually becomes a relatively straightforward procedure.

Late Retransplantation

Retransplantation of the liver is indicated in selected patients with failure of their previous transplant, either acutely or chronically [37,38]. Various causes may lead to failure of a previous liver transplant, including early hepatic artery thrombosis, chronic rejection, nonanastomic biliary strictures, and recurrence of the original disease [38]. When the need for retransplantation is urgent and occurs within a few weeks after primary liver transplantation (i.e. primary nonfunction or hepatic artery thrombosis) the retransplant procedure can be relatively quick and simple. However, in case of a "late" retransplantation (>3–6 months) after primary transplantation, the original liver graft may have become firmly attached to the surrounding organs and structures due to adhesions and fibrous reaction [37,39]. This is particularly true for patients who need retransplantation for chronic rejection or intrahepatic bile duct strictures. In the latter group, patients have frequently been treated with percutaneous biliary catheters, leading to perihepatic adhesions and fibrous tissue formation. Apart from the intra-abdominal adhesions, patients may have received steroids for several years, resulting in more friable blood vessels and weakening of the tissue strength in general. This can complicate a late retransplant procedure and increases the risk for postoperative complications, such as wound-healing complications and infections.

■ **REFERENCES**

1. Bilbao I, Armadans L, Lazaro JL, et al. Predictive factors for early mortality following liver transplantation. Clin Transplant 2003;17(5):401–411.

2. Lerut J, Mazza D, van Leeuw V, et al. Adult liver transplantation and abnormalities of splanchnic veins: experience in 53 patients. Transpl Int 1997;10(2):125–132.

3. Ramos E, Dalmau A, Sabate A, et al. Intraoperative red blood cell transfusion in liver transplantation: influence on patient outcome, prediction of requirements, and measures to reduce them. Liver Transpl 2003;9(12):1320–1327.

4. Gayowski T, Marino I, Doyle H, et al. A high incidence of native portal vein thrombosis in veterans undergoing liver transplantation. J Surg Res 1996;60(2):333–338.

5. Yerdel M, Gunson B, Mirza D, et al. Portal vein thrombosis in adults undergoing liver transplantation: risk factors, screening, management, and outcome. Transplantation 2000;69(9):1873–1881.

6. Filipponi F, Pisati R, Cavicchini G, et al. Cost and outcome analysis and cost determinants of liver transplantation in a European National Health Service hospital. Transplantation 2003;75(10):1731–1736.

7. Manzanet G, Sanjuan F, Orbis P, et al. Liver transplantation in patients with portal vein thrombosis. Liver Transpl 2001;7(2):125–131.

8. Cappadonna C, Johnson L, Lu A, et al. Outcome of extra-anatomic vascular reconstruction in orthotopic liver transplantation. Am J Surg 2001;182(2):147–150.

9. Gerunda GMR, Neri D, Angeli P, et al. Cavoportal hemitransposition: a successful way to overcome the problem of total portosplenomesenteric thrombosis in liver transplantation. Liver Transpl 2002;8(1):72–75.

10. Tzakis A, Kirkegaard P, Pinna A, et al. Liver transplantation with cavoportal hemitransposition in the presence of diffuse portal vein thrombosis. Transplantation 1998;65(5):619–624.

11. Varma C, Mistry B, Glockner J, et al. Cavoportal hemitransposition in liver transplantation. Transplantation 2001;72(5):960–963.

12. Charco R, Margarit C, Lopez-Talavera J, et al. Outcome and hepatic hemodynamics in liver transplant patients with portal vein arterialization. Am J Transplant 2001;1(2):146–151.

13. Stange B, Glanemann M, Nussler N, et al. Indication, technique, and outcome of portal vein arterialization in orthotopic liver transplantation. Transplant Proc 2001;33(1–2):1414–1415.

14. Ott R, Bohner C, Muller S, et al. Outcome of patients with pre-existing portal vein thrombosis undergoing arterialization of the portal vein during liver transplantation. Transpl Int 2003;16(1):15–20.

15. Kato T, Levi D, DeFaria W, et al. Liver transplantation with renoportal anastomosis after distal splenorenal shunt. Arch Surg 2000;135(12):1401–1404.

16. Brown RS, Rush SH, Rosen HR, et al. Liver and intestine transplantation. Am J Transplant 2004;4:81–92.

17. Wojcicki M, Haagsma E, Gouw A, et al. Orthotopic liver transplantation for porto-systemic encephalopathy in an adult with congenital absence of the portal vein. Liver Transpl 2004;10(9):1203–1207.

18. Muralidharan V, Imber C, Leelaudomlipi S, et al. Arterial conduits for hepatic artery revascularisation in adult liver transplantation. Transpl Int 2004;17(4): 163–168.

19. Figueras J, Pares D, Aranda H, et al. Results of using the recipient's splenic artery for arterial reconstruction in liver transplantation in 23 patients. Transplantation 1997;64(4):655–658.

20. Menon K, Shah V, Kamath P. The Budd–Chiari syndrome. N Engl J Med 2004; 350(6):578–585.

21. Klein A, Molmenti E. Surgical treatment of Budd–Chiari syndrome. Liver Transpl 2003;9(9):891–896.

22. Olzinski A, Sanyal A. Treating Budd–Chiari syndrome: making rational choices from a myriad of options. J Clin Gastroenterol 2000;30(2):155–161.

23. Srinivasan P, Rela M, Prachalias A, et al. Liver transplantation for Budd–Chiari syndrome. Transplantation 2002;73(6):973–977.

24. Miyamoto S, Polak W, Geuken E, et al. Liver transplantation with preservation of the inferior vena cava. A comparison of conventional and piggyback techniques in adults. Clin Transplant 2004;18(6):686–693.

25. Min A, Atillasoy E, Schwartz M, et al. Reassessing the role of medical therapy in the management of hepatic vein thrombosis. Liver Transpl Surg 1997;3(4):423–429.

26. Peeters P, Sieders E, de Jong K, et al. Comparison of outcome after pediatric liver transplantation for metabolic diseases and biliary atresia. Eur J Pediatr Surg 2001;11(1):28–35.

27. Abou Jaoude M, Almawi W. Liver transplantation in patients with previous porta-systemic shunt. Transplant Proc 2001;33(5):2723–2725.

28. Jenkins R, Gedaly R, Pomposelli J, et al. Distal splenorenal shunt: role, indications, and utility in the era of liver transplantation. Arch Surg 1999;134(4):416–420.

29. Clavien P, Selzner M, Tuttle-Newhall J, et al. Liver transplantation complicated by misplaced TIPS in the portal vein. Ann Surg 1998;227(3):440–445.

30. Everson G, Taylor M, Doctor R. Polycystic disease of the liver. Hepatology 2004;40(4):774–782.

31. Gustafsson B, Friman S, Mjornstedt L, et al. Liver transplantation for polycystic liver disease – indications and outcome. Transplant Proc 2003;35(2):813–814.

32. Chen M. Surgery for adult polycystic liver disease. J Gastroenterol Hepatol 2000;15(11):1239–1242.

33. Pirenne J, Aerts R, Yoong K, et al. Liver transplantation for polycystic liver disease. Liver Transpl 2001;7(3):238–245.

34. Swenson K, Seu P, Kinkhabwala M, et al. Liver transplantation for adult polycystic liver disease. Hepatology 1998;28(2):412–415.

35. Ben-Haim M, Roayaie S, Ye M, et al. Hepatic epithelioid hemangioendothelioma: resection or transplantation, which and when? Liver Transpl Surg 1999;5(6): 526–531.

36. Lerut J, Orlando G, Sempoux C, et al. Hepatic haemangioendothelioma in adults: excellent outcome following liver transplantation. Transpl Int 2004;17(4):202–207.

37. Facciuto M, Heidt D, Guarrera J, et al. Retransplantation for late liver graft failure: predictors of mortality. Liver Transpl 2000;6(2):174–179.

38. Sieders E, Peeters P, TenVergert EM, et al. Retransplantation of the liver in children. Transplantation 2001;71(1):90–95.

39. Lerut J, Bourlier P, de Ville de Goyet J, et al. Improvement of technique for adult orthotopic liver retransplantation. J Am Coll Surg 1995;180(6):729–732.

Surgical Aspects of Living Donor Transplantation

**Zakiyah Kadry and
Pierre-Alain Clavien**

IVING DONOR liver transplantation (LDLT) is being increasingly used since the first such procedure in the late 1980s for pediatric patients and since the early 1990s after the first right lobe LDLT was performed for an adult patient in Japan [1,2]. With an increasing number of patients benefiting from this procedure, transplant physicians have had to develop their baseline knowledge and experience in all aspects of LDLT, including preoperative workup, intraoperative technique, and the postoperative care of both donors and recipients of LDLT. More patients initially underwent LDLT in Asia and Japan but data from both the European Liver Transplant Registry (ELTR) and the United Network for Organ Sharing (UNOS) have shown an increasing use of LDLT, particularly in adult patients, in the last few years [3,4]. According to UNOS, the number of LDLT procedures reached 511 in 2001, up from 36 in 1993 [3], but decreased in 2002 to 358, probably due to concerns generated by the widely publicized donor death in New York as well as the accumulation of data on donor morbidity and mortality [3,5–7]. However, in view of the large number of patients worldwide who have so far received a liver transplant from a living donor as well as the continued critical organ shortage that will likely result in more centers performing LDLT in order to expand their donor pool and address their waiting list mortality, experience in the care of both donors and recipients of LDLT has become essential.

LDLT requires expertise in both hepatobiliary surgery and liver transplantation. The experience derived from liver resections performed for oncologic indications has been modified in order to apply to the liver transplant setting and the approach to a living donor operation needs to take into account a number of factors that play an important role in the maintenance of priority to donor safety while allowing the necessary criteria for successful transplantation in the recipient. As a result, detailed anatomic planning and volume measurements are essential for this operation. A graft of adequate size with optimal portal and arterial inflow, complete outflow, as well as good biliary drainage is necessary for success in the recipient. In the donor, however, safety is the highest priority and volume measurements need to take into consideration an adequate remnant liver volume in order to avoid postoperative liver insufficiency or dysfunction, while vascular and biliary anatomic mapping is aimed at not compromising these structures in the donor.

GENERAL TECHNICAL CONSIDERATIONS

The pretransplant evaluation of living donors is a multilevel process involving the early recognition of general medical contraindications as well as a detailed psychosocial workup (see Chapters 4 and 12). General donor requirements by most transplant centers are age between 18 and 60 years; ABO blood group compatibility; absence of previous major abdominal surgery; absence of major medical problems such as diabetes mellitus; severe or uncontrolled hypertension; hepatic, cardiac, renal, or pulmonary disease; presence of a demonstrable significant long-term relationship with the recipient; and normal laboratory values such as liver function tests, serum electrolytes, full blood count, and hepatitis A, B, and C serologies [8–11]. General medical and psychosocial contraindications need to be identified early in the donor workup; this chapter, however, will restrict itself to technical issues related to the surgical aspects of LDLT.

Preoperative radiological volume calculations are performed by most transplant centers that undertake LDLT [9–14]. The calculated liver volume using imaging techniques have been shown to differ from intraoperatively measured liver volumes by approximately 3.9–12.5% [13]. Total liver volume has been described as having a relatively constant relation to body weight, ranging between 2% and 2.7% in healthy subjects [14,15]. Outcomes in LDLT are reported in terms of graft-to-recipient weight ratio (GRWR) or graft volume to estimated standard liver volume (ESLV). Both computed and magnetic resonance volumetric analyses allow a preoperative calculation of the volume of the future graft for the recipient and of the remnant liver in the potential donor [14,16]. In terms of outcomes, there appears to be a reduction in overall LDLT recipient survival with smaller graft sizes having a GRWR <0.8%. Kiuchi et al. [17] from the University of Kyoto published their 1- and 3-year actuarial graft survival rates in elective LDLT stratified according to GRWR and showed that the best survival occurred in the group with a GRWR between >1.0% and <3.0%.Lo et al. [18] also reported a 95% survival rate using grafts greater than 40% of ESLV compared with a survival of 40% with graft volumes less than 40% ESLV. Todo et al. [19] published overall results of LDLT from Japan for the period extending from 1991 to 1999 involving 20 centers and 308 adult LDLT procedures. The cumulative 1- and 3-year patient survival rates were stratified according to the ratio of graft volume to standard calculated recipient liver volume (GV/SV). Their results further corroborate the fact that small-for-size grafts (GV/SV of <30% or GRWR <0.6) appear to result in inferior survival compared with larger grafts [19].

In donors, on the other hand, remnant liver volumes <30% of their original total liver volume, or having >15% hepatic steatosis, have been shown to result in a greater prevalence of prolonged cholestasis and infection in the donor [20,21]. The ELTR has also reported a higher incidence of prolonged post-operative liver insufficiency or dysfunction in donors as manifested by abnormal coagulation factors when larger liver volumes are harvested, with right lobe donors having 2.4% incidence of such dysfunction as compared with a 0–0.5% in left liver donors [4].

Estimations of the degree of liver steatosis form an integral part of the LDLT workup. In volume estimations performed prior to LDLT, each percent steatosis is considered to reduce the functional liver mass by an equal percent and is thus subtracted from the total liver volume. This is based on the precept that fat is not functional and therefore does not contribute to the overall hepatic mass. Most centers perform a preoperative liver biopsy to estimate the degree of hepatic steatosis, but some recommend estimations based on donor body mass index or using radiological means to estimate the degree of liver steatosis in view of the 1% risk for serious complication and the need to hospitalize up to 5% of patients from complications associated with liver biopsies [22,23]. The importance, however, of an accurate estimate of the degree of donor liver steatosis is emphasized by the first reported donor death in Japan, which was due to undiagnosed nonalcoholic steatohepatitis. This ultimately resulted in a low remnant residual liver volume estimate of 28% and liver failure in the donor [24].

Recipient LDLT graft function in the early postoperative period appears to be influenced also by the severity of the original liver disease and the degree of portal hypertension; these can negatively impact outcome if a low graft volume is used. Small-for-size syndrome (SFSS) has been described most frequently with low GRWR; it is characterized by prolonged cholestasis, reduced liver synthetic function with persistent prolonged coagulopathy, intractable ascites, decreased bile production, an increased risk for septic complications and is associated with high mortality. Ben-Haim et al. [25] described a 12.5% incidence of SFSS that occurred only in advanced pretransplant Child B or C cirrhotics [25]. Makuuchi et al. [26] also found a higher mortality rate (40%) and prolonged hospitalization in patients with higher MELD scores when reviewing their results in 48 left lobe recipients. More specifically, Shimamura et al. [27] from Sapporo examined portal vein flow in 35 LDLT patients and found higher peak serum bilirubin levels as well as longer hospitalizations in patients with a portal vein flow >260 ml/min/100 g liver graft tissue. Portal venous hyperperfusion has been observed in animal models of SFSS using partial liver grafts [28]. In the experimental animal model, histopathological changes were most marked in the 20–30% partial liver grafts and consisted of almost immediate moderate to severe periportal/septal edema and hemorrhage progressing to rupture and thrombosis of the periportal sinusoids with hepatocyte necrosis and apoptosis in zones 1 and 2 [28]. Ito et al. [29] described poorer outcomes in adult living donor recipients with a GRWR <0.8 in whom the mean portal vein pressure was >20 mmHg early in the first postoperative week, with a significantly worse survival of 38.5% at 6 months, compared with an 84.5% 6-month survival in LDLT patients with portal vein pressures <20 mmHg in the first four postoperative days.

Hepatic arterial buffer response is a term developed in the early 1980s to describe the physiologic regulation of liver blood flow. This basically consists of an inverse response of the hepatic artery to changes in portal vein flow [30,31]. The hepatic arterial buffer response can be seen when doubling the portal vein flow to the liver, resulting in maximal constriction of the hepatic artery. Lowering the portal vein flow on the other hand results in increasing dilation of the hepatic artery in order to maintain vascular perfusion of the liver [30]. Initial observations of this physiologic effect of portal vein flow on hepatic arterial perfusion have been attributed to Child in 1954, to Betz in 1863, and to Gad in 1873 [30]. The term ''hepatic arterial buffer response'' describing this physiologic reflex was eventually coined by Lautt in 1981 [30,31], and present studies looking at intraoperative hepatic arterial and portal blood flows in living donors appear to confirm the same findings in the LDLT setting [27,32–37]. With this observed physiologic response, a variety of flow modification maneuvers have been described in the setting of LDLT in an attempt to improve small-for-size graft outcomes, ameliorate hepatic arterial perfusion, and avoid having to use larger right lobe grafts, which carry an increased donor risk [32,34–37]. Troisi et al. [32,34–38] described splenic artery ligation as a means to reduce high portal vein flow and avoid SFSS, while other authors have recommended inflow modification by creating side-to-side mesocaval, distal splenorenal, or end-to-side portacaval shunts or splenectomy. A lower incidence of SFSS with favorable graft outcomes has been reported by applying these techniques with lower GRWR LDLT grafts.

SFSS is believed to be multifactorial in origin [36]. Although graft size and the degree of patient disease are both assumed to play an important role in the development of SFSS in LDLT, other factors such as recipient and donor age, latent disease in the graft (e.g. underestimated steatosis, ethanol injury), length of warm and cold ischemia, and technical issues such as inadequate outflow reconstructions are all assumed to also impact early graft function and can contribute to the development of SFSS [36]. In terms of graft volume, dual-graft implantation in a single recipient involving the use of either two left liver grafts or a right lobe with a left lateral liver graft from two separate donors has been described in the literature in an attempt to increase the transplanted liver mass and thus avoid an SFSS. This has been mainly implemented in countries where cadaveric liver organs are in short supply [39,40]. Use of marginal LDLT grafts, with a risk for the development of SFSS, should be limited, especially if cadaveric liver transplantation is available. Technical issues such as venous outflow reconstructions are discussed later in this chapter.

■ RIGHT LOBE LIVER TRANSPLANTATION

The use of right lobe grafts involves the harvesting of segments, 5 to 8 inclusive, and is used in adult LDLT as it provides a sufficient functional liver volume needed for an adequate GRWR in the adult recipient. The right liver, however, also represents 60–70% of the total liver volume, and ensuring donor safety is of utmost importance. Technical issues specific to right lobe LDLT relate to the venous drainage of this graft as well as to variations in vascular and biliary anatomy.

The anterior segments, 5 and 8 of the right lobe graft, drain into the middle hepatic vein. With the accrual of experience in right lobe LDLT, it became apparent that congestion caused by inadequate drainage of these two segments can impact significantly graft function and surgical outcome. The group from Tokyo has reported intraoperative clamping of the donor middle hepatic vein and right hepatic artery, with the flow pattern of the anterior sector of the future right lobe being observed by Doppler ultrasonography [41]. In cases of inversion of the portal vein hepatofugal flow, a hepatic venous reconstruction of the right lobe graft is considered necessary. Surgical methods devised to ensure adequate segment 5 and 8 outflow have included the use of venous jump grafts and the harvesting of the right lobe with both the middle and the right hepatic veins [41–48]. The main concern with the inclusion of the middle hepatic vein with the right lobe graft is the development of congestion of segment 4 in the donor. As a result, anatomic criteria contraindicating the harvesting of the middle hepatic vein have been suggested by Belghiti et al. and include the following: the presence of a long common trunk of the middle and left hepatic veins, which would preclude harvesting the middle hepatic vein at its origin; direct drainage of segment 2 and 3 tributaries directly into the middle hepatic vein; and finally a pretransplant estimate of a small remnant liver volume in the donor with a predominant drainage of segment 4 through the middle hepatic vein [46]. By using these criteria, the same group reported no increased morbidity with the harvesting of the middle hepatic vein in their personal series of right donor hepatectomies, with no significant difference in intraoperative blood loss, transaminase, and bilirubin levels as well as donor remnant liver regeneration when compared with patients where the middle hepatic vein was preserved in the donor [46]. Venous jump grafts have been used by some groups to ensure adequate venous drainage of segments 5 and 8 of the right lobe graft, without the risk of segment 4 congestion of the remnant donor liver. Criticisms of this method include technical difficulties when numerous venous branches draining segments 5 and 8 are present, an increased risk of thrombosis of the jump grafts with resultant graft dysfunction, and concerns of prolongation of warm-ischemia time associated with the construction of jump grafts. However, ensuring overall adequate venous drainage of the right lobe graft as a whole is important. Other than congestion of the anterior segments, outflow stenosis has been described in the long-term follow-up of right lobe LDLT recipients and several different approaches have been reported to overcome this problem [49–51]. These have included use of a single wide anastomosis of the donor right hepatic vein to a wide oval cavotomy of the vena cava including the stump of the recipient right hepatic vein, venous patch reconstructions of the donor hepatic veins, or even a double vena cava technique using cryopreserved venous grafts (vena cava or iliac vein branch) [49–51]. In the latter, side holes are made on the cryopreserved vena cava graft to which the donor right and significant short hepatic veins are anastomosed in the backtable in association with a separate cryopreserved vein graft for middle hepatic vein tributaries [49]. The recipient vena cava is then sideclamped and longitudinally incised for anastomosis with the similarly incised cryopreserved vena cava to which the various venous tributaries of the right lobe graft were reconstructed at the backtable. Although such techniques allow a wide connection and greatly simplify the final venous anastomosis between the recipient and the donor graft, long-term follow-up is necessary to check on patency, thrombosis, and stricture rates of such venous grafts.

Other vascular anomalies that can be dealt with ex situ during the backtable reconstruction are the presence of a double right portal vein as well as the presence of two hepatic graft arterial branches. In the case of a double right portal vein, harvesting of the right lobe with the two portal branches on a common patch should not be performed as this can significantly increase the risk of stenosis of the main portal vein in the donor, with resultant thrombosis. The two separate portal vein branches can always be reconstructed on the backtable using a segment of recipient portal vein with its preserved right and left branches [48]. In the case of two arterial branches to the right lobe graft, a backtable arterioplasty using a reversed trunk of recipient hepatic artery can be performed, with the two anastomoses involving the recipient gastroduodenal and common hepatic arteries to the two separate donor vessels [48,52]. The presence of high-grade celiac artery stenosis in the potential donor has been quoted as a contraindication to right lobe living donation [53]. This has been safely performed, however, in cases of isolated and asymptomatic high-grade celiac artery stenosis as long as retrograde vascularization of the donor liver is maintained by careful preservation of the pancreaticoduodenal arcade and the gastroduodenal artery [53].

Biliary complications in right lobe LDLT have been the Achilles heel of this procedure. The reported incidence in recipients of a right lobe graft varies between 8% and 40% [54–57], with the risk increasing if more than one biliary anastomosis is required. In 53% of cases, variations in the biliary tree anatomy, mainly related to the level of insertion of the right posterior segment tributaries, can result in more than one biliary duct orifice on the right lobe allograft [55,58]. Several biliary reconstructions have been described in the recipient of a right lobe graft, such as hepaticojejunostomy, direct end-to-end or end-to-side duct-to-duct anastomoses, or cystic duct and main hepatic duct of the recipient to the donor graft bile ducts [54,59–61]. Although Roux-en-Y hepaticojejunostomy has been considered as the gold standard by most centers, the duct-to-duct biliary anastomosis does offer the advantage of providing easy endoscopic access for both diagnostic and therapeutic purposes. The overall incidence of biliary complications in right lobe LDLT has been reported to vary between 8% and 30% [54,59,61].

Biliary tract complications have also been reported in donors of right liver grafts. These range between a 3% and an 8% incidence, with bile leaks and bilomas forming the major part [4,62,63]. This is partly attributed to technical issues such as disruption of the segment 4 arterial branch, which arises from the right hepatic artery in 15–30% of cases and which should be preserved in a right lobe donor hepatectomy if segment 4 biliary radical ischemia is to be avoided. Biliary stenoses have also been described involving either the donor left hepatic or the main bile duct and have been reported to occur in up to 1–2% of cases [4,62]. In 4% of cases, donor biliary complications have required surgical intervention, endoscopic retrograde cholangiopancreatography, or percutaneous catheter drainage of a biloma [62].

■ LEFT LOBE LIVER TRANSPLANTATION

The left liver graft consists of liver segments 2, 3, and 4 and due to its smaller volume, it is generally reserved for adults weighing less than 60 kg. Two recipient complications associated with left liver LDLT include volume mismatch with a risk of development of SFSS and a risk for graft rotation with resultant venous kinking affecting the venous return from the graft.

In terms of the graft size mismatch, use of an extended left liver graft with the inclusion of segment 1 or caudate lobe has been described as a means of improving the left liver graft volume [64–67]. The increment in liver volume using the extended left liver graft has been estimated to be approximately 5.9–12% [64,65,67]. Technical points related to the procurement of a left liver graft with the caudate lobe include preservation of the thickest and largest vein draining segment 1, division of the portal vein at the portal bifurcation without dissection of its transverse portion in order to maintain the portal caudate lobe branches, isolation of any aberrant left hepatic artery up to the celiac axis, inclusion of the middle hepatic vein with the extended left lobe graft, division of the liver parenchyma at 1 cm to the right of the middle hepatic vein up to the center of the vena cava, and continuation of the transection behind the hilar plate, taking care not to injure any small vessels of the caudate lobe [64]. Takayama et al. [64] recommend the use of the extended left liver graft with the caudate lobe when the predicted graft volume to recipient standard liver volume ratio is expected to be <33%. In situations where the drainage of the caudate lobe into the vena cava is close to the orifices of the left and middle hepatic veins, reconstruction is recommended, and in 20% of cases where there are two caudate short hepatic veins, reconstruction and maintenance of only one such vein is required for recipient graft implantation [65]. When venous drainage of the caudate lobe is not preserved, the caudate lobe has been shown to not regenerate proportionally with the left liver [65,68]. Other technical refinements include the reconstruction of the caudate portal vein branch, which in 30% of cases has been described to originate from the main portal vein rather than its left branch [69].

■ RIGHT POSTERIOR SEGMENT OR LATERAL SECTOR LIVER GRAFTS

Right posterior or lateral sector liver grafts consist of segments 6 and 7 of the right liver. They are much less commonly used due to the technical difficulties associated with the harvesting of such grafts. Right posterior segment grafts have been implemented in situations where the left lobe volume, including the caudate lobe, is too small for safe left liver LDLT in the recipient and the remnant donor liver volume is estimated to be less than 30% of the standard liver volume, thus precluding full right lobe donation [48,70–72]. Thus the indications for procurement of a posterior segment graft include the presence of a donor right liver volume >70% of the estimated total donor liver volume and an estimated volume of the two right lateral or posterior segments that is greater than that of the left liver [70,72]. Also, it is recommended that the right posterior graft should be more than 40% of the recipient's standard liver volume [72].

One of the advantages of the right posterior graft is that the risk of graft rotation is much less than that of a left liver graft, with easy positioning and complete venous drainage [48]. Disadvantages of the right posterior segment graft relate to anatomical variations in vascular and biliary anatomy, which can either preclude or increase the risk of right posterior segment harvesting [70]. Intrahepatic branching of the relevant portal vein, hepatic artery, and biliary drainage of segments 6 and 7 can make procurement of these two segments difficult [70]. Sugawara et al. [71] describe the use of right posterior segment grafts in 6 out of 32 adult LDLT procedures in their institution; complications included a 50% bile leak rate with increased donor blood loss ranging from 427 to 1100 mL, requiring 0–600 mL of autologous blood transfusion. The same group considers that there are no anatomic variations of the bile duct that contraindicate right posterior segment procurement.

In conclusion, experience with right posterior or lateral sector liver grafts is limited with few reported cases. The Tokyo group describes 19 such LDLT grafts as of August 2004, with 18 patients being alive and having normal graft function, while the group from the Asan Medical Center in Seoul, Korea, reports three such cases [70,72]. The technique does offer an expansion of the donor pool in countries where cadaveric liver transplantation is not readily available, and also requires expertise in both liver transplantation and hepatobiliary surgery.

■ REFERENCES

1. Strong RW, Lynch SV, Ong TH, et al. Successful liver transplantation from a living donor to her son. N Engl J Med 1990; 322:1505–1507.

2. Yamaoka Y, Washida M, Honda K, et al. Liver transplantation using a right lobe graft from a living donor. Transplantation 1994;57:1127–1130.

3. OPTN/SRTR. The OPTN/SRTR annual report. Chapter 7: Liver and intestine transplantation, 2003 http://www.optn.org/AR2003/default.htm.

4. www.eltr.org.

5. Miller C, Florman S, Kim-Schluger L, et al. Fulminant and fatal gas gangrene of the stomach in a healthy live liver donor. Liver Transpl 2004;10(10):1315–1319.

6. Brown RS, Jr, Russow MW, Lai M, et al. A survey of liver transplantation from living adult donors in the United States. N Engl J Med 2003;348(9):818–825.

7. Lo CM, Fan ST, Liu CL, et al. Complications and long-term outcome in living liver donors: a survey of 1508 cases in five Asian centers. Transplantation 2003; 75(3S):S12–S15.

8. Fan ST. Donor safety in living donor liver transplantation. Liver Transpl 2000;6(2): 250–251.

9. Trotter JF, Wachs M, Trouillot T, et al. Evaluation of 100 patients for living donor liver transplantation. Liver Transpl 1993;6(3):290–295.

10. Trotter JF, Wachs M, Everson GT, et al. Adult-to-adult transplantation of the right hepatic lobe from a living donor. N Engl J Med 2002;346(14):1074–1082.

11. Pomfret EA, Pomposelli JJ, Lewis D, et al. Live donor adult liver transplantation using right lobe grafts: donor evaluation and surgical outcome. Arch Surg 2001;136(4):425–433.

12. Chen YS, Cheng YF, de Villa VH, et al. Evaluation of living liver donors. Transplantation 2003;75(3 suppl):S16–S19.

13. Settmacher U, Theruvath T, Pascher A, et al. Living-donor liver transplantation – European experiences. Nephrol Dial Transplant 2004;19(suppl 4):iv16–iv21.

14. Kamel IR, Kruskal JB, Warmbrand G, et al. Accuracy of volumetric measurements after virtual right hepatectomy in potential donors undergoing living adult liver transplantation. Am J Roentgenol 2001;176(2):483–487.

15. Henderson JM, Heymsfield SB, Horowitz J, et al. Measurement of liver and spleen volume by computed tomography. Radiology 1981;141:525–527.

16. Cheng YF, Chen CL, Chen TY, et al. Single imaging modality evaluation of living donors in liver transplantation: magnetic resonance imaging. Transplantation 2001;72(9):1527–1533.

17. Kiuchi T, Kasahara M, Uryuhara K, et al. Impact of graft size mismatching on graft prognosis in liver transplantation from living donors. Transplantation 1999;67(2):321–327.

18. Lo CM, Fan ST, Liu CL, et al. Minimum graft size for successful living donor liver transplantation. Transplantation 1999;68(8):1112–1116.

19. Todo S, Furukawa H, Jin MB, et al. Living donor liver transplantation in adults: outcome in Japan. Liver Transpl 6(6 suppl 2):S66–S72.

20. Fan ST, Lo CM, Liu CL, et al. Safety of donors in live donor liver transplantation using right lobe grafts. Arch Surg 2000;135(3):336–340.

21. Marcos A, Ham JM, Fisher RA, et al. Single-center analysis of the first 40 adult-to-adult living donor liver transplants using the right lobe. Liver Transpl 2000;6(3):296–301.

22. Iwasaki M, Takada Y, Hayashi M, et al. Noninvasive evaluation of graft steatosis in living donor liver transplantation. Transplantation 2004;78(10):1501–1505.

23. Rinella ME, Alonso E, Rao S, et al. Body mass index as a predictor of hepatic steatosis in living liver donors. Liver Transpl 2001;7(5):409–414.

24. Akabayashi A, Slingsby BT, Fujita M. The first donor death after living-related liver transplantation. Transplantation 2004;77(4):634–639.

25. Ben-Haim M, Emre S, Fishbein TM, et al. Critical graft size in adult-to-adult living donor liver transplantation: impact of the recipient's disease. Liver Transpl 2001;7(11):948–953.

26. Sugawara Y, Makuuchi M, Kanelo J, et al. MELD score for selection of patients to receive a left liver graft. Transplantation 2003;75(4):573–574.

27. Shimamura T, Tanigichi M, Jin MB, et al. Excessive portal venous inflow as a cause of allograft dysfunction in small-for-size living donor liver transplantation. Transplant Proc 2001;33(1–2):1331.

28. Kelly DM, Demetris AJ, Fung JJ, et al. Porcine partial liver transplantation: a novel model of the "small-for-size" liver graft. Liver Transpl 2004;10(2):253–263.

29. Ito T, Kiuchi T, Yamamoto H, et al. Changes in portal venous pressure in the early phase after living donor liver transplantation: pathogenesis and clinical implications. Transplantation 2003;75(8):1313–1317.

30. Lautt WW. The 1995 Ciba-Geigy award lecture. Intrinsic regulation of hepatic blood flow. Can J Physiol Pharmacol 1996;74(3):223–233.

31. Lautt WW. Mechanism and role of intrinsic regulation of hepatic arterial blood flow: hepatic arterial buffer response (Part 1). Am J Physiol 1985;249(5):G549–G556.

32. Troisi R, Cammu G, Militerno G, et al. Modulation of portal graft inflow: a necessity in adult living-donor liver transplantation? Ann Surg 2003;237(3):429–436.

33. Marcos A, Olzinski AT, Ham JM, et al. The interrelationship between portal and arterial blood flow after adult to adult living donor liver transplantation. Transplantation 2000;70(12):1697–1703.

34. Troisi R, de Hemptinne B. Clinical relevance of adapting portal vein flow in living donor liver transplantation in adult patients. Liver Transpl 2003;9(9):S36–S41.

35. Takada Y, Ueda M, Ishikawa Y, et al. End-to-side portocaval shunting for a small-for-size graft in living donor liver transplantation. Liver Transpl 2004;10(6):807–810.

36. Kiuchi T, Tanaka K, Ito T, et al. Small-for-size graft in living donor liver transplantation: how far should we go? Liver Transpl 2003;9(9):S29–S35.

37. Boillot O, Delafosse D, Mechet I, et al. Small-for-size partial liver graft in an adult recipient; a new transplant technique. Lancet 2002; 359(9304):406–407.

38. Masetti M, Siniscalchi A, Pietri LT, et al. Living donor liver transplantation with left liver graft. Am J Transplant 2004;4(10):1713–1716.

39. Kaihara S, Ogura M, Kasahara F, et al. A case of adult-to-adult living donor liver transplantation using right and left lateral lobe grafts from 2 donors. Surgery 2002;131(6):682–684.

40. Lee S, Hwang S, Park K, et al. An adult-to-adult living donor liver transplant using dual left lobe grafts. Surgery 2001;129(5):647–650.

41. Sano K, Makuuchi M, Miki K, et al. Evaluation of hepatic venous congestion: proposed indication criteria for hepatic vein reconstruction. Ann Surg 2002;236(2): 241–247.

42. Lee S, Park K, Hwang S, et al. Congestion of right liver graft in living donor liver transplantation. Transplantation 2001;71(6):812–814.

43. Ghobrial RM, Hsieh CB, Lerner S, et al. Technical challenges of hepatic venous outflow reconstruction in right lobe adult living donor liver transplantation. Liver Transpl 2001;7(6):551–555.

44. Lee KW, Lee DS, Lee HH, et al. Interposition vein graft in living donor liver transplantation. Transplant Proc 2004;36(8):2261–2262.

45. Kornberg A, Heyne J, Schotte U, et al. Hepatic venous outflow reconstruction in right lobe living-donor liver graft using recipient's superficial femoral vein. Am J Transplant 2003;3(11):1444–1447.

46. Scatton O, Belghiti J, Dondero F, et al. Harvesting the middle hepatic vein with a right hepatectomy does not increase the risk for the donor. Liver Transpl 2004; 10(1):71–76.

47. Lo CM. Technique of right hepatectomy with the inclusion of the middle liver vein. Transplant Proc 2003;35(3):956.

48. Belghiti J, Kianmanesh R. Surgical techniques used in adult living donor liver transplantation. Liver Transpl 2003;9(10 suppl 2):S29–S34.

49. Sugawara Y, Makuuchi M, Akamatsu N, et al. Refinement of venous reconstruction using cryopreserved veins in right liver grafts. Liver Transpl 2004;10(4): 541–547.

50. Sugawara Y, Makuuchi M, Imamura H, et al. Outflow reconstruction in extended right liver grafts from living donors. Liver Transpl 2003;9(3):306–309.

51. Kinkhabwala MM, Guarrera JV, Leno R, et al. Outflow reconstruction in right hepatic live donor liver transplantation. Surgery 2003;133(3):243–250.

52. Marcos A, Killackey M, Orloff MS, et al. Hepatic arterial reconstruction in 95 adult right lobe living donor liver transplants: evolution of anastomotic technique. Liver Transpl 2003;9(6):570–574.

53. Kadry Z, Furrer K, Selzner M, et al. Right living donor hepatectomy in the presence of celiac artery stenosis. Transplantation 2003;75(6):769–772.

54. Kadry Z, Cintorino D, Foglieni CS, et al. The pitfall of the cystic duct biliary anastomosis in right lobe living donor liver transplantation. Liver Transpl 2004;10(12):1549–1550.

55. Egawa H, Inomata Y, Uemoto S, et al. Biliary anastomotic complications in 400 living related liver transplantations. World J Surg 2001;25(10):1300–1307.

56. Sugawara Y, Makuuchi M, Sano K, et al. Duct-to-duct biliary reconstruction in living-related liver transplantation. Transplantation 2002;73(8):1348–1350.

57. Kawachi S, Shimazu M, Wakabayashi G, et al. Biliary complications in adult living donor liver transplantation with duct-to-duct hepaticocholedochostomy or Roux-en-Y hepaticojejunostomy biliary reconstruction. Surgery 2002;132(1): 48–56.

58. Smadja C, Blumgart LH. The biliary tract and the anatomy of biliary exposure. In Blumgart LH, ed., Surgery of the liver and biliary tract. New York: Churchill Livingstone, 1994:11–24.

59. Suh KS, Choi SH, Yi NJ, et al. Biliary reconstruction using the cystic duct in right lobe living donor liver transplantation. J Am Coll Surg 2004;199(4):661–664.

60. Liu CL, Lo CM, Chan SC, et al. Safety of duct-to-duct biliary reconstruction in right-lobe live-donor liver transplantation without biliary drainage. Transplantation 2004;77(5):726–732.

61. Malago M, Testa G, Hertl M, et al. Biliary reconstruction following right adult living donor liver transplantation end-to-end or end-to-side duct-to-duct anastomosis. Langenbecks Arch Surg 2002;387(1):37–44.

62. Pomfret EA. Early and late complications in the right-lobe adult living donor. Liver Transpl 2003;9(10 suppl 2):S45–S49.

63. Beavers KL, Sandler RS, Shrestha R. Donor morbidity associated with right lobectomy for living donor liver transplantation to adult recipients: a systematic review. Liver Transpl 2002;8(2):110–117.

64. Takayama T, Makuuchi M, Kubota K, et al. Living-related transplantation of left liver plus caudate lobe. J Am Coll Surg 2000;190(5):635–638.

65. Sugawara Y, Makuuchi M, Kaneko J, et al. New venoplasty technique for the left liver plus caudate lobe in living donor liver transplantation. Liver Transpl 2002; 8(1):76–77.

66. Sugawara Y, Makuuchi M, Takayama T. Left liver plus caudate lobe graft with complete revascularization. Surgery 2002;132(5):904–905.

67. Hwang S, Lee SG, Ha TV, et al. Simplified standardized technique for living donor liver transplantation using left liver graft plus caudate lobe. Liver Transpl 2004; 10(11):1398–1405.

68. Ikegami T, Nishizaki T, Yanaga K, et al. Changes in the caudate lobe that is transplanted with extended left lobe liver graft from living donors. Surgery 2001; 129(1):86–90.

69. Kokudo N, Sugawara Y, Kaneko J, et al. Reconstruction of isolated caudate portal vein in left liver graft. Liver Transpl 2004;10(9):1163–1165.

70. Hwang S, Lee SG, Lee YJ, et al. Donor selection for procurement of right posterior segment graft in living donor liver transplantation. Liver Transpl 2004;10(9):1150–1155.

71. Sugawara Y, Makuuchi M, Takayama T, et al. Right lateral sector graft in adult living-related liver transplantation. Transplantation 2002;73(1):111–114.

72. Sugawara Y, Makuuchi M. Right lateral sector graft as a feasible option for partial liver transplantation. Liver Transpl 2004;10(9):1156–1157.

Anesthesia

Kerri M. Robertson and Marco Piero Zalunardo

IMPROVED medical evaluation and care of patients with end-stage liver disease (ESLD) and the acceptance of liver transplantation as lifesaving therapy have resulted in the identification of as many as 10–15 000 potential liver transplant candidates in the USA each year. Recipient 1-year survival rates exceed 90%, and as such an increasing number of liver transplant patients have subsequent non-transplant-related surgery. It is inevitable that with increasing frequency anesthesiologists with minimal transplant experience will be requested to participate in the perioperative care of these patients.

■ ANESTHETIC MANAGEMENT OF THE TRANSPLANT CANDIDATE PRIOR TO LIVER TRANSPLANTATION

Perioperative care of potential liver transplant recipients requires an understanding of the physiological processes, metabolic function, and drug disposition in the liver; evaluation and interpretation of liver test results; systemic manifestations and medical management of the major complications of ESLD; identification of risk factors for patients with compensated cirrhosis; and knowledge of the effects of anesthesia on the diseased liver [1–4] (Table 17.1).

Physiological Characteristics

Total hepatic blood flow (HBF) at 1.5 L/min represents about 25–30% of the cardiac output, with contributions from the hepatic artery and portal vein being 25% and 75%, respectively. Under normal conditions, each blood source provides the liver with 50% of its oxygen supply. The portal venous system is

Table 17.1 *Anesthetic Considerations for Patients with Liver Disease*

Physiological processes, biological function, and drug disposition

Interpretation of liver function study results

Acute versus compensated chronic liver failure

Systemic manifestations of ESLD

Major consequences of cirrhosis

  Portal hypertension and complications: variceal hemorrhage, splenomegally,
    spontaneous bacterial peritonitis, sepsis, ascites, hepatorenal syndrome,
    encephalopathy

  Portopulmonary hypertension

  Coagulopathy

  Cholestasis, jaundice

Impact of anesthesia on liver function

  Limited functional reserve

  Hepatic blood flow

  Drug clearance

  Anesthesia-induced hepatitis

  Postoperative jaundice

Risk factors for decompensation in patients with cirrhosis

essentially a passive vascular bed where flow is dependent on perfusion pressure, cardiac output, and resistance in the splanchnic vasculature. Reductions in portal inflow are usually associated with reciprocal vasodilatation of the hepatic artery, thereby maintaining hepatic oxygen supply and total HBF. The liver vasculature also has a vital role as a blood reservoir able to "squeeze" 500–700 cc of blood into the systemic circulation with sympathetic stimulation.

Metabolic Function

Hepatic failure may result in impairment of numerous complex metabolic functions that may significantly impact anesthetic care. The liver plays a critical role in maintaining a normal blood glucose level; hypoglycemia frequently results from failure of gluconeogenesis, insufficient insulin degradation, and a depletion of glycogen stores. Most patients with chronic liver disease are undernourished and fat stores are diminished with impairment of lipid transport and the integrity of cellular membranes.

Ammoniagenesis and removal by urea formation are often impaired, as are interconversions between nonessential amino acids and the formation of plasma proteins. Hypoalbuminemia is very common; albumin is responsible for maintaining a normal plasma oncotic pressure and is the principal binding and transport protein for a large number of drugs. All coagulation factors, with the exception of the von Willebrand factor, are produced by the liver. Cholinesterase is also manufactured in the liver.

Drug Disposition

Most intravenous anesthetic agents are lipid-soluble and undergo biotransformation in the liver to inactive or ionized water-soluble metabolites, which are then excreted in the bile or urine. Mechanisms of altered drug pharmacokinetics in patients with advanced liver disease include impaired hepatocyte function (decreased intrinsic clearance due to impaired cytochrome P450 metabolism and excretory function), decreased HBF, and changes in the apparent volume of distribution. The concentration of the pharmacologically active, unbound fraction of a highly protein-bound drug may be increased, warranting a reduction in drug dosage of 20–50%, depending on the degree of hypoalbuminemia and acidosis. The pharmacodynamic effect produced by interaction between a drug and its receptors is also unpredictable as a result of generalized debilitation, loss of muscle mass, and altered drug sensitivity. In addition, if there is concomitant renal insufficiency, accumulation of drugs or their active metabolites may occur if they are predominantly dependent on the kidney for elimination. These drugs should have their maintenance dosing reduced by 30–50%. Markedly reduced plasma cholinesterase activity may in theory produce prolongation of block and/or clinical toxicity to succinylcholine, mivacurium, and ester-linked local anesthetics.

Although elimination of volatile anesthetic agents depends on minute ventilation and lung perfusion, varying degrees of hepatic biotransformation (halothane 20–45%, enflurane 2.5–8.5%, sevoflurane 3–5%, isoflurane <1%, and desflurane <0.1%) may produce toxic metabolites. Essentially, all anesthetic agents must be titrated cautiously to the desired effect, as alterations in drug disposition make drug handling and clinical response unpredictable.

Liver Tests

Laboratory evaluation of liver function is complicated by the liver's large functional reserve; routine laboratory values may be normal in the presence of significant underlying disease. Abnormality in the results of four common laboratory tests may loosely reflect hepatic dysfunction.

Prothrombin time (PT) measures activity of the extrinsic coagulation pathway requiring fibrinogen, prothrombin, and factors V, VII, and X. Slight changes may reflect severe liver dysfunction as only 20–30% of normal factor activity is required for coagulation. An international normalized ratio (INR) >1.5 if not corrected within 24 h with vitamin K administration implies severe liver disease.

Albumin is produced in the liver and represents the best measure of chronic hepatic synthetic dysfunction, if one excludes increased losses in the urine or gastrointestinal (GI) tract. As a result of its long half-life of 20 days, 3–4 weeks of severe liver dysfunction are required before a significant change in serum level becomes apparent. A serum albumin concentration of 2.5 g/dL clinically impacts colloid oncotic pressure, placing the patient at risk for increased third-space fluid shifts and alterations in protein–drug binding.

Bilirubin is primarily the end product of hemoglobin metabolism. Uptake and transport of unconjugated bilirubin into hepatocytes is followed by conjugation with glucuronide and excretion into bile canaliculi. A total bilirubin concentration greater than 1.5 mg/dL is abnormal, and jaundice is clinically apparent above serum levels of 3.0 mg/dL. Conjugated hyperbilirubinemia reflects hepatocellular dysfunction, intrahepatic cholestasis, or biliary obstruction. If the increase in total bilirubin concentration is primarily unconjugated, hemolysis or defects in uptake, transport, or conjugation are the most likely causes.

Serum ammonia level represents the balance between ammoniagenesis primarily in the gut and kidney and the synthesis of urea by the liver. Since the reserve capacity of the normal liver for urea synthesis is great, elevation of the serum ammonia level usually indicates significant loss of hepatic function. Increased production of ammonia may be seen with hypokaleuria, increased protein intake, decreased bowel transit, or colonic deprivation.

■ TRANSPLANT CANDIDATE WITH ACUTE LIVER FAILURE

The differentiation of acute fulminant liver failure versus an acute exacerbation of chronic liver disease is important with regard to therapeutic and prognostic implications, as not all acute liver failure patients are the same (see Chapter 13). Fulminant hepatic failure is rapidly progressive liver failure with the onset of encephalopathy within 8 weeks of the onset of jaundice in patients without a previous history of liver disease. The mortality rate for intra-abdominal surgery in patients with severe acute hepatic disease approaches 100%. Therefore, all elective surgery should be postponed until the inflammatory process has resolved, as indicated by normal liver function studies. The recovery period may take up to 4 months in patients with severe acute viral hepatitis. For the majority of fulminant failure patients, survival ultimately depends on medical stabilization and urgent liver transplantation.

If emergency surgery is unavoidable, one should proceed cautiously, starting with a detailed comprehensive preoperative evaluation including the cause of liver disease, assessment of hepatic impairment, systemic manifestations, and coexisting illness. Careful attention should be given to fluid replacement and correction of electrolytes (hyponatremia), acidosis, hypoglycemia, and coagulation factor abnormalities. Arterial blood pressure and oxygen saturation should be monitored and the airway protected from aspiration by elective endotracheal intubation in patients with marked confusion or coma. Continuing management of cerebral edema, renal failure, and sepsis may be required (see Chapter 13).

Anesthetic management utilizing maximal monitoring and the fewest agents should be chosen. The goal is to preserve hepatic function by maintaining adequate pulmonary ventilation and cardiovascular homeostasis including cardiac output, blood volume, and perfusion pressure. A reduction in HBF and/or cellular ischemia may result from arterial hypotension, hypovolemnia, hypoxia, hypercarbia, hypocarbia, and sympathetic adrenergic stimulation. Excessive airway pressures may increase intrathoracic pressure, thereby impeding venous return and reducing cardiac output.

Premedication may include a histamine-receptor blocker, metoclopramide, and sodium citrate. Sedatives, especially benzodiazepines (e.g. midazolam), should be omitted. Provided that the patient is hemodynamically stable, the "best" general anesthesia for the liver would include preoxygenation, rapid sequence induction with cricoid pressure, and endotracheal intubation after the administration of fentanyl, propofol or thiopental, and succinylcholine. Potentially hepatotoxic agents should be avoided. All volatile anesthetic agents potentially decrease HBF but are relatively safe if the mean arterial blood pressure and cardiac output are maintained. Isoflurane is the best choice. Drug handling may be extremely variable, so all drug dosages should be reduced and titrated to the desired effect. All opioids may accumulate. Cisatracurium besylate is ideal for muscle relaxation being an intermediate acting drug relatively independent of renal or hepatic function for elimination. Titration of the muscle relaxant using a transcutaneous nerve stimulator is desirable. A strategy for renal protection is crucial [5] (Table 17.2). Patients with encephalopathy grade 3 or 4 and raised intracranial pressure (ICP) will require ICP monitoring and therapeutic intervention (see Chapter 13). The cerebral perfusion pressure should be kept above 60 mmHg, with the arterial pressure transducer positioned at the level of the head.

Neurological and ventilatory function should be evaluated prior to extubation. Patients should be fully awake to reduce the risk of aspiration. Narcotic analgesics administered for postoperative pain relief may worsen hypoxemia by causing pulmonary shunting and alveolar hypoventilation. Postoperative surveillance and care should take place in an intensive care setting. Clinical indicators of suboptimal liver function include persistent hypothermia,

Table 17.2 *Strategic Plan for Optimizing Renal Function and Prevention of Hepatorenal Syndrome [5]*

Initial management

1. Homeostatic environment (electrolytes, acid–base status, hematocrit)
2. Cardiovascular stability (euvolemia, mean arterial pressure > 60 mmHg)
3. Identify intrinsic renal parenchymal disease
4. Treat bacterial infections and complications related to liver disease, i.e. ascites, dilutional hyponatremia, and variceal bleeding
5. Avoid nephrotoxic agents, e.g. NSAID or aminoglycosides

Optimize renal perfusion

1. Intravascular volume expansion
2. Drug therapy (splanchnic vasoconstriction or renal vasodilators): vasopression analogs, α-adrenergic agonists, endothelin antagonists, antioxidants

Strategies

1. Transjugular intrahepatic portosystemic shunt
2. Spontaneous bacterial peritonitis: albumin and antibiotic therapy
3. Severe alcoholic hepatitis: pentoxifylline
4. Plasma expansion after large-volume paracentesis

Renal support

1. Hemodialysis
2. Continuous arteriovenous or venovenous hemofiltration
3. Liver transplantation

coagulopathy, hypocapnia, acidosis, hyperglycemia (later, hypoglycemia), renal insufficiency, hemodynamic instability, acute respiratory distress syndrome (ARDS), and delay in postoperative awakening.

■ TRANSPLANT CANDIDATE WITH CHRONIC LIVER DISEASE

Patients with cirrhosis have a reduced life expectancy. A large natural history study from Innsbruck University showed that the estimated 1- and 5-year survival rates were 95% and 75% for patients with Child–Pugh class B and 85% and 50% for patients with Child–Pugh class C, respectively (see Chapter 1). After the onset of the first major medical complication (ascites, variceal bleeding, jaundice, or encephalopathy), survival rates for these patients were significantly reduced. Given the findings of Gines et al. [6] regarding a median survival rate in compensated versus uncompensated cirrhotics of 8.9 versus 1.6

years, the probability of decompensation may be relatively low, but once decompensation occurs, mortality rates are high.

Child's classification has traditionally been used as a predictive index for operative mortality rate in patients undergoing portosystemic shunting procedures. The high perioperative mortality risk of 10%, 31%, and 76% for Child's class A, B, and C patients, respectively, is also predictive of operative outcome for hepatobiliary procedures and is generally associated with outcome for nonoperative patients. The most current model for end-stage liver disease (MELD) in adults uses a scoring system based on total bilirubin, serum creatinine and INR. It is an accurate predictor of 3-month mortality and a continuous measurement of disease severity, independent of complications of portal hypertension and etiology of liver disease. Anesthesia and surgery are known to have decompensatory effects on patients with cirrhosis. Multivariate factors that are associated with perioperative complications and mortality are listed in Table 17.3 [7].

Cholelithiasis occurs twice as often in patients with cirrhosis as in the general population [8]. Despite advances in anesthetic care over the past two decades, the high rates of mortality (7–20%) and morbidity (5–23%) associated with cholecystectomy in patients with liver disease have not decreased substantially. Open gallbladder surgery in the cirrhotic patient has been reported

Table 17.3 *Subset Risk Factors Associated with Perioperative Complications in Cirrhotic Patients [7]*

Male gender

High Child–Pugh score

Ascites

Cirrhosis other than primary biliary cirrhosis (especially cryptogenic cirrhosis)

Elevated serum creatinine

Chronic renal failure

Chronic obstructive pulmonary disease

Congestive heart failure

Ischemic heart disease

Insulin-dependent diabetes

Emergency case

Preoperative infection

Preoperative upper gastrointestinal bleeding

High American Society of Anesthesiologists (ASA) physical status rating

High surgical severity score

Intraoperative hypotension

to be associated with a 25% perioperative mortality rate. Many of the patients who died experienced postoperative bleeding, renal failure, and sepsis [9]. Ziser et al. reported the overall 30-day perioperative mortality rate for cirrhotic patients undergoing anesthesia and operation to be as high as 11.6%, with a complication rate of 30.1%. Pneumonia was the most frequent postoperative complication [7]. In 1986, the 30-day mortality rate following laparotomy and liver biopsy in patients with severe hepatic disease and ascites or PT more than 2.5 seconds greater than the control value was reported to exceed 80–90% [10].

Despite the introduction of laparoscopic surgery for cholecystectomy (LC) in the late 1980s and its reported advantages, many surgeons do not consider patients with Child–Pugh class C cirrhosis as candidates due to an unacceptably high risk of morbidity and mortality. This practice is consistent with the 1992 National Institutes of Health (NIH) consensus statement on LC, which states:

Most patients with symptomatic gallstones are candidates for LC, if they are able to tolerate general anesthesia and have no serious cardiopulmonary disease or other comorbid conditions that preclude operation. Patients who are usually not candidates for LC include those with generalized peritonitis, septic shock from cholangitis, severe acute pancreatitis, end-stage cirrhosis of the liver with portal hypertension, severe coagulopathy unresponsive to treatment, known cancer of the gallbladder, and chole-cysto-enteric fistulas [11].

A recent meta-analysis (1993–2001) comparing patients with cirrhosis undergoing laparoscopic cholecystectomy versus an open technique (OC) showed the advantage of less intraoperative blood loss, shorter operative time, and reduced length of hospitalization in the LC group. Patients with Child–Pugh class A or B cirrhosis compared with patients without cirrhosis had higher conversion rates, operative times, bleeding complications (26.4% vs. 3.1%), and overall morbidity (20.86% vs. 7.99%). No mortality was observed in the OC group. The overall

Table 17.4 *Cardiovascular, Pulmonary, and Renal Complications of Advanced Cirrhosis*

Cardiovascular
  Hyperdynamic circulation
    Increased cardiac index and stroke volume
    Decreased systemic vascular resistance
    Low to normal mean arterial pressure (widened pulse pressure)
    Increased heart rate
  Central hypovolemia
    Increased circulating blood volume
    Decreased effective plasma volume
    Increased sympathetic tone

Table 17.4 *Continued*

Hyporesponsiveness of the vasculature to pressor therapy

Flow-dependent oxygen consumption

Hepatic and splanchnic vasculature

    Portal hypertension

    Portal–systemic collateral circulation

    Decreased hepatic blood flow

Alcoholic cardiomyopathy (reduced LVEF)

Cirrhotic cardiomyopathy (impaired cardiac contractility, defective excitation
    contraction coupling, systolic and diastolic function, prolonged QTc interval,
    autonomic dysfunction, impaired beta-adrenergic function and postreceptor
    defect, decreased responsiveness to catecholamines, conductance abnormalities)

Arrythmias

Pulmonary

  Arterial hypoxemia ($PaO_2 < 70\,mmHg$)

    Hepatopulmonary syndrome

    Portopulmonary hypertension

    Impaired hypoxic pulmonary vasoconstriction

    Increased pulmonary blood flow

  Parenchymal abnormalities

    Restrictive ventilatory pattern due to ascites-limiting diaphragmatic excursion,
      pleural effusions, or chest wall deformity due to osteoporosis

    Obstructive airway disease, emphysema, bronchitis–bronchiectasis

    Interstitial lung disease (infection, pneumonitis, pulmonary edema)

Renal

  Renin–angiotensin–aldosterone activation: impaired sodium handling, water
    excretion, potassium metabolism, and concentrating ability

  Impaired renal acidification

  Prerenal insufficiency (ascites or diuretics)

  Acute renal failure (acute liver failure, biliary obstruction, sepsis)

  Hepatorenal syndrome

Glomerulopathies

mortality rate after LC in patients with cirrhosis was 0.28%, but in the small subset of Child–Pugh class C cirrhosis patients it was as high as 17% [12]. One contributory factor to the high incidence of multisystem organ failure in patients with severe chronic liver disease (Table 17.4) may be the release of inflammatory mediators induced by hepatic ischemia during surgery, which is more pronounced after OC compared with LC [13].

Patients with Child's class B and C cirrhosis are also at very high risk for complications and mortality with cardiac surgery. Contributory factors include risk of bleeding from hemodilution of clotting factors during cardiopulmonary bypass, platelet abnormalities and anticoagulation with heparin; renal dysfunction; and prolonged surgery and further hepatic deterioration, which is seen in 3% of adults undergoing cardiac surgery, compared with a mortality rate in patients with preexisting liver dysfunction of 11.4% [14].

Anesthesia, Surgery, and Liver Function

During anesthesia all factors inducing arterial hypotension should be avoided. General anesthesia and surgery decrease HBF and jeopardize oxygen supply to the liver. Intraoperative reductions in the arterial blood pressure and cardiac output decrease portal blood flow. Contributing factors include anesthetic drugs (inhalational anesthetics, vasodilators, beta-blockers, alpha-1-agonists, histamine-receptor-2 (H$_2$) blockers, and vasopressin), hypovolemia, ventilatory mode, hypoxema, hypercarbia, and acidosis. Surgical manipulation in the right upper quadrant can reduce HBF up to 60% from sympathetic activation or direct compression of the vena cava and splanchnic vessels. Compensatory vasodilatation of the hepatic artery in response to decreased portal inflow is diminished by volatile anesthetic agents in a dose-related manner, and consequently blood flow becomes pressure-dependent. Isoflurane has the least detrimental effect on liver blood flow. A simultaneous decrease in the liver's metabolic demand tends to balance the oxygen supply-to-uptake ratio. With cirrhosis, the reciprocal flow relationship between the portal vein and the hepatic artery is not well maintained. The cirrhotic patient may be at increased risk of ischemic injury to the liver secondary to preexisting impaired perfusion as well as multiorgan system failure from the release of cellular inflammatory mediators. Halothane anesthesia should be avoided as it is accompanied by the most prominent decrease in hepatic blood and oxygen supply and postoperative hepatic dysfunction. Nitrous oxide use may be undesirable because of its sympathomimetic effects, propensity to cause bowel distension, and limiting effect on increasing the inspiratory concentration of oxygen.

In general, outcome is less influenced by the choice of anesthetic agents than by the urgency or type of operative procedure and severity of underlying chronic liver disease. When administering drugs to patients with chronic liver disease, we must appreciate the substantially changed pharmacokinetics. All drug dosages should be decreased and carefully titrated until the desired effect is achieved. Experts currently recommend that in patients with chronic liver disease, isoflurane alone or in combination with small doses of fentanyl be used as the method of choice provided adequate pulmonary ventilation, cardiac output, and arterial pressure are maintained.

■ POSTOPERATIVE LIVER DYSFUNCTION

Because of the liver's large functional reserves, clinically significant acute liver dysfunction following anesthesia and surgery is uncommon and chiefly limited to patients with preexisting hepatic disease, massive blood transfusion, hepatic oxygen deprivation (hypoxia, anemia, decreased arterial pressure or cardiac output, and decreased HBF), infection, and drug toxicity.

■ SYSTEMIC MANIFESTATIONS OF END-STAGE LIVER DISEASE

ESLD is associated with unique systemic physiological alterations [15] (Table 17.4). Cardiovascular considerations include selection of monitoring and drug choice for induction and pressor support as dictated by a hyperdynamic circulation, fixed low total systemic vascular resistance (SVR), and compensatory rise in cardiac output, impaired circulatory reserve, and diminished response to catecholamine infusions. High-risk patients are those with alcoholic cardiomyopathy and dysrhythmias, congestive heart failure from fluid and electrolyte imbalances, and moderate to severe pulmonary hypertension.

Arterial hypoxemia usually responds to supplemental oxygen and positive pressure ventilation. Depressed airway reflexes, delayed gastric emptying, hiatus hernia, and massive ascites increase the risk of aspiration. Postoperative pulmonary edema, atelectasis, and pneumonia are common.

Renal function may be impaired; the kidneys are very susceptible to insult and prone to failure. Fluid and electrolyte imbalances are secondary to diuretic therapy, hypoalbuminemia, and portal hypertension causing generalized ascites, progressive edema, hypovolemia, hyponatremia, and hypokalemic metabolic alkalosis.

The patient is at major risk of GI hemorrhage from esophageal and/or gastric varices and peptic ulcer disease. Severe obstructive jaundice increases the risk of renal failure, neurotoxicity, and bradyarrhythmias. Bleeding is a potential risk from vitamin K deficiency, impaired hepatic synthesis of coagulation factors, bone marrow suppression, and splenic platelet sequestration. Malnutrition can lead to immunosuppression, which puts the patient at risk for infectious pulmonary complications.

With severe liver disease, patients may also have evidence of fibrinolysis, disseminated intravascular coagulation, or abnormal fibrinogen synthesis. Nutritional deficiencies lead to hypoglycemia, protein malnutrition, poor ventilatory reserve, and infection. Central nervous system (CNS) manifestations depend on the acuity of presentation, ranging from depressed mental status and confusion to acute cerebral edema in the fulminant liver failure patient.

Table 17.5 *Cardiac Evaluation of Adults with End-Stage Liver Disease*

Examination	Indication
1. Cardiac history, clinical examination, ECG, pulmonary function studies, chest X-ray, SaO_2, and PaO_2	All patients
2. Screening risk factors for CAD	All patients
3. Exercise stress test (ECG)	Inadequate examination for most patients (ascites, lethargy, beta-blockade)
4. Contrast enhanced transthoracic echocardiography	All patients
5. Transthoracic echocardiography while on waiting list	All patients every 12 months. MELD score > 20, patients with pulmonary hypertension, or pathological finding in the screening echocardiography, repeat every 6 months
6. Right heart catheterization	Patients with pulmonary hypertension; hypoxemia and severe intrapulmonary shunting (hepatopulmonary syndrome); assessment of right ventricular function (RV systolic pressure > 50 mmHg or abnormal RV size and function); morbid obesity (BMI ≥ 30 and MELD > 15 or BMI ≥ 30 and CPAP for sleep apnea or BMI ≥ 30 and diabetes)
7. Coronary arteriography	Patients with documented coronary artery disease or symptoms suggestive of myocardial ischemia; evidence of ischemic wall motion abnormalities on dobutamine stress echocardiography; left bundle block; pacemaker; diabetes mellitus and age > 40 years; age > 50 years and > 2 risk factors for CAD
8. Dobutamine stress echocardiogram or myocardial perfusion scintigraphy	Risk factors for CAD; diabetes mellitus; age > 45 years; ejection fraction < 50%

■ CARDIOVASCULAR RISK FACTORS AND PERIOPERATIVE COMPLICATIONS

Recent studies indicate that the prevalence of coronary artery disease (CAD) in patients with cirrhosis ranges from 2.5% to 27%; this exceeds the 2.5% prevalence in a healthy population. For many years it was believed that cirrhosis was cardioprotectant as a result of lower serum cholesterol levels, peripheral vasodilatation reducing the incidence of systemic hypertension, greater estrogen levels preventing atherosclerosis, and the effect of alcohol elevating high-density lipoprotein levels and lowering cardiovascular mortality. The theory that cirrhosis has a protective effect on coronary circulation appears to be no longer valid [16]. As more patients in their sixties and seventies are wait-listed and given the high rates of morbidity and mortality in patients with CAD who undergo liver transplantation, detection and treatment of CAD in the potential recipient is essential (Table 17.5). Diabetes mellitus is likely the most predictive risk factor.

Screening for CAD in patients with cirrhosis includes history and physical examination, ECG, SpO_2, PaO_2, and in most centers, a two-dimensional (2-D) echocardiogram for left ventricular dysfunction (LVEF $< 50\%$), valvular pathology, estimation of pulmonary artery pressure, and exclusion of severe intrapulmonary shunting. Further studies for specific evaluation of CAD and inducible ischemia include functional studies (stress thallium nuclear imaging, dobutamine stress echocardiography (DSE), and stress single-photon emission computed tomographic (SPECT) imaging), and cardiac catheterization. DSE is the preferred screening tool for patients at risk for perioperative cardiac events related to obstructive CAD; however, the predictive value of this noninvasive test for ischemic events or detecting cardiomyopathy is controversial [17–21]. Both Plevak and Plotkin recommend following the guidelines of the American College of Cardiology and the American Heart Association, which combine clinical predictors of active heart disease, functional capacity, surgery-specific risk, and the presence or lack of recent coronary evaluation to identify patients likely to benefit from noninvasive testing [18,22,23].

■ PORTOPULMONARY HYPERTENSION AND HEPATOPULMONARY SYNDROME

The bane of every anesthesiologists' existence is inserting a pulmonary artery catheter for invasive hemodynamic monitoring and finding that the patient has a mean pulmonary artery pressure (mPAP) > 25 mmHg. To proceed, delay and treat, or cancel surgery is problematic in patients with increased mPAP. One must differentiate between reactive pulmonary hypertension due to light general anesthesia or metabolic/respiratory acidosis, volume overload, high cardiac output, left-sided heart disease, cardiomyopathy, valvular heart disease, interstitial or obstructive lung disease, chronic thromboembolism, or pulmonary vasoconstriction with vasoproliferation. Up to 20% of cirrhotic patients are at risk of developing pulmonary hypertension. The current diagnostic criteria for portopulmonary hypertension include portal hypertension (ascites, varices, splenomegally), mPAP > 25 mmHg, pulmonary capillary wedge pressure < 15 mmHg, and pulmonary vascular resistance (PVR) < 240 dynes s cm^{-5}. In patients with mPAP of 35–40 mmHg and preserved right ventricular function, an attempt to reduce the mPAP < 35 mmHg and PVR < 240 dynes s cm^{-5} is ideal and consideration should be given to continuing the surgery. For mPAP > 45 mmHg and PVR < 240 dynes s cm^{-5}, surgery should be deferred and pulmonary vasodilator epoprostenol initiated as the patient has a poor prognosis and is at increased risk of intraoperative death from acute right heart failure [20,24–27].

The frequency of hepatopulmonary syndrome in patients with liver disease is reported to be between 4% and 29% [28,29]. Patients with liver disease may develop progressive and refractory hypoxemia due to abnormal intrapulmonary vascular dilatation causing anatomical shunting and ventilation–perfusion abnormalities [30]. These patients are at risk for systemic arterial embolization causing stroke, intracranial hemorrhage, or brain abscess. The prognosis of the hepatopulmonary syndrome is poor, and mortality rates of 41% within 2–5 years have been reported [31,32].

CENTRAL PONTINE MYELINOLYSIS

Central pontine myelinolysis (CPM) is a frequently symmetric noninflammatory demyelinating disorder within the brainstem pons. In at least 10% of patients, demyelination also occurs in extrapontine areas. Clinical manifestations are characterized by postoperative confusion and/or weakness or a ''locked-in'' syndrome after transplantation [33]. The most frequent findings are delirium, pseudobulbar palsy, and spastic quadriplegia, which may result in permanent neurologic deficits. CPM occurs inconsistently as a complication of severe and prolonged hyponatremia, particularly when the sodium is corrected too rapidly, and has been reported to be present in 29% of postmortem examinations of liver transplant patients. Risk factors included serum sodium less than 120 mEq/L for more than 48 h, aggressive IV fluid therapy with hypertonic saline solutions, and hypernatremia during treatment. Empirical data show that CPM is likely to occur when the total perioperative increase in sodium concentration is above 15–20 mEq/L [34]. Cirrhotic patients treated with potent diuretics are at a special risk for low sodium plasma concentrations; therefore, major surgical procedures with the potential for large-volume blood loss, fluid shifts, or metabolic acidosis are not recommended in patients with a very low preoperative sodium concentration.

■ ANESTHETIC MANAGEMENT FOR LIVER TRANSPLANTATION

Monitoring

Monitoring for liver transplantation significantly exceeds the routine standard care for major abdominal surgery. Together with invasive arterial blood pressure measurement and central venous access with a multiple lumen catheter, the insertion of a pulmonary artery catheter is mandatory in most cases. Following the practice guidelines of the American Society of Anesthesiologists (ASA) Task Force on Perioperative Transesophageal Echocardiography (TEE), TEE monitoring in liver transplantation is recommended as an accurate intraoperative tool for diagnosis and management of hemodynamic disturbances. ICP monitoring has been discussed earlier and also in Chapter 13. Use of a rapid transfusion device and cell saver may be useful when massive blood loss is anticipated. Institutional preference dictates use of a femoral arterial and venous line in addition to a radial arterial line and central line placed in the neck.

Anesthesia Induction and Maintenance

There is no routine drug set listed in most reviews on anesthetic management of liver transplantation, but a slight trend for maintenance of anesthesia with inhalational agents may be seen, especially using isoflurane [35]. Experimental data show that flow velocity is enhanced with isoflurane and hepatic arterial autoregulation and oxygen delivery are effectively maintained [36,37]. There is little scientific information about the use of sevoflurane or desflurane. Rapid sequence IV induction with cricoid pressure and endotracheal intubation after the administration of fentanyl, propofol or thiopental (rarely etomidate), and succinylcholine is routine for patients euvolemic with serum potassium levels in the normal range. A larger volume of distribution, which may necessitate a larger initial dose of drug and close monitoring of subsequent doses, should be anticipated. Pseudocholinesterase deficiency may cause prolongation of the action of succinylcholine, which is of limited clinical significance. Muscle relaxation with cisatracurium or vecuronium is advantageous in patients with renal impairment. An infusion of octreotide may reduce venous pressures in patients with portal hypertension. Intravascular volume expansion with colloid, crystalloid, or blood products and drug therapy including renal vasodilators (dopamine) or splanchnic vasoconstrictors (vasopressin analogues) may be utilized to optimize renal perfusion. Of interest, clonidine 4 μg/kg IV during induction has been reported to significantly reduce the intraoperative requirements for intravenous fluids and blood products without compromising circulatory stability. Improvement in immediate reperfusion-induced hemodynamic disturbances was also observed [38].

Hemodynamic Management

Maintaining hemodynamic stability during liver dissection, the anhepatic phase, and on reperfusion depends on the surgical technique (classic caval clamping verus. caval preservation), the use of venovenous bypass, autologous backwash of the donor liver, metabolic abnormalities, and surgical hemostasis. Cross-clamping of the inferior vena cava (IVC) causes a marked reduction of venous return to the heart, resulting in a decrease in cardiac output, decrease in PAP, and compensatory increase in heart rate and SVR. This effect is less pronounced in patients with ESLD and venous collateral circulation, which partially maintains preload. Hypotension is treated by gentle fluid administration and pressor support (norepinephrine, dopamine, epinephrine, phenylephrine), as needed. Flooding the patient with intravenous crystalloid or colloid may have disastrous consequences on reperfusion. If the piggyback technique with caval preservation is used or venovenous bypass is initiated prior to caval cross-clamping, venous return may be maintained and less reduction in cardiac output seen. In the scenario of right ventricular failure, milrinone, dobutamine, or epinephrine infusions with nitric oxide or prostaglandin E_1 are indicated to support cardiac output and reduce pulmonary artery pressure. The goal for cold-ischemia time of the donor liver (storage time in cold preservation solution) is under 15 h and of the warm-ischemia time (time from liver up into the surgical field until reperfusion in the recipient) of < 90 min. Reactivation of hepatitis C in the new liver may be less if the warm-ischemia time can be kept under 35 min [39].

Extreme hemodynamic changes may occur immediately after reperfusion of the transplanted liver, including hypotension, bradycardia, supraventricular and ventricular arrhythmias, variable cardiac output, and occasionally cardiac arrest (0–5%). The incidence of this postreperfusion syndrome may be as high as 30% [40]. Immediately after reperfusion, left ventricular function may be impaired and pulmonary capillary wedge pressure, central venous pressure (CVP), and PAP usually increase with a reduction in SVR, while TEE monitoring shows a stable or even decreased left ventricular end-diastolic volume. These contradictory findings may be due to a period of deteriored left ventricular compliance or "cardioplegia" on reperfusion [41,42].

Hemostatic Management

During the hepatectomy, the effects of fibrinolysis, thrombocytopenia, coagulation factor and fibrinogen deficiency on clinical bleeding are not always predictable and transfusion requirements are variable. Portal hypertension with venous collaterals, adhesions from prior operations, and lack of surgical hemostasis (especially a hole in the IVC) contribute to the complexity of massive blood loss and hemostatic management. Thromboelastography and other useful on-site devices have been developed for coagulation monitoring, and rapid infusion devices are available to allow intravenous transfusion up to 2 L/min. Intraoperative use of aprotinin may significantly reduce blood transfusion requirements, and prophylactic use of aprotinin has been reported to ameliorate the postreperfusion syndrome in liver transplantation, as reflected by a significant reduction in vasopressor requirements [43,44]. However, reports on fatal pulmonary thromboembolism bring into question the unreflected routine use of aprotinin in all liver transplant recipients [45]. Tranexamic and epsilon-aminocaproic acid have been used as antifibrinolytic agents during liver transplantation, but their effect on transfusion requirements is controversial [46]. Calcium is an important coenzyme in the coagulation cascade. During the hepatectomy and anhepatic phases of liver transplantation, acute ionized hypocalcemia may develop, especially when large amounts of fresh frozen plasma have been transfused. In many transplant centers, continuous calcium infusions and magnesium supplements are routine therapy.

Target-directed transfusion goals are used for replacement of blood products, if the patient is actively bleeding with adequate surgical hemostasis during the hepatectomy phase. Following reperfusion, ideally the hematocrit should be maintained at 27–29% to minimize the risk of hepatic artery thrombosis due to the increase in blood viscosity. It is not possible to correct the PT with administration of FFP. Partial thromboplastin time (PTT) may be prolonged due to residual heparin used during the donor procurement procedure, which clears within 5 min of reperfusion or venous congestion of the recipient bowel producing heparinoid-like substances. Many transplant centers use the normalization of the PT and platelet count as indicators of recovery of donor liver graft function. Administration of cryoprecipitate for fibrinogen < 100 mg/dL prior to transport to the ICU is common practice.

◼ ANESTHETIC MANAGEMENT AFTER LIVER TRANSPLANTATION

Preoperative patient evaluation after liver transplantation requires an understanding of:

- Functional evaluation of the liver
- Early: diagnosis of rejection or infection (cytomegalovirus (CMV) or bacterial)
- Late: ischemia risk, detection of chronic rejection or infection, drug-induced liver toxicity, universal recurrence of hepatitis C
- Minimal physiological and pharmacological problems of denervation
- The significance of residual physiologic alterations of ESLD
- Coexisting systemic disease
- Optimizing patient and graft function
- Immunosuppression-related complications, toxicities, and adverse effects
- Choices for anesthetic techniques and monitoring
- Postoperative care and rejection surveillance

GRAFT FUNCTION

Recovery of cytochrome P450-dependent microsomal enzyme activity starts immediately after reperfusion of the graft. Morphine, fentanyl, propofol, muscle relaxants, and amide-linked local anesthetic agents appear to be well handled by the newly transplanted liver [47–49]. By the second postoperative week the patient's coagulation profile should have normalized and synthetic function restored. In contrast, liver test results may remain elevated with changes in trends over time of aspartate aminotransferase (AST), gamma glutamyl transpeptidase (GGT), and alkaline phosphatase more important than absolute values.

Elective surgery should be postponed in the presence of rejection. Pre-operative assessment should include specific inquiry about new onset of jaundice, change in urine or stool color, pruritis, right upper quadrant tenderness, fever, malaise, weight gain, and ankle edema. Laboratory evaluation of graft function should include standard liver tests: AST, alanine amino transferase (ALT), albumin, and PT/INR (hepatocellular injury); and bilirubin, alkaline phosphatase, and GGT (cholestasis). A liver biopsy may be needed for definitive diagnosis. Deterioration of graft function may also indicate the presence of infection, recurrence of the primary disease process (especially hepatitis C), or a toxic effect of immunosuppression.

PHYSIOLOGICAL ADAPTATIONS AND COEXISTING SYSTEMIC DISEASE

Liver transplantation does not fully correct many of the unique systemic physiological alterations associated with ESLD. Total liver blood flow is increased, despite the return of portal pressures to normal, with persistence of portal–systemic collaterals evident 4 years after transplantation [50]. Portal venous inflow is still under the influence of the normal vasomotor tone of the superior mesenteric artery, whereas the hepatic artery is denervated; this may be the main cause of the increase in hepatic perfusion. The potential long-term effect of persistently elevated liver blood flow on various metabolic pathways in the liver or disposition of high hepatic extraction drugs is unknown [51]. The patient may be at risk for intraoperative hemorrhage due to the presence of residual portal–systemic collaterals, mild to moderate coagulopathy, and a clinical impression of a decreased capacity of the denervated hepatic vasculature to constrict and shunt blood centrally in response to systemic hypotension.

Reported changes in the systemic hemodynamic status appear more controversial. Arterial hypertension and increased total SVR are consistent findings. Cardiac index has been observed to remain high in the presence of good liver function and subsequently return to a more normal value [52,53]. The persistence of a high output state is generally well tolerated. Significant increases in peripheral vascular resistance, due to the combined effect of reversal of the pretransplantation vasodilatation and the vasoconstrictor effect of cyclosporine and FK 506 may be particularly detrimental in patients with evidence of coexisting cardiomyopathy or valvular insufficiency. Myocardial ischemia may occur in patients with underlying CAD or in those with coronary spasm or accelerated arteriosclerotic disease secondary to cyclosporine and steroid therapy.

The most common pulmonary complication following liver transplantation is infection, with no evidence of the significant airway obstruction or bronchiolitis obliterans seen in bone marrow transplant recipients and heart–lung transplantation patients. Pulmonary hypertension in association with cirrhosis may occur in up to 20% of patients receiving liver transplants. Resolution of the pulmonary hypertension has been observed in survivors over a period of 13 months after liver transplantation [54]. Approximately 50% of all liver transplant candidates have some form of abnormal arterial oxygenation, frequently PaO_2 less than 70 mmHg. Hepatopulmonary syndrome, defined as the triad of hepatic dysfunction, pulmonary vascular dilatation, and abnormal arterial oxygenation (frequently severe hypoxemia with $PaO_2 < 50$ mmHg), affects up to 45% of these patients [55]. Normalization in arterial PaO_2 has been demonstrated from 1 to 9 months after transplantation in patients with a type 1 angiographic pattern, responsive to 100% oxygen [56].

■ IMMUNOSUPPRESSION

Immunosuppressive protocols for liver transplant patients generally include varying combinations of drugs. The regimen in an individual patient reflects prior rejection episodes and side-effects. Immunosuppressive agents must be continued perioperatively, with consideration given to the general recommendations listed in Table 17.6 (see also Chapters 29 and 30).

Cyclosporine A

Interactions between cyclosporine A and any drug that is a substrate for cytochrome P450 are possible (see Chapter 30). Very few animal and human studies of possible drug interactions between cyclosporine A and anesthetic agents have appeared in the literature. Isoflurane decreases the rate of absorption of cyclosporine A by reducing gastric emptying and absorption from the proximal small bowel. Oral doses of cyclosporine A should be given 4–7 h preoperatively; most formulations contain olive oil, castor oil, or corn oil and represent a significant risk if regurgitation and aspiration occur [57,58]. In addition, the desired therapeutic blood levels may not be achieved if given outside this time interval. Cyclosporine A has been shown to prolong non-depolarizing neuromuscular blockade, which is thought to be secondary to a combined effect of inhibition of calcium entry into the muscle cell by the parent drug and nonspecific interference by polyoxethylated castor oil with drug binding, effectively increasing the concentration of nondepolarizing drug at the neuromuscular junction [58]. The interaction of cyclosporine and depolarizing muscle relaxants has not been studied in humans. Cyclosporine A has been reported to increase analgesia produced by fentanyl in a dose-dependent manner and to increase pentobarbital hypnosis [59]. Insufficient corroborating data exist to determine the clinical significance of these findings.

It is essential to appreciate the potential interactions between cyclosporine A and anesthetic agents; many of the latter drugs cause liver enzyme induction, which may alter cyclosporine A levels 7–10 days later or potentiate cyclosporine A-related side-effects.

Table 17.6 *Recommendations for Immunosuppressive Therapy in the Surgical Patient*

1. Continue immunosuppressive therapy (aspiration risk and reduced bioavailability if taken immediately prior to surgery).
2. Monitor patient for adverse effects attributable to specific drugs.
3. Consider all patients as susceptible to life-threatening infections.
4. Supplement with steroids for stress of surgery.
5. Consider possible anesthetic drug interactions.
6. Optimize renal function.

Tacrolimus

Tacrolimus (FK 506) was introduced into clinical trials in 1990 and has a pharmacokinetic profile similar to that of cyclosporine with P450 liver enzyme metabolism except that it does not require bile acids for solubilization and absorption. Neurological complications of high blood levels include seizures and CPM, dysarthria, and motor disturbances; these resolve with dose reduction. Headache and insomnia are common complaints that are dose-related. Recently, a tacrolimus-induced pain syndrome has been described as a post-transplant complication [60].

Steroids

There is a long-standing debate regarding whether a history of exogenous steroid administration, followed by surgical stress with no supplementation, precipitates acute adrenal insufficiency. Recommendations for perioperative steroid coverage take into consideration the route of administration, total dose, interval from last dose to surgery, duration of therapy, magnitude of perceived surgical stress, and presence of glucose intolerance. In reality, few patients with suppressed adrenal function and no steroid supplement develop hypotension after surgery. Patients on chronic corticosteroid therapy may develop osteoporosis and increased potential for traumatic fractures; careful positioning is necessary.

■ ANESTHESIA AND MONITORING

Virtually any anesthetic technique can be utilized successfully in liver transplant patients if liver function is stable and coagulation is within normal limits [61]. The "healthy" transplanted liver is no more susceptible to potentially hepatotoxic drugs than the liver in a normal patient [62]. Routine immunosuppressive therapy should be continued, with monitoring for signs of toxicity and adverse effects. Choice of anesthetic technique depends on surgical considerations, minimization of additional insult or physiological trespass to the liver, presence of absolute or relative contraindications for regional anesthesia, and individual preference.

Standardized routine monitoring is usually sufficient in most cases. One must weigh the risk–benefit ratio of invasive procedures (arterial or central venous catheter) versus the increased risk of infection in transplant recipients. Attention to aseptic techniques and the use of prophylactic antibiotics are essential. Patients receiving cyclosporine may demonstrate prolonged recovery from nondepolarizing muscle relaxants; therefore blockade monitoring is necessary. Hypertension and renal insufficiency should be anticipated in all patients. The elevated blood pressure is often relatively refractory to medical therapy and may require vasodilators, angiotensin-converting enzyme (ACE) inhibitors, calcium channel blockers, and beta-blockade for control. As a result, the depth of anesthesia or responses to noxious stimuli may be difficult to assess when using blood pressure and heart rate responses as an accurate guide to anesthetic requirements. Bispectral index (BIS®) monitoring is a helpful adjunct to determine when the patient has achieved a sufficient level of hypnosis, and given an appropriate dose of narcotic, one then manages hypertension with pharmacological agents.

■ REGIONAL ANESTHESIA

In considering the advisability of regional anesthesia, documentation of any existing neurological deficit is prudent, as is prevention of hypomagnesemia, which potentiates cyclosporine-induced neurotoxicity. Care with patient positioning must be taken. An additional concern is the possibility of a concurrent viral or opportunistic CNS infection, which frequently has few clinical findings and is reported in approximately 5–10% of transplant patients. Continuation of aspirin, azathioprine, and dipyridamole in the preoperative period can affect platelet adhesiveness. In the absence of evidence of overt platelet dysfunction, however, most clinicians do not consider use of these drugs a contraindication for regional anesthesia. Continuing evidence of portal hypertension and the possible presence of large venous collaterals may be a relative contraindication for placement of a catheter in the epidural space, with increased risk of vessel penetration and possible hematoma formation [29]. Peripheral nerve block may pose less risk than a spinal or epidural technique if the nerve sheaths are located in a manually compressible space.

■ INTRAOPERATIVE CHALLENGES

As mentioned, resuscitation situations require large-bore intravenous access. Transfusion practices should take into consideration the Rhesus titer and the CMV status of the patient. Institutional practices vary from (1) administering only CMV-negative blood products to all transplanted patients or identifying the CMV-negative recipient who has received a CMV-negative organ, (2) white cell filtering of the blood and platelets to prevent transmission of CMV carried in the leukocytes, and (3) irradiation to destroy T cells, which provoke graft-versus-host disease. The target transfusion hematocrit should not exceed 30%, and the judicious use of antifibrinolytic therapy would seem wise to prevent the rare but potentially lethal complication of hepatic artery thrombosis.

Hypertension may necessitate intra-arterial blood pressure monitoring and aggressive medical intervention. Persistent hypertension may be a clue to blood levels of cyclosporine or FK 506 that are elevated above therapeutic target levels. It is vital to maintain a good urine output perioperatively, because further renal insults from drugs or periods of low cardiac output may be additive and can cause the patient to become rapidly anuric. Nonsteroidal anti-inflammatory drugs (NSAIDs) should be avoided for postoperative analgesia as they potentially worsen cyclosporine-induced renal insufficiency. Many of these patients suffer from chronic pain syndromes, which are managed with Tylenol R, oxycodone, codeine, or maintenance methadone and as such, a consultation for postoperative pain management may be necessary.

An adrenal crisis is life-threatening, and primarily a diagnosis of exclusion. Supplemental high-dose steroid therapy has little associated morbidity and should be administered perioperatively to cover maximal stress requirements equivalent to cortisol 200–500 mg/day. Hyperglycemia due to steroid administration, cyclosporine, and surgical stress is predictable and should be monitored and treated with insulin as needed. Numerous medical problems inherent in acute and chronic liver failure may require continuing therapy or recognition and treatment.

■ REFERENCES

1. Gelman S. Anesthesia and the liver. In Barash P, Cullen B, Stoelting R, eds., Clinical anesthesia, 3rd ed. Philadelphia, PA: Lippincott-Raven, 1997:1003–1024.

2. Maze M, Bass N. Anesthesia and the hepatobiliary system. In Miller RD, ed., Anesthesia, 5th ed. Philadelphia, PA: Churchill Livingstone, 2000:1960–1972.

3. Parks D, Skinner K, Gelman S, et al. Hepatic physiology. In Miller RD, ed., Anesthesia, 5th ed. Philadelphia, PA: Churchill Livingstone, 2000:647–662.

4. Sladen R. Anesthetic concerns for the patient with renal or hepatic disease. ASA Refresher Course Lecture 1997;271:1–7.

5. Gines P, Guevara M, Arroyo V, et al. Hepatorenal syndrome. Lancet 2003;362(9398):1819–1827.

6. Gines P, Quintero E, Arroyo V, et al. Compensated cirrhosis: natural history and prognostic factors. Hepatology 1987;7(1):122–128.

7. Ziser A, Plevak DJ, Wiesner RH, et al. Morbidity and mortality in cirrhotic patients undergoing anesthesia and surgery. Anesthesiology 1999;90(1):42–53.

8. Tuech JJ, Pessaux P, Regenet N, et al. Laparoscopic cholecystectomy in cirrhotic patients. Surg Laparosc Endosc Percutan Tech 2002;12(4):227–231.

9. Aranha GV, Sontag SJ, Greenlee HB. Cholecystectomy in cirrhotic patients: a formidable operation. Am J Surg 1982;143(1):55–60.

10. Aranha GV, Greenlee HB. Intra-abdominal surgery in patients with advanced cirrhosis. Arch Surg 1986;121(3):275–277.

11. National Institutes of Health Consensus Development Conference Statement on Gallstones and Laparoscopic Cholecystectomy. Am J Surg 1993;165(4):390–398.

12. Puggioni A, Wong LL. A metaanalysis of laparoscopic cholecystectomy in patients with cirrhosis. J Am Coll Surg 2003;197(6):921–926.

13. Lausten SB, Ibrahim TM, El-Sefi T, et al. Systemic and cell-mediated immune response after laparoscopic and open cholecystectomy in patients with chronic liver disease. A randomized, prospective study. Dig Surg 1999;16(6):471–477.

14. Michalopoulos A, Alivizatos P, Geroulanos S. Hepatic dysfunction following cardiac surgery: determinants and consequences. Hepatogastroenterology 1997;44(15): 779–783.

15. Robertson K. Transplantation. In Gambling D, Douglas MJ, eds., Obstetric anesthesia and uncommon disorders. Philadelphia, PA: WB Saunders, 1998:145–170.

16. Keeffe BG, Valantine H, Keeffe EB. Detection and treatment of coronary artery disease in liver transplant candidates. Liver Transpl 2001;7(9):755–761.

17. Donovan CL, Marcovitz PA, Punch JD, et al. Two-dimensional and dobutamine stress echocardiography in the preoperative assessment of patients with end-stage liver disease prior to orthotopic liver transplantation. Transplantation 1996;61(8): 1180–1188.

18. Plotkin JS, Johnson LB, Rustgi V, et al. Coronary artery disease and liver transplantation: the state of the art. Liver Transpl 2000;6(4 suppl 1):S53–S56.

19. Williams K, Lewis JF, Davis G, et al. Dobutamine stress echocardiography in patients undergoing liver transplantation evaluation. Transplantation 2000;69(11): 2354–2356.

20. Krowka MJ, Mandell MS, Ramsay MA, et al. Hepatopulmonary syndrome and portopulmonary hypertension: a report of the multicenter liver transplant database. Liver Transpl 2004;10(2):174–182.

21. Moller S, Henriksen JH. Cirrhotic cardiomyopathy: a pathophysiological review of circulatory dysfunction in liver disease. Heart 2002;87(1):9–15.

22. Plevak DJ. Stress echocardiography identifies coronary artery disease in liver transplant candidates. Liver Transpl Surg 1998;4(4):337–339.

23. Eagle KA, Brundage BH, Chaitman BR, et al. Guidelines for perioperative cardiovascular evaluation for noncardiac surgery. Report of the American College of Cardiology/American Heart Association Task Force on Practice Guidelines

(Committee on Perioperative Cardiovascular Evaluation for Noncardiac Surgery). J Am Coll Cardiol 1996;27(4):910–948.

24. Swanson KL, Wiesner RH, Krowka MV. Natural History of Hepatopulmonary syndrome: impact of liver transplantation. Hepatology 2005; 41 (5): 1122–9.

25. Arguedas MR, Abrams GA, Krowa MJ. Fallon MB. Prospective evaluation of outcomes and predictons of mortality in patients with Hepatopulmonary syndrome undergoing liver transplantation. Hepatology 2003; 37 (1): 192–7.

26. Ramsay MA, Spikes C, East CA, Lynch K, Hein HA, Ramsay KJ, Klintmacm GB. The perioperative management of portopulmonary hypertension with nitric oxide and eprostenol. Anesthesiology 1999; 90 (1): 299–301.

27. Minder S, Fischler M, Muellhaupt B, et al. Intravenous iloprost bridging to orthotopic liver transplantation in portopulmonary hypertension. Eur Respir J 2004;24(4): 703–707.

28. Naeije R. Hepatopulmonary syndrome and portopulmonary hypertension. Swiss Med Wkly 2003;133(11–12):163–169.

29. Mazzeo AT, Lucanto T, Santamaria LB. Hepatopulmonary syndrome: a concern for the anesthetist? Pre-operative evaluation of hypoxemic patients with liver disease. Acta Anaesthesiol Scand 2004;48(2):178–186.

30. Hoeper MM, Krowka MJ, Strassburg CP. Portopulmonary hypertension and hepatopulmonary syndrome. Lancet 2004;363(9419):1461–1468.

31. Krowka MJ, Dickson ER, Cortese DA. Hepatopulmonary syndrome. Clinical observations and lack of therapeutic response to somatostatin analogue. Chest 1993;104(2):515–521.

32. Krowka MJ, Plevak DJ, Findlay JY, et al. Pulmonary hemodynamics and perioperative cardiopulmonary-related mortality in patients with portopulmonary hypertension undergoing liver transplantation. Liver Transpl 2000;6(4):443–450.

33. Estol CJ, Faris AA, Martinez AJ, et al. Central pontine myelinolysis after liver transplantation. Neurology 1989;39(4):493–498.

34. Wszolek ZK, McComb RD, Pfeiffer RF, et al. Pontine and extrapontine myelinolysis following liver transplantation. Relationship to serum sodium. Transplantation 1989;48(6):1006–1012.

35. Carton EG, Plevak DJ, Kranner PW, et al. Perioperative care of the liver transplant patient (Part 2). Anesth Analg 1994;78(2):382–399.

36. Gelman S, Fowler KC, Smith LR. Liver circulation and function during isoflurane and halothane anesthesia. Anesthesiology 1984;61(6):726–730.

37. Grundmann U, Zissis A, Bauer C, et al. In vivo effects of halothane, enflurane, and isoflurane on hepatic sinusoidal microcirculation. Acta Anaesthesiol Scand 1997;41(6):760–765.

38. De Kock M, Laterre PF, Van Obbergh L, et al. The effects of intraoperative intravenous clonidine on fluid requirements, hemodynamic variables, and support during liver transplantation: a prospective, randomized study. Anesth Analg 1998;86(3):468–476.

39. Baron PW, Sindram D, Higdon D, et al. Prolonged rewarming time during allograft implantation predisposes to recurrent hepatitis C infection after liver transplantation. Liver Transpl 2000;6(4):407–412.

40. Aggarwal S, Kang Y, Freeman JA, et al. Postreperfusion syndrome: cardiovascular collapse following hepatic reperfusion during liver transplantation. Transplant Proc 1987;19(4 suppl 3):54–55.

41. de la Morena G, Acosta F, Villegas M, et al. Ventricular function during liver reperfusion in hepatic transplantation. A transesophageal echocardiographic study. Transplantation 1994;58(3):306–310.

42. De Wolf AM. Does ventricular dysfunction occur during liver transplantation? Transplant Proc 1991;23(3):1922–1923.

43. Molenaar IQ, Begliomini B, Martinelli G, et al. Reduced need for vasopressors in patients receiving aprotinin during orthotopic liver transplantation. Anesthesiology 2001;94(3):433–438.

44. Porte RJ, Molenaar IQ, Begliomini B, et al. Aprotinin and transfusion requirements in orthotopic liver transplantation: a multicentre randomised double-blind study. EMSALT Study Group. Lancet 2000;355(9212):1303–1309.

45. Fitzsimons MG, Peterfreund RA, Raines DE. Aprotinin administration and pulmonary thromboembolism during orthotopic liver transplantation: report of two cases. Anesth Analg 2001;92(6):1418–1421.

46. Molenaar IQ, Legnani C, Groenland TH, et al. Aprotinin in orthotopic liver transplantation: evidence for a prohemostatic, but not a prothrombotic effect. Liver Transpl 2001;7(10):896–903.

47. Kelley SD, Cauldwell CB, Fisher DM, et al. Recovery of hepatic drug extraction after hypothermic preservation. Anesthesiology 1995;82(1):251–258.

48. Magorian T, Wood P, Caldwell J, et al. The pharmacokinetics and neuromuscular effects of rocuronium bromide in patients with liver disease. Anesth Analg 1995;80(4):754–759.

49. Pitter JF, Morel DR, Mentha G, et al. Vecuronium neuromuscular blockade reflects liver function during hepatic autotransplantation in pigs. Anesthesiology 1994;81:168–175.

50. Chezmar JL, Redvanly RD, Nelson RC, et al. Persistence of portosystemic collaterals and splenomegaly on CT after orthotopic liver transplantation. Am J Roentgenol 1992;159(2):317–320.

51. Henderson JM. Abnormal splanchnic and systemic hemodynamics of end-stage liver disease: what happens after liver transplantation? Hepatology 1993;17(3): 514–516.

52. Gadano A, Hadengue A, Widmann JJ, et al. Hemodynamics after orthotopic liver transplantation: study of associated factors and long-term effects. Hepatology 1995;22(2):458–465.

53. Hadengue A, Lebrec D, Moreau R, et al. Persistence of systemic and splanchnic hyperkinetic circulation in liver transplant patients. Hepatology 1993;17(2):175–178.

54. Koneru B, Ahmed S, Weisse AB, et al. Resolution of pulmonary hypertension of cirrhosis after liver transplantation. Transplantation 1994;58(10):1133–1135.

55. Krowka MJ, Cortese DA. Hepatopulmonary syndrome: an evolving perspective in the era of liver transplantation. Hepatology 1990;11(1):138–142.

56. McCloskey JJ, Schleien C, Schwarz K, et al. Severe hypoxemia and intrapulmonary shunting resulting from cirrhosis reversed by liver transplantation in a pediatric patient. J Pediatr 1991;118(6):902–904.

57. Brown MR, Brajtbord D, Johnson DW, et al. Efficacy of oral cyclosporine given prior to liver transplantation. Anesth Analg 1989;69(6):773–775.

58. Sharpe MD. Cyclosporin potentiates vecuronium blockade and prolongs recovery time in humans. Can J Anaesth 1992;39:A126.

59. Cirella VN, Pantuck CB, Lee YJ, et al. Effects of cyclosporine on anesthetic action. Anesth Analg 1987;66(8):703–706.

60. Malat GE, Dupuis RE, Kassman B, et al. Tacrolimus-induced pain syndrome in a pediatric orthotopic liver transplant patient. Pediatr Transplant 2002;6(5):435–438.

61. Alhashemi JA, Gelb AW, Sharpe MD. Anesthesia for the transplanted patient. In Sharpe MD, Gelb AW, eds., Anesthesia and transplantation. Boston, Oxford, Auckland, Johannesburg, Melbourne, New Delhi: Butterworth Heinemann, 1999:323–336.

62. Black AE. Anesthesia for pediatric patients who have had a transplant. Int Anesthesiol Clin 1995;33(2):107–123.

Recovery in the Immediate Postoperative Period

Julie S. Hudson and Judith W. Gentile

THE PURPOSE of this chapter is to describe the liver transplant recipient's course during the first 6 months after transplantation in order to provide a frame of reference for referring physicians, patients, and family members. As in most of clinical medicine, there is considerable individual variation; "typical" rarely defines a real patient. Variables such as the preoperative diagnosis, the model for end-stage liver disease (MELD) score, degree of debility at the time of transplantation, comorbid illnesses, and operative complexity each influence the rate at which a patient will progress during recovery. For the purpose of description, there are three sequential stages at which recovery can be assessed: in the intensive care unit (ICU), in the inpatient transplantation unit, and as an outpatient following discharge from hospital.

■ THE INTENSIVE CARE UNIT

Immediately following liver transplantation, the patient returns to an ICU. In some institutions with large liver transplant programs, there may be specific ICUs for liver transplant patients; in most programs patients are initially cared for in a general surgical or medical ICU. Most patients with an uncomplicated course in the operating room remain in the ICU for approximately 24 h before being transferred to an inpatient liver transplant unit.

The patient gradually awakens from anesthesia, as it is not reversed, during the first 8 h in the ICU. This is often a time of elation as they have survived the surgery and at long last have a new liver. This realization, fortified by the preparation and teaching they received while awaiting a donor, helps the patient and family members cope with the stressful environment of the ICU.

However, some patients who are transplanted because of fulminant hepatic failure lapse into coma before they are aware of the need for a liver transplant. For these patients, awakening in an ICU can be a terrifying experience. Often a psychiatrist, the nurse coordinators, and social workers on the transplant team are needed to assist the patient and family to adapt to this sudden and overwhelming change in their lives.

Fifteen to twenty percent of liver transplant patients are taken back to the operating room during the transplant admission. The reasons for reoperation include postoperative bleeding, vascular, and biliary complications (see Chapters 20 and 21). The patient and family may interpret reoperation only as a setback in the patient's recovery. Communication between the transplant team and the patient and family can help to reassure them. The need for surgery at this early phase does not delay long-term wound healing and recovery. The reason surgery is required is more predictive of effect on postoperative outcome.

While in the ICU, the patient is monitored with frequent laboratory work and hemodynamic assessment. Vital signs, intake, output, physical changes in drain output, bile production, and signs of postoperative bleeding are recorded hourly. The intensity of the ICU routine is balanced by visits from family and close friends. Many patients and family members are attentive to changes in the patient's condition and, particularly, to the laboratory results during the time in the ICU. Most are unaware that rising transaminases and bilirubin in the 48 h immediately after transplantation may not be ominous signs as long as the prothrombin time, serum lactate, bile production, or other measures of hepatic function are stable or improving. It is especially important during this time to allow opportunities to ask questions and vent anxiety. The relationship the transplant coordinator (TC) established during the pretransplant phase builds trust and offers comfort during this time.

Surprisingly, despite the extensive surgery, postoperative pain is usually not a major complaint; an exception to this occurs in patients who had been using (or abusing) analgesics on a regular basis prior to surgery. Most patients use minimal amounts of narcotics, especially when self-administered by patient-controlled analgesia programs. In some transplant centers narcotics are not regularly used; intravenous diphenhydramine, supplemented when necessary by narcotics, prevents depression of the respiratory drive and hastens weaning from analgesics.

By the end of the second postoperative day, most transplant patients will have only one intravenous line, a Foley catheter, a biliary T-tube (unless the biliary anastomosis was by Roux-en-Y), and, possibly, one surgical drain. The patient usually has been out of bed to a chair but has not resumed an oral diet. The move to the transplant unit frequently is a psychological boost for the patient and the family. For some the abrupt decrease in the intensity of care and monitoring is threatening, especially for those who have required prolonged ICU admission. Many patients and family members require reassurance that neither the patient nor the liver graft will suddenly decompensate.

■ THE INPATIENT TRANSPLANT UNIT

Most transplant centers have geographically defined inpatient units for each specific organ transplant population. A nursing staff specially trained to monitor liver transplant recipients at all stages of postoperative care provides the backbone of the liver transplant unit; the nurse-to-patient ratio in the unit is generally better than in a regular acute care unit. The advantage of geographical localization of liver transplant patients also includes the increased expertise and experience of the clerical, dietary, physical therapy, and pharmacy personnel. A continuing education program for the staff of the liver transplant unit, supported by members of the transplant team, maintains these advantages.

One of the important objectives while the patient is in the liver transplant unit is education of the patient and family with respect to health practices posttransplantation. Transplant nurse coordinators, pharmacists, physical therapists, and dieticians spend time instructing the patient and family during this phase of recovery. The focus is on medications, signs and symptoms of infection, rejection, diet, and general rules of health maintenance after discharge (Table 18.1). Patients are also instructed in the care of the operative wound, the T-tube, and any drains that remain. It is vital that the patient and family have a good knowledge of medications and care issues at the time of discharge.

The average patient spends a week in the liver transplant unit before being discharged from the hospital. Some patients are discharged in as few as 5 days, necessitating early independence and providing limited time for education. The more debilitated patient pretransplant (i.e. chronic disease with MELD score >30) may have a complicated recovery requiring several weeks in hospital. Discharge to a rehabilitation center or home with intensive therapy may be necessary.

During the time on the transplant unit, the patient progresses to independent ambulation. Once bowel function resumes, medications are changed to oral dosing, and diet is advanced as tolerated. Patients may experience complications during this phase of recovery; acute cellular rejection is common during this early phase (Chapter 19) as is postoperative infection (Chapter 25). If the patient experiences acute rejection, discharge may be delayed 2–3 days. Continuation of intravenous infusions of antibiotics or antirejection drugs for an outpatient under the supervision of a home health agency has become

Table 18.1   *Health Practices Posttransplantation*

Daily care
>   Temperature (report >101°F)
>   Daily weight (report >4 lb/week)
>   Incisional staples for 3 weeks
>   T-tube for 4–6 months
>   No submersion of staples or tubes in water (bath, pool)

Symptoms of rejection
>   Fever >100.5°F
>   Jaundice
>   Clay-colored stool, dark urine
>   RUQ pain (Right Upper Quadrant)
>   Fatigue

General restrictions
>   No driving for 4 weeks or as long as narcotics are required
>   No heavy lifting for 3 months
>   May return to work after 8–12 weeks

Medications
>   Gradual dose reduction over time
>   Do not take prior to laboratory work
>   Regular dosing time to avoid missing doses
>   Bring updated list to clinic visits
>   Reorder prescriptions before supply exhausted
>   Report vomiting or diarrhea over 24 h if unable to take medications

Symptoms of infection
>   Fever >101°F
>   Chills
>   Erythema, discharge, pain at wound or drain
>   Symptoms specific to organ system (cough, spitum, dysuria)

General guidelines
>   Resume sexual activity whenever comfortable
>   May need to consider birth control or safe sexual practice
>   Frequent hand washing for protection from infections
>   Wash fruits/vegetables
>   Cook all foods thoroughly
>   Dental antibiotic prophylaxis for first 6 months

normal practice. Coordination of care and collaboration with the local physician are crucial for successful outcomes.

Prior to discharge from the hospital, the patient and family are instructed in follow-up care routines and expectations. Directions to the liver transplant clinic, appointment times, and contact telephone numbers for the liver transplant team members are given. This time of separation from the hospital and the transplant team is often anxiety-producing for patients and families. The transplant nurse coordinator and social worker begin to address this anxiety several days before discharge. Patients are discharged when there is no evidence of a new complication, liver tests are normal or improving, antirejection medications are in the therapeutic range, and the patient has learned the fundamentals of post-transplantation health maintenance (Table 18.1).

If the patient's home (or that of a friend or family member) is within an hour's travel time of the transplant center, most programs will allow discharge to that location. Otherwise, the patient and family are requested to stay in the vicinity of the transplant center in a hotel, or comparable accommodation, for at least another week to 10 days. Some transplant centers have special transplant homes for patients and families, similar in concept to the Ronald MacDonald Houses for pediatric patients.

During this initial outpatient period, the patient is seen in the liver transplant clinic two or three times a week for medical supervision, laboratory evaluation, wound care, and medication adjustment. These visits are opportunities for reinforcement of teaching, especially concerning medications. Routine laboratory tests include liver tests, electrolytes, complete blood count, prothrombin time, and trough levels of cyclosporine, tacrolimus, or sirolimus. The dose of the immunosuppressive medications is adjusted according to blood values. Diuretics, antihypertensives, and other drugs are also added or adjusted as necessary. It is not unusual for patients to spend several hours at a clinic visit while being assessed and waiting for laboratory results. This can be tiring for both patients and family members; some of the time may be spent in a support group session or other educational activities if available.

Most patients are ready to return home within 3 weeks after their liver transplant. By this point, their incisional staples, as well as all surgical drains, with the exception of the T-tube, have been removed. For patients who have a T-tube placed during their transplant, it remains in the common bile duct for several months while the duct-to-duct anastamosis heals. During this time the T-tube provides convenient access to the biliary system if needed to evaluate a change in liver tests. Between 3 and 6 months, the patient will return to the transplant center to have the T-tube removed. Removal of the T-tube is usually accomplished in the transplant clinic. In approximately 10% of patients, T-tube removal is associated with a bile leak that requires endoscopic sphincterotomy and placement of a biliary stent.

When the patient returns home, the transplant center team will communicate with the local physician to coordinate the patient's care. At times, more than one local physician will participate in the post-transplant care; it is important to define which physician has the primary responsibility in order to ensure that care continues without interruption. For the first 2–3 months, the patient will return for regular visits to the liver transplant clinic. As time progresses, and particularly after the T-tube is removed, a greater portion of the care is shifted to the patient's local physician. A transplant center physician and nurse coordinator remain "on-call" and available to the primary care physician at all times.

It is the responsibility of the transplant team to ensure that the local physician is knowledgeable about the specific concerns surrounding long-term management of the transplant recipient. At the time the patient returns home, a member of the transplant team, who is often the nurse coordinator, will communicate to the local physician about individual care issues.

Most blood tests used to follow liver transplant recipients are standardized; the tests can be done locally and the results faxed or phoned to the transplant center the next day. It is important that the information arrives at the transplant center in a timely fashion so that adjustments in medications or arrangements for radiologic interventions and liver biopsies can be made without delay.

Transplant centers that measure trough levels of cyclosporine, tacrolimus, or sirolimus in-house often prefer that the same hospital laboratory continues to perform these tests for some time after the patient returns to his local area. As part of the planning for the return home, the transplant nurse coordinators instruct the local area phlebotomy site and the patient regarding how to ship the specimen back to the transplant center. Overnight delivery of the sample permits the assay to be performed the next day and facilitates adjustments in the patient's immunosuppressant dose. When the relationship between the patient's dose of cyclosporine, tacrolimus, or sirolimus and the trough blood levels has stabilized, it is often acceptable to perform the assay locally. Many transplant centers allow patients with stable trough levels to begin using commercial laboratories at the time of discharge to their community.

Liver biopsies are done in some transplant programs at fixed intervals; other transplant programs only do liver biopsies "for cause" such as abnormal liver tests. It is preferable for the patient to have a liver biopsy done at the transplant center, especially in the early post-transplant period.

The essential parts of successful post-transplantation care are cooperation and communication. The patient, the local physician, and the transplant team each have important roles to play. The relative contribution of each part of the care group is determined by a number of factors, chief among which is the patient's course. A committed patient with an uncomplicated post-transplant course who is easily reintegrated into normal life will have little need of the kind of expertise unique to the transplant center. This patient will be seen at least once a year at the transplant center for ongoing evaluation of transplant-specific issues such as immunosuppressive changes, long-term complications of transplantation and immunosuppression, and recurrence of original disease (Chapter 24). Attention to health maintenance issues as well as treatment for chronic medical problems (hypertension, diabetes, etc.) are best managed by the local primary care physician.

The patient with persistent complications, on the other hand, may experience repeated admissions to the transplant center and many outpatient procedures and clinic visits. Such a patient may not see the local physician for many months at a time. In each case, communication and understanding between the transplant team and the local care team is essential.

Role of the Transplant Coordinator

The TC serves as a facilitator during the entire transplant process beginning with the referral of the patient to the transplant center. He or she is usually the first person to meet the patient and the family at the transplant center and most often will have had prior telephone contact with them. The TC is the person who will schedule the patient's evaluation and collate the results of laboratory tests for the medical team, and is responsible for maintaining a current MELD score. If the decision is made to transplant the patient, the TC will notify the United Network for Organ Sharing (UNOS) database and confirm the ABO blood type. The TC usually has an advanced degree in nursing; some have additional training as nurse or practitioner or may be certified in a nursing specialty area pertinent to organ transplantation.

It is the primary focus of the TC to ensure continuity of information flow between the transplant team, the patient, the patient's family, and the referring physician, applying the knowledge derived from training and especially experience with liver transplantation. The goal is to forge a bond between the TC and the patient and the patient's family such that there is no hesitation to ask questions about the liver transplantation process. The TC is the cheerleader, confessor, and interpreter during the patient's complex journey through the transplant process and beyond.

Rejection

▼   ▼   ▼   ▼   ▼   ▼   ▼   ▼   ▼

Bradley H. Collins and Dev M. Desai

■ **INTRODUCTION**

Despite the recent introduction of novel immunosuppressive therapy, 20–40% of liver transplant recipients will develop at least one episode of acute cellular rejection within the first year following transplantation [1,2]. Although much less common, chronic rejection is virtually always progressive and consideration of retransplantation is usually necessary (Chapters 1 and 24). The purpose of this chapter is to outline immunosuppressive therapy protocols utilized for liver transplant recipients, describe the types of rejection encountered, and review the evaluation and treatment of liver allograft rejection.

■ **LIVER TRANSPLANT IMMUNOLOGY**

When compared with other solid organ transplants, the liver has always been considered "privileged" with respect to the recipient's immune system. Nevertheless, recent data show that acute rejection of allografts liver may occur with equal or greater frequency than other organs; however, the sequelae of these episodes of rejection are not as significant because of the protective mechanisms and the regenerative capacity of the liver [3,4]. In addition, of the commonly transplanted allografts, the liver is the only organ that consistently permits aggressive weaning of immunosuppressive therapy to a single agent or in selected cases, all immunotherapy. The recent advent of new small molecule and biologic immunotherapeutic agents has permitted drug combinations capitalizing on the unique properties of individual immunosuppressive agents, thus permitting customization of the immunosuppressive therapy regimen to the individual recipients. The benefits of reducing immunosuppressive therapy exposure to minimize the long-term side-effects of immunosuppression cannot be overstated.

ABO Blood Groups

Liver transplants are most commonly performed between matching ABO blood types. Decades ago it was noted that unlike the kidney and heart, the liver could be transplanted across ABO-incompatible blood groups without immediate graft loss [5]. Although the short-term function of these grafts was good, long-term complications occurred, including a greater incidence of biliary complications, rejection episodes, and hepatic artery thrombosis. Both biliary epithelial cells and vascular endothelial cells contain donor blood group antigens that sustain chronic injury when exposed to the recipient's anti-ABO antibodies.

Children under 1 year of age in receipt of ABO-incompatible grafts have the best outcomes with over 75% 1-year survival compared with less than 22% in adults at 1 year [6]. Adjunctive therapies such as plasmapheresis, splenectomy, intravenous immunoglobulin (IVIg) and anti-B lymphocyte agents such as rituximab (anti-CD20 monoclonal antibody) have been reported as single cases or in small case series to reduce hemolysis, acute humoral graft rejection, and graft loss [7]. Despite these improvements, liver transplantation across incompatible blood groups is still reserved for critically ill patients in whom no other options exist.

ABO-compatible, but unmatched, donor–recipient combinations (i.e. an O liver into an A recipient or a B liver into an AB recipient) are more commonly employed. Recipients of these grafts frequently develop a transient hemolytic syndrome that is the result of passenger lymphocytes in the liver that produce antibodies to the recipient's own red cells. This clinical entity usually resolves spontaneously in several days to a few weeks, and these patients generally recover without untoward effects.

The Crossmatch

Although crossmatching is the standard of care among patients undergoing kidney and pancreas transplantation, the test is not required before proceeding with liver transplantation. Before performing kidney or pancreas transplantation, an in vitro crossmatch is performed between the donor's lymphocytes and the recipient's serum by means of flow cytometry or cellular cytotoxicity assary. A positive crossmatch confirms the presence of anti-human leukocyte antigen (anti-HLA) antibodies in the recipient's serum that are capable of binding to allograft endothelial cells. Once bound to the vascular endothelium of the transplanted organ, these antibodies provoke an antibody-dependent complement-mediated cytotoxicity (ADCC), resulting in a rapid and destructive immune response known as hyperacute rejection. Hyperacute rejection leads to vascular thrombosis and rapid graft destruction within a matter of minutes to hours.

Before the advent of the University of Wisconsin organ preservation solution (Viaspan, Dupont Inc., Wilmington, DE), it was not practical to perform prospective crossmatching for liver transplantation, because of the rapidity with which the liver had to be transplanted. Liver allografts were transplanted without prospective crossmatches and, unlike renal allografts, liver allograft and patient survival were excellent. In fact, there is only one report of hyperacute rejection of a liver allograft; in this case the anti-HLA antibody titer was exceedingly high at 1:30 000 [8]. When retrospective crossmatching has been performed in liver transplant recipients, it was determined that positive crossmatches did not correlate with early graft dysfunction or loss but were associated with a higher incidence of early acute cellular rejection [9]. More recently, in a single-center retrospective analysis of more than 440 patients over 13 years, Doran et al. demonstrated a statistically significant decrease in graft survival at 3 and 12 months among those liver allograft recipients with a positive cytotoxic crossmatch. Furthermore, they also demonstrated that a positive flow cytometry crossmatch predicted both acute and chronic allograft rejection [10]. It is not certain whether these retrospective results (over one decade) are applicable in the current immunosuppressive therapy era since there has been continued improvement in allograft survival and reduction in acute rejection rates despite a lack of prospective crossmatching prior to liver transplantation.

Occasionally a liver transplant recipient will present as a clinical dilemma wherein it is possible that rejection is playing a role in the clinical picture. A patient may also present with recurrent episodes of acute rejection. Requesting the HLA laboratory to perform a retrospective crossmatch may be helpful in these circumstances. If the crossmatch is positive, the recipient may require more potent immunosuppressive therapy or adjunctive therapies such as antilymphocyte antibodies, IVIg, and/or plasmapheresis.

■ IMMUNOSUPPRESSION PROTOCOLS

Standard

Although the incidence of acute hepatic allograft rejection is greater than that observed among other solid organ recipients, it is also the case that maintenance immunosuppression requirements are much less. In fact, many transplant centers have adopted a double immunosuppressive agent protocol that includes the calcineurin inhibitor tacrolimus (FK 506) and prednisone. A number of centers are utilizing the mammalian target of rapamycin (mTOR) inhibitor sirolimus rather than tacrolimus, in combination with prednisone. Because it is not nephrotoxic, sirolimus is usually reserved for those recipients with baseline renal insufficiency or in whom renal dysfunction develops postoperatively [11]. After several months, these centers often aggressively wean the patient from the steroids until they are discontinued. Liver transplant recipients are then maintained on monotherapy comprising only tacrolimus or sirolimus. One advantage of such a protocol is that patients are spared some of the long-term adverse effects of prednisone including bone density loss, cataract formation, avascular necrosis, and weight gain. Prednisone has some side-effects in common with tacrolimus (see Chapter 29). Certain liver allograft recipients do not qualify for steroid withdrawal therapy because it is thought that to do so would increase the risk of recurrent disease in the transplanted liver. Their original disease processes are usually those that are immunologically mediated including autoimmune hepatitis, primary sclerosing cholangitis, and primary biliary cirrhosis.

One current controversy in the field of liver transplantation is whether induction immunotherapy is necessary. Induction agents are administered to the recipient a few hours before transplantation and induce a state of immunosuppression. Examples include rabbit antithymocyte globulin (RATG), OKT3, and the IL-2 receptor antagonists basiliximab and daclvzimab. Induction therapy has been shown to decrease the incidence of early acute rejection, but the long-term effects on rejection prevention are far less conclusive [12]. Because reversal of acute hepatic allograft rejection is achieved in virtually all cases, the routine use of induction therapy may not be warranted. Worrisome side-effects of induction immunotherapy include infections and an increased incidence of certain malignancies. An accepted indication for induction therapy is among patients with impaired renal function for whom initiation of calcineurin inhibitor therapy must be delayed to spare the kidneys.

A basic immunosuppression protocol is outlined in Table 19.1. Institutions that utilize triple-drug protocols employ some combination of calcineurin inhibitor (cyclosporine or tacrolimus), antimetabolite (mycophenolate mofetil or azathioprine), and prednisone. Double-drug protocols are usually based on tacrolimus or sirolimus and prednisone. The doses of calcineurin inhibitors and sirolimus are determined by serum trough levels. Mycophenolate mofetil dosing is standard unless the patient develops side-effects such as gastrointestinal complaints or leukopenia. The dose of azathioprine is standard unless the patient develops leukopenia at which point it is decreased. A detailed description of the mechanisms of action, dosing, and side-effects of these agents is found in Chapter 29.

Hepatitis C

Over the last several years, chronic hepatitis C virus (HCV) liver disease has emerged as the most common indication for liver transplantation. Patients

Table 19.1 *Immunosuppression Protocol (Duke University Medical Center Maintenance Agents)[a]*

Prednisone
- Patients administered 20 mg/day orally beginning on postoperative day 5
- 15 mg/day postoperative weeks 2 to 4
- 10 mg/day postoperative weeks 4 to 8
- 7.5 mg/day postoperative weeks 8 to 10
- 5 mg/day postoperative weeks 10 to 12
- Monthly taper by 1 mg/month until prednisone discontinued
- Postoperative taper accelerated as clinically indicated such as recipients with hepatitis C
- Recipients transplanted for autoimmune hepatitis, primary biliary cirrhosis, and primary sclerosing cholangitis remain on 5 mg/day

FK 506 (tacrolimus)
- Administered orally BID to achieve a serum trough level of approximately 10–12 ng/mL for the first 3 months, 8–10 ng/mL for months 3–6, and 5–8 ng/mL after 6 months

Cyclosporine
- An alternative to FK 506
- Administered orally BID to achieve a target trough level of 200–250 ng/mL for the first several days postoperatively, then 150–200 ng/mL for the first 6 months, and then 100–150 ng/mL after 6 months

Sirolimus
- Oral loading dose of 5–10 mg (higher dose reserved for African American recipients)
- Then, once-daily dosing to achieve a trough serum level of 5–10 ng/mL (usually requires 1–5 mg/day)

Mycophenolate mofetil
- Reserved for patients who develop multiple episodes of acute rejection, resistant rejection, or chronic renal insufficiency
- Usual dose 500 mg orally BID, but may be decreased if patient develops gastrointestinal side-effects such as diarrhea, gastritis, or abdominal pain

Azathioprine
- An alternative to mycophenolate mofetil
- Occasionally utilized for patients with recurrent autoimmune disease
- Usual dose 1–2 mg/kg orally per day

[a]Maintenance agents usually initiated within a day or two of transplantation. The initiation of the calcineurin inhibitors tacrolimus and cyclosporine is often delayed in patients with acute and/or chronic renal insufficiency. In those cases, recipients are often temporized with an induction antibody.

transplanted for HCV liver disease are excellent candidates for steroid with-drawal protocols because it is believed that a partially competent recipient immune system plays a role in slowing the course of recurrent hepatitis, an increasing cause of liver allograft loss. Some centers utilize aggressive induction protocols in this patient population so as to minimize the risk of subsequent acute cellular rejection [2]. It is thought that the regimen required to reverse acute allograft rejection is more likely to result in clinically significant, recurrent HCV liver disease than induction therapy administered prior to transplantation. Large multicentered trials will be required to more definitively answer this question.

■ HYPERACUTE REJECTION AND PRIMARY NONFUNCTION

Hyperacute acute rejection is a fulminant immune reaction in the recipient that occurs in the presence of preformed antibodies to antigens (ABO and HLA) present on donor endothelial and parenchymal cells. Complement fixation, inflammatory cellular infiltration, and microangiopathy are seen and the trans-planted organ is destroyed in rapid order. Although hyperacute liver allograft rejection can be induced in experimental animal models, its clinical relevance in liver transplantation remains controversial [13,14]. Rodent and primate models of hyperacute liver rejection have required presensitization of animals with multiple allogeneic skin grafts, which result in high titers of anti-MHC (HLA-equivalent) antibodies; these are significantly higher than levels that are encountered clinically.

There have been clinical reports of fulminant hepatic failure consistent with hyperacute rejection in the early posttransplant period in recipients receiving ABO-incompatible allografts [15]. Humoral components have been identified in these grafts including IgM, IgG, and complement deposits; how-ever, the contribution of preservation injury or ischemic damage is difficult to ascertain. Additionally, since hyperacute rejection is directed predominantly at the vascular endothelium, it has been suggested that early portal vein or hepatic artery thrombosis may be immunologic and not secondary to technical complications.

Clinical features of hyperacute rejection are indistinguishable from those of primary graft nonfunction and early portal or hepatic vascular thrombosis. They include hepatic coma, profound coagulopathy, acidosis, and elevated liver test concentrations. Since portal vein and hepatic artery thrombosis can also present in this manner Doppler sonographic evaluation of these vessels should be performed to rule out vascular thrombosis, which may be amenable to surgical intervention. Otherwise, the only treatment is urgent retransplantation.

The vast majority of livers transplanted across a positive crossmatch or ABO barrier do not undergo hyperacute rejection. The mechanism for this relative resistance is not certain. However, the liver likely avoids antibody-mediated injury by absorbing and rapidly processing bound antibodies. In contrast to other transplanted solid organs, the liver does not contain end-arteries, but instead is composed of fenestrated sinusoids fed by portal venous and hepatic arterial flow, which can reciprocally compensate for compromised flow in either system. Moreover, the Kupffer cells and macrophages that line hepatic sinusoids have a great capacity for removing antibody complexes.

The liver's resistance to antibody-mediated injury has led many investigators to propose that hyperacute hepatic allograft rejection does not occur, and that this phenomenon is really primary nonfunction, a syndrome marked by failure of the liver to function upon revascularization. Primary nonfunction can be a mortal immediate complication of liver transplantation. The diagnosis is predominantly clinical: lack of bile production, encephalopathy and coma, persistent or worsening coagulopathy, markedly elevated liver tests, and metabolic acidosis in the presence of a patent portal vein and hepatic artery. Liver biopsies early after reperfusion in organs with primary nonfunction demonstrate hepatocyte swelling, and apoptosis as well as centrilobular hemorrhage and necrosis [16]. Numerous donor and recipient risk factors for primary nonfunction have been identified through retrospective multivariate analysis. Important donor factors include steatosis (>30%), serum sodium concentration (>160 mmol/L), donor age greater than 50, and cold preservation time longer than 12 h; in the recipient, retransplantation, and poor medical condition (renal failure, etc.). As organ procurement and preservation techniques have improved, the incidence of primary nonfunction has decreased significantly [17].

■ ACUTE CELLULAR REJECTION

Twenty to forty percent of patients will experience acute cellular rejection within the first year of liver transplantation [2]. Recipients are most often affected within the first week of transplantation, and the incidence decreases as a function of time. Late episodes of acute rejection, i.e. those occurring after the first year, are most likely the result of decreased immunosuppression such as occurs with skipped doses of immunosuppressive therapy. The clinician's index of suspicion for medication noncompliance should be heightened in these instances. New medications should be initiated with caution in transplant recipients. There are a number of commonly prescribed agents that induce the cytochrome P_{450} system, thus enhancing the metabolism of calcineurin inhibitors. Blood levels of cyclosporine or tacrolimus may plummet, resulting in an unexpected episode of acute rejection (see Chapter 30).

An association has been identified between hepatitis C and acute cellular rejection [18]. The mechanism of increased incidence of rejection in hepatitis C-positive recipients has not been elucidated, although both viral stimulation of the immune system and the upregulation of allograft antigens have been postulated as potential etiologies. In addition, the use of interferon to diminish the hepatitis C viral load has been shown to increase the incidence of rejection [19]. Interferon is a known stimulator of the immune system, and it has been hypothesized that it increases the expression of donor antigens, thus promoting a host immune response and rejection. Others have theorized that interferon therapy leads to viral elimination and so enhances the liver's metabolic capacity [20]. This then leads to increased metabolism of immunosuppressive agents, which results in a reduction in the overall state of immunosuppression, thus favoring the development of acute rejection.

Mechanism

Histologic analysis of the acutely rejecting liver demonstrates a cellular inflammatory infiltrate directed against biliary epithelial cells as well as the endothelial cells of the portal and hepatic veins. T-lymphocytes are the primary offenders. In addition to having a direct cytotoxic effect on the transplanted liver, the T cells also serve to attract other effector cells including macrophages. Eosinophils are usually present also, but their role in the pathogenesis of rejection is not known.

Symptoms

Patients with acute cellular rejection frequently present with nonspecific complaints. Symptoms may include, but are not limited to, generalized malaise, decreased appetite, and right upper quadrant pain. Many patients with documented acute cellular rejection progress along the normal postoperative course and are asymptomatic.

Physical Findings

Physical signs including jaundice and low-grade fever are occasionally observed. Patients with T-tubes may note a decrease in bile volume. The character of the bile may change from a thick, dark green, viscous liquid to a thinner, lighter quality. Clinicians must always keep in mind that patients with rejection may present without signs or symptoms, so the index of suspicion must remain high; additional assessment is always warranted if laboratory indicators are present.

Laboratory Evaluation

Following orthotopic liver transplantation, serum biochemical tests are obtained according to protocol. Immediately after transplantation while the patient is recovering in the intensive care unit, liver biochemical parameters and function tests are assayed frequently, as are levels of immunosuppressants (see Chapter 18). Immunosuppressant levels are monitored to facilitate drug dosage adjustment in order to optimize immunosuppression. Once the patient has stabilized, laboratory studies are obtained daily until discharge. After discharge, the liver tests are obtained at least weekly until liver function and immunosuppressive therapy drug levels are optimal. Thereafter, the frequency of liver chemistries and immunosuppressive agent assays varies according to clinical indications but is not less than monthly.

In general, immediately following liver transplantation, liver tests are abnormal because of preservation and reperfusion injury during implantation. In the absence of primary allograft nonfunction or vascular complication (hepatic artery or portal vein thrombosis), these laboratory parameters stabilize over the ensuing few days. In most patients, the first indication of a problem is either increased liver test concentrations or failure of liver tests to return to normal, with plateauing in an abnormally elevated range. Either event should prompt a workup for complications, including rejection.

The target tissues of the host's cellular immune response are the biliary epithelial cells and endothelial cells of the portal and hepatic venous systems. The cannilicular enzymes (alkaline phosphatase and γ-glutamyl transpeptidase) are usually first to increase when an acute rejection episode occurs. In more severe grades of rejection, the offending cells may spill into the adjacent parenchyma, resulting in hepatocyte injury or death. In these cases, the serum aminotransferase concentrations are elevated also, usually signaling a severe episode of acute cellular rejection. Any patient with an elevated bilirubin should be evaluated for obstruction of the biliary system (see later).

While elevation of hepatic biochemical parameters is a hallmark of acute cellular rejection, it is not pathognomonic and must be differentiated from other etiologies of hepatic inflammation, such as recurrent viral hepatitis and recurrent or de novo autoimmune hepatitis. An adjunctive method to help differentiate between acute rejection presumably due to insufficient immunosuppression and recurrent hepatitis virus infection, exacerbated by overimmunosuppression, is to measure global immune cell function. The Food and Drug Administration (FDA) recently approved an immune cell function assay (Cylex Inc., Columbia, MD) that measures T lymphocyte intracellular adenosine triphosphate (ATP) levels [21]. Since ATP is the cellular energy source, low levels of ATP would indicate depressed T cell function, thus overimmunosuppression would suggest an etiology of liver inflammation other than acute cellular rejection.

Radiographic Studies

Because a number of posttransplant clinical conditions are associated with elevated liver enzymes and function tests, a complete evaluation of recipients is indicated, including radiographic evaluation of the transplanted liver. Ultrasound (US) is a rapid and relatively inexpensive method of evaluating multiple aspects of a transplanted liver. Doppler interrogation of the blood vessels supplying (hepatic artery and portal vein) and draining (hepatic veins) the liver can be informative. Elevated liver tests in the presence of patent blood vessels should increase the clinician's suspicion for rejection (Chapter 20).

US may be also useful in determining whether the etiology of elevated liver tests is due to biliary obstruction. Dilation of both the intra- and the extrahepatic bile ducts can be identified using US. If dilatation is present additional evaluation of the biliary tree should be performed prior to liver biopsy. A T-tube cholangiogram may be performed if the tube is present. Endoscopic retrograde or percutaneous biliary cholangiography may be necessary, as dictated by the clinical situation (Chapter 21).

Diagnosis

Elevated hepatic enzymes and function tests are not specific for acute rejection. The single, most informative diagnostic test of liver graft rejection is liver biopsy. Once abnormalities of the hepatic vascular and biliary systems have been ruled out as potential causes of elevated liver tests, a biopsy should be performed. Because the risk of liver biopsy is so small, the threshold for use of this technique for diagnosis should be very low indeed. There are few indications for the empiric treatment of rejection without histologic confirmation of the diagnosis. Disease processes such as recurrent HCV liver disease and cytomegalovirus disease are worsened by the doses of immunosuppressive therapy used to treat rejection; therefore, it is imperative to rule out other etiologies of elevated liver function tests prior to embarking on a treatment course.

The value of a pathologist trained in liver transplant pathology is immeasurable and cannot be overstated. The multitude of potential diagnoses and the subtleties that separate them are often only discernible by the trained and highly experienced eye. Recurrent HCV liver disease and acute rejection share many histological characteristics. It is important to have sufficient confidence in the pathologist's abilities so that one can commit a patient to the high doses of immunsuppressive therapy necessary to treat rejection.

There are multiple techniques for obtaining a specimen from a transplanted liver. The method selected for biopsy is dictated by the patient's clinical condition. The most common technique is percutaneous biopsy of the right lobe with a 16- or 18-gauge biopsy device. The procedure can be performed safely either at the bedside or in the clinic. Some clinicians prefer a US-guided technique to minimize the incidence of inadvertent injury to other organs or the liver's vascular supply. US is also useful for obtaining a biopsy from a specific location in the liver (e.g. right vs. left lobe).

Percutaneous biopsy of a transplanted liver is safer than a native liver biopsy because the risk of postbiopsy bleeding is less. Following transplantation, the liver becomes encased by adhesions that serve to effect hemostasis at the level of the liver capsule. As with certain pretransplant patients, some liver transplant recipients are not good candidates for percutaneous biopsy. Within the first few days of transplantation prior to the adhesion response, when patients may still have ascites and coagulopathy, the risk of bleeding associated with percutaneous biopsy may be too high. In these instances, liver biopsy via the transjugular approach may be most appropriate.

An open-needle biopsy is an alternative to the transjugular route. This requires a brief trip to the operating room where a small portion of the incision is reopened. The biopsy is then performed directly with a needle device or biopsy gun, hemostasis is achieved with electrocautery, and the incision is closed. A few centers perform a Williams' window at the time of transplantation [22]. This is a small opening in the midline portion of the incision overlying the liver through which the liver can be biopsied at the bedside. Hemostasis of the biopsy site is achieved with pressure applied by a finger. The window can be utilized for several weeks until the wound granulates. For a patient with an abnormal coagulation profile who requires liver biopsy, partial or complete correction with fresh frozen plasma, cryoprecipitate, and platelets should be considered.

Once obtained, the transplant liver biopsy specimen should be placed on a saline-soaked piece of gauze and transported immediately to the pathology laboratory, where the specimen is then placed in 10% formalin solution and processed for hematoxylin and eosin staining. Frozen sections are not useful in the diagnosis of acute rejection, so the specimens are formalin-fixed and processed routinely. Some rapid processing techniques exist that can provide a permanent fixed slide within 4–6 h; however, most centers require 24 h to complete the process. If the index of suspicion is high, all tests are negative, and the patient has no indication of an acute infectious process, some clinicians will initiate treatment for rejection prior to waiting for 24 h for final biopsy results. This is a common practice in kidney and pancreas transplantation. However, unlike both kidney and pancreas, the liver tolerates acute rejection well due to its regenerative capacity; therefore, waiting a day until the diagnosis is confirmed is generally not associated with decreased reversibility. The advantage of delaying treatment is a decreased risk of infection associated with unnecessary administration of excess amounts of immunosuppressive therapy.

A patient who undergoes a liver biopsy by the percutaneous route should be kept on bedrest for 4–6 h. Vital signs should be checked every 15 min for the first hour, every 30 min for the second hour, and then hourly for the last 2 h. The hematocrit should also be determined at the end of bedrest. Any worrisome changes in vital signs or a significant decrease in hematocrit should prompt an emergent US scan to assess for hematoma formation. Observational therapy may be sufficient in combination with correction of abnormal coagulation parameters; however, operative intervention may be necessary.

Treatment

The initial form of treatment for acute cellular rejection is corticosteroid bolus therapy (Table 19.2). A number of protocols are available, but the general theme is the same. A typical protocol includes daily intravenous methylprednisolone with the typical dose for adults ranging from 500 to 1000 mg/day. The duration of therapy is based on the patient's clinical response, and typically lasts between 3 and 5 days. If the patient is doing well otherwise,

Table 19.2 *Management of Acute Cellular Rejection (Duke University Medical Center)*

Initial episode

Methylprednisolone

• 500 mg IV administered daily for 3 days

Recurrent episode

• Methylprednisolone (if previous episode successfully treated)
• 500 mg IV administered daily for 5 days

Steroid-resistant episodes

Rabbit antithymocyte globulin

• 1.5 mg/kg IV daily for a total of 5–7 doses
• Dose reduction necessary if leukopenia or thrombocytopenia develops

OKT3

• An alternative to rabbit antithymocyte globulin
• 5 mg IV/day for 7–10 days
• Side-effects common during the initial doses (fever, rigors, etc.) secondary to cytokine release syndrome; patients should be pretreated with acetaminophen and prednisone

outpatient management of acute rejection is indicated. Daily infusions of steroids and serum biochemistries can be performed in the clinic. If the patient has any change in his/her clinical condition, such as elevated temperature or abdominal pain, then inpatient management is more appropriate. Patients will often exhibit a leukocytosis with the early doses of steroids due to demargination of white blood cells.

While recipients are treated for rejection, their liver biochemical parameters are assessed on a daily basis. Successful therapy is marked by a decrease in liver test concentrations. Although values may not normalize immediately, there should be a steady and sustained decline by the time the course of steroid therapy is completed. If the rejection has caused significant liver injury, it may take several additional days to weeks for the inflammatory changes to resolve. Clinicians should be aware that patients may have multiple episodes of acute rejection within a given period of time. Each should be managed as outlined earlier so long as there is resolution after each course of steroids.

If there is no improvement in liver tests with a steroid pulse or, if the numbers plateau, then additional evaluation may be necessary. In particular, Doppler US scan should be repeated to reassess the hepatic vasculature. If these studies are negative, then further liver biopsy is indicated to evaluate for continuing rejection.

Steroid-Resistant Rejection

Approximately 5–10% of acute cellular rejection episodes do not respond to pulsed steroid therapy. Treatment of steroid-resistant rejection episodes in the cyclosporine era was managed by conversion to tacrolimus; however, now that tacrolimus has replaced cyclosporine as the primary maintenance immunosuppressive agent, steroid-resistant rejection generally requires use of an antilymphocyte agent [23].

There are numerous antilymphocyte antibody preparations available currently, and newer agents are on the horizon. Two agents, Minnesota antilymphocyte globulin (ALG or MALG) and antithymocyte gamma globulin (ATGAM, equine source) are no longer used clinically and in general, are not commercially available. The aforementioned OKT3, a monoclonal antibody generated in mice with specificity for the CD3 component of the T cell receptor, is a potent agent that results in removal of all CD3-bearing lymphocytes from the circulation within minutes of administration. This drug is administered intravenously in bolus fashion at a dose of 2.5–10 mg/day for 7–14 days, and results in a cytokine release syndrome that produces flu-like symptoms in recipients lasting between 24 and 48 h [24]. The most worrisome acute side-effect of OKT3 is the sudden development of severe pulmonary edema, occurring in approximately 2% of patients [24]. Treatment usually requires prompt endotracheal intubation. Because of the severity of this complication, all recipients of OKT3 should receive a chest radiograph to rule out preexisting pulmonary disease prior to commencement of therapy. Diuretics should be administered before dosing if the patient is volume-overloaded. Hemodialysis may be necessary if the patient has renal dysfunction.

As with pulsed corticosteroid therapy, the efficacy of OKT3 therapy is monitored by the response in the biochemical parameters. It is also prudent to follow absolute CD3 counts, (<10 CD3$^+$ cells/mL being the target) as a means to document effective clearance of rejection-causing T lymphocytes. Occasionally the daily dose may need to be doubled if the CD3 count does not initially fall to <10 cells/mL. The use of OKT3 can be problematic. In addition to severe and potentially life-threatening side-effects of the cytokine release syndrome, tachyphylaxis may result from repeated use because of formation of antimurine antibodies. Furthermore, there is an increased incidence of early-onset, severe recurrent HCV liver disease and graft loss in recipients transplanted for HCV cirrhosis as well as an increased risk of posttransplant lymphoproliferative disorder (PTLD) in all patients receiving OKT3. The incidence of PTLD may be proportional to the cumulative lifetime dose [25]. Since there are numerous short- and long-term complications associated with the use of OKT3, another antilymphocyte preparation, RATG, is being increasingly utilized [26]. RATG is a polyclonal antibody preparation that does not activate T cells and, thus, the degree of cytokine release is significantly lower. Tachyphylaxis has not been described as a clinically significant problem, thus permitting repeated usage of RATG for treatment of acute cellular rejection.

The anti-interleukin-2 receptor antibodies (basiliximab and dacluzimab) have been utilized for induction immunotherapy, but they have not been effective for the treatment of rejection. The newest antilymphocyte agent, alemtuzumab (Campath-1H, Berlex Inc., Montvail, NJ), is a humanized monoclonal antibody that recognizes CD52, a small glycoprotein highly expressed on T and B lymphocytes, as well as on natural killer cells. Campath-1H is FDA-approved for the treatment of leukemia, and has been used as an induction agent in kidney, pancreas, and liver transplantation [27,28]. Its use for the treatment of steroid-resistant rejection has not been formally evaluated; however, because of its ability to deplete T lymphocytes, it may be an effective agent in that regard and warrants evaluation.

Most episodes of acute rejection of a transplanted liver can be reversed with either pulsed steroid therapy or antithymocyte/lymphocyte antibody preparations. Refractory acute rejection is an extremely rare indication for retransplantation. Once a patient has developed recurrent acute cellular rejection or steroid-resistant rejection, a change in their maintenance immunosuppression is warranted. Conversion to tacrolimus from cyclosporine may be necessary. The addition of mycophenolate mofetil, sirolimus, or azathioprine to the standard two-drug regimen has also been utilized in this population of patients.

■ CHRONIC REJECTION

Chronic rejection is an immunologic process that usually begins within a year of liver transplantation and has been documented as early as the first month. A combination of cellular and humoral immune mechanisms has been implicated. As with acute cellular rejection, the immune attack is apparently focused on biliary epithelial cells; in addition, muscular arteries (arterioles) are also targets. Chronic rejection is also referred to as both vanishing bile duct syndrome and ductopenic rejection in the literature. These names reflect the characteristic histologic feature of this entity, namely a paucity or almost complete absence of bile ducts. An additional histologic feature is foamy macrophage invasion of the intimal and subintimal regions of muscular arteries, which results in an arteriopathy. Obliteration of the arterial lumen probably also contributes to the loss of bile ducts since the blood supply is based solely on hepatic arterial vasculature.

A number of risk factors have been identified that are likely associated with the development of chronic liver allograft rejection. A history of at least one episode of acute rejection is present in almost all of those who eventually develop chronic rejection. Patients who are inadequately treated for an acute rejection episode are believed to be particularly at risk [29]. Inadequate immunosuppression in the early posttransplant phase may play a role. Patients whose etiology of native liver failure has an immunologic component are thought to be at higher risk, e.g. autoimmune hepatitis. A strong association between cytomegalovirus infection and the development of chronic rejection has been identified. African Americans are at higher risk than Caucasians. The strongest predictor for the development of chronic rejection is a previous history of transplantation for chronic rejection. Patients transplanted for chronic rejection have a recurrence rate that approaches 90% [30].

The development of chronic allograft rejection is insidious and the initial stages are not associated with specific symptoms or signs. As the disease progresses, patients develop a picture of cholestatic liver test abnormalities and hyperbilirubinemia that do not improve with steroid bolus therapy. With time, the cholestasis worsens and, without treatment, ultimately results in graft destruction and death of the patient unless retransplantation is performed.

The diagnosis of chronic liver allograft rejection is confirmed histologically (Chapter 22). The pathologist searches for a loss of bile ducts in at least 50% of portal triads. Unfortunately, this histologic finding occurs late in the course of the disease. Identification of the arteriopathy is rarely made on needle biopsy, because the affected arterioles are medium-sized vessels that are centrally located. Although rarely performed for this indication, a wedge biopsy will more consistently yield this result. Traditionally, the arteriopathy is not confirmed until the liver is examined after explantation at the time of retransplantation or at autopsy.

Over the last decade, there have been fundamental changes in the management of chronic liver allograft rejection. Medical therapy has been utilized with some success. Tacrolimus has a definite role in reversing chronic rejection. Many studies have demonstrated that conversion from cyclosporine to tacrolimus can salvage a significant number of grafts. Factors that are predictive of success include mild to moderate cholestasis at the time of diagnosis (serum bilirubin <10 mg/dL) as well as intervention prior to the loss of 50% of bile ducts [31]. Patients in whom the diagnosis is made at least 3 months after transplantation had a greater rate of recovery [31]. Theoretically, the antifibrotic properties of the mTOR inhibitor sirolimus would be beneficial in the prevention or treatment of chronic rejection. It is premature to assess the efficacy of sirolimus in the prevention of chronic rejection; however, there are initial reports of its use as rescue therapy for chronic rejection.

Fortunately, the incidence of chronic rejection is decreasing. This is likely the result of improved immunosuppressants, prompt and aggressive treatment of acute rejection, and effective prophylaxis for cytomegalovirus disease. The loss of liver transplants to chronic rejection is also decreasing because of earlier diagnosis and medical intervention.

■ SUMMARY

Although acute rejection occurs in approximately 30% of liver transplant recipients, the incidence of graft loss due to rejection has decreased significantly. The dramatic improvement in organ and recipient survival in all organ systems coincides with the introduction of calciunerin inhibitor-based immunosuppression protocols in the 1980s. Cyclosporine, tacrolimus, and the recently introduced sirolimus are the primary agents on which current protocols are based. The advantages of tacrolimus include the ability to wean posttransplant immunosuppression to a single agent as well to prevent and treat chronic rejection. Sirolimus is a renal sparing agent that also may prove efficacious in the treatment of chronic rejection.

The successful treatment of rejection demands a high index of suspicion, early evaluation with biopsy, and an aggressive, thorough course of treatment. Adopting these practices will continue to yield improvements in allograft function and, ultimately, increases in patient survival.

■ REFERENCES

1. Data reports. www.unos.org. Accessed January 26, 2005.

2. Sellers MT, McGuire BM, Haustein, SV, et al. Two-dose daclizumab induction therapy in 209 liver transplants: a single-center analysis. Transplantation 2004;78: 1212–1217.

3. Vincenti F, Kirkman R, Light S, et al. Interleukin-2-receptor blockade with daclizumab to prevent acute rejection in renal transplantation. Daclizumab Triple Therapy Study Group. N Engl J Med 1998;338:161–165.

4. Cantarovich D, Giral-Classe M, Hourmant M, et al. Low incidence of kidney rejection after simultaneous kidney–pancreas transplantation after antithymocyte globulin induction and in the absence of corticosteroids: results of a prospective pilot study in 28 consecutive cases. Transplantation 2000;69:1505–1508.

5. Gordon RD, Iwatsuki S, Esquivel CO, et al. Liver transplantation across ABO blood groups. Surgery 1986;100:342–348.

6. Egawa H, Fumitaka O, Buhler L, et al. Impact of recipient age on outcome of ABO-incompatible living-donor liver transplantation. Transplantation 2004;77:403–411.

7. Monteiro I, McLoughlin LM, Fisher A, et al. Rituximab with plasmapheresis and splenectomy in ABO-incompatible liver transplantation. Transplantation 2003;76: 1648–1649.

8. Ratner L, Phelan D, Brunt E, et al. Probable antibody-mediated failure of two sequential ABO-compatible hepatic allografts in a single recipient. Transplantation 1993;55:814–819.

9. Gordon RD, Fung JJ, Markus B, et al. The antibody crossmatch in liver transplantation. Surgery 1986;100:705–715.

10. Doran TJ, Geczy AF, Painter D, et al. A large, single center investigation of the immunogenetic factors affecting liver transplantation. Transplantation 2000;69: 1491–1498.

11. Fairbanks KD, Eustace JA, Fine D, et al. Renal function improves in liver transplant recipients when switched from a calcineurin inhibitor to sirolimus. Liver Transpl 2003;9:1079–1085.

12. Eckhoff DE, McGuire B, Sellers M, et al. The safety and efficacy of a two-dose daclizumab (zenapax) induction therapy in liver transplant recipients. Transplantation 2000;69:1867–1872.

13. Knechtle SJ, Kolbeck PC, Tsuchimoto S, et al. Hepatic transplantation into sensitized recipients. Demonstration of hyperacute rejection. Transplantation 1987;43:8–12.

14. Merion RM, Colletti LM. Hyperacute rejection in porcine liver transplantation: clinical characteristics, histopathology, and disappearance of donor-specific lymphocytotoxic antibody from serum. Transplantation 1990;49:861–868.

15. Bird G, Friend P, Donaldson P, et al. Hyperacute rejection in liver transplantation: a case report. Transplant Proc 1989;21:3742–3744.

16. Abraham S, Furth EE. Quantitative evaluation of histological features in "time-zero" liver allograft biopsies as predictors of rejection or graft failure: receiver-operating characteristic analysis application. Hum Pathol 1996;27:1077–1084.

17. D'Alessandro AM, Kalayoglu M, Sollinger HW, et al. Current status of organ preservation with University of Wisconsin solution. Arch Pathol Lab Med 1991;115:306–310.

18. McTaggart RA, Terrault NA, Vardanian AJ, et al. Hepatitis C etiology of liver disease is strongly associated with early acute rejection following liver transplantation. Liver Transpl 2004;10:975–985.

19. Saab S, Kalmaz D, Gajjar NA, et al. Outcomes of acute rejection after interferon therapy in liver transplant recipients. Liver Transpl 2004;10:859–867.

20. Kugelmas M, Osgood MJ, Trotter JF, et al. Hepatitis C virus therapy, hepatocyte drug metabolism, and risk for acute cellular rejection. Liver Transpl 2003;9:1159–1165.

21. Kowalski R, Post D, Schneider MC, et al. Immune cell function testing: an adjunct to therapeutic drug monitoring in transplant patient management. Clin Transplant 2003;17:77–88.

22. Williams JW, Vera SR, Peters TG. A technique for safe, frequent biopsy of the liver after hepatic transplantation. Surg Gynecol Obstet 1986;162:592–594.

23. Millis JM, Woodle ES, Piper JB, et al. Tacrolimus for primary treatment of steroid-resistant hepatic allograft rejection. Transplantation 1986;61:1147–1165.

24. Anonymous. Immunomodulators. In Drug evaluations, 6th ed. Chicago IL, Am Med Assoc 1986;11147–11165.

25. Swinnen LJ, Costanzo-Nordin MR, Fisher SG, et al. Increased incidence of lympho-proliferative disorder after immunosuppression with the monoclonal antibody OKT3 in cardiac-transplant recipients. N Engl J Med 1990;323:1723–1728.

26. Bijleveld CG, Klompmaker IJ, van den Berg AP, et al. Incidence, risk factors, and outcome of antithymocyte globulin treatment of steroid-resistant rejection after liver transplantation. Transpl Int 1996;9:570–575.

27. Knechtle SJ, Fernandez LA, Pirsch JD, et al. Campath-1H in renal transplantation: the University of Wisconsin experience. Surgery 2004;136:754–760.

28. Marcos A, Eghtesad B, Fung JJ, et al. Use of alemtuzumab and tacrolimus mono-therapy for cadaveric liver transplantation: with particular reference to hepatatitis C virus. Transplantation 2004;78:966–971.

29. Wiesner RH, Ludwig J, Krom RA, et al. Treatment of early cellular rejection following liver transplantation with intravenous methylprednisolone. The effect of dose on response. Transplantation 1994;58:1053–1056.

30. van Hoek B, Wiesner RH, Krom RA, et al. Severe ductopenic rejection following liver transplantation: incidence, time of onset, risk factors, treatment, and outcome. Semin Liver Dis 1992;12:41–50.

31. Sher LS, Cosenza CA, Michel J, et al. Efficacy of tacrolimus as rescue therapy for chronic rejection in orthotopic liver transplantation: a report of the U.S. Multicenter Liver Study Group. Transplantation 1997;64:258–263.

Vascular Complications

▼　▼　▼　▼　▼　▼　▼　▼　▼

**Paul Suhocki, S. Ravi Chari,
and Richard L. McCann**

K NOWLEDGE of hepatic vascular anatomy and its variations is critical during the preoperative workup of the recipient, the donor, and the transplant procedures. In the early and late periods following transplantation, vascular thrombosis or stenosis can cause significant morbidity and mortality and must be included in the list of etiologies for altered liver function and biliary complications. This chapter discusses hepatic vascular anatomic variations and their effect on organ recovery and implantation. Causes and treatment of vascular abnormalities that develop after transplantation are also addressed.

■ HEPATIC VASCULAR ANATOMY

The liver has a dual vascular supply from the hepatic artery and the portal vein. The hepatic artery provides 25% of the blood supply to the liver and about half of the oxygen supply. The common hepatic artery arises from the celiac trunk and passes transversely, superior to the pancreas, toward the liver. This vessel divides in the porta hepatis to supply the left and right lobes of the liver. In about 15–20% of individuals, the right hepatic artery arises from the superior mesenteric artery rather than from the proper hepatic artery. In another 20–25% of cases, either a branch of the left hepatic artery or the entire left hepatic artery arises from the left gastric artery, also a branch of the celiac trunk. An accessory right hepatic artery may arise from the left hepatic artery. This variant is especially important in split-liver transplantation and has been reported as being present in 2 of 37 split-liver procedures [1]. The entire hepatic arterial supply arises from the superior mesenteric artery in 2.5% and from the aorta in 2% of individuals [2]. While ligation of part or even the entire

323

▼

arterial supply to the liver is usually well tolerated in the nontransplant patient, failure to restore the complete arterial revascularization is poorly tolerated in the cold preserved liver. Complete nonfunction of the graft, biliary leak or strictures, and hepatic abscess can result.

The portal vein supplies 75% of hepatic blood flow and about half of the oxygen. The portal vein is formed by the confluence of the superior mesenteric vein and the splenic vein behind the pancreas. High in the porta hepatis, it bifurcates into the right and left portal veins. Gradual thrombosis of the portal vein may occur in the setting of liver cirrhosis. Portal vein thrombosis (PVT) has been reported to have a 16% prevalence in the pretransplant patient [3]. The etiology of this is unclear but may be related to decreased or bidirectional portal venous blood flow secondary to increased postsinusoidal resistance. When PVT occurs, an abundance of collateral venous drainage develops. Although development of PVT may be clinically subtle, it must be recognized preoperatively since it impacts negatively on the technical success of liver transplantation and graft survival. Depending on the degree of extension of the thrombus into the mesenteric bed, liver transplantation may not be feasible or may require portal venous reconstruction.

The liver drains into three major hepatic veins and 10–50 smaller caudate veins that open into the inferior vena cava. Knowledge of the hepatic vein anatomy is critical for the preparation of reduced size, split-, and living-related grafts and for the percutaneous creation of a transjugular intrahepatic porto-systemic shunt (TIPS) (see Chapter 3). Pretransplant hepatic vein thrombosis (Budd–Chiari syndrome) is uncommon and is consistently associated with ascites. Documentation of a patent vena cava in the recipient is important to determine the feasibility of liver transplantation. Hepatic veins can also be used for venous reconstruction at the time of implantation (piggyback tech-nique), particularly in pediatric patients (see Chapters 14 and 31).

■ PREOPERATIVE IMAGING STUDIES

Adequate visualization of all hepatic vessels is mandatory prior to listing patients for liver transplantation. Most biliary and vascular complications occurring immediately postoperatively occur due to technical problems and the failure to recognize anatomic variation [4]. In patients who have undergone TIPS placement, the inferior vena cava (IVC) and the main portal vein are closely evaluated for the degree of extension of the stent into these vessels. The stent may interfere with clamping of the vessels and the creation of venous anastomoses. Very low positioning of the stent in the main portal vein may necessitate creation of an interpositional vascular graft during transplantation.

A noninvasive and relatively inexpensive method of evaluating the hepatic vasculature preoperatively is Duplex ultrasonography (real-time imaging with

Doppler analysis of blood flow). This technique evaluates the portal vein for patency, direction of flow, and the presence of thrombus. The hepatic veins, IVC, and hepatic arteries are also examined. Preoperative assessment of IVC patency and location is particularly important in the pediatric population. There is a high incidence of hepatic vascular anomalies associated with biliary atresia, the most common cause for transplantation in this group [5] (see Chapter 24). Body habitus and overlying bowel gas may cause inadequate sonographic evaluation of the hepatic vasculature, most frequently of the main portal vein, splenic vein, and proximal hepatic artery. In addition, the hyperechoic properties of the cirrhotic liver impair the ability of ultrasound to reliably assess the parenchyma for the presence of malignant lesions.

Although the historic gold standard, transcatheter angiography is falling from favor as a tool for evaluating the hepatic vasculature in the liver transplant patient. Transcatheter angiography is an invasive procedure that carries the attendant risks of catheter-induced arterial injury and contrast agent-associated renal impairment and allergic reaction. The superior imaging now being provided by state-of-the-art magnetic resonance imaging (MRI) has resulted in conventional arteriography being used only for patients in whom MRI is contraindicated. Contrast-enhanced MR angiography combined with true fast imaging with steady-state precession provides excellent visualization of the entire hepatic vasculature [6] (Fig. 20.1). MRI has the added benefit of assessing the liver parenchyma for the presence of malignant lesions. Improvements in MR cholangiopancreatography show promise for optimal visualization of the biliary tree as well.

Vascular Considerations in the Donor Operation

Most donors have normal portal veins and a normal vena cava. However, arterial anomalies occur frequently and impact greatly on transplantation of the organ. Adequate arterial inflow to all segments of the liver is important in preventing the development of biliary strictures that can place the allograft and the patient in jeopardy (Fig. 20.2). The common anomalous origins of the right and left hepatic arteries already described should be routinely searched for during dissection of the donor. In the era of multiorgan harvesting, the liver transplant surgeon recovering a liver with anomalous arterial supply should not hesitate to sacrifice use of the pancreas from transplantation if a complete arterial supply of the liver cannot be obtained. A donor organ with anomalous hepatic arterial supply often requires vascular reconstruction prior to implantation. For example, a donor aberrant right hepatic artery can be anastomosed to the stump of the donor splenic artery at the time of the recipient operation. This permits only one anastomosis between the donor celiac trunk and the recipient hepatic artery.

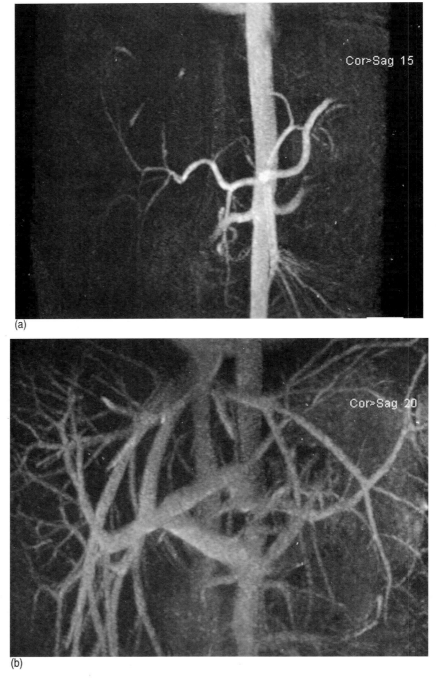

Fig. 20.1 *Maximum-intensity three-dimensional projections (3D MIP) following gadolinium injection during magnetic resonance imaging (MRI) demonstrate (a) the abdominal aorta, hepatic arteries, and other mesenteric arteries and (b) the hepatic veins and portal veins.*

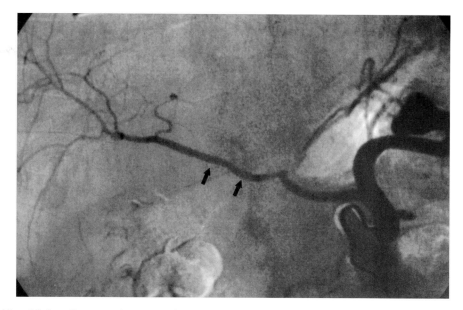

Fig. 20.2 *Contrast injection during selective catheterization of the celiac artery in a posttransplant patient demonstrates flow into the right hepatic artery only (arrows). The anomalous left hepatic artery arising separately from the right hepatic artery was missed during organ procurement and was not anastomosed to the recipient artery.*

Additional vessels should be routinely obtained at the time of the donor procedure. The most suitable vessels for reconstruction of the recipient portal vein are the donor iliac veins. The donor iliac artery between the aorta and the inguinal ligament should also be harvested in the event that hepatic arterial reconstruction with a vascular conduit is required. Unused iliac arteries should be stored in the cold for about a week following the transplant procedure; these grafts can be used for arterial reconstruction in case of hepatic artery thrombosis (HAT) during the immediate postoperative period.

Vascular Considerations in the Recipient Operation

The most common strategy for liver transplantation is the orthotopic procedure (see Chapter 14). In the recipient, the segment of the IVC between the renal veins and the diaphragm, containing the entry of the hepatic veins, is excised along with the native liver. The new liver is then installed along with a corresponding segment of donor vena cava so that individual hepatic vein anastomoses are not required. It is only necessary to anastomose the sleeve of vena cava at the diaphragm and just above the renal veins. The portal veins are usually joined in end-to-end fashion (see Chapter 14).

Sometimes it is preferable to leave the recipient vena cava intact. The donor vena cava may be anastomosed to the recipient vena cava in a piggyback, end-to-side or side-to-side fashion [7]. In the case of the piggyback technique, the upper end of the donor vena cava is anastomosed to the recipient hepatic veins. The lower end of the donor vena cava is closed. With the end-to-side technique, the upper end of the donor vena cava is anastomosed to the side of the recipient vena cava. The lower end of the donor vena cava is closed. With the side-to-side anastomosis, the upper and lower ends of the donor vena cava are closed after cavotomy of the donor and recipient vena cavae and side-to-side anastomosis is performed.

It is important that the vascular connections be constructed expeditiously in order to minimize the amount of anaerobic rewarming of the donor organ while it is being installed. Flow is usually restored to the liver after construction of the portal vein anastomosis. The length of the portal vein is critical and its anastomosis must be technically exact to avoid constriction and kinking. After the organ is supplied with adequate portal venous blood, the hepatic arterial anastomosis can be constructed without the liver experiencing irreversible ischemia. Some authors advocate arterialization of the liver allograft before construction of the portal vein anastomosis. This has been found to be associated with less hepatocellular injury, less reperfusion injury, and better endothelial cell function in donor pig livers [8].

Vessel length is less critical for arterial reconstruction but the anastomosis must be technically exact to avoid HAT. The reported incidence of HAT ranges from 4% to 26%. This variability reflects the different methods of diagnosis used and the relative number of pediatric recipients within these studies. Immunologic phenomena may play a role in the development of HAT. Other possible contributors include technical problems, rejection episodes, and cold-ischemic injury. The use of arterial conduits, retransplantation, ABO mismatch, and elevated hematocrit have been proposed as risk factors.

Conduits may be required if satisfactory lengths of recipient and donor vessels are not available. If PVT is present in the recipient, mesenteric venous drainage must be provided from the superior mesenteric vein to the transplant portal vein. This often requires a bridging venous conduit placed anteriorly to the duodenum and pancreas [9]. The most frequent graft used is the donor iliac vein. If this is not available, femoral vein or jugular vein from the recipient may be utilized. Because of the high degree of portal hypertension in these patients, this type of revascularization is often a formidable task. A rare complication of TIPS is downward migration of the metallic stent into the lower segment of the portal vein. This segment of the recipient portal vein must be resected during orthotopic liver transplantation (OLT). The portal vein is then reconstructed with donor iliac vein interposition [10]. It may be necessary to create a "pants graft" to connect the recipient splenic vein and superior mesenteric vein individually to the donor portal vein [11]. The middle colic vein has been used to provide portal inflow to the graft in a patient with PVT discovered at the time of OLT [12].

Conduits to bridge the hepatic artery are more commonly used. If the recipient hepatic artery is small or the flow is poor or absent, a conduit between the donor hepatic artery and the aorta (supraceliac and suprarenal aorta) is necessary. The most convenient graft is obtained from the donor iliac artery, but recipient saphenous veins can also be used successfully. Use of the recipient inferior epigastric artery as an interpositional vascular graft has been reported [13].

Vascular Complications following Transplantation

Although vascular complications are seen less frequently than biliary complications following transplantation, they are a source of significant morbidity and mortality. They occur in 1–10% and cause poor graft function, sometimes requiring retransplantation [14]. The most common are arterial complications, which account for 5% [15]. Doppler ultrasound is considered an efficient screening method for detecting vascular complications. Because vascular complications can be asymptomatic, Kok et al. [16] recommend performing routine liver Doppler ultrasound at 24 h and then every 3 days for the first 2 weeks, with special attention to the first day. They suggest that daily Doppler ultrasound be performed only in high-risk patients, such as in young children, following complex vascular reconstruction or following thrombectomy.

MRI of the hepatic vasculature is performed when Doppler ultrasound findings are equivocal or suggest that an abnormality may be present in the hepatic artery or portal vein. Although arteriography is the gold standard, three-dimensional spoiled gradient-echo MRI with injection of gadolinium contrast material may be used to evaluate the hepatic artery, portal vein, hepatic veins and IVC following liver transplantation [17,18]. Arterial catheterization is not necessary for this study. Also, gadolinium's lack of nephrotoxicity offers an advantage over iodinated contrast in liver transplant patients, many of whom have some degree of renal insufficiency related to cyclosporine or tacrolimus.

Hepatic Artery Thrombosis

One of the most serious complications in the immediate postoperative period is HAT [19]. Factors contributing to the development of HAT include technical difficulties, prolonged cold-ischemia time, pediatric recipient, whole-liver allograft, positive crossmatch, and the use of an aortic conduit [20]. Other factors include transient deficiency of anticoagulant factors protein C, protein S, or antithrombin III; increased thrombin activity; and elevated levels of plasminogen activator inhibitor-1 [21]. Cytomegalovirus (CMV)-seronegative patients receiving a seropositive allograft may be at risk for early HAT [22]. The clinical presentation of HAT is variable. It is usually associated with a dramatic rise in serum transaminases but its occurrence can be subtle. Any decrease in the volume of bile output, change in the character of the bile, or persistent elevation of the prothrombin time or bilirubin levels should trigger tests to rule out HAT. Monitoring of hepatic artery patency using Duplex sonography is routinely performed at many centers. This is particularly important in the pediatric population where the incidence of HAT is high and the clinical manifestation is often silent.

The sensitivity of Duplex sonography in detecting HAT is greater than 90%. It has the added advantage of detecting other anomalies such as bile duct dilatation, bile lakes, areas of infarction, and hepatic abscesses. In the absence of Doppler flow in the hepatic artery and with clinical and laboratory presentation suggestive of HAT, no further tests are necessary. Immediate reoperation and revascularization by thrombectomy or the use of a conduit is mandatory. The single most important factor in graft outcome is the length of time that the liver lacks hepatic arterial blood supply. With equivocal Doppler ultrasound findings, absence of clinical presentation consistent with HAT, or occurrence more than 2 weeks postoperatively, arteriography should be performed for confirmation of HAT. HAT within a month of transplantation usually warrants reoperation and an attempt at revascularization [23]. In case of persistent graft failure, urgent retransplantation is required to prevent death.

The management of late HAT (occurring later than 2 months postoperatively) is more controversial and depends on the presence of associated diseases. In the presence of severe liver impairment with persistent elevated bilirubin or diffuse biliary stricture, retransplantation without prior attempt at revascularization is usually the best option. Reoperation may disrupt spontaneous revascularization of the graft in the porta hepatis and from adherent tissues. This can result in rapid liver failure. Transcatheter thrombolytic therapy for HAT is contraindicated in the immediate postoperative period because of the risk of bleeding complications but successful infusion of urokinase into the hepatic artery months after transplantation has been reported [24]. Tissue plasminogen activator can also be used. Once clot lysis has occurred, the cause of thrombosis should be looked for. Percutaneous balloon angioplasty or vascular stenting of stenoses has been of help in avoiding revision or retransplantation in selected cases [25]. Long-term success of vascular or surgical revascularization is based on the level of graft function at the time of the intervention [26]. While HAT is usually catastrophic, there have been reported cases of grafts, mostly in children, which have continued to function well following HAT. This is probably due to the development of sufficient extra-hepatic collateral arterial supply [27].

Hepatic Artery Stenosis

Besides complete occlusion of the hepatic artery, stenosis with impaired flow can also be the source of significant morbidity and mortality. Hepatic artery stenosis is associated with cholangiographic abnormalities in more than 60% of cases [26]. The diagnosis requires confirmation by arteriography. During the early postoperative course, management of symptomatic hepatic artery stenosis follows the same guidelines used for HAT. Urgent surgical revascularization is mandatory. If a stenosis is discovered 1 month or more after OLT, management depends again on the liver reserve and associated anomalies. Measuring a pressure gradient across the stenosis with a catheter and pressure transducer during arteriography can help determine if the stenosis is physiologically significant and whether intervention is necessary. There are no studies, however, that have determined what constitutes an abnormal hepatic artery pressure gradient. Percutaneous balloon angioplasty can be performed to treat the stenosis, with an 80–100% success rate. The restenosis rate is 30–60% [14].

The need for and timing of retransplantation should be based on the severity of associated conditions and the local expertise with invasive radiological vascular and biliary interventions. In our experience, about half of the patients with hepatic artery stenosis and biliary strictures can be treated successfully without reoperation (Fig. 20.3).

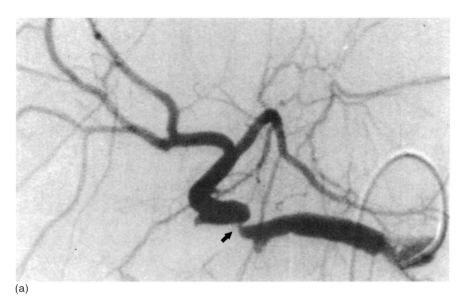

(a)

Fig. 20.3 *(a) Contrast injection during selective catheterization of the common hepatic artery demonstrates a stenosis (arrow) at the anastomosis with the donor hepatic artery.*

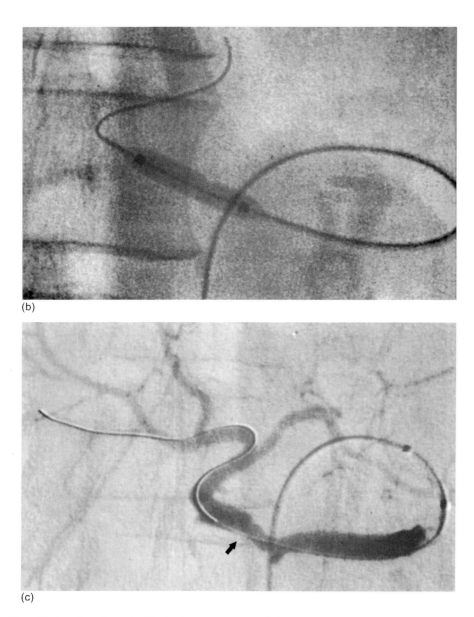

(b)

(c)

Fig. 20.3 *Continued. (b) A 6-mm-diameter balloon traverses the stenosis and is inflated to 12 atm; (c) Repeat contrast injection of the common hepatic artery demonstrates a normal arterial anastomosis (arrow).*

Mycotic Aneurysm of the Hepatic Artery

A devastating late vascular complication of liver transplantation is mycotic aneurysm at the arterial anastomosis (Fig. 20.4). This is a confusing term since the aneurysm is usually the result of bacterial and not fungal infection. Mycotic

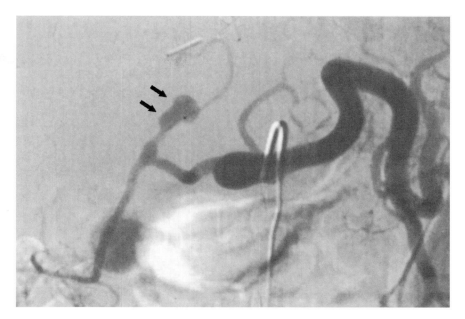

Fig. 20.4 *Contrast injection during selective catheterization of the celiac artery demonstrates a mycotic aneurysm (arrows) of the common hepatic artery, with diminished flow in the hepatic artery branches.*

aneurysm of the hepatic artery often is associated with biliary tract complications and local infection. The infection involves the hepatic arterial anastomosis and a false aneurysm develops. This mycotic aneurysm is often fatal. Ligation of the hepatic artery carries an extremely high morbidity and mortality, particularly early after transplantation. Excision of the aneurysm and immediate revascularization with donor iliac artery or autogenous saphenous vein has been associated with an 88% survival [28].

Portal Vein Thrombosis

With increased surgical expertise with the transplant procedure and prevention of a redundant portal vein, PVT has become rare. PVT usually occurs in patients with preexisting partial PVT and inadequate restoration of the portal flow. As with HAT, early PVT is a dramatic complication that is diagnosed by Doppler ultrasound. It requires immediate revascularization or retransplantation to prevent death of the patient. In the later postoperative course, PVT usually has a similar presentation as in the nontransplant patients. Venous collaterals due to prehepatic portal hypertension occur with upper gastrointestinal bleeding as the most common initial presentation. The diagnosis usually is easily made by Duplex sonography. MR portal venography is indicated to delineate the extent of the clot. In the presence of good liver reserve, a shunt procedure such as a splenorenal (Warren) or mesocaval shunt will correct the portal hypertension. With poor liver reserve or venous anatomy unsuitable for reconstruction, retransplantation should be considered. PVT has been treated nonoperatively by infusing urokinase directly into the portal vein or the superior mesenteric artery [29,30]. This means of treatment should be reserved for patients who are in the later postoperative course and who are not bleeding from varices.

Interposition grafts are used to reduce tension on the portal vein anastomosis in reduced-size hepatic transplants. This lowers the rate of portal venous thrombosis in children and adolescents. These conduits are prone to delayed stenosis, a problem that is difficult to manage surgically. Such portal vein stenoses can be treated percutaneously with balloon angioplasty, followed by metallic stent placement when balloon angioplasty alone fails [31].

Hepatic Vein Occlusion or Stenosis

This is a rare complication following transplantation and is almost always associated with a hypercoagulable state. It is also seen in patients with preoperative Budd–Chiari syndrome or in those who received a right lobe graft from a living donor. In the latter case, the graft does not include the middle hepatic vein for the safety of the donor. Since the hepatic venous outflow from segments V and VIII usually drains into the middle hepatic vein, varying degrees of hepatic venous congestion may occur in these segments. Hepatic venous congestion may also occur in segments VI and VII if the right inferior accessory hepatic vein is ligated or if its anastomosis is stenotic. Areas of hepatic venous congestion may be detected on dual-phase computed tomography as zones of variable attenuation [32].

While partial hepatic vein occlusion may be well tolerated or even asymptomatic, complete hepatic venous outflow obstruction is catastrophic and requires immediate retransplantation. Hepatic vein occlusion in the late course of liver transplantation in patients with good liver reserve and major ascites can be treated successfully with a mesocaval shunt (see Chapter 4). Late hepatic vein stenosis or occlusion can also be treated percutaneously with a metallic stent [33].

IVC Stenosis or Thrombosis

IVC stenosis or occlusion is currently seen in less than 2% of patients [34]. Depending on the level of caval occlusion, the patient may present with truncal edema or symptoms of hepatic venous outflow obstruction. Patients require long-term anticoagulation. Surgical repair is difficult; percutaneous balloon angioplasty or stenting has proven useful in this setting and results in rapid improvement in patient symptoms [35–37].

Spleen-Related Problems

Severe thrombocytopenia is sometimes seen in the patient with persistent splenomegaly and platelet sequestration following liver transplantation. This can be treated via the splenic artery with partial particulate embolization of the spleen to decrease the splenic volume [38].

Reduced hepatic arterial perfusion posttransplantation may be caused by steal of arterial flow from the celiac artery by an enlarged spleen. This situation has been called "splenic artery steal syndrome" [39]. Blood flow to the hepatic artery is increased by coil embolization of the splenic artery or its branches.

Splenic artery aneurysms are seen in 7–17% of patients with cirrhosis. Rupture typically occurs in aneurysms greater than 15 mm in diameter. The aneurysm is treated surgically during liver transplantation when seen preoperatively [40]. Transcatheter coil embolization of the aneurysm is performed if the diagnosis is made after transplantation [41].

■ CONCLUSIONS

Vascular complications after liver transplantation represent an important source of morbidity and mortality. Prevention continues to be based on meticulous surgical technique. Early diagnosis is critical to graft salvage, and surgical intervention is the mainstay of management in the early postoperative period. However, in the late postoperative period, nonsurgical percutaneous interventions can maintain organ viability and extend patient survival.

■ REFERENCES

1. Rela M, McCall J, Karani J, et al. Accessory right hepatic artery arising from the left: implications for split liver transplantation. Transplantation 1998;66:792–794.

2. Kadir S, ed. Diagnostic angiography. Philadelphia, PA: WB Saunders, 1986.

3. Cherqui D, Duvoux C, Rahmouni A, et al. Orthotopic liver transplantation in the presence of partial or total portal vein thrombosis: problems in diagnosis and management. World J Surg 1993;17:669–674.

4. Deshpande R, Heaton N, Rela M. Surgical anatomy of segmental liver transplantation. Br J Surg 2002;89:1078–1088.

5. Morton M, James E, Wiesner R, et al. Applications of duplex ultrasonography in the liver transplant patient. Mayo Clin Proc 1990;65:360–372.

6. Carr J, Nemcek A, Abecassis M, et al. Preoperative evaluation of the entire hepatic vasculature in living liver donors with use of contrast-enhanced MR angiography and true fast imaging with steady-state precession. J Vasc Interv Radiol 2003;14:441–449.

7. Navarro F, Le Moine M, Fabre J, et al. Specific vascular complications of orthotopic liver transplantation with preservation of the retrohepatic vena cava: review of 1361 cases. Transplantation 1999;68:646–650.

8. As A, Lotz Z, Tyler M, et al. Impact of early arterialization in the liver allograft. Transplant Proc 1999;31:406–407.

9. Stieber A, Zetti G, Todo S, et al. The spectrum of portal vein thrombosis in liver transplantation. Ann Surg 1991;213:199–206.

10. Farney A, Gamboa P, Payne W, et al. Donor iliac vein interposition during liver transplantation in a patient with a migrated transjugular intrahepatic portosystemic shunt. Transplantation 1998;65:572–574.

11. Clavien P, Selzner M, Tuttle-Newhall J, et al. Liver transplantation complicated by misplaced TIPS in the portal vein. Ann Surg 1998;227:440–445.

12. Rudroff C, Scheele J. The middle colic vein: an alternative source of portal inflow in orthotopic liver transplantation complicated by portal vein thrombosis. Clin Transplant 1998;12:538–542.

13. Nakatsuka T, Takushima A, Harihara Y, et al. Versatility of the inferior epigastric artery as an interpositional vascular graft in living-related liver transplantation. Transplantation 1999;67:1490–1492.

14. Vignali C, Cioni R, Petruzzi P, et al. Role of interventional radiology in the management of vascular complications after liver transplantation. Transplant Proc 2004;36:552–554.

15. Sanchez-Bueno F, Hernandez Q, Ramirez P, et al. Vascular complications in a series of 300 orthotopic liver transplants. Transplant Proc 1999;31:2409–2410.

16. Kok T, Slooff M, Thijn C, et al. Routine Doppler ultrasound for the detection of clinically unsuspected vascular complications in the early postoperative phase after orthotopic liver transplantation. Transpl Int 1998;11:272–276.

17. Stafford-Johnson D, Hamilton B, Dong Q, et al. Vascular complications of liver transplantation: evaluation with gadolinium-enhanced MR angiography. Radiology 1998;207:153–160.

18. Glockner J, Forauer A, Solomon H, et al. Three-dimensional gadolinium-enhanced MR angiography of vascular complications after liver transplantation. Am J Roentgenol 2000;174:1447–1453.

19. Langnas A, Marujo W, Stratta R, et al. Vascular complications after orthotopic liver transplantation. Am J Surg 1991;161:82–83.

20. Eid A, Lyass S, Venturero M, et al. Vascular complications post orthotopic liver transplantation. Transplant Proc 1999;31:1903–1904.

21. Schuetze S, Linenberger M. Acquired protein S deficiency with multiple thrombotic complications after orthotopic liver transplant. Transplantation 1999;67:1366–1369.

22. Madalosso C, de Souza NJ, Ilstrup D, et al. Cytomegalovirus and its association with hepatic artery thrombosis after liver transplantation. Transplantation 1998;66:294–297.

23. Sakamoto Y, Harihara Y, Nakatsuka T, et al. Rescue of liver grafts from hepatic artery occlusion in living-related liver transplantation. Br J Surg 1999;86:886–889.

24. Hidalgo E, Abad J, Cantarero J, et al. High-dose intra-arterial urokinase for the treatment of hepatic artery thrombosis in liver transplantation. Hepatogastroenterology 1989;36:529–532.

25. Vorwerk D, Gunther R, Klever P, et al. Angioplasty and stent placement for treatment of hepatic artery thrombosis following liver transplantation. J Vasc Interv Radiol 1994;5:309–311.

26. Orons P, Zajko A. Angiography and interventional procedures in liver transplantation. Radiol Clin North Am 1995;33:541–558.

27. Yedlicka JJ, Halloran J, Payne W, et al. Angiogenesis after hepatic arterial occlusion in liver transplant patients. J Vasc Interv Radiol 1991;2:235–240.

28. Bonham C, Kapur S, Geller D, et al. Excision and immediate revascularization for hepatic artery pseudoaneurysm following liver transplantation. Transplant Proc 1999;31:443.

29. Yankes J, Uglietta J, Grant J, et al. Percutaneous transhepatic recanalization and thrombolysis of the superior mesenteric vein. Am J Roentgenol 1988;151:289–290.

30. Poplausky M, Kaufman J, Geller S, et al. Mesenteric venous thrombosis treated with urokinase via the superior mesenteric artery. Gastroenterology 1996;110: 1633–1635.

31. Funaki B, Rosenblum J, Leef J, et al. Percutaneous treatment of portal venous stenosis in children and adolescents with segmental hepatic transplants: long-term results. Radiology 2000;215:147–151.

32. Kim B, Kim T, Kim J, et al. Hepatic venous congestion after living donor liver transplantation with right lobe graft: two-phase CT findings. Radiology 2004;232:173–180.

33. Sze D, Semba C, Razavi M, et al. Endovascular treatment of hepatic venous outflow obstruction after piggyback technique liver transplantation. Transplantation 1999;68:446–449.

34. Glanemann M, Settmacher U, Stange B, et al. Caval complications after orthotopic liver transplantation. Transplant Proc 2000;32:539–540.

35. Raby N, Karani J, Thomas S, et al. Stenoses of vascular anastomoses after hepatic transplantation: treatment with balloon angioplasty. Am J Roentgenol 1991;157:167–171.

36. Rose B, Van-Aman M, Simon D, et al. Transluminal balloon angioplasty of infrahepatic caval anastomotic stenosis following liver transplantation. Cardiovasc Intervent Radiol 1988;11:79–81.

37. Simo G, Echenagusia A, Camunez F, et al. Stenosis of the inferior vena cava after liver transplantation: treatment with Gianturco expandable metallic stents. Cardiovasc Intervent Radiol 1995;18:212–216.

38. Sockrider C, Boykin K, Green J, et al. Partial splenic embolization for hypersplenism after liver transplantation. Transplant Proc 2001;33:3472–3473.

39. Uflacker R, Selby J, Chavin K, et al. Transcatheter splenic artery occlusion for treatment of splenic artery steal syndrome after orthotopic liver transplantation. Cardiovasc Intervent Radiol 2002;25:300–306.

40. Heestand G, Sher L, Lightfoote J, et al. Characteristics and management of splenic artery aneurysm in liver transplant candidates and recipients. Am Surg 2003;69:933–940.

41. Lupattelli T, Garaci F, Sandhu C, et al. Endovascular treatment of giant splenic aneurysm that developed after liver transplantation. Transpl Int 2003;16:756–760.

Biliary Complications following Liver Transplantation

**Lucas McCormack and
Peter Bauerfeind**

■ INTRODUCTION

Biliary complications are an important and frequent problem after orthotopic liver transplantation (OLT), with an incidence of 9–33% (Table 21.1). The lack of a standardized assessment of perioperative complications is a serious limitation to an analysis of the real incidence of biliary complications after OLT [1]. Some authors identify a complication only when an intervention is needed and asymptomatic patients usually are not investigated.

The rate of biliary problems is greater in adult-to-adult living donor liver transplantation (LDLT) than in cadaveric transplantation and pediatric LDLT [2–4]. The posttransplant biliary anatomy will determine the methods used to evaluate and treat potential biliary complications. This chapter discusses the current surgical techniques used for biliary tract reconstruction and the multidisciplinary management of early and long-term biliary complications.

■ PATHOGENESIS AND BILIARY RECONSTRUCTION

Many factors are involved in the generation of biliary complications after OLT: severe acute rejection associated with ABO incompatibility, chronic ductopenic rejection, prolonged graft cold preservation time, and donor duct ischemia. However, technical problems and ischemia are the most important underlying causes of biliary complications after OLT.

Biliary complications secondary to technical failures occur usually during the first 3 months after OLT [5] (Table 21.2). Options include choledochocholedochostomy (CC) with or without externalized T-tube and Roux-en-Y choledochojejunostomy (RY) (see Chapter 14). Of all the biliary complications in patients with CC with T-tube, almost 80% are related to T-tube removal [6]. To

339

Table 21.1 *Biliary Complications after Liver Transplantation Reported in Literature*

Authors	Year	Number of OLTs	Donor Type	Global BC (%)	Bile Leaks (%)	Biliary Stenosis (%)
Golling et al. [57]	1998	179	Cadaveric	15.1	10.1	5
Rabkin et al. [58]	1998	227	Cadaveric	30	19	12
Margarit et al. [5]	2001	224	Cadaveric	17	5.3	4
Davidson et al. [59]	1999	100	Cadaveric	31	17.5	13.5
Scatton et al. [6]	2001	180	Cadaveric	24.4	6.6	
Roumilhac et al. [46]	2003	216	Cadaveric	—	—	13.8
Fondevila et al. [60]	2003	46	Living[a]		23.9	32.6
Malago et al. [20]	2004	74	Living[a]	23	16.2	6.8
Kling et al. [21]	2004	68	Living[b]	33	20	17
Miller et al. [4]	2001	109	Living	—	15.5	8.2
Yersiz et al. [15]	2003	71	Right graft[c]	10	7	1.4
		94	Left graft[c]	9	7.4	1
Pekolj et al. [61]	2001	300	Cadaveric and living	17.3	5	9

[a]Adult-to-adult living donor liver transplantation.
[b]Adult-to-pediatric living donor liver transplantation.
[c]Series of cadaveric in situ split-liver transplantation.
OLT, orthotopic liver transplantation; BC, biliary complication.

reduce the incidence of this complication, removal of the T-tube is delayed for a minimum of 3 months to allow the T-tube tract to mature. Immunosuppression and the patient's general status are likely responsible for any delay in the formation of a fibrous tract between the biliary duct and the skin after T-tube placement. The increased biliary pressure in the biliary tract after OLT may also be a contributing factor to fistula development [7]. Many centers have advocated, when it is feasible, to do a direct biliary–biliary anastomosis without stenting to avoid this complication.

Unfortunately, biliary anastomosis is very sensitive to ischemic injury. Because the blood supply to the major bile ducts is by branches of the hepatic artery, many patients with hepatic artery thrombosis (HAT) develop biliary leaks because of dehiscence of the biliary anastomosis or ischemic strictures. It has been suggested that more than 20% of the strictures are associated with HAT and that Patients with HAT are at high risk for strictures and retransplantation [8]. Tzakis et al. [9] described three types of presentation of HAT within the first 3 months of OLT: fulminant hepatic necrosis, biliary leak, and relapsing bacteremia with intermittent sepsis due to acute cholangitis [9]. Late HAT has been reported to cause biliary tree necrosis, biliary leak, intrahepatic biloma, and liver abscess [10]. Arterial hypoperfusion of the liver as observed in stenosis of

Table 21.2 *Timing of Biliary Complication in the Liver Transplant Recipient*

Early (<3 months)	Late (>3 months)
Anastomotic biliary leak	Anastomotic stricture
Anastomotic stricture	Nonanastomotic stricture
Redundant bile duct (kinking)	Bile leak at T-tube removal
Bile leaks on the cut surface of reduced liver	Oddi's sphincter dysfunction
Mucocele of the cystic duct	Recurrent biliary stone or sludge
Extrahepatic bile duct necrosis	
Bile leak at T-tube exit	
Obstruction of T-tube stent	
Cholangitis after T-tube cholangiography	
Residual biliary stone or sludge	
Oddi's sphincter dysfunction	

the hepatic artery or in arterial steal syndrome may also lead to ischemic biliary lesions in liver transplant recipients. If untreated, these lesions may progress to cause sectorial or diffuse biliary strictures, sepsis, and graft loss [11–14].

In reduced-size grafts, complications relating to the bile ducts are the main cause of morbidity, with an incidence of 10–32% [2,15–21]. Multiple reasons for the higher rate of biliary complications in these patients have been proposed: bile leaks on the cut surface of the donor liver, small biliary duct size, excessive periductal dissection in the donor resulting in relative ischemia of the native bile duct, and increased complexity of biliary reconstructions in cases of two or more biliary anastomosis [3,22]. Additionally, inadvertent ligation of small bile ducts in the graft may lead to bile obstruction in that segment of the liver. The orifices and the patency of the bile duct branches to each segment in the graft must be examined to avoid surgical problems [23]. The optimal approach to biliary reconstruction in adult-to-adult LDLT remains to be defined [4]. Marcos et al. [24] favor the RY technique, believing that this provides extra-arterial inflow to the duct. Azoulay et al. [25] proposed a tension-free duct-to-duct anastomosis with or without stent if the viability of the native bile ducts is confirmed by the presence of active arterial bleeding from both cut ends. However, an RY must be performed if these conditions are not fulfilled. The rate of anastomotic strictures seems to be higher with right liver grafts but this must be confirmed in a large series [3].

Nonanastomotic biliary strictures (NABS) often result from an ischemic insult to the biliary tree of the donor liver. Most of the patients with NABS have hepatic artery problems: HAT, stenosis of the arterial anastomosis, or arterial steal syndrome due to a shift of hepatic blood flow into the splenic or the gastroduodenal artery [12,26]. Other factors that may influence the formation of NABS are ABO incompatibility, prolonged cold preservation time of the graft, or disease of the recipient's bile ducts such as primary sclerosing cholangitis. Arterial occlusion secondary to intimal hyperplasia and endothelial injury has probably a multifactorial origin including increased atherogenic risk of many liver recipients, arterial hypertension, hypercholesterolemia, obesity, diabetes, and arteriosclerosis. These factors are related in some cases to the advanced age of recipients or to the side-effects of immunosuppressive treatment. Furthermore, Margarit et al. [5] reported that an additional risk factor for development of late HAT is donor age. Since older donors of 60 years or even up to the 80 years are accepted due to the scarcity of donors, this last factor could become important in the future.

■ CLINICAL PRESENTATION

Most of the biliary complications occur within the first 3 months after OLT, as is shown in Table 21.2 [27]. Depending on the time of the appearance, biliary complications can be classified as early (before 3 months) or late after OLT. Those related to surgical technique usually occur early after OLT [5]. A prompt diagnosis is essential to avoid long-term graft and patient morbidity and mortality [28]. In one large study, nearly half of 83 patients subsequently recognized to have biliary complications were initially treated for rejection at least one time before recognition of the underlying biliary pathology. This patient population had a significantly high biliary tract-related mortality rate [29].

Hepatic necrosis with fulminant hepatic failure and extrahepatic necrosis of the biliary tree are common early presentations of HAT. However, most of the biliary complications are presented with infectious symptoms such as fever, cholangitis, or abdominal pain, which need abdominal ultrasonography in most of the cases to diagnose the problem. Some patients are asymptomatic except for elevated liver function tests and undergo abdominal ultrasound (US) after a routine assessment of the biochemistry.

The laboratory diagnosis of biliary complications includes elevation of bilirubin, alkaline phosphatase, and white blood cell count. The differential diagnosis of elevation in these laboratory findings early after OLT includes sepsis, preservation damage of the graft, graft injury secondary to ischemia, and rejection.

Since steroids and immunosuppressants may mask significant complications, abnormalities in the liver test function should prompt consideration of a biliary problem even in the face of minimal clinical symptoms. Unless there is a strong clinical and histological evidence for another diagnosis, visualization of the biliary anatomy is mandatory.

A bile leak should be considered when a recipient develops bile-straining of the abdominal drainage immediately after surgery or in patients with intra-abdominal fluid collections. Biliary drains are another important source of problems early or late after OLT. One of the most frequent T-tube-related biliary complications is the bile leak, which occurs after T-tube removal even if it is delayed more than 3 months after OLT. It usually presents as acute and severe abdominal pain immediately after T-tube removal.

A biliary stricture should be considered when a patient a few months after OLT has fever, jaundice, abdominal pain, or histological findings of biliary obstruction. Several reports showed that anastomotic strictures are more common in RY than in CC and in pediatric compared with adult OLT [30,31].

One of the most common presentations is asymptomatic cholestasis. However, asymptomatic patients who have a normal cholangiogram 3 months after OLT are unlikely to have biliary tract disease and should initially be considered for liver biopsy.

Some complications seen in CC such as those associated with the T-tube, mucocele formation with obstruction, redundant bile duct, and those related to the Oddi's sphincter dysfunction are not seen in patients with an RY reconstruction.

■ DIAGNOSTIC TOOLS AND IMAGING

The first image modality that should be used when a biliary complication is suspected should be abdominal ultrasonography. Alternatively, a cholangiogram can be done depending on the type of biliary reconstruction performed in the OLT, the status of each patient, and the preference of each liver transplant team. In patients with acute cholangitis, the cholangiogram must be followed by a minimally invasive drainage of the bile ducts using catheters or stents. Abdominal evaluation with computed tomography (CT) or magnetic resonance imaging (MRI) will provide complete evaluation of the abdominal cavity in order to exclude other postoperative complications. Additional diagnostic tools are hepatobiliary radionuclide scintigraphy (HBRS) and liver biopsy. In all the cases of biliary tree complication after OLT, problems related to the hepatic artery should be excluded and treated. Usually the Doppler US is enough but in case of unclear findings, an angiogram of the liver to assess patency and flow of the hepatic artery must be performed.

Although there is no standardized algorithm for the diagnosis of bile duct complication our proposal is described in Fig. 21.1.

Transabdominal Ultrasound

This noninvasive method is used routinely in the early postoperative period to exclude vascular complications (e.g. HAT) after OLT. In the evaluation of the biliary system, the finding of dilated bile ducts suggests obstruction, and

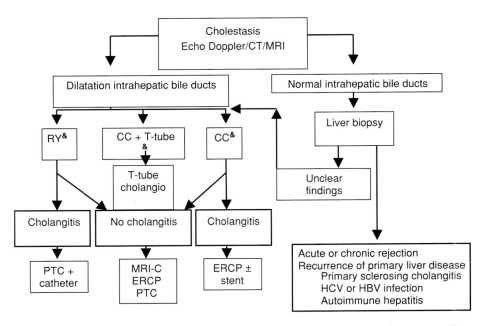

Fig. 21.1 *Algorithm for the diagnosis of bile duct complications in liver transplant recipients. Ampersand symbol (&) represents the type of biliary reconstruction performed during liver transplantation; RY, Roux-en-Y choledochojejunostomy; CC, choledochocholedochostomy; Echo, echography; CT, computed tomography; MRI, magnetic resonance imaging; MRI-C, magnetic resonance imaging cholangiography; PTC, percutaneous transhepatic cholangiography; ERC, endoscopic retrograde cholangiography; HCV, hepatitis C virus; and HBV, hepatitis B virus.*

identification of a subhepatic or perihepatic fluid collection may be associated with bile leak [32]. Unfortunately, the sensitivity of US in detection of biliary complication after OLT has been described to be as low as 54% [32]. A negative US examination finding, therefore, does not rule out biliary tract disease in liver transplant recipients; if there is significant clinical suspicion, further investigation with visualization of the bile ducts must be done [33]. An important adjunct to US is the measurement of the flow in the hepatic vessels with real-time Doppler analysis. In the presence of abnormal Doppler findings suggesting hepatic artery or portal vein thrombosis, contrast angiography must be performed to confirm the diagnosis.

Abdominal CT and MRI Scans

When US is limited by the presence of intra-abdominal gas or in patients with inadequate scanning technique due to abdominal pain, abdominal CT or MRI may provide better information with respect to biliary tree problems. These imaging tools are noninvasive and provide information about dilatation of the bile ducts and intra-abdominal fluid collection. Furthermore, they can exclude other coexisting complications (e.g. small bowel perforation). Contrast-enhanced CT permits evaluation of the vascular supply to the liver and indirect evaluation of the intra- and extrahepatic biliary system. In patients with kidney failure after OLT, the use of gadolinium-enhanced MRI offers similar images with lower toxicity for the kidneys [34,35]. Advantages of these methods over US are better objective evaluation of the abdominal cavity, less operator dependency, and images that are easier to read and understand, allowing for open discussion in a multidisciplinary manner. An additional advantage of MRI in patients with high suspicion of biliary complications is the possibility to complement the study with a cholangiogram, permitting direct evaluation of the biliary tree.

Cholangiography

In patients with CC over a T-tube, a cholangiogram through the T-tube is the study of choice. Unfortunately, T-tube-C is directly related to an increased risk of infection despite the use of prophylactic antibiotics; thus this should not be used as a first procedure [6,36]. If there is no T-tube and the suspicion of a biliary complication is high, endoscopic retrograde cholangiography (ERC) or MRI cholangiography (MRI-C) can be good options. The RY reconstruction prevents easy endoscopic access to the biliary tree; in these patients the investigation of posttransplant biliary anatomy relies on MRI-C or percutaneous transhepatic cholangiography (PTC). In asymptomatic patients with biochemical abnormalities that are not easily explained by acute cellular rejection or viral infection in the late phase after OLT, MRI-C for the detection of delayed biliary complications after OLT offers excellent assessment of the biliary tree [37]. A noninvasive approach in these patients avoids the risk of bleeding, acute pancreatitis, or ascending cholangitis [6]. Minimally invasive diagnostic tools should be reserved for patients in whom interventions in the biliary tree are required. It is accepted that endoscopic and percutaneous access not only are useful and reliable methods for diagnosis but can also be safely used for dilatation and stenting. ERC allows the endoscopic sphincterotomy when indicated but has the additional risk of ascending cholangitis, pancreatitis, or duodenal perforation. In patients with coagulopathy, endoscopic or percutaneous are contraindicated because of the risk of profuse bleeding. Since the percutaneous approach is done through the liver parenchyma, there is a higher risk of hemorrhagic complications.

PTC is most easily performed in the presence of biliary dilatation. If there is no dilatation of the bile ducts, PTC requires an increased number of punctures through the liver; the chance of bleeding in these patients is higher. However, the percutaneous approach is clearly indicated when ERC access is not possible, e.g. in patients with RY reconstruction and for the treatment of lesions located in the bile ducts high within the liver (e.g. intrahepatic ischemic stenosis), which cannot be reached from below via an endoscope.

Hepatobiliary Scintigraphy

HBRS using technetium-99m can detect both bile leaks and biliary obstruction after OLT [38]. The leak appears as tracer activity outside the confines of the biliary tract and obstruction as a failure of the tracer to progress out of the biliary system to the duodenum or small bowel. A 1997 prospective study comparing HBRS with ERC for detection of early biliary complications after OLT showed sensitivity and specificity for bile leak of 50% and 79% and for biliary stricture of 62% and 64%, respectively [39]. In a 2002 retrospective study, the sensitivity and specificity of the HBRS for diagnosis of biliary complications were each 100% for bile leak in patients with suspected bile leak or biloma, and of 93% and 88% for biliary obstruction [40]. Although HBRS is an accurate diagnostic modality in the evaluation of biliary complications after OLT, it has limitations as a means of differential diagnosis of nonbiliary complications. Additionally, the information provided is inferior to direct visualization of the biliary tree in determining the exact location and caliber of biliary strictures or leaks. In most of the liver transplant programs, the use of HBRS has been replaced by the other diagnostic tools mentioned earlier.

Liver Biopsy

In those patients with abnormal liver function test results in absence of bile duct dilatation, liver biopsy is often indicated to exclude acute rejection, recurrence of the primary liver disease, or viral hepatitis. In liver transplant recipients, cholangitis or bile duct obstruction caused by biliary complications can be difficult to differentiate from acute cellular rejection (see Chapter 22). When there is any doubt about the interpretation of the histological findings (e.g. intrahepatic biliary thrombus), cholangiography must be performed. Misinterpretation of the biopsy may delay appropriate treatment in cases of biliary complication. Moreover, inappropriate treatment with administration of steroid boluses and other potent immunosuppressive drug may adversely affect the healing of bile leaks and impair treatment of biliary infection.

■ MANAGEMENT OF BILE LEAK

Leaks occurring initially after OLT are usually related to anastomotic complications and may result in focal or generalized peritonitis. Other sites of early leaks include the T-tube exit site, aberrant bile ducts, and the surface of the liver in reduced-liver, split-liver, or living donor's liver grafts [4,15,16,20,21]. Delayed leaks related to T-tube removal occur in some patients who develop acute abdominal pain and are sometimes associated with intra-abdominal fluid collection.

Early identification and treatment of bile leaks are important. An infected biloma resulting from a persistent bile leak can compromise surgical repair of the biliary tract or may result in pseudoaneurysm or mycotic aneurysm of the adjacent hepatic artery. Surgical repair of the bile leak should be delayed until infection is controlled. Moreover, the presence of a bile leak not related with a T-tube requires assessment of the hepatic arterial flow by Doppler US and/or contrast angiography.

The appropriate therapy for a bile leak depends on the clinical presentation, the location of the leak, and the existence of hepatic artery problems. HAT or stenosis should be corrected prior to addressing the biliary leak. Our proposal of the algorithm for the management of bile leaks after OLT is showed in Fig. 21.2.

When bilious drainage develops in an asymptomatic patient after OLT, the first rule of treatment is not to remove the abdominal drain until the leak stops completely. In patients developing a leak, abdominal imaging must be done to

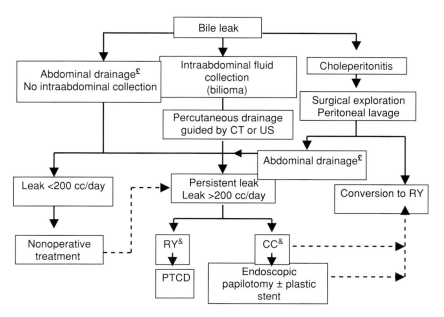

Fig. 21.2 *Algorithm for the management of bile leaks after liver transplantation. Pound symbol (£) represents intraoperative placement during the liver transplantation and ampersand symbol (&) the type of biliary reconstruction performed during liver transplantation.*

determine if there is a biloma or diffuse coleperitoneum. Most bilomas can be treated with US or CT-guided percutaneous catheter drainage under local anesthesia. Bilomas usually result from small, self-limited bile leaks, which form collections. Due to the small size without downstream obstruction these leaks most often close spontaneously; the fluid collection can be successfully treated via abdominal drainage. In cases of persistent leak through the drain or in bile leaks of more than 200 cc/day, a percutaneous or endoscopic papilotomy with placement of a plastic stent must be considered. If minimal invasive management fails, surgical revision must be considered.

In patients who develop diffuse peritonitis, an explorative laparotomy with peritoneal lavage and possible anastomotic revision must be performed. In case of ongoing copious bile leak resulting from anastomotic CC disruption, the strategy must be to convert to an RY. Primary repair of the CC leak is contraindicated because of the local inflammation and the poor arterial supply at the site of the anastomosis. In case of a leak from an RY, the anastomosis should be taken down and the hepatic duct shortened to the level of brisk capillary bleeding before performing the new RY. Attempts to place additional stitches in the primary anastomosis will increase the size of the fistula, with a consequent increment in the bile leak. Sometimes a small, well-contained bile leak can be treated successfully by placement of a T-tube or a transcystic drain above the anastomosis and a subhepatic drain at the site of the leak. In all cases, distal biliary obstruction preventing resolution of the leak should be excluded with a preoperative or an intraoperative cholangiogram or with surgical exploration at the time of laparotomy.

Management of bile leaks from the T-tube exit site rarely requires reoperation. When such leaks occur in the early postoperative phase, reopening the T-tube to external drainage should be the initial treatment. If T-tube drainage fails, a transpapillary stent may be inserted endoscopically beside the T-tube, bridging the area of the leak; this can be performed without additional sphincterotomy [41]. The stent can be removed after 2–4 weeks, but if there is a continued leakage the duct must be restented for an additional 4–6 weeks.

A leak along the T-tube tract immediately after T-tube removal is the most common biliary complication in patients with CC over a T-tube. Typically the patient develops acute abdominal pain and sometimes hypotension within the first minutes after the T-tube is withdrawn. To reduce the incidence and the severity of this complication, several recommendations have been proposed. The first few is to delay the removal of the T-tube to at least 90 days after OLT. Also, intravenous access should be obtained prior to removal and a cholangiogram should be made with prophylactic antibiotics in order to assess CC anastomosis and the bile flow through the papilla prior to removal of the T-tube. Patients must be observed in bed and vital signs monitored for 2 h after T-tube removal. In case of acute abdominal pain, analgesic drugs may be administered to control the symptoms. An abdominal CT or US must be performed to assess the need for percutaneous drainage of any eventual intra-abdominal fluid collection. In case of a biloma or persistence of abdominal pain, an ERC must be performed with placement of an internal stent bridging the sphincter of Oddi. If there is any associated biliary stenosis the stent should be placed across the involved area. Most stents can be removed after 4–6 weeks.

■ MANAGEMENT OF BILE STRICTURES

Biliary stenoses are usually classified depending on the location either in nonanastomotic (NABS) or in anastomotic biliary strictures (ABS). As shown in Fig. 21.3, the management of these patients is completely different.

Nonanastomotic Biliary Strictures

Strictures secondary to ischemia are usually multiple, but solitary intrahepatic regional strictures can occur. Cholangiographic findings of NABS range from mucosa irregularities to focal narrowing of the lumen with proximal ductal

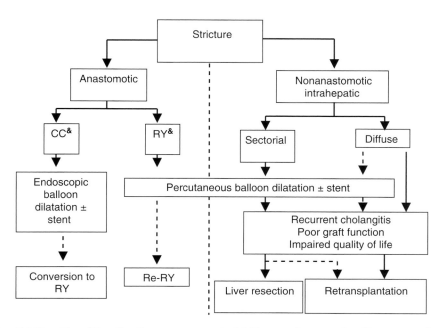

Fig. 21.3 *Algorithm for the management of biliary strictures after liver transplantation based on the location. Ampersand symbol (&) represents the type of biliary reconstruction performed during liver transplantation.*

dilatation. Additionally, ischemic damage to the bile ducts may be associated with extrahepatic bile leaks and intrahepatic bilomas.

Management depends on location, severity, number, and liver function. Options range from observation to endoscopic or percutaneous approaches, liver resection, or retransplantation. The assessment of the arterial supply to the liver in the presence of NABS is very important to define pathogenesis and treatment. Correction of arterial problems prior to treatment of the biliary problem is essential to achieve optimal results. Angioplasty of the hepatic artery must be performed if a hepatic artery stenosis is identified. Percutaneous embolization of the splenic artery represents a safe therapeutic option for patients with arterial steal syndrome after OLT. If this treatment fails, splenectomy, surgical ligation, or banding of the splenic and gastroduodenal artery to improve graft perfusion have been described [12].

Asymptomatic segmental strictures with isolated elevation of the alkaline phosphatase or gamma-glutamyl transpeptidase can be observed. Correction of the underlying ischemic arterial problem without any biliary intervention can usually solve the problem.

In patients with jaundice but good liver function, endoscopic or percutaneous dilatation of a single or dominant stricture followed by stenting with a plastic endoprosthesis is usually recommended [42]. Since these strictures are usually located above the hilium, the percutaneous approach plays an important role in their management [43]. In patients with biliary sepsis, infected biloma, or in those with transpapillary stents, adequate antibiotic treatment is indicated. Most patients need repeated dilatations and require stenting for several months. In a series with endoscopic management, patients with NABS compared with ABS require more endoscopic interventions and are associated with a higher incidence of cholangitis and choledocholithiasis [44]. After 3 years the success rate after endoscopic treatment was lower in patients with NABS (73% vs. 90%) [44]. However, the success rate reported by others has not been as promising with a recurrent rate of 50% after stent removal [45]. Longer follow-up with a larger patient series is necessary to assess the effectiveness of this minimal-invasive treatment.

Because metal stents tend to remain patent longer than plastic stents, some have suggested that use of these stents might benefit patients with biliary strictures. However, we do recommend this approach since metal stents eventually occlude and frequently require invasive procedures to manage their obstruction [46].

The use of hepatic resection as a graft-saving procedure has been advocated for the treatment of complications after OLT, such as segmental HAT with ischemic biliary stenosis. When liver resection is done early after OLT, the reported mortality rate is very high [47]. Mortality in patients undergoing delayed liver resection 3 months after OLT is lower compared with those undergoing early liver resections (22% vs. 66%) [47]. This approach may avoid retransplantation in selected cases of biliary strictures localized in one hemi-liver in patients without cholangitis and with otherwise excellent performance status [48].

In patients with poor graft function, deterioration of the patient's quality of life, or recurrent cholangitis, retransplantation should be considered (Fig. 21.3) [49]. Palliative stenting may help the patient as a bridge until a new donor is available. However, nonoperative management of these patients avoids colon-ization of the bile ducts until the next liver transplant. Retransplantation must be considered before the patient's general condition deteriorates too, at which the success of the OLT is compromised. When retransplantation becomes necessary, better nutritional status and lower levels of immunosuppression during the time on the waiting list will make them better candidates.

Anastomotic Biliary Strictures

These strictures result from a combination of surgical technique, local ische-mia, and scar tissue formation. The choice of treatment depends on the type of biliary reconstruction performed at the time of OLT and the local preferences in each liver transplant program. In a 1995 survey, only 29% of the transplant centers in the USA chose reoperation as a first choice of treatment, whereas 45% use endoscopic and 22% percutaneous management of the anastomotic strictures after OLT [50].

Long-term surgical results are considered superior to those obtained with endoscopic or percutaneous techniques, but are still accompanied by a higher short-term morbidity. Surgical treatment late after OLT can be technically difficult with a particular risk of damaging the hepatic artery. In general, surgery remains the last solution in case of failure of minimally invasive treatment, but it remains unclear how much time we should give to these new approaches before surgical repair is attempted. Therefore, endoscopic or percutaneous balloon dilatation should be the first choice in the treatment of ABS after OLT. However, patency after this initial treatment is only 70% after 1 year [46]. Failure of balloon dilatation is a reason to propose endoscopic plastic nonexpandable retrograde stents, which are removed after 3–12 months. These stents require periodic replacement every 3 or 4 months to avoid stent occlu-sion and cholangitis. Long-term outcome after all stents were removed (mean: 54 months) for 22 patients with ABS after CC treated endoscopically shows a successful rate of 90% [51].

A 2003 study of patients who underwent percutaneous balloon dilatation and stenting of ABS showed that the patency of the anastomosis after one session is as low as 58% [46]. Further percutaneous intervention increases the patency to 88% at 60 months after the first treatment is made [46]. The early recurrence of the stricture after balloon dilatation suggests the presence of fibrosis, which requires stent placement.

Metallic expandable stents were used in 12 patients but 58% of them experienced obstruction of the stent [46]. The main pitfall of the expandable stents seems to be the mucosal hyperplasia between the metal wires causing obstruction and gallstones, requiring surgical intervention. Moreover, metallic stent placement may be a complicating factor for further surgical procedures because it can be difficult to remove due to the mucosal ingrowth into the wall of the bile duct.

Success of the percutaneous technique, with low morbidity and mortality, has been demonstrated even in small-size recipients with nondilated intrahepatic bile ducts [52]. This minimally invasive approach permits dilatation and stenting of the ABS with some rate of success [53]. Use of an internal–external stent in biliary–enteric stenosis allows the anastomosis to remain patent. After 6 weeks, partial withdrawal of the stent and cholangiogram can show whether the stenosis has opened up or not. If the stenotic part is still narrow, further dilatation and stenting at the same time can be performed for another 6 weeks [53]. In a recent series of percutaneous dilatation of biliary strictures after living-related pediatric liver transplantation, the success rate was 100% with preserved graft function [21]. For anastomotic strictures in RY patients, percutaneous catheterization of the intestinal loop of the hepatojejunostomy seems to offer a novel and promising approach [54].

If the endoscopic or percutaneous transhepatic approaches fail, surgical conversion of CC to an RY or "redo" of the hepatojejunostomy is the next step. In case of poor liver function or complete obstruction of the hepatic artery, retransplantation should be considered.

■ OTHER BILIARY COMPLICATIONS

Sphincter of Oddi Dysfunction

Diffuse dilatation of the donor and recipient bile duct after CC reconstruction in the absence of any documented mechanical obstruction may be caused by Oddi's sphincter dysfunction [28]. Delayed passage of the biliary contrast medium through the papilla during a cholangiogram in a patient without evidence of stricture suggests the diagnosis. Diffuse dilatation of the common bile duct with elevation of liver tests after T-tube clamping and resolution when the T-tube is unclamped are also suggestive [55]. The pathogenesis is probably related to a papillary dyskinesia caused by either devascularization or denervation of the ampulla of Vater during total hepatectomy.

Transpapillary stenting with or without sphincterotomy has been reported as a successful treatment [55]. The majority of patients in our experience do well after 1–3 months of stenting alone. In situations in which cholestasis persists after sphincterotomy or where there is recurrent cholangitis, conversion of the CC to an RY may be necessary.

Stones and Sludge

Stones and sludge are relatively infrequent after liver transplantation but are associated with high morbidity. A retrospective review of 4100 cholangiograms in 1650 patients after OLT showed a prevalence of bile duct filling defects of 5.7% ($n = 94$) categorized as sludge or cast in 53 grafts (56%), stones in 32 (34%), and necrotic debris in 9 (10%) [56]. Debris and bile duct necrosis are related to ischemia from hepatic artery occlusion; ischemic pathogenesis can also explain some cases of sludge after OLT [5]. Necrotic debris and sludge were associated with hepatic artery occlusion in 78% and 30% of the cases, respectively [56]. Bile duct stones most frequently occur in the setting of biliary strictures, suggesting that bile stasis is an important factor.

The treatment of posttransplant cholecholithiasis or sludge often requires more than one endoscopic or percutaneous procedure and typically utilizes a combination of dilatation, stenting, lithotripsy, and sphincterotomy. Surgical treatment for debris or stone removal may be necessary [5].

Mucocele of the Cystic Duct

This infrequent complication occurs when the cystic duct of the donor is ligated at both ends. Continued endothelial secretion causes enlargement of the cyst duct and extrinsic compression of the extrahepatic bile duct. Surgery usually is required to solve the problem.

Redundant Bile Duct

Bile flow obstruction due to the kinking of a redundant bile duct is a technical complication that can occur after CC reconstruction. While some centers are in favor of surgical correction, others prefer an endoscopic approach. The latter involves placing an endoscopic stent to stretch the bile duct at the site of the CC. Scar tissue around the bile duct prevents recurrence of kinking, and the stent can be removed safely after 6 weeks. If the stent cannot be placed or fails, the CC must be converted to an RY.

Cholangitis

The use of T-tube in OLT is directly related to an increased risk of infection and cholangitis [6]. Cholangitis following iatrogenic contamination of the biliary tree at the time of T-tube or endoscopic cholangiography can occur despite the use of prophylactic antibiotics. Biliary stenosis producing obstruction of the bile flow in patients without preservation of the sphincter of Oddi after RY reconstruction may be implicated in the development of ascending cholangitis. Management of acute cholangitis is similar to that recommended to nontransplant patients. The principle is to relive obstruction and to identify and treat the organism causing the infection. Preferably, endoscopic or percutaneous drainage is the first choice of treatment in these immunosuppressed patients. However, some patients require surgical treatment for the underlying bile duct stenosis. Before any intervention in the biliary system, the arterial flow to the graft must be assessed with a Doppler US and/or an angiogram of the liver to exclude hepatic artery problems.

■ SUMMARY

Biliary complications are still frequent problems after OLT. The type of biliary reconstruction will determine the type of complication and the diagnostic and therapeutic procedures that can be employed. A prompt diagnosis is essential to avoid long-term graft and patient morbidity and mortality. Although the management remains controversial, minimally invasive measures play a fundamental role in the diagnosis and treatment of early and late biliary complications after OLT. Most of these complications can be managed nonoperatively with conservative treatment. However, severe diffuse strictures related to hepatic artery problems remain the most challenging biliary complication; these complications are likely to fail conservative treatment and require retransplantation. Indications for surgical treatment, particularly retransplantation, include recurrent cholangitis despite conservative treatments, impaired quality of life, and poor graft function.

■ REFERENCES

1. Clavien PA, Camargo CA, Jr, Croxford R, et al. Definition and classification of negative outcomes in solid organ transplantation. Application in liver transplantation. Ann Surg 1994;220(2):109–120.

2. Broelsch CE, Frilling A, Testa G, et al. Early and late complications in the recipient of an adult living donor liver. Liver Transpl 2003;9(10 suppl 2):S50–S53.

3. Broelsch CE, Frilling A, Testa G, et al. Living donor liver transplantation in adults. Eur J Gastroenterol Hepatol 2003;15(1):3–6.

4. Miller CM, Gondolesi GE, Florman S, et al. One hundred nine living donor liver transplants in adults and children: a single-center experience. Ann Surg 2001;234(3): 301–311; discussion 311–312.

5. Margarit C, Hidalgo E, Lazaro JL, et al. Biliary complications secondary to late hepatic artery thrombosis in adult liver transplant patients. Transpl Int 1998; 11(suppl 1):S251–S254.

6. Scatton O, Meunier B, Cherqui D, et al. Randomized trial of choledochocholedo-chostomy with or without a T tube in orthotopic liver transplantation. Ann Surg 2001;233(3):432–437.

7. Thune A, Friman S, Persson H, et al. Raised pressure in the bile ducts after orthotopic liver transplantation. Transpl Int 1994;7(4):243–246.

8. Bhatnagar V, Dhawan A, Chaer H, et al. The incidence and management of biliary complications following liver transplantation in children. Transpl Int 1995;8(5): 388–391.

9. Tzakis AG, Gordon RD, Shaw BW, Jr, et al. Clinical presentation of hepatic artery thrombosis after liver transplantation in the cyclosporine era. Transplantation 1985;40(6):667–671.

10. Gunsar F, Rolando N, Pastacaldi S, et al. Late hepatic artery thrombosis after orthotopic liver transplantation. Liver Transpl 2003;9(6):605–611.

11. Abbasoglu O, Levy MF, Vodapally MS, et al. Hepatic artery stenosis after liver transplantation – incidence, presentation, treatment, and long term outcome. Trans-plantation 1997;63(2):250–255.

12. Nussler NC, Settmacher U, Haase R, et al. Diagnosis and treatment of arterial steal syndromes in liver transplant recipients. Liver Transpl 2003;9(6):596–602.

13. Vogl TJ, Pegios W, Balzer JO, et al. [Arterial steal syndrome in patients after liver transplantation: transarterial embolization of the splenic and gastroduodenal arter-ies]. Rofo Fortschr Geb Rontgenstr Neuen Bildgeb Verfahr 2001;173(10):908–913.

14. Denys AL, Qanadli SD, Durand F, et al. Feasibility and effectiveness of using coronary stents in the treatment of hepatic artery stenoses after orthotopic liver transplantation: preliminary report. Am J Roentgenol 2002;178(5):1175–1179.

15. Yersiz H, Renz JF, Farmer DG, et al. One hundred in situ split-liver transplanta-tions: a single-center experience. Ann Surg 2003;238(4):496–505; discussion 506–507.

16. Renz JF, Emond JC, Yersiz H, et al. Split-liver transplantation in the United States: outcomes of a national survey. Ann Surg 2004;239(2):172–181.

17. Brown RS, Jr, Russo MW, Lai M, et al. A survey of liver transplantation from living adult donors in the United States. N Engl J Med 2003;348(9):818–825.

18. Bak T, Wachs M, Trotter J, et al. Adult-to-adult living donor liver transplantation using right-lobe grafts: results and lessons learned from a single-center experience. Liver Transpl 2001;7(8):680–686.

19. Todo S, Furukawa H, Jin MB, et al. Living donor liver transplantation in adults: outcome in Japan. Liver Transpl 2000;6(6 suppl 2):S66–S72.

20. Malago M, Testa G, Frilling A, et al. Right living donor liver transplantation: an option for adult patients: single institution experience with 74 patients. Ann Surg 2003;238(6):853–862; discussion 862–863.

21. Kling K, Lau H, Colombani P. Biliary complications of living related pediatric liver transplant patients. Pediatr Transplant 2004;8(2):178–184.

22. Azoulay D, Marin-Hargreaves G, Castaing D, et al. Ex situ splitting of the liver: the versatile Paul Brousse technique. Arch Surg 2001;136(8):956–961.

23. Harihara Y, Makuuchi M, Takayama T, et al. A simple method to avoid a biliary complication after living-related liver transplantation. Transplant Proc 1998;30(7):3199.

24. Marcos A, Ham JM, Fisher RA, et al. Surgical management of anatomical variations of the right lobe in living donor liver transplantation. Ann Surg 2000;231(6): 824–831.

25. Azoulay D, Marin-Hargreaves G, Castaing D, et al. Bismuth H. Duct-to-duct biliary anastomosis in living related liver transplantation: the Paul Brousse technique. Arch Surg 2001;136(10):1197–1200.

26. Orons PD, Sheng R, Zajko AB. Hepatic artery stenosis in liver transplant recipients: prevalence and cholangiographic appearance of associated biliary complications. Am J Roentgenol 1995;165(5):1145–1149.

27. Lemmer ER, Spearman CW, Krige JE, et al. The management of biliary complications following orthotopic liver transplantation. S Afr J Surg 1997;35(2):77–81.

28. Mazariegos GV, Molmenti EP, Kramer DJ. Early complications after orthotopic liver transplantation. Surg Clin North Am 1999;79(1):109–129.

29. Greif F, Bronsther OL, Van Thiel DH, et al. The incidence, timing, and management of biliary tract complications after orthotopic liver transplantation. Ann Surg 1994;219(1):40–45.

30. Shaked A. Use of T tube in liver transplantation. Liver Transpl Surg 1997;3(5 suppl 1):S22–S23.

31. Gaber A, Thistlethwaite J, Busse H. Improved results of preservation of hepatic grafts preflushed with albumin and prostaglandins. Transplant Proc 1988;20:992.

32. Zemel G, Zajko AB, Skolnick ML, et al. The role of sonography and transhepatic cholangiography in the diagnosis of biliary complications after liver transplantation. Am J Roentgenol 1988;151(5):943–946.

33. Hussaini SH, Sheridan MB, Davies M. The predictive value of transabdominal ultrasonography in the diagnosis of biliary tract complications after orthotopic liver transplantation. Gut 1999;45(6):900–903.

34. Eubank WB, Wherry KL, Maki JH, et al. Preoperative evaluation of patients awaiting liver transplantation: comparison of multiphasic contrast-enhanced 3D

magnetic resonance to helical computed tomography examinations. J Magn Reson Imaging 2002;16(5):565–575.

35. Goyen M, Barkhausen J, Debatin JF, et al. Right-lobe living related liver transplantation: evaluation of a comprehensive magnetic resonance imaging protocol for assessing potential donors. Liver Transpl 2002;8(3):241–250.

36. Ben-Ari Z, Neville L, Davidson B, et al. Infection rates with and without T-tube splintage of common bile duct anastomosis in liver transplantation. Transpl Int 1998;11(2):123–126.

37. Norton KI, Lee JS, Kogan D, et al. The role of magnetic resonance cholangiography in the management of children and young adults after liver transplantation. Pediatr Transplant 2001;5(6):410–418.

38. Shah AN. Radionuclide imaging in organ transplantation. Radiol Clin North Am 1995;33(3):473–496.

39. Kurzawinski TR, Selves L, Farouk M, et al. Prospective study of hepatobiliary scintigraphy and endoscopic cholangiography for the detection of early biliary complications after orthotopic liver transplantation. Br J Surg 1997;84(5):620–623.

40. Kim JS, Moon DH, Lee SG, et al. The usefulness of hepatobiliary scintigraphy in the diagnosis of complications after adult-to-adult living donor liver transplantation. Eur J Nucl Med Mol Imaging 2002;29(4):473–479.

41. Thuluvath PJ, Atassi T, Lee J. An endoscopic approach to biliary complications following orthotopic liver transplantation. Liver Int 2003;23(3):156–162.

42. Gopal DV, Pfau PR, Lucey MR. Endoscopic management of biliary complications after orthotopic liver transplantation. Curr Treat Options Gastroenterol 2003;6(6):509–515.

43. Almogy G, Bloom A, Verstandig A, et al. Hepatic artery pseudoaneurysm after liver transplantation. A result of transhepatic biliary drainage for primary sclerosing cholangitis. Transpl Int 2002;15(1):53–55.

44. Rizk RS, McVicar JP, Emond MJ, Rohrmann CA, Jr, Kowdley KV, Perkins J, et al. Endoscopic management of biliary strictures in liver transplant recipients: effect on patient and graft survival. Gastrointest Endosc 1998;47(2):128–135.

45. Petersen BD, Timmermans HA, Uchida BT, et al. Treatment of refractory benign biliary stenoses in liver transplant patients by placement and retrieval of a temporary stent-graft: work in progress. J Vasc Interv Radiol 2000;11(7):919–929.

46. Roumilhac D, Poyet G, Sergent G, et al. Long-term results of percutaneous management for anastomotic biliary stricture after orthotopic liver transplantation. Liver Transpl 2003;9(4):394–400.

47. Catalano G, Urbani L, Biancofiore G, et al. Hepatic resection after liver transplantation as a graft-saving procedure: indication criteria, timing and outcome. Transplant Proc 2004;36(3):545–546.

48. Honore P, Detry O, Hamoir E, et al. Right hepatic lobectomy as a liver graft-saving procedure. Liver Transpl 2001;7(3):269–273.

49. Gopal DV, Corless CL, Rabkin JM, et al. Graft failure from severe recurrent primary sclerosing cholangitis following orthotopic liver transplantation. J Clin Gastroenterol 2003;37(4):344–347.

50. Vallera RA, Cotton PB, Clavien PA. Biliary reconstruction for liver transplantation and management of biliary complications: overview and survey of current practices in the United States. Liver Transpl Surg 1995;1(3):143–152.

51. Morelli J, Mulcahy HE, Willner IR, et al. Long-term outcomes for patients with post-liver transplant anastomotic biliary strictures treated by endoscopic stent placement. Gastrointest Endosc 2003;58(3):374–379.

52. Lorenz JM, Funaki B, Leef JA, et al. Percutaneous transhepatic cholangiography and biliary drainage in pediatric liver transplant patients. Am J Roentgenol 2001;176(3):761–765.

53. Chan KL, Tso WK, Fan ST, et al. Balloon dilatation for postoperative vascular and biliary stenoses in pediatric liver transplantation. Transplant Proc 1998;30(7):3200–3202.

54. Castaing D, Azoulay D, Bismuth H. Percutaneous catheterization of the intestinal loop of hepatico-jejunostomy: a new possibility in the treatment of complex biliary diseases. Gastroenterol Clin Biol 1999;23(8–9):882–886.

55. Clavien PA, Camargo CA, Jr, Baillie J, et al. Sphincter of Oddi dysfunction after liver transplantation. Dig Dis Sci 1995;40(1):73–74.

56. Sheng R, Ramirez CB, Zajko AB, et al. Biliary stones and sludge in liver transplant patients: a 13-year experience. Radiology 1996;198(1):243–247.

57. Golling M, von Frankenberg M, Ioannidis P, et al. Impact of biliary reconstruction on postoperative complications and reinterventions in 179 liver transplantations. Transplant Proc 1998;30(7):3180–3181.

58. Rabkin JM, Orloff SL, Reed MH, et al. Biliary tract complications of side-to-side without T tube versus end-to-end with or without T tube choledochocholedochostomy in liver transplant recipients. Transplantation 1998;65(2):193–199.

59. Davidson BR, Rai R, Kurzawinski TR, et al. Prospective randomized trial of end-to-end versus side-to-side biliary reconstruction after orthotopic liver transplantation. Br J Surg 1999;86(4):447–452.

60. Fondevila C, Ghobrial RM, Fuster J, et al. Biliary complications after adult living donor liver transplantation. Transplant Proc 2003;35(5):1902–1903.

61. Pekolj J, Acuña Barrios J, Mattera J, et al. Manejo de las complicaciones biliares en 300 transplantes hepaticos. Rev Argent Cir 2001;107(5):143–146.

The Role of Histopathology

▼ ▼ ▼ ▼ ▼ ▼ ▼ ▼ ▼

Mary K. Washington and M. David N. Howell

22

I N THIS chapter, the application of histopathologic analysis of liver biopsy tissue for the management of the liver transplant recipient is summarized. The opening section focuses on general information regarding the selection of patients for biopsy, the handling of biopsy tissue, the spectrum of histologic studies applied in liver biopsy analysis, and the histologic evaluation of donor livers prior to implantation. Subsequent sections present a histologic overview of problems prevalent in the early (0–7 days), mid (1 week to 2 months), and late (more than 2 months) posttransplant intervals. This scheme is intended to provide a useful reference to the differential diagnosis of transplant dysfunction at different times during the patient's clinical course. The divisions, however, are of necessity somewhat inexact; inclusion of a pathologic process in one of the three chronological sections does not preclude its occurrence in another. For further information, the reader is directed to two recent book chapters [1,2].

■ BIOPSY OF THE LIVER ALLOGRAFT: WHEN, WHY, HOW

Biopsies are performed to determine the cause of liver allograft dysfunction and to assess response to therapy. Some programs have established posttransplant biopsy protocols, with biopsies performed at set intervals; these vary among institutions. The argument has been made that day 5 protocol biopsies may help to document early rejection episodes that may not be clinically evident [3], and that protocol biopsies are justified because serum liver tests have poor sensitivity and specificity in diagnosis of graft dysfunction [4]. However, there is no compelling evidence that patient outcome is improved with use of early protocol biopsies [5], and the topic remains controversial.

Protocol 10-year biopsies have been shown to demonstrate a high prevalence of subclinical histologic changes such as chronic rejection and recurrent disease, and may be useful in adjusting therapy [6]. In any case, biopsy prior to treatment for presumed acute rejection is of critical importance, as post-therapy biopsy may not be diagnostic.

Liver biopsy can be done safely in the transplant patient; most studies report similar rates of complications as for the nontransplant patient. Bleeding is the most common serious complication, with 0.1–0.24% of patients suffering postbiopsy hemorrhage, often requiring transfusion and selective arterial embolization [7]. Surgery is rarely needed [7]. Rates of bleeding complications appear similar for suction needle (0.22%) and cutting needle (0.14%) [7]. Transjugular liver biopsy may be used effectively in liver transplant patients, yielding diagnostic tissue in up to 87% of procedures [8]. Some centers report slightly higher complication rates with automatic cutting needle biopsy (0.8–3.6%) [7,9]. Some studies suggest that the rate of infectious complications is higher in patients with Roux-en-Y anastomosis, ranging up to 9.8–12.5% [10,11], but other investigators have not confirmed this finding [7].

Although it may seem counterintuitive, needle biopsy is often preferable to wedge biopsy for histologic evaluation despite the smaller amount of tissue obtained with needle biopsies. Increased subcapsular fibrosis is a common finding, and wedge biopsy may overestimate the amount of fibrous tissue in the liver and give a false impression of bridging fibrosis. Thus, needle biopsies may reflect more accurately the overall changes in the liver, although inadequate sampling is always a possibility for irregularly distributed lesions. While fine needle aspiration biopsy has been advocated for diagnosis of acute rejection [12], this technique has not received wide acceptance because of limitations in demonstration of alternative diagnoses.

Guidelines for adequacy of biopsies have been published, but vary considerably depending on the condition being evaluated. For example, recent guidelines for the diagnosis of acute allograft rejection recommend a sample containing at least five portal triads [13], while many investigators recommend a sample containing at least 20 triads for a diagnosis of chronic rejection [14,15]. In general, the larger the sample available for study, the better.

Handling of Liver Biopsy Specimens

Tissue handling of the liver biopsy specimen is in part dictated by clinical differential diagnosis. Most of the biopsy should be submitted in fixative, 10% buffered formalin at most institutions, for paraffin embedment and routine histologic studies. In all cases, sections of the formalin-fixed, paraffin-embedded tissue are stained with hematoxylin and eosin (H&E); in many instances, such sections are sufficient for diagnosis. Additional useful stains include Masson trichrome, to demonstrate connective tissue, and periodic acid–Schiff stain with diastase digestion, helpful in demonstrating bile duct damage.

In selected cases, it is prudent to set aside small portions of the biopsy for special studies that may be needed. On rare occasions, reservation of a small piece of fresh frozen tissue may be warranted (e.g. for molecular diagnostic studies or immunofluorescence microscopy for deposits of complement components). If viral infection is suspected, a small portion of the biopsy (1–2 mm of the tissue core) may be submitted in glutaraldehyde for electron microscopy. This procedure is expensive, however, and may yield false-negative results owing to the focal nature of many viral infections. Culture of biopsy tissue for bacteria, fungi, and/or viruses is rarely indicated; the presence of these infectious agents can generally be detected by histologic examination of the biopsy and performance of other clinical tests (e.g. blood cultures).

Ancillary Staining Techniques

In addition to routine histochemical stains, special staining procedures, including immunohistologic staining and in situ hybridization, are used occasionally in the tissue diagnosis of liver allograft dysfunction. A growing panel of antibodies reactive with T cell, B cell, and monocyte/macrophage markers can be applied to formalin-fixed, paraffin-embedded tissues using the immunoperoxidase technique. These are useful in distinguishing rejection (usually T cell predominant) from posttransplant lymphoproliferative disorder (PTLD) (usually B cell predominant).

Several studies have suggested the possible utility of immunohistologic T cell subset analysis in the diagnosis of liver allograft rejection [16,17]. Acute and/or chronic rejection of liver transplants has also been associated with altered expression of adhesion molecules and matrix proteins [18,19], markers of cell proliferation and programmed cell death [20–22], complement components and inhibitors [23], granzymes [24], leukocyte costimulatory molecules [25], lymphokines/chemokines and their receptors [26,27], and major histocompatibility complex (MHC) molecules [28,29], as assessed by immunohistochemistry and other staining methods. Such analyses are currently employed primarily as research tools.

Immunohistologic staining and in situ hybridization are also useful in the diagnosis of allograft infections, particularly with viruses. Immunoperoxidase stains for hepatitis B surface and core antigens, cytomegalovirus (CMV), herpes simplex virus, varicella zoster virus, and adenovirus can all be performed on formalin-fixed, paraffin-embedded tissue. Immunoperoxidase stains and in situ hybridization for Epstein–Barr virus (EBV) components are also of great value in the diagnosis of PTLD. Immunoperoxidase staining and in situ hybridization methods for detection of hepatitis C have also been described [30], but their diagnostic utility has yet to be firmly established.

Evaluation of the Donor Liver

Biopsy of the donor liver helps eliminate borderline unsuitable organs for donation and establishes a baseline for evaluating histologic changes in the graft in subsequent biopsies. Frozen section examination is desirable for the evaluation of potential cadaveric donor livers with an abnormal gross appearance, or when there is an unfavorable history in the donor; for most "back-table" biopsies, routine tissue handling and processing is sufficient. It is difficult to predict subsequent function of the organ, but most studies have indicated a higher incidence of primary nonfunction when grafts with severe macrovesicular steatosis are used, with "severe" defined as greater than 50–60% of hepatocytes containing fat [31]. Moderate steatosis (fat droplets in 16–45% of hepatocytes) was associated with increased postoperative alanine amino transferase (ALT) and prothrombin time in one prospective study [32], and fatty change up to 25% or more has been shown to be an independent predictive factor for outcome after transplantation in a multivariate analysis [33]. Microvesicular fat does not appear to carry the same association with primary nonfunction [34]. The pathogenesis of the increased incidence of graft failure in steatotic livers is not known, but is postulated to be due to greater susceptibility to ischemic injury [31]. Other exclusion criteria reported include diffuse centrilobular ischemic necrosis, portal inflammation expanding every portal triad, marked periductal fibrosis, and granulomas [32]. Most donor livers have only minor changes such as mild portal fibrosis, often seen in older donors, and mild steatosis.

The major role for pretransplantation liver biopsy in evaluation of the donor for living donor liver transplantation is determination of hepatic steatosis. However, an appreciable number of such biopsies (roughly 40%) will show other histologic abnormalities of uncertain significance, such as lymphocytic inflammation in portal tracts, mild fibrosis, and increased iron [35].

■ EARLY POSTTRANSPLANT PERIOD (0–7 DAYS)

Procurement/Preservation/Reperfusion Injury

Procurement/preservation/reperfusion injury are terms used to describe non-immunologic injury of the liver allograft that occurs during harvesting and implantation. Most of the damage to the allograft has been attributed to cold preservation or to ischemic injury in the donor or at the time of transplantation. On biopsies of the donor liver taken 1–2 weeks after transplantation, centrilobular pallor, ballooning degeneration of hepatocytes, and canalicular cholestasis are features associated with this type of injury (Fig. 22.1). Spotty hepatocyte necrosis and mitotic figures in hepatocytes are often identified. The presence of sinusoidal neutrophils and hepatocellular necrosis in liver biopsies taken immediately after reperfusion correlates with the development of histologic procurement injury in the early postoperative period [36]. The changes of preservation injury typically resolve in the immediate posttransplant period, and rarely are severe enough to interfere with graft function.

Technical Complications

Ischemic complications, usually hepatic artery thrombosis with or without portal vein thrombosis, generally develop in the immediate postoperative period, but may also occur late after transplantation [37]. Hepatic artery thrombosis is relatively rare in adults, seen in less than 5% of patients in most series, but is more common in pediatric liver transplant patients, possibly because of the technically more difficult vascular anastomoses [38]. Late hepatic artery thrombosis may be relatively asymptomatic but often results in biliary complications [39]. Pathologic changes due to vascular occlusion may be irregularly distributed in the liver, and biopsy may be misleadingly

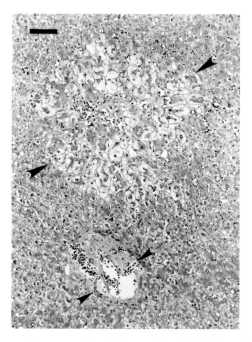

Fig. 22.1 *Procurement/preservation injury. Centrilobular pallor and ballooning degeneration of hepatocytes are present (large arrowheads). The portal (small arrowheads) and midzonal areas are normal in appearance. (H&E stain; bar = 100 μm.)*

negative. Changes associated with ischemic injury range from centrilobular pallor, hepatocyte necrosis, and cholestasis to large infarcts that may become secondarily infected, resulting in abscess formation.

Biliary stricture may be an early or a late complication, but generally becomes clinically evident 1 week to 2 months following transplantation. Strictures occurring in the large extra- or intrahepatic bile ducts may be related to ischemic injury to the bile ducts, whose blood supply derives from the hepatic artery. Appearance on biopsy is identical to that of large duct obstruction occurring in the nontransplanted liver, with portal edema, centrilobular canalicular cholestasis, neutrophils in portal areas and within bile duct epithelium, and bile ductular proliferation. Similar changes can be seen in occasional patients with postoperative ascending cholangitis.

Antibody-Mediated (Humoral) Allograft Rejection

Acute humoral allograft rejection is mediated by the binding of antidonor antibodies, usually directed against MHC or ABO blood group antigens, to the endothelium of graft blood vessels. Though it is a well-documented phenomenon in renal and cardiac allografting, and has been demonstrated in animal models of liver transplantation [40], it is fortunately rare in clinical hepatic transplantation [14,41], occurring most frequently in the setting of ABO-incompatible allografts. The reasons underlying this rarity are not entirely clear, but may include the unique structure of the hepatic sinusoidal microvasculature, the paucity of expression of relevant target antigens, and/or the enormous surface area of the hepatic vascular bed.

The histologic stigmata of humoral rejection include vascular platelet/fibrin thrombi and congestion, neutrophil margination and tissue infiltration, endothelial cell swelling and necrosis, and perivascular hemorrhage and edema. In extreme cases, some of these changes may be present in hepatic sinusoids and thus represented in percutaneous hepatic biopsies. Frequently, however, they are confined to medium-sized or large arteries, and are only detected in transplant hepatectomies or tissues sampled postmortem. The vascular compromise produced by humoral rejection can give rise to a variety of sequelae, including hemorrhagic infarcts and centrilobular ischemic damage. Bile duct injury, with consequences including cholestasis, ductular proliferation, and cholangitis-like changes, has also been reported in ABO-incompatible hepatic allografts [42,43]; periportal edema and necrosis have been described as early stigmata [44].

Many of the histologic features of humoral rejection, including vascular thrombosis, hemorrhage, and tissue necrosis, can be seen in association with nonimmune processes, particularly occlusions of graft vascular anastomoses. The diagnosis of humoral rejection requires careful clinicopathological exclusion of alternative etiologies for graft dysfunction such as thrombosis of the hepatic artery. Vascular deposits of antibody and complement components in humoral rejection are surprisingly difficult to detect by conventional immunostaining methods. Recently, however, staining for C4d has emerged as a reliable marker for humoral rejection in renal and cardiac allografts [45]. Application of this technique to liver transplant biopsies has as yet been limited [46].

■ MID-POSTTRANSPLANT PERIOD (1 WEEK TO 2 MONTHS)

Acute Cellular Allograft Rejection

Acute cellular rejection occurs most frequently in the period between 5 and 21 days posttransplantation, though its onset may be as early as 3–4 days or as late as several years following transplantation. In some cases, late-onset acute cellular rejection may be potentiated by concomitant viral infections or low maintenance immunosuppression [47]. Though the diagnosis is often straightforward, difficulties occasionally arise in patients with viral hepatitis, rejection superimposed on other forms of tissue injury, partially treated rejection, or mixtures of acute and chronic rejection.

Inflammatory Cells in Acute Cellular Rejection

Hepatic allografts undergoing acute rejection are typically infiltrated by a mixture of inflammatory cells including a majority population of mononuclear cells and lesser numbers of granulocytes (Figs 22.2 and 22.3). Though the proportions of the various cell types may vary somewhat, several useful generalizations can be made.

T lymphocytes are central to the pathogenesis of acute cellular rejection. They are invariably present to some degree in acute rejection episodes, and frequently constitute over 50% of the inflammatory infiltrate [16,17]. In most biopsies, a spectrum of T cells representing different stages of activation is present, including small lymphocytes, activated lymphocytes, and blasts; inflammatory cells undergoing mitosis may also be encountered.

The infiltrating T lymphocyte population typically includes both CD4+ (primarily helper/inducer) and CD8+ (primarily cytotoxic) T cells. CD4+ T cells mediate graft injury by elaborating cytokines, which activate other effector cells, including monocytes/macrophages. CD8+ T cells presumably cause graft damage by direct cytolytic attack on graft cells. The relative importance of the two T cell subtypes to the rejection process is currently unclear; most investigators now feel that both play a role.

Monocytes/macrophages also play a major role in cellular rejection, both as lymphokine-stimulated effectors of graft damage and as antigen-presenting

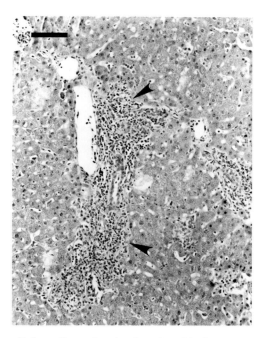

Fig. 22.2 *Acute cellular allograft rejection. In this low-power view, a primarily portal inflammatory infiltrate is seen (arrowheads). (H&E stain; bar = 100 μm.)*

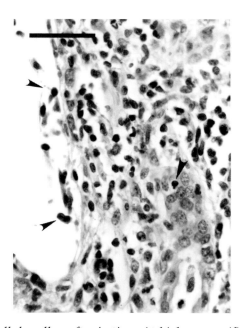

Fig. 22.3 *Acute cellular allograft rejection. At higher magnification, inflammatory attack on portal vein endothelium, or "endothelialitis" (small arrowheads) and on bile duct epithelium (large arrowhead) is seen. The inflammatory infiltrate consists primarily of mononuclear leukocytes. (H&E stain; bar = 100 μm.)*

cells (APCs) in the generation of T cell responses. Cells of monocyte/macrophage lineage are invariably present to some degree in acute cellular rejection, and often represent a sizable minority of the total population of inflammatory cells. In patients with resolving, partially treated, or ongoing rejection, monocytes/macrophages and Kupffer cells may also phagocytize cellular debris produced by the death of liver cells and other inflammatory cells. In biopsies obtained from such patients, mononuclear phagocytes may be the predominant inflammatory cell population.

A third cell type whose presence is associated strongly with acute cellular rejection is the eosinophil. Though eosinophils typically constitute less than 20% of the total inflammatory cell infiltrate, their distinctive appearance makes them a useful and easily visible histologic marker. In some studies of inflammatory cells infiltrating hepatic allografts, acute rejection has had a greater statistical correlation with eosinophils than with any other cell type [48,49]. The role played by eosinophils in the rejection process is unclear; some investigators have suggested that they function as an effector cell in immune response [50].

Tissue eosinophils can also be encountered in pathologic processes other than rejection, including allergic and drug reactions, parasitic infections, and paraneoplastic syndromes. In the absence of other typical stigmata of rejection, the presence of large numbers of eosinophils in a transplant biopsy should prompt a search for such alternative causes of eosinophilia.

A variety of other cell types are often present as minority populations in acute cellular rejection. B lymphocytes are frequently present in small numbers, but generally constitute less than 10% of the total infiltrate. The detection of greater numbers of B lymphocytes, particularly if some of the cells have atypical cytologic features, may signal the presence of PTLD. Moderate numbers of plasma cells are sometimes encountered in liver biopsies from patients with acute rejection, particularly in biopsies performed several months post-transplantation; the significance of these cells is unclear. Neutrophils are also a common component of the inflammatory infiltrate in acute cellular rejection, usually comprising less than 20% of the infiltrate. If neutrophils are more prevalent, and particularly if they are seen within bile ducts, an alternative diagnosis such as ascending cholangitis should be entertained.

Tissue Injury in Acute Cellular Rejection

A majority of the inflammatory cells in hepatic allografts undergoing acute cellular rejection are usually found in portal tracts (Figs 22.2 and 22.3). Typically, the inflammation expands the tracts, often to a considerable degree. In higher grades of rejection, inflammatory cells may spill out into the surrounding lobular parenchyma, in some cases damaging or obscuring the limiting plate. This phenomenon is sometimes described as "piecemeal necrosis," though the degree of interface inflammation and hepatocyte injury is generally less than that associated with chronic active hepatitis [51].

Within portal areas, inflammation is generally focused on two target structures: portal vein endothelium and bile duct epithelium [51,52]. In the former process, often designated "endothelialitis" (or "endotheliitis"), inflammatory cells adhere to, infiltrate, and undermine the venous endothelium, with associated endothelial cell swelling, vacuolization, nuclear reactive changes, and in severe cases, necrosis and sloughing (Fig. 22.3). This inflammatory attack generally spares adjacent hepatic arteries unless the grade of rejection is unusually severe. In bile duct inflammation, inflammatory cells cluster around ducts and infiltrate between adjacent epithelial cells or between the epithelium and its basement membrane, with associated epithelial cell injury.

The presence of significant portal inflammation in the absence of endothelialitis and associated tissue damage should prompt a search for pathologic processes other than rejection, such as PTLD and viral hepatitis. Hepatitis C infection can also cause significant inflammatory injury to bile ducts (see later).

A second major target of cellular liver allograft rejection is the centrilobular parenchyma, including the endothelium of terminal hepatic venules and the surrounding perivenular tissue ("central venulitis") [53](Fig. 22.4). This form of inflammation is often seen in combination with portal inflammatory infiltrates, but is occasionally the predominant inflammatory pattern in liver transplant biopsies. It is often accompanied by hydropic change, acidophilic necrosis, and/or dropout of hepatocytes; edema and vascular congestion are also frequently seen. In contrast to the "cookie cutter" pattern of abrupt transition and symmetry seen in centrilobular ischemic injury, the centrilobular damage in cellular rejection frequently has a ragged, asymmetric border. Ischemic or toxic centrilobular injury can also be distinguished from centrilobular rejection by the relative paucity of inflammation in the former processes. Though centrilobular inflammatory changes in rejection were initially reported in patients treated with tacrolimus (FK 506) [54], they are also encountered occasionally in patients not receiving this drug [53]. Centrilobular alterations during an initial bout of acute rejection have been associated with an increased frequency of recurrent acute rejection and development of chronic ductopenic rejection [55].

Though inflammatory cells are frequently present in the hepatic lobules during episodes of cellular rejection, lobular inflammatory infiltrates are generally less impressive than those found in portal and central vein regions. Scattered acidophil bodies and hepatocyte reactive changes can also be seen. The presence of large numbers of zone 2 inflammatory cells, especially in conjunction with extensive hepatocyte damage, should raise the suspicion of viral hepatitis as an alternative or additional diagnosis. Similarly, it is not uncommon to encounter mild cholestasis as a histologic component of cellular

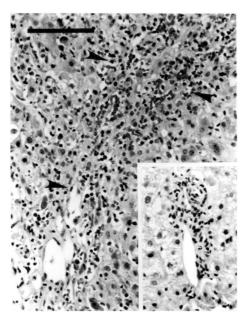

Fig. 22.4 *Acute cellular allograft rejection, centrilobular pattern in patients treated with tacrolimus. Extensive inflammation and architectural disruption are present adjacent to a central vein (arrowheads). A portal triad from the same biopsy (inset) is minimally inflamed. (H&E stain; bar = 100 μm.)*

rejection. Extensive cholestasis, however, should prompt a search for other etiologies, including extrahepatic biliary obstruction, sepsis, or drug toxicity.

Grading of Acute Cellular Allograft Rejection

A variety of systems have been proposed for the grading of acute rejection in liver allografts. Assignment of an overall level of severity for rejection in a given biopsy is complicated by the complex architecture of the hepatic parenchyma, the existence of variable patterns of rejection, and the somewhat subjective nature of the available histologic criteria. Nonetheless, several grading systems have been shown to have reasonably good intra- and interobserver reproducibility as well as prognostic value [13,52,56,57]. General features of some of the more popular schemas are discussed below; further information can be obtained from several reviews [13,14,41,57].

In several systems, including the National Institute of Diabetes and Digestive and Kidney Diseases (NIDDK) system [56] and the "Minnesota" system of Snover et al. [52], rejection is graded as mild, moderate, or severe (with corresponding numerical grades of 1, 2, and 3) based on semiquantitative analysis of histologic features. The "Pittsburgh" system of Demetris et al. [51] has a fourth category of "indeterminate" rejection, assigned a grade of 1;

this offsets the numerical grades for mild, moderate, and severe rejection to 2, 3, and 4. A diagnosis of rejection generally requires the presence of at least two of the following three features delineated by Snover et al. [52]: predominantly mononuclear portal inflammation, bile duct inflammation/injury, and portal or central venular endothelialitis. In mild rejection, these changes are limited in intensity and often involve only a subset of portal triads. Moderate rejection is diagnosed when more intense inflammation, bile duct injury, and/or endothelialitis are present in a majority of portal tracts. The criteria for severe rejection vary among systems, but include paucity of bile ducts; extension of inflammation into lobules or inflammatory linkage of portal triads; centrilobolar inflammation; hepatocyte ballooning, dropout, or necrosis, particularly in centrilobular areas; and arteritis.

In a somewhat more quantitative approach described by Dousset et al. [58] ("European" system), each of the three items in Snover's triad of portal inflammation, bile duct inflammation/injury, and endothelialitis is graded on a scale of 0 to 3; the grades are summed to yield an aggregate score of 0 to 9. In a similar system published by Datta Gupta et al. [57] ("Royal Free Hospital" system), these three features plus eosinophil infiltrates are likewise graded on a 0 to 3 scale, yielding a total range of 0–12. In each case, the authors provide ranges that can be used to convert the numerical scores into descriptive diagnoses of mild, moderate, or severe rejection.

In 1995, participants in the Third Banff Conference on Allograft Pathology produced a consensus document describing a grading schema for liver transplant rejection. Published in 1997, the Banff system includes both a global assessment of rejection as indeterminate, mild, moderate, or severe based on features similar to the NIDDK system and a semiquantitative scoring of portal, bile duct, and venular inflammation ("rejection activity index") similar to that employed in the European system [13]. The Banff schema has become the grading system of choice at a majority of transplant centers.

Differential Diagnosis

Though the clinicopathological diagnosis of acute cellular rejection is often straightforward, several clinical situations frequently pose diagnostic challenges. The following is a short summary of the most prevalent diagnostic problems.

Rejection versus Other Processes

The histologic manifestations of acute cellular allograft rejection, though generally distinctive, overlap to some degree with those of other processes, including viral and autoimmune hepatitis. Portal inflammatory infiltrates composed primarily of mononuclear cells, a cardinal feature of cellular rejection, are also typical of hepatitis C virus (HCV) infection, chronic hepatitis B virus infection, and autoimmune hepatitis. In addition, hepatitis C infection is occasionally accompanied by bile duct inflammation and injury. Other features of viral hepatitis, including lobular inflammation, hepatocyte necrosis, and cholestasis, can also be encountered in rejection.

Histologic features of acute rejection useful in distinguishing it from viral hepatitis include endothelialitis and centrilobular tissue damage. In contrast, biopsies from patients with hepatitis C infection may contain portal inflammatory cell aggregates or follicles; hepatocytes frequently exhibit macro- or microvesicular steatosis, and occasionally contain material resembling Mallory's hyalin [59]. Irregularity of the limiting plate, lobular inflammation, hepatocyte necrosis, and reactive changes of hepatocytes (nuclear variability, multinucleation, mitoses) are more prevalent in viral and autoimmune hepatitis than in rejection.

Rejection Plus Other Processes

Documentation of acute cellular rejection in a hepatic transplant biopsy does not guarantee the absence of additional pathological processes. In the early posttransplant period, combinations of rejection with resolving procurement/preservation/reperfusion injury or sequelae of surgical complications can be seen. At later time points, rejection and infection, particularly with viruses, sometimes occur together.

Several factors may contribute to the coexistence of rejection and other forms of tissue injury. In occasional patients, particularly those with viral hepatitis as a primary illness, maintenance immunosuppressive therapy may be insufficient to prevent rejection but sufficiently potent to allow progression of infection. Patients with documented cellular rejection treated with bolus steroids or other forms of antirejection therapy are at even greater risk for infectious complications, which may supervene before resolution of the rejection episode. Conversely, viral infection and other forms of nonimmune allograft damage may facilitate rejection by recruiting inflammatory cells to the graft, eliciting cytokine production, and inducing the expression of target antigens for rejection in graft tissues.

Diagnosis of rejection in combination with other forms of allograft pathology is most difficult for superimposed processes that share histologic features with rejection, particularly viral hepatitis. The differential diagnostic points discussed earlier are often useful in this setting. For example, if a transplant biopsy exhibits extensive endothelialitis in addition to typical features of hepatitis C infection, a dual diagnosis of cellular rejection and viral hepatitis should be entertained. A thorough review of the patient's clinical history, including primary disease, posttransplant interval, and laboratory tests for the presence of viral genomic material, is also crucial in resolving such diagnostic dilemmas.

Treated Rejection

Liver transplant biopsies are occasionally performed to monitor the progress of antirejection therapy, particularly if the therapy has not elicited the anticipated response in clinical or biochemical measures of hepatic function. Since an individual biopsy represents a single time point in a dynamic clinical process, it is frequently difficult to determine whether observed inflammatory changes are ongoing, in the process of resolution, or undergoing recrudescence. Comparison of sequential biopsies, particularly if one has been obtained before the institution of antirejection therapy, is often helpful in resolving this issue. Incomplete response to a course of antirejection therapy is best judged by persistence of portal and/or centrilobular inflammation, endothelialitis, and inflammatory attack on bile ducts.

Successful antirejection therapy typically induces a progressive decrease in the number of graft-infiltrating inflammatory cells, particularly T cells and eosinophils, over a period of several days. Debris produced by the breakdown of dying inflammatory cells is sometimes difficult to distinguish from the breakdown products of hepatic parenchymal elements damaged by ongoing rejection. Cellular fragments are ingested by phagocytic cells, including macrophages and neutrophils; it is not unusual for such cells, particularly macrophages, to persist in the graft after a majority of the T cells have disappeared. As inflammatory cells die, the infiltrate often appears less densely packed; interstitial spaces vacated by dying inflammatory cells may mimic the edema of aggressive, ongoing rejection.

Acute and Chronic Rejection

In their pure forms, acute cellular rejection and chronic rejection of liver transplants have histologic features that are sufficiently distinct to preclude confusion in the vast majority of cases. Interpretation may be difficult, however, when acute and chronic rejection processes coexist in the same transplant. On occasion, the pathologist will be faced with the task of estimating the relative contributions of acute and chronic rejection in a hepatic transplant biopsy; the distinction is by no means trivial, since the therapeutic approaches to the two forms of injury differ.

As detailed below, chronic rejection typically involves atrophy and obliteration of bile ducts accompanied by minimal overt inflammation. Paucity of identifiable bile ducts can also be a feature of aggressive acute rejection, however. In mixed forms of rejection, the relative contribution of acute and chronic processes to bile duct dropout may be difficult to gauge.

Opportunistic Infections

Infections are common in the posttransplant period, generally occurring in the first 2 months, and are a common cause of early posttransplant death [60]. While bacterial and fungal infections often involve other organs systems and do not require liver biopsy for diagnosis, viral infections may directly affect the liver allograft and may require biopsy to differentiate from rejection. The most important viruses for the pathologist to recognize in biopsies from this patient population are CMV, herpes simplex and varicella, and adenovirus, which all produce nuclear inclusions that may be identified on histopathologic examination.

Cytomegalovirus

CMV infection is not uncommon in the posttransplant period, with some centers reporting incidences of over 20% [61]. CMV infection posttransplant may be primary or a reactivation of a latent infection; both types of infection rarely occur before the third week after transplantation. Clinically, CMV infection of the allograft may mimic acute rejection, with patients presenting with fever and abnormal liver function tests.

The characteristic pattern of well-developed CMV hepatitis is the presence of small clusters of neutrophils (microabscesses) associated with injured hepatocytes (Fig. 22.5). We have found that numerous microabscesses (>9) within a biopsy but not the size of the microabscesses correlates with CMV infection [62]. In some cases, the inflammatory cells are mononuclear, with lymphocytes and activated Kupffer cells forming a small aggregate around a necrotic hepatocyte. Portal tracts do not contain large numbers of inflammatory cells, and there is generally only spotty hepatocyte necrosis. Nuclear inclusions may be identified in endothelial cells, hepatocytes, and bile duct epithelial cells (Fig. 22.5).

In early CMV infection, the classic enlarged cell with nuclear and cytoplasmic inclusions may be impossible to identify on standard H&E sections, and immunoperoxidase stains for an early CMV antigen, using multiple tissue sections, may be necessary for confirmation of suspected infection (Fig. 22.6). Immunostaining techniques using monoclonal antibodies for CMV appear to be more sensitive than DNA in situ hybridization and cell culture techniques [63], and may offer the first evidence of CMV as the etiology of graft dysfunction. It has been suggested that a positive immunostain for CMV, in the absence of clinical signs of CMV hepatitis, may precede the development of overt infection

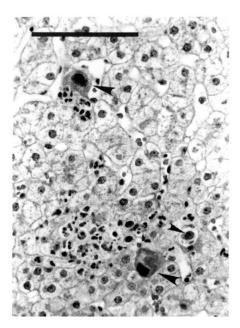

Fig. 22.5 *Cytomegalovirus (CMV) infection. Two cytomegalic cells with intranuclear inclusions are present (large arrowheads). The adjacent parenchyma contains clusters of neutrophils with occasional necrotic hepatocytes (small arrowhead). (H&E stain; bar = 100 μm.)*

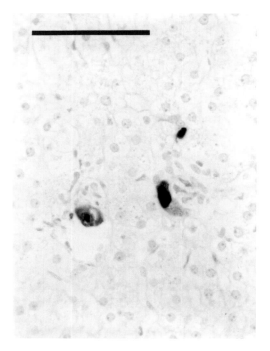

Fig. 22.6 *Cytomegalovirus (CMV) infection. Immunoperoxidase stain for CMV performed on same biopsy illustrated in Fig. 22.5. Staining, primarily nuclear, is seen in three cells. (Bar = 100 μm.)*

[63]. Polymerase chain reaction (PCR) may be used on formalin-fixed, paraffin-embedded tissue or fresh tissue, but does not appear to offer measurable advantage over immunohistochemical staining as a diagnostic technique [64], and is not available in all centers. PCR using nested primers for CMV, while offering excellent sensitivity and negative predictive value, is probably overly sensitive for use as a diagnostic test for relevant clinical disease [64].

Herpes Simplex Virus

Hepatitis due to herpes simplex often occurs earlier in the posttransplant period than does CMV hepatitis, with 50% occurring within 3 weeks of transplantation [61]. Patchy, randomly distributed areas of hepatocyte necrosis, coalescing into larger areas of geographic coagulative necrosis in severe cases, are seen. Ground glass nuclear inclusions may be identified in viable hepatocytes at the periphery of necrotic areas. Occasional multinucleated hepatocytes with nuclear inclusions are seen (Fig. 22.7). Immunoperoxidase staining for herpes simplex is helpful in confirming the infection. Herpes zoster infection involving the liver allograft is relatively rare, with only one case reported in 101 consecutive liver transplant cases in one series [61]. Histologically, zoster infection resembles herpes simplex hepatitis. Similarly,

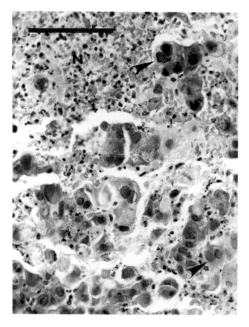

Fig. 22.7 *Herpes simplex virus infection. Numerous hepatocytes with "ground glass" nuclei are present; occasional multinucleate cells are seen (arrowheads). An adjacent area of necrosis (N) is present. (H&E stain; bar = 100 μm.)*

immunoperoxidase stain for herpes zoster antigen is helpful in confirming the diagnosis. Human herpesvirus-6 infections have been reported in solid organ transplant patients and may be associated with acute rejection or coinfection with CMV; liver biopsies show a lymphocytic infiltrate [65].

Adenovirus

Adenovirus hepatitis is rare in the adult liver transplant patient, but is somewhat more common in the pediatric transplant population and in children with primary immunodeficiencies. We have not seen a case of adenovirus hepatitis in any of our liver transplant patients, the vast majority of whom are adults. The histologic pattern is that of patches of hepatocyte necrosis, randomly distributed throughout the lobule. At the edge of the necrotic foci, viable hepatocytes contain intranuclear inclusions, resulting in a dark, homogeneously staining nucleus (smudge cell). Inflammatory reaction is minimal. Immunoperoxidase stains are available for confirmation of diagnosis, and electron microscopy shows characteristic 65–90 nm viral particles.

Epstein–Barr Virus and Posttransplant Lymphoproliferative Disorder

EBV infections are common in liver transplant recipients and are usually seen in the first 3 months following transplantation. In children, infection is often primary and more likely to be symptomatic, but in adults it generally represents reactivation of latent virus [66]. The histologic appearance ranges from alterations seen in infectious mononucleosis to a dense mononuclear inflammatory infiltrate indistinguishable from malignant lymphoma in PTLD (Fig. 22.8).

In the milder forms of EBV hepatitis, portal tracts contain a polymorphous mononuclear inflammatory infiltrate, with some enlarged atypical lymphocytes intermixed with smaller lymphocytes and plasma cells. An increased number of lymphocytes is seen in the sinusoids, sometimes in linear arrays described as resembling "strings of pearls." Hepatocyte necrosis is minimal relative to the degree of inflammation, and bile ducts are not infiltrated by lymphocytes.

PTLD occurs in 2.2–3.6% of adult patients [67] and up to 10% of pediatric recipients [66], often in the setting of more intensive immunosuppression [66]. The diagnosis should be suspected when a diffuse proliferation of lymphocytes is encountered; in contrast to cellular rejection, eosinophils are few in number. The lesions of PTLD are heterogeneous in histologic appearance, phenotype, and clonality. A widely accepted classification scheme recognizes three subtypes: plasmacytic hyperplasia, in which the proliferating cells are polyclonal and polymorphic, often including mixtures of small and large

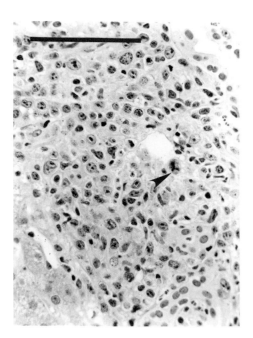

Fig. 22.8 *Posttransplant lymphoproliferative disorder (PTLD). A portal triad is expanded by a population of atypical lymphoid cells with irregular nuclear features, including prominent, often multiple nucleoli. An aberrant, tripolar mitosis is present (arrowhead). (H&E stain; bar = 100 μm.)*

lymphocytes, immunoblasts, and plasma cells; polymorphic B cell hyperplasia/lymphoma, in which the proliferating cells are variable in morphology but generally monoclonal; and immunoblastic lymphoma/multiple myeloma, in which the proliferating cells are monoclonal, monomorphic in appearance, and often have alterations in proto-oncogenes or tumor suppressor genes [68]. Tumors with features of Burkitt's lymphoma have also been described in a few patients [69]. The monomorphic lesions generally behave as malignant lymphomas, whereas the polymorphic lesions may regress upon diminution of immunosuppression. PTLD in liver transplant recipients often presents as systemic illness, but is localized to the liver or porta hepatis in occasional patients; in the latter instance, the presenting symptoms may be those of extrahepatic biliary obstruction [67]. The proliferating cells in liver-localized PTLD have been shown in some cases to be of donor origin [67].

Ancillary histologic tests are of great value in the diagnosis of PTLD. The proliferating cells are almost invariably B lymphocytes, though rare cases of T cell lymphoma have been described [70]; these phenotypes can be detected by immunoperoxidase staining. In most cases of B cell PTLD, EBV antigens or genomic material can be detected by immunohistochemistry or in situ hybridization, though EBV-negative lymphoproliferative processes have been reported in a minority of patients [71]. Clonality may be determined by immunoglobulin gene rearrangement studies [68].

Fungal and Bacterial Infection

Bacterial infection is common in the postoperative period, but liver biopsy is generally not indicated for diagnosis, as most infections involve organs other than the liver. It should be remembered, however, that a distinctive but not pathognomonic pattern of cholestasis is sometimes associated with sepsis and may be confused with large bile duct obstruction. In cholestasis associated with sepsis, inspissated bile is present in periportal cholangioles as well as in centrilobular areas, but is often not seen in the interlobular bile ducts. Small collections of neutrophils may be present in the parenchyma. Biliary studies may be necessary to exclude biliary stricture, however. Disseminated fungal infection may involve the liver, with candida and aspergillus the most important pathogens; nearly all such infections occur in hospitalized patients. Liver biopsy is seldom indicated for diagnosis.

Drug Reactions

In the early postoperative period, patients often receive many drugs with potentially hepatotoxic effects. If the patient receives total parenteral nutrition (TPN) for prolonged periods of time, changes similar to those described for TPN in the nontransplant patient may be seen. Changes attributed to TPN include steatosis, canalicular cholestasis, and portal fibrosis with bile ductular proliferation.

Immunosuppressive agents are also implicated as a cause of liver injury, although many confounding factors are usually present and it is difficult to implicate a specific agent as the cause of liver dysfunction. For instance, hepatotoxic effects of azathioprine are relatively rare, but include cholestatic hepatitis, centrilobular hemorrhagic necrosis, and peliosis hepatis [72]; veno-occlusive disease has also been described in renal transplant patients [73]. Azathioprine is also one of the agents associated with nodular regenerative hyperplasia, a rare cause of noncirrhotic portal hypertension, described in a few liver transplant patients posttransplant [74]. Sinusoidal dilatation and centrilobular hepatocyte degeneration mimicking hepatic outflow obstruction have been attributed to toxic effects of azathioprine and may be a result of damage to endothelial cells lining sinusoids and central veins [72]. In short, the histologic features are not specific, but it is important to suspect azathioprine as the cause of graft dysfunction to prevent irreversible injury to the graft.

Cyclosporine therapy is often associated with a mild elevation of serum bilirubin and may be associated with the formation of biliary sludge and calculi in renal and cardiac transplant recipients [72], but the histologic features of hepatic injury attributable to this agent are not well documented. Collections of foamy material in hepatocytes have been reported in suspected cyclosporine hepatotoxicity [75]. Corticosteroid therapy may produce changes in the liver allograft similar to those in nontransplanted livers, such as steatosis and bland cholestasis.

■ LATE POSTTRANSPLANT PERIOD (MORE THAN 2 MONTHS)

Recurrent Disease

Information regarding recurrence of disease has slowly accumulated, as more and more patients have undergone liver transplantation and have been followed for a number of years. In general, the risk of recurrence depends on the nature of the original disease.

Hepatitis B

Recurrence is uncommon in patients transplanted for fulminant acute hepatitis B. However, the risk of recurrence is very high in the untreated patient with chronic infection, particularly in patients with evidence of active viral replication. Antiviral therapy and hepatitis B immune globulin have shown efficacy in preventing hepatitis B reactivation after transplantation, with long-term survival comparable with that seen in other indications for liver transplantation [76]. Recurrent hepatitis B progresses through an acute hepatitis phase, develops into chronic active hepatitis, and progresses to cirrhosis, often with accelerated progression compared with the original disease [77]. The histologic appearance of each stage is similar to hepatitis B in the nontransplant liver in most cases; however, an unusual pattern of injury termed "fibrosising cholestatic hepatitis" has been observed in a few cases [78]. Serial liver biopsies in patients with recurrent hepatitis B surviving more than 60 days posttransplantation indicated that hepatitis B core antigen was detectable 2–5 weeks following transplantation. Acute viral hepatitis developed after about 150 days, and evolved into chronic active hepatitis after an average of 242 days. Cirrhosis developed in five patients, detected after a mean of 942 days [79]. Rarely, hepatocellular carcinoma has developed in the transplanted liver.

Hepatitis C

If sensitive PCR techniques are used, active hepatitis C viral replication can be detected in virtually all patients following transplantation for chronic hepatitis C infection. Indeed, levels of HCV RNA in serum are 10- to 20-fold higher following transplantation [80]. Approximately two-thirds of these patients will have histologic evidence of hepatitis [81]. Histologically evident recurrent hepatitis progresses to the chronic phase within 1–2 years in most patients, and is associated with reduction in graft and patient survival [82].

Distinguishing recurrent hepatitis C from other causes of graft dysfunction can be a formidable challenge in the posttransplantation period, and serial biopsies may be necessary. Histologically evident recurrence in the liver graft begins with spotty hepatocyte necrosis (Fig. 22.9), with a variable mononuclear inflammatory response and lobular disarray. As the disease evolves into the chronic phase, portal tract mononuclear inflammatory infiltrates, with a variable degree of lobular hepatitis, are seen (Fig. 22.10). The portal tract infiltrates may contain dense nodular lymphoid aggregates, as seen in hepatitis C in the nontransplant patient. Steatosis is often seen in hepatitis C infection, but cannot be used as a meaningful diagnostic feature in this group, as fat accumulation may be related to nutritional factors or drug therapy. Ballooning degeneration may be seen in recurrent hepatitis C, and when centrilobular in location, may be confused with ischemic injury. Rarely, marked centrilobular cholestasis may occur, and atypical features such as bile ductular proliferation and neutrophilic portal inflammatory infiltrate mimicking obstruction have been reported. Patients with this severe cholestatic form of recurrent hepatitis C have persistently higher levels of HCV RNA than those with noncholestatic

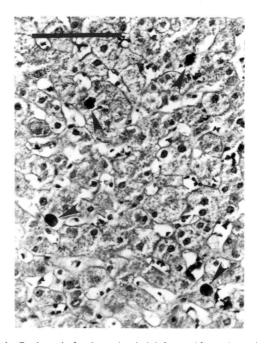

Fig. 22.9 *Hepatitis C virus infection. An initial manifestation of recurrent hepatitis C is spotty hepatocyte necrosis (arrowheads). (H&E stain; bar = 100 μm.)*

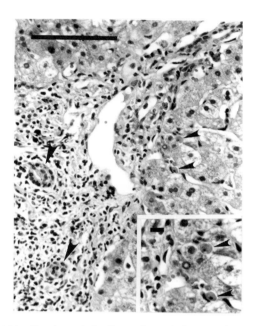

Fig. 22.10 *Hepatitis C virus infection. A portal tract is expanded by a dense infiltrate of mononuclear inflammatory cells, some of which encroach on bile duct epithelium (large arrowheads). Piecemeal necrosis of hepatocytes adjacent to the limiting plate is also present (small arrowheads, inset). (H&E stain; main figure bar = 100 μm, inset bar = 10 μm.)*

recurrent disease [83]; emergence of new viral quasispecies may also be a factor [84].

Autoimmune Hepatitis

Recurrence of autoimmune hepatitis, as evidenced by interface hepatitis, lobular mononuclear inflammation and necrosis, and portal lymphoplasmacytic inflammatory infiltrate, has been reported in up to 30% of patients undergoing liver transplantation for this disorder [85]. Autoantibodies persist after transplantation, although usually in lower titers. Disease recurrence is typically detected 1–3 years after transplantation and may be severe, leading to graft cirrhosis, although generally the recurrent disease is readily controlled with increased dosages of corticosteroids. Serological and histological features of autoimmune hepatitis may develop de novo following liver transplantation [86].

Primary Biliary Cirrhosis

Recurrent primary biliary cirrhosis (PBC) is difficult to diagnose based on clinical grounds, because serologic abnormalities, such as antimitochondrial antibodies and elevated IgM, persist in the PBC patient posttransplantation [87]. In a blinded study of protocol biopsies from asymptomatic patients, the diagnosis of recurrent PBC was made based on portal inflammation, portal lymphoid aggregates, and bile duct injury [87]. Because many of these features are nonspecific, and may be seen in other disease entities such as cellular rejection and hepatitis C infection, the prevalence of recurrent PBC has been difficult to determine, but is estimated at 20% [88]. The finding of portal tract granulomas associated with bile duct injury (florid duct lesion) (Fig. 22.11) is regarded as definitive evidence of recurrent disease. The natural history of recurrent PBC is unknown; disease progression is likely to be slow, and graft survival is probably not affected.

Primary Sclerosing Cholangitis

Although the question of recurrence of primary sclerosing cholangitis (PSC) (Fig. 22.12) has been a controversial topic, evidence is accumulating that the disease recurs in up to 20% of patients [89]. Evaluation of recurrence is complicated by the observation that a lesion resembling sclerosing cholangitis, with marked periductal fibrosis and features suggestive of large duct obstruction,

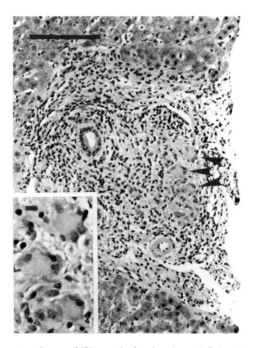

Fig. 22.11 *Recurrent primary biliary cirrhosis. A portal tract contains granulomatous inflammation (florid duct lesion); multinucleate giant cells (arrowheads) are illustrated at higher magnification in the inset. (H&E stain; main figure bar = 100 μm, inset bar = 10 μm.)*

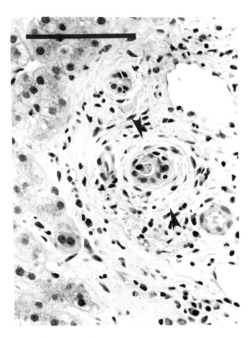

Fig. 22.12 *Recurrent primary sclerosing cholangitis (PSC). Bile ducts are surrounded by concentric layers of fibroblasts and collagen (arrowheads). (H&E stain; bar = 100 μm.)*

may occur following liver transplantation in patients transplanted for other liver diseases [90]. Numerous factors, such as ischemic injury to bile ducts following hepatic artery thrombosis or stenosis, prolonged graft ischemia, chronic vascular rejection with ductopenia, and use of ABO-incompatible grafts, have been associated with this lesion [90]. However, when patients with these risk factors are stringently excluded, nonanastomotic strictures of the biliary tree and fibrous cholangitis on liver biopsy have been reported in 20% of patients transplanted for PSC. Histologic recurrence was documented over 3 years after transplantation in most of the reported cases. Recurrence of PSC did not affect overall patient and graft survival in this study of 120 patients transplanted for PSC [89].

Steatohepatitis

Cirrhosis associated with nonalcoholic steatohepatitis (NASH) is an uncommon, but not rare, indication for orthotopic liver transplantation, representing the cause for transplantation in 2.9% of patients in one large series [91]. In addition to transplants performed in patients with biopsy-proven NASH, a sizable percentage of patients transplanted for cryptogenic cirrhosis, estimated at a third or more, are thought to have "burned-out" steatohepatitis based on clinicopathologic criteria [92,93].

A variety of manifestations of nonalcoholic fatty liver disease, including steatosis, recurrent NASH, and cirrhosis, can occur in liver transplants performed in patients with NASH or cryptogenic cirrhosis. Recurrence of NASH in transplants was first documented in the mid to late 1990s [94,95], and has since been reported to occur in as many as 33% of patients with known NASH or cryptogenic cirrhosis as their primary disorders [91–93]. Steatohepatitis is distinguished from uncomplicated steatosis by the presence of ballooning degeneration of hepatocytes in areas of fatty change, typically accompanied by pericellular fibrosis (Fig. 22.13). Neutrophils are sometimes seen in association with injured hepatocytes in areas of steatohepatitis, but their presence is not considered obligatory for the diagnosis. They are absent in many cases of transplant steatohepatitis, possibly owing to the use of maintenance immunosuppression.

The presence of steatosis, with or without associated hepatocyte injury, fibrosis, or inflammation, in a liver transplant biopsy is by no means pathognomonic for recurrent nonalcoholic fatty liver disease. Other possible causes include ethanol ingestion, de novo or recurrent hepatitis C, and steatosis in the donor liver. Correlation with clinical history and previous biopsies is essential in sorting out these possibilities. Anecdotal reports suggest that recurrence of

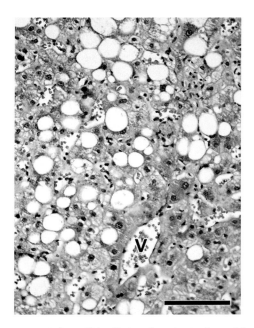

Fig. 22.13 *Recurrent steatohepatitis. Extensive steatosis and hepatocyte ballooning degeneration are seen in the vicinity of a terminal hepatic venule (V). (H&E stain; bar = 100 μm.)*

NASH in obese transplant recipients may be avoided or ameliorated by recipient weight loss [94] or gastric bypass surgery [96].

Chronic Allograft Rejection

Chronic allograft rejection is a relatively late complication of liver transplantation, generally occurring 6 weeks to 6 months following transplantation, though earlier and later onsets occur occasionally [15]. Chronic rejection has two major sites of attack in the liver: interlobular bile ducts and the intimal layers of muscular arteries. The bile duct damage generally takes the form of epithelial atrophy with nuclear pyknosis followed by total disappearance of ducts: a process frequently termed "vanishing bile duct syndrome" (Fig. 22.14). The loss of ducts is typically accompanied by only mild inflammation unless it is complicated by some other process (e.g. ongoing acute rejection, hepatitis). In advanced cases, marked canalicular cholestasis is often present. Bile duct dropout is most easily quantified by comparing the number of duct profiles in a biopsy with the number of hepatic artery/arteriole profiles. The latter number is generally fairly constant, though it may be decreased in advanced cases of arteriopathic rejection (see later).

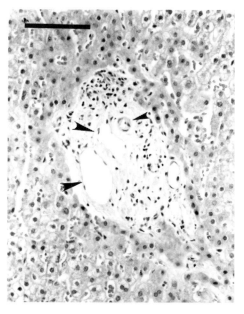

Fig. 22.14 *Chronic allograft rejection: vanishing bile duct syndrome. This portal tract lacks a bile duct; portal vein (large arrowheads) and hepatic artery (small arrowhead) are clearly visible. Minimal inflammation is present. (H&E stain; bar = 100 μm.)*

The arterial changes in chronic rejection, referred to variously as "obliterative arteriopathy," "obliterative endarteritis," and "foam cell arteriopathy," are characterized by progressive expansion of the intima of larger hepatic arteries. The thickened intimal layer often contains large numbers of foamy histiocytes, and may virtually obliterate the arterial lumen (Fig. 22.15). Similar changes can be seen in portal veins [97]. Arteries directly affected by obliterative arteriopathy are generally not represented in percutaneous needle biopsies. Several forms of secondary damage can be seen in such biopsies, however, including atrophy and disappearance of smaller arteries and arterioles, ballooning degeneration or dropout of centrilobular hepatocytes, and perivenular sclerosis [14,15,41,98,99].

Initial published guidelines for the evaluation of liver transplant rejection required loss of bile ducts in 50% of portal triads for a diagnosis of chronic rejection [41]. More recent studies have stressed the importance of identifying earlier lesions [14,15,98–100]. An update of the International Banff Schema for Liver Transplant Rejection published in 2000 [99] proposed a subdivision of features of chronic rejection into "early" (potentially reversible) changes (e.g. ductal degenerative changes, bile duct loss in a minority of portal tracts, early centrilobular ischemic damage) and "late" (presumably irreversible) changes (e.g. loss of a majority of ducts with degenerative changes in the remainder, obliteration of terminal hepatic venules with bridging fibrosis).

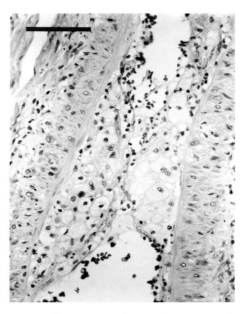

Fig. 22.15 *Chronic allograft rejection: foam cell arteriopathy. The intima of this muscular hilar artery is expanded by foamy phagocytic cells, markedly narrowing the lumen. (H&E stain; bar = 100 μm.)*

The pathogenesis of chronic rejection is poorly understood: both humoral and cell-mediated alloimmune mechanisms have been posited to play a role, and nonimmune processes such as CMV infection have also been suggested as possible contributing factors [15]. It is also unclear whether vanishing bile duct syndrome and arteriopathic rejection are etiologically connected or represent unrelated events. The two processes are frequently seen together, but each can occur in the absence of the other. Vanishing bile duct syndrome has been attributed variously to direct alloimmune attack on bile ducts and to ischemic damage secondary to obliterative arteriopathy; it is possible that both mechanisms contribute to chronic bile duct injury [15].

■ REFERENCES

1. Hubscher SG, Portmann BC. Transplantation pathology. In MacSween RNM, Burt AD, Portmann BC, et al., eds., Pathology of the liver, 4th ed. Edinburgh, UK: Churchill Livingstone, 2002:885–941.

2. Demetris AJ, Crawford JM, Malesnik M, et al. Transplantation pathology of the liver. In Odze RD, Goldblum JR, Crawford JM, eds., Surgical pathology of the GI tract, liver, biliary tract, and pancreas. Philadelphia, PA: WB Saunders, 2004:909–966.

3. Brunt EM, Peters MG, Flye WW, et al. Day-5 protocol liver allograft biopsies document early rejection episodes and are predictive of recurrent rejection. Surgery 1992;111:511–517.

4. Neuberger J, Wilson P, Adams D. Protocol liver biopsies: the case in favour. Transplant Proc 1998;30:1497–1499.

5. Bartlett AS, Ramadas R, Furness S, et al. The natural history of acute histologic rejection without biochemical graft dysfunction in orthotopic liver transplantation: a systematic review. Liver Transpl 2002;8:1147–1153.

6. Sebagh M, Rifai K, Feray C, et al. All liver recipients benefit from the protocol 10-year liver biopsies. Hepatology 2003;37:1293–1301.

7. Van Thiel DH, Gavaler JS, Wright H, et al. Liver biopsy: its safety and complications seen at a liver transplant center. Transplantation 1993;55:1087–1090.

8. Azoulay D, Raccuia JS, Roche B, et al. The value of early transjugular liver biopsy after liver transplantation. Transplantation 1996;61:406–409.

9. Chezmar JL, Keith LL, Nelson RC, et al. Liver transplant biopsies with a biopsy gun. Radiology 1991;179:447–448.

10. Bubak ME, Porayko MK, Krom RAF, et al. Complications of liver biopsy in liver transplant patients: increased sepsis associated with choledochojejunostomy. Hepatology 1991;14:1063–1065.

11. Larson AM, Chan GC, Wartelle CF, et al. Infection complicating percutaneous liver biopsy in liver transplant recipients. Hepatology 1997;26:1406–1409.

12. Kwekkeboom J, Zondervan PE, Kuijpers MA, et al. Fine-needle aspiration cytology in the diagnosis of acute rejection after liver transplantation. Br J Surg 2003;90:246–247.

13. Banff schema for grading liver allograft rejection: an international consensus document. Hepatology 1997;25:658–663.

14. Batts KP. Acute and chronic hepatic allograft rejection: pathology and classification. Liver Transpl Surg 1999;5(suppl 1):S21–S29.

15. Wiesner RH, Batts KP, Krom RAF. Evolving concepts in the diagnosis, pathogenesis, and treatment of chronic hepatic allograft rejection. Liver Transpl Surg 1999;5:388–400.

16. McCaughan GW, Davies JS, Waugh JA, et al. A quantitative analysis of T-lymphocyte populations in human liver allografts undergoing rejection: the use of monoclonal antibodies and double immunolabeling. Hepatology 1990;12:1305–1313.

17. Ibrahim S, Dawson DV, Killenberg P, et al. The pattern and phenotype of T-cell infiltration associated with human liver allograft rejection. Hum Pathol 1993;24:1365–1370.

18. Bacchi CE, Marsh CL, Perkins JD, et al. Expression of vascular cell adhesion molecule (VCAM-1) in liver and pancreas allograft rejection. Am J Pathol 1993;142:579–591.

19. Demirci G, Hoshino K, Nashan B. Expression patterns of integrin receptors and extracellular matrix proteins in chronic rejection of human liver allografts. Transpl Immunol 1999;7:229–237.

20. Ray MB, Schroeder T, Michaels SE, et al. Increased expression of proliferating cell nuclear antigen in liver allograft rejection. Liver Transpl Surg 1996;2:337–342.

21. Afford SC, Hubscher S, Strain AJ, et al. Apoptosis in the human liver during allograft rejection and end-stage liver disease. J Pathol 1995;176:373–380.

22. Rivero M, Crespo J, Mayorga M, et al. Involvement of the Fas system in liver allograft rejection. Am J Gastroenterol 2002;97:1501–1506.

23. Conti F, Grude P, Calmus Y, et al. Expression of the membrane attack complex of complement and its inhibitors during human liver allograft transplantation. J Hepatol 1997;27:881–889.

24. Kuijf ML, Kwekkeboom J, Kuijpers MA, et al. Granzyme expression in fine-needle aspirates from liver allografts is increased during acute rejection. Liver Transpl 2002;8:952–956.

25. Bartlett AS, McCall JL, Ameratunga R, et al. Analysis of intragraft gene and protein expression of the costimulatory molecules, CD80, CD86 and CD154, in orthotopic liver transplant recipients. Am J Transplant 2003;3:1363–1368.

26. Conti F, Calmus Y, Rouer E, et al. Increased expression of interleukin-4 during liver allograft rejection. J Hepatol 1999;30:935–943.

27. Goddard S, Williams A, Morland C, et al. Differential expression of chemokines and chemokine receptors shapes the inflammatory response in rejecting human liver transplants. Transplantation 2001;72:1957–1967.

28. Hubscher SG, Adams DH, Elias E. Changes in the expression of major histocompatibility complex class II antigens in liver allograft rejection. J Pathol 1990;162:165–171.

29. Creput C, Durrbach A, Menier C, et al. Human leukocyte antigen-G (HLA-G) expression in biliary epithelial cells is associated with allograft acceptance in liver–kidney transplantation. J Hepatol 2003;39:587–594.

30. Qian X, Guerrero RB, Plummer TB, et al. Detection of hepatitis C virus RNA in formalin-fixed paraffin-embedded sections with digoxigenin-labeled cRNA probes. Diagn Mol Pathol 2004;13:9–14.

31. Strasberg SM, Howard TK, Molmenti EP, et al. Selecting the donor liver: risk factors for poor function after orthotopic liver transplantation. Hepatology 1994;20:829–838.

32. Markin RS, Wisecarver JL, Radio SJ, et al. Frozen section evaluation of donor livers before transplantation. Transplantation 1993;56:1403–1409.

33. Zamboni F, Franchello A, David E, et al. Effect of macrovesicular steatosis and other donor and recipient characteristics on the outcome of liver transplantation. Clin Transpl 2001;15:53–57.

34. Fishbein TM, Fiel MI, Emre S, et al. Use of livers with microvesicular fat safely expands the donor pool. Transplantation 1997;64:248–251.

35. Ryan CK, Johnson LA, Germin BI, et al. One hundred consecutive hepatic biopsies in the workup of living donors for right lobe liver transplantation. Liver Transpl 2002;8:1114–1122.

36. Gaffey MJ, Boyd JC, Traweek ST, et al. Predictive value of intraoperative biopsies and liver function tests for preservation injury in orthotopic liver transplantation. Hepatology 1997;25:184–189.

37. Gunsar F, Rolando N, Pastacaldi S, et al. Late hepatic artery thrombosis after orthotopic liver transplantation. Liver Transpl 2003;9:605–611.

38. Stevens LH, Emond JC, Piper JB, et al. Hepatic artery thrombosis in infants: a comparison of whole livers, reduced-size grafts, and grafts from living-related donors. Transplantation 1992;53:396–399.

39. Stange BJ, Glanemann M, Nuessler NC, et al. Hepatic artery thrombosis after adult liver transplantation. Liver Transpl 2003;9:612–620.

40. Knechtle S, Kolbeck PC, Tsuchimoto S, et al. Hepatic transplantation into sensitized recipients. Transplantation 1987;43:169–172.

41. International Working Party, World Congresses of Gastroenterology 1994. Terminology for hepatic allograft rejection. Hepatology 1995;22:648–654.

42. Farges O, Kalil AN, Samuel D, et al. The use of ABO-incompatible grafts in liver transplantation: a life-saving procedure in highly selected patients. Transplantation 1995;59:1124–1133.

43. Minamiguchi S, Sakurai T, Fujita S, et al. Living related liver transplantation: histopathologic analysis of graft dysfunction in 304 patients. Hum Pathol 1999;30: 1479–1487.

44. Haga H, Egawa H, Shirase T, et al. Periportal edema and necrosis as diagnostic histological features of early humoral rejection in ABO-incompatible liver transplantation. Liver Transpl 2004;10:16–27.

45. Michaels PJ, Fishbein MC, Colvin RB. Humoral rejection of human organ transplants. Springer Semin Immunopathol 2003;25:119–140.

46. Krukemeyer MG, Moeller J, Morawietz L, et al. Description of B lymphocytes and plasma cells, complement, and chemokines/receptors in acute liver allograft rejection. Transplantation 2004;78:65–70.

47. Cakaloglu Y, Devlin J, O'Grady J, et al. Importance of concomitant viral infection during late liver allograft rejection. Transplantation 1995;59:40–45.

48. Foster PF, Sankary HN, Williams JW, et al. Morphometric inflammatory cell analysis of human liver allograft biopsies. Transplantation 1991;51:873–876.

49. Ben-Ari Z, Booth JD, Gupta SD, et al. Morphometric image analysis and eosinophil counts in human liver allografts. Transpl Int 1995;8:346–352.

50. de Groen PC, Kephart GM, Gleich GJ, et al. The eosinophil as an effector cell of the immune response during hepatic allograft rejection. Hepatology 1994;20:654–662.

51. Demetris AJ, Qian S, Sun H, et al. Liver allograft rejection: an overview of morphologic findings. Am J Surg Pathol 1990;14(suppl 1):49–63.

52. Snover DC, Freese DK, Sharp HL, et al. Liver allograft rejection: an analysis of the use of biopsy in determining outcome of rejection. Am J Surg Pathol 1987;11:1–10.

53. Tsamandas AC, Jain AB, Felekouras ES, et al. Central venulitis in the allograft liver: a clinicopathologic study. Transplantation 1997;64:252–257.

54. Demetris AJ, Fung JJ, Toso S, et al. Conversion of liver allograft recipients from cyclosporine to FK506 immunosuppressive therapy – a clinicopathologic study of 96 patients. Transplantation 1992;53:1056–1062.

55. Lovell MO, Speeg KV, Halff GA, et al. Acute hepatic allograft rejection: a comparison of patients with and without centrilobular alterations during first rejection episode. Liver Transpl 2004;10:369–373.

56. Demetris AJ, Seaberg EC, Batts KP, et al. Reliability and predictive value of the National Institute of Diabetes and Digestive and Kidney Diseases liver transplant-

ation database nomenclature and grading system for cellular rejection of liver allografts. Hepatology 1995;21:408–416.

57. Datta Gupta S, Hudson M, Burroughs AK, et al. Grading of cellular rejection after orthotopic liver transplantation. Hepatology 1995;21:46–57.

58. Dousset B, Hubscher SG, Padbury RTA, et al. Acute liver allograft rejection – is treatment always necessary? Transplantation 1993;55:529–534.

59. Lefkowitch JH, Schiff ER, Davis GL, et al. Pathological diagnosis of chronic hepatitis C: a multicenter comparative study with chronic hepatitis B. Gastroenterology 1993;104:595–603.

60. Markin RS, Hollins S, Wood RP, et al. Main autopsy findings in liver transplant patients. Mod Pathol 1989;2:339–344.

61. Kusne S, Dummer JS, Singh N, et al. Infections after liver transplantation: an analysis of 101 consecutive cases. Medicine 1988;67:132–143.

62. Lamps LW, Pinson CW, Raiford DS, et al. The significance of microabscesses in liver transplant biopsies: a clinicopathologic study. Hepatology 1998;28:1532–1537.

63. Paya CV, Holley KE, Wiesner RH, et al. Early diagnosis of cytomegalovirus hepatitis in liver transplant recipients: role of immunostaining, DNA hybridization, and culture of hepatic tissue. Hepatology 1990;12:119–126.

64. Brainard JA, Greenson JK, Vesy CJ, et al. Detection of cytomegalovirus in liver transplant biopsies: a comparison of light microscopy, immunohistochemistry, duplex PCR, and nested PCR. Transplantation 1994;57:1753–1757.

65. Lautenschlager I, Hockerstedt K, Linnavuori K, et al. Human herpesvirus-6 infection after liver transplantation. Clin Infect Dis 1998;26:702–707.

66. Cox KL, Lawrence-Miyasaki LS, Garcia-Kennedy R, et al. An increased incidence of Epstein–Barr virus infection and lymphoproliferative disorder in young children of FK506 after liver transplantation. Transplantation 1995;59:524–529.

67. Nuckols JD, Baron PW, Stenzel TT, et al. The pathology of liver-localized posttransplant lymphoproliferative disease: a report of three cases and a review of the literature. Am J Surg Pathol 2000;24:733–741.

68. Knowles DM, Cesarman E, Chadburn A, et al. Correlative morphologic and molecular genetic analysis demonstrates three distinct categories of posttransplantation lymphoproliferative disorders. Blood 1995;85:552–565.

69. Pasquale MA, Weppler D, Smith J, et al. Burkitt's lymphoma variant of posttransplant lymphoproliferative disease (PTLD). Pathol Oncol Res 2002;8:105–108.

70. Costes-Martineau V, Delfour C, Obled S, et al. Anaplastic lymphoma kinase (ALK) protein expressing lymphoma after liver transplantation: case report and literature review. J Clin Pathol 2002;55:868–871.

71. Nelson BP, Nalesnik MA, Bahler DW, et al. Epstein–Barr virus-negative post-transplant lymphoproliferative disorders: a distinct entity? Am J Surg Pathol 2000;24:375–385.

72. Kowdley KV, Keeffe EB. Hepatotoxicity of transplant immunosuppressive agents. Gastroenterol Clin North Am 1995;24:991–1001.

73. Sterneck M, Wiesner R, Ascher N, et al. Azathioprine hepatotoxicity after liver transplantation. Hepatology 1991;14:806–810.

74. Gane E, Portmann B, Saxena R, et al. Nodular regenerative hyperplasia of the liver graft after liver transplantation. Hepatology 1994;20:88–94.

75. Wisecarver JL, Earl RA, Haven MC, et al. Histologic changes in liver allograft biopsies associated with elevated whole blood and tissue cyclosporine levels. Mod Pathol 1992;5:611–616.

76. Lo CM, Fan ST, Liu CL, et al. Prophylaxis and treatment of recurrent hepatitis B after liver transplantation. Transplantation 2003;75:S41–S44.

77. Martin P, Munoz SJ, Friedman LS. Liver transplantation for viral hepatitis: current status. Am J Gastroenterol 1992;87:409–418.

78. Davies SE, Portmann BC, O'Grady JG, et al. Hepatic histological findings after transplantation for chronic hepatitis B virus infection, including a unique pattern of fibrosing cholestatic hepatitis. Hepatology 1991;13:150–157.

79. Todo S, Demetris AJ, Van Thiel D, et al. Orthotopic liver transplantation for patients with hepatitis B virus-related liver disease. Hepatology 1991;13:619–626.

80. Chazouilleres O, Kim M, Combs C, et al. Quantitation of hepatitis C virus RNA in liver transplant recipients. Gastroenterology 1994;106:994–999.

81. Shuhart MC, Bronner MP, Gretch DR, et al. Histological and clinical outcome after liver transplantation for hepatitis C. Hepatology 1997;26:1646–1652.

82. Alonso O, Loinaz C, Abradelo M, et al. Changes in the incidence and severity of recurrent hepatitis C after liver transplantation over 1990–1999. Transplant Proc 2003;35:1836–1837.

83. Doughty AL, Spencer JD, Cossart YE, et al. Cholestatic hepatitis after liver transplantation is associated with persistently high serum hepatitis C virus RNA levels. Liver Transpl Surg 1998;4:15–21.

84. Pessoa MG, Bzowej N, Berenguer M, et al. Evolution of hepatitis C virus quasispecies in patients with severe cholestatic hepatitis after liver transplantation. Hepatology 1999;30:1513–1520.

85. Hubscher SG. Recurrent autoimmune hepatitis after liver transplantation: diagnostic criteria, risk factors, and outcome. Liver Transpl 2001;7:285–291.

86. Kerkar N, Hadzic N, Davies ET, et al. De novo autoimmune hepatitis after liver transplantation. Lancet 1998;351:409–413.

87. Hubscher SG, Elias E, Buckels JAC, et al. Primary biliary cirrhosis: histologic evidence of disease recurrence after liver transplantation. J Hepatol 1993;18:173–184.

88. Faust TW. Recurrent primary biliary cirrhosis, primary sclerosing cholangitis, and autoimmune hepatitis after transplantation. Liver Transpl 2001;7:S99–S108.

89. Graziadei IW, Wiesner RH, Batts KP, et al. Recurrence of primary sclerosing cholangitis following liver transplantation. Hepatology 1999;29:1050–1056.

90. Sebagh M, Farges O, Kalil A, et al. Sclerosing cholangitis following human orthotopic liver transplantation. Am J Surg Pathol 1995;19:81–90.

91. Charlton M, Kasparova P, Weston S, et al. Frequency of nonalcoholic steatohepatitis as a cause of advanced liver disease. Liver Transpl 2001;7:608–614.

92. Contos MJ, Cales W, Sterling RK, et al. Development of nonalcoholic fatty liver disease after orthotopic liver transplantation for cryptogenic cirrhosis. Liver Transpl 2001;7:363–373.

93. Ayata G, Gordon FD, Lewis WD, et al. Cryptogenic cirrhosis: clinicopathologic findings at and after liver transplantation. Hum Pathol 2002;33:1098–1104.

94. Kim WR, Poterucha JJ, Porayko MK, et al. Recurrence of nonalcoholic steatohepatitis following liver transplantation. Transplantation 1996;62:1802–1805.

95. Carson K, Washington MK, Treem WR, et al. Recurrence of nonalcoholic steatohepatitis in a liver transplant recipient. Liver Transpl Surg 1997;3:174–176.

96. Duchini A, Brunson ME. Roux-en-Y gastric bypass for recurrent nonalcoholic steatohepatitis in liver transplant recipients with morbid obesity. Transplantation 2001;72:156–159.

97. Jain D, Robert ME, Navarro V, et al. Total fibrous obliteration of main portal vein and portal foam cell venopathy in chronic hepatic allograft rejection. Arch Pathol Lab Med 2004;128:64–67.

98. Blakolmer K, Seaberg EC, Batts K, et al. Analysis of the reversibility of chronic liver allograft rejection: implications for a staging schema. Am J Surg Pathol 1999;23:1328–1339.

99. Demetris A, Adams D, Bellamy C, et al. Update of the International Banff Schema for Liver Allograft Rejection: working recommendations for the histopathologic staging and reporting of chronic rejection. An international panel. Hepatology 2000;31:792–799.

100. Sebagh M, Blakolmer K, Falissard B, et al. Accuracy of bile duct changes for the diagnosis of chronic liver allograft rejection: reliability of the 1999 Banff schema. Hepatology 2002;35:117–125.

▼ ▼ ▼ ▼ ▼ ▼ ▼ ▼ ▼ ▼

Chronic Medical Problems in the Transplant Recipient

Medical Problems after Liver Transplantation

23

**Eberhard L. Renner and
Jean-François Dufour**

W ITH LONG-TERM survival after liver transplantation having become the rule, the care for medical problems potentially arising over time in the liver transplant recipient has gained increasing importance. Medical management must aim at minimizing long-term morbidity and mortality and, thus, at optimizing long-term quality of life and survival.

Conceptually, long-term medical problems occurring in the liver transplant recipient can be divided into (1) medical problems that are related to the liver transplant and/or immunosuppression per se and (2) medical problems that are unrelated to transplant/immunsuppression, i.e. are encountered in a similar frequency in an age- and sex-matched nontransplant population. The latter will not be dealt with herein. Within the former, medical problems may arise in connection with overall too little or too much immunosuppression, i.e. rejection (Chapter 19), infections (Chapter 25), and tumors (Chapters 25, 27, and 29), or with recurrent underlying liver disease (Chapter 24). Other medical problems are associated with, and/or facilitated by, commonly used immunosuppressive agents. These include obesity, arterial hypertension, dyslipidemia, diabetes mellitus, cardiovascular risk, gout, osteoporosis, and kidney failure. With the exception of the latter (Chapter 26), these, as well as some issues regarding skin disorders and family planning, are discussed in this chapter.

■ OBESITY

Weight gain is common after liver transplantation. In a cohort of 774 adult liver transplant recipients from three centers, body mass index (BMI) (corrected for ascites) increased from $24.8\,kg/m^2$ pretransplantation to $27.0\,kg/m^2$ in the first and to $28.1\,kg/m^2$ in the second posttransplant year, with little change thereafter [1]. Moreover, 21.6% of nonobese liver transplant recipients became obese (BMI $\geq 30\,\text{kg/m}^2$) within 2 years after grafting [1]. Thus, an overall posttransplant prevalence of obesity (BMI $\geq 30\,\text{kg/m}^2$) of around 20% [2] and of overweight (BMI $\geq 25\,\text{kg/m}^2$) of up to 60% was found in some series [3]. These prevalence rates are likely to increase further in the future due to increasing numbers of obese patients being transplanted for cirrhosis related to nonalcoholic fatty liver disease and the increasing prevalence of overweight and obesity in the general population. Transplant-specific risk factors for postoperative weight gain include therapy with steroids [1] and presumably the choice of calcineurin inhibitor [1,2]. While prevalence rates of overweight and obesity post liver transplant were slightly – albeit not always statistically significantly – higher than in the normal population [1,4], they likely contribute to the increased incidence of diabetes mellitus, arterial hypertension, dyslipidemia and thus, cardiovascular risk in these patients (cf. later). In addition, overweight/obesity is a risk factor for nonalcoholic fatty liver disease including its potentially progressive variant, i.e. nonalcoholic steatohepatitis, which has been reported to occur de novo in the graft [5]. The risk of developing health problems according to BMI and waist circumferences, as published by Health Canada [6], is summarized in Table 23.1A,B.

Given the high rate of developing overweight/obesity post liver transplant, it seems reasonable to consider routine prophylactic counseling on diet [7,8] and regular exercising [9,10] for all transplant recipients (and their partners) within 3 months posttransplant. Lifestyle measures should be reinforced

Table 23.1 *Classification/Terminology and Health Risk*

A:

Classification	BMI[a] Category (kg/m^2)	Risk of Developing Health Problems
Underweight	<18.5	Increased
Normal weight	18.5–24.9	Least
Overweight	25.0–29.9	Increased
Obese	≥30.0	
Class I	30.0–34.9	High
Class II	35.0–39.9	Very high
Class III	≥40.0	Extremely high

B:

Waist Circumference (cm)	Risk of Developing Health Problems
Men ≥102	Increased
Women ≥88	Increased

[a]BMI values are age- and gender-independent and may not be correct for all ethnic groups.

and repeat therapeutic counseling offered once BMI increases to $\geq$25.0 kg/m^2. The potential benefit of other measures in the morbidly obese (BMI $\geq$ 40.0 kg/m^2), including orlistat and bariatric surgery, has not been assessed in the post-liver-transplant setting. Such measures, however, bear a risk of interfering with absorption and/or metabolism of immunosuppressive drugs.

■ DYSLIPIDEMIA

Dyslipidemia is common after liver transplantation. Thus, hypercholesterol-emia has been reported in one-third to two-third of the liver transplant recipients and hypertrygliceridemia in some 10–50% of liver transplant recipients [2,11], with many, but not all of these patients, having mixed hyperlipidemia. Compared with other solid organ transplant recipients, both prevalence and extent of dyslipidemia are generally less in patients with a liver transplant. Thus, in a comparative study, serum cholesterol levels averaged 180 mg/dL in liver transplant compared with 226 mg/dL in kidney transplant recipients [12].

Transplant-specific risk factors for development of posttransplant dyslipidemia include antirejection medications, in particular steroids [12], calcineurin inhibitors (with tacrolimus likely, but debatably, causing somewhat less hypercholesterolemia than cyclosporine) [13,14], and sirolimus, which typically leads to more pronounced elevation of triglycerides than cholesterol [15].

Although not formally proven beyond doubt, it seems reasonable to assume that, as in the non-liver-transplant population, cardiovascular risk increases in liver transplant recipients with increasing duration and severity of dyslipidemia (cf. later). Thus, for assessment of cardiovascular risk and for determining thresholds for therapeutic interventions in dyslipidemia, current guidelines and recommendations proposed for the nontransplant population by the respective experts/associations should be followed. The National Cholesterol Education Program Adult Treatment Panel III Guidelines from the USA stratify patients according to their 10-year risk of experiencing a coronary event (Table 23.2) and propose the intervention thresholds outlined in Table 23.3 [16]. The typical adult liver transplant recipient is in his/her mid-fifties, hypertensive, and/or diabetic (cf. later); many liver transplant recipients therefore fall into at least the moderately high-risk group.

Of the currently available low-density lipid (LDL)–cholesterol-lowering drugs (i.e. HMG-CoA reductase inhibitors or statins), pravastatin and cerivastatin have been formally shown to be safe in liver transplant patients in controlled clinical trials [17,18]. Pravastatin is not prone to drug interactions with calcineurin inhibitors since it has little affinity to the cytochrome P450

Table 23.2 *ATP III Risk Categories*

Risk Category (10-Year Risk for Coronary Event)	Definition
High (>20%)	Coronary heart disease (CHD) (history of myocardial infarction, unstable angina, stable angina, coronary artery procedures (angioplasty or bypass surgery), or evidence of clinically significant myocardial ischemia) or CHD risk equivalents (clinical manifestations of noncoronary forms of atherosclerotic disease (peripheral arterial disease, abdominal aortic aneurysm, carotid artery disease with transient ischemic attacks or stroke of carotid artery origin) or >50% obstruction of a carotid artery, diabetes, and ≥2 risk factors with 10-year risk for hard CHD >20%)
Moderately high (10–20%)[a]	≥2 of the following risk factors: • Cigarette smoking
Moderate (<10%)[a]	• Arterial hypertension (BP ≥140/90 or on antihypertensive medication) • Low HDL cholesterol (<40 mg/dL, i.e. <1.03 mmol/L) • Family history of premature CHD (CHD in male first-degree relative <55 years of age; CHD in female first-degree relative <65 years of age) • Age (men ≥45 years, women ≥55 years)
Low[b]	0–1 of the above risk factors

[a]Calculator available at www.nhlbi.nih.gov/guidelines/cholesterol.
[b]Almost all people with 0 or 1 risk factor have a 10-year risk <10%; a 10-year risk assessment is thus not necessary.
From Grundy SM, Cleeman JI, Merz NB, et al. [16].

system, in particular CYP3A4. Apart from myopathy and other potential side-effects, statins lead to dose-dependent, reversible hepatic toxicity (alanine amino transferase (ALT) elevation) in approximately 1–3% of patients; close monitoring of liver enzymes is therefore advisable when starting liver transplant recipients on statins [19]. It remains to be determined whether HMG-CoA reductase inhibitors exert beneficial effects beyond lowering

Table 23.3 *ATP III LDL–Cholesterol Goals and Intervention Thresholds for Therapeutic Lifestyle Intervention (TLC) and Drug Therapy in Different Risk Categories (Modified from Ref. [16])*

Risk Category	LDL–Cholesterol Goal	Intervention Threshold		
		Lifestyle	Drug Therapy[a]	
High	<100 mg/dL (<2.59 mmol/L) (optional: <70 mg/dL (<1.81 mmol/l))[b]	≥100 mg/dL (≥2.59 mmol/L)[c]	≥100 mg/dL (≥2.59 mmol/L) (<100 mg/dL (<2.59 mmol/L): consider drug options)[d]	
Moderately high	<130 mg/dL (<3.36 mmol/L)[e]	≥130 mg/dL (≥3.36 mmol/L)[c]	≥130 mg/dL (≥3.36 mmol/L) (100–129 mg/dL (2.59–3.35 mmol/L): consider drug options)[f]	
Moderate	<130 mg/dL (<3.36 mmol/L)	≥130 mg/dL (≥3.36 mmol/L)	≥160 mg/dL (≥4.14 mmol/L)	
Low	<160 mg/dL (<4.14 mmol/L)	≥160 mg/dL (≥4.14 mmol/L)	≥190 mg/d (≥4.91 mmol/L) (160–189 mg/dL) (4.14–4.90 mmol/L: LDL-lowering drug optional)	

[a]When LDL-lowering drug therapy is employed, it is advised that intensity of therapy be sufficient to achieve at least 30–40% reduction in LDL–cholesterol levels.

[b]Very high risk favors the optimal LDL–cholesterol goal of <70 mg/dL, and in patients with high triglyceride, non-HDL–cholesterol <100 mg/dL.

[c]Any person at high or moderately high risk who has a lifestyle-related risk factor (e.g. obesity, physical inactivity, elevated triglycerides, low HDL–cholesterol, or metabolic syndrome) is a candidate for therapeutic lifestyle changes to modify these risk factors regardless of LDL–cholesterol level.

[d]If baseline LDL–cholesterol is <100 mg/dL, institution of an LDL-lowering drug is a therapeutic option on the basis of available clinical trials. If a high-risk person has high triglycerides or low HDL–cholesterol, combining a fibrate or nicotinic acid with an LDL-lowering drug can be considered.

[e]Optimal LDL goal <100 mg/dL.

[f]For moderately high-risk persons, when LDL–cholesterol level is 100–129 mg/dL, at baseline or on lifestyle therapy, initiation of an LDL-lowering drug to achieve an LDL–cholesterol level <100 mg/dL is a therapeutic option on the basis of available trial results.

LDL–cholesterol in liver transplant recipients such as immunomodulatory effects reported from heart and kidney transplant recipients [20] and the stimulation of bone formation observed in postmenopausal women [21–23].

■ ARTERIAL HYPERTENSION

Arterial hypertension is common in liver transplant recipients. Some 40–80% of liver transplant recipients develop arterial hypertension, within months to years after transplant [11,24–28]. Thus, compared with a normal population, age-adjusted prevalence rates of arterial hypertension have been reported to be increased to 3.07 (95% confidence interval (CI) 2.35–3.93) and 1.55 (95% CI 0.98–1.81] in long-term survivors ($\geq$5 years) after liver transplantation in an American and a Spanish Center, respectively [4,11].

Risk factors for developing arterial hypertension are prevalent in liver transplant recipients and include immunosuppressive therapy with steroids and calcineurin inhibitors, obesity, and the metabolic syndrome [29,30]. Both glucocorticoids and cyclosporine promote sodium and water retention by the kidney, the former via a mineralocorticoid side-effect and the latter via sympathetic nerve-mediated renal vasoconstriction [31,32]. The reversible cyclosporine-mediated renal vasoconstriction together with a more chronic calcineurin inhibitor-associated interstitial nephropathy adds up to calcineurin inhibitor nephrotoxicity (cf. Chapter 26), which predisposes further to arterial hypertension. This may lead to a vicious cycle, with increasing hypertension again aggravating further kidney dysfunction. Moreover, calcineurin inhibitors seem to have direct vasoconstrictive effects. Thus, cyclosporine has been shown to induce in human vascular smooth muscle cells in vitro upregulation of angiotensin II receptors and sensibilization to angiotensin-mediated Ca-dependent contraction [33], as well as upregulation of vasopressin receptors [34].

As in the nontransplant population, arterial hypertension likely adds to the cardiovascular risk of these patients [30], which is already elevated by the high prevalence of obesity, dyslipidemia, and diabetes. According to the Seventh Report of the Joint National Committee on Prevention, Detection, Evaluation, and Treatment of High Blood Pressure [30] the definitions and thresholds for intervention given in Table 23.4 apply.

Pharmacotherapy of arterial hypertension in the liver transplant recipient is in principle not different from that in the nontransplant patient and there is a multitude of drugs available (for review cf. [30]). The following summarizes a few issues specific to liver transplant recipients that are worth mentioning: steroid withdrawal has been shown to decrease blood pressure in liver transplant recipients [35,36].

Table 23.4 *High Blood Pressure – Definition and Threshold for Intervention[a]*

Category[a]	Blood Pressure[b]		Intervention
	Systolic[c]	Diastolic[c]	
Normal	<120	<80	—
Prehypertension[d]	120–139	80–89	Lifestyle modification[e]
			Consider 24 h blood pressure monitoring[f]
Hypertension[g]	≥140	≥90	Lifestyle modification[e]
			Drug therapy[h]
IF diabetic[g]	>130	>80	Lifestyle modification[e]
or			Drug therapy[h]
Impaired kidney function[g] (GFR <60 mL/min/1.72 m²)			
or			
Albuminuria[g] (>300 mg/d or >200 mg/g creatinin)			

[a]Modified from Ref. [30]; applies to adults aged 18 and older; the classification is based on the average of ≥2 properly measured, seated blood pressure readings on each of ≥2 office visits.
[b]In mmHg.
[c]Diastolic blood pressure is a more potent cardiovascular risk factor than systolic blood pressure until the age of 50 years; thereafter, systolic blood pressure is more important [30]. Thus, treatment of systolic hypertension warrants attention, especially in those ≥50 years old.
[d]Prehypertension is not a disease category, but identifies subjects at high risk of developing hypertension.
[e]Prehypertensive subjects should be advised to practice lifestyle modification in order to reduce their risk of developing hypertension; lifestyle modification is an indispensable part of therapy in hypertensive subjects. Lifestyle modification includes dietary measures in order to decrease overweight/obesity and ideally to reach/ maintain a body mass index of 18.5–24.9 kg/m², reduction of sodium intake to 6 g NaCl a day, regular aerobic physical activity, and moderation of alcohol consumption. Each of these is able to reduce blood pressure by 2 to up to 20 mmHg [30].
[f]A loss of the physiologic nighttime decrease in blood pressure or nighttime hypertension is common in liver transplant recipients [88,89]. Office blood pressure measurements may therefore underestimate average blood pressure in these patients and 24 h ambulatory blood pressure monitoring should be liberally utilized if prehypertension develops.
[g]Many liver transplant recipients fall in this category. In (nontransplant) patients with diabetes or chronic kidney disease (defined as glomerular filtration rate <60 mL/min/1.72 m² or albuminuria >300 mg/d or >200 mg/g creatinin) rigorous blood pressure control decreases progression of chronic kidney disease (for detail cf. Ref. [30]). Thus, the recommended blood pressure limits are lower than in the absence of these comorbidities.
[h]Start pharmacotherapy, if lifestyle modification does not reduce blood pressure below 140/90 (130/80 for subjects with diabetes or chronic kidney disease); for choice of drugs cf. Ref. [30] and text.

Many patients on calcineurin inhibitors have increased uric acid plasma levels. Concomitant use of thiazide diuretics may further inCTEUSE hyperuricemia in such patients and precipitate gout attacks.

Many patients on calcineurin inhibitors have increased plasma potassium levels. Concomitant use of ACE inhibitors and AT-II blockers may further the risk of clinically relevant hyperkalemia.

Calcium channel blockers interfere with calcineurin inhibitor metabolism (inhibition of or competition for CYP3A4) and may lead to elevated cyclosporine and tacrolimus plasma levels. This is of clinical relevance for the nondihydropyridines diltiazem and verapamil, less so for the dihydropyridines, except nicardipine. Moreover, dihydropyridine calcium channel blockers have been shown to protect against calcineurin inhibitor-mediated nephrotoxicity [37,38] and to lower calcineurin inhibitor-induced hyperuricemia [38]. Dihydropyridine calcium channel blockers such as amlodipine or nifedipin may therefore be considered as first-choice antihypertensive pharmacotherapy in the liver transplant recipients. Their most common side-effect, peripheral edema, may be counteracted and the antihypertensive effect increased by adding a low dose of a thiazide.

■ DIABETES MELLITUS

Diabetes is common in liver transplant recipients. Conceptually, one distinguishes diabetes already present prior to liver transplantation from diabetes developing de novo only after liver transplantation, i.e. new-onset posttransplant diabetes. Prevalence rates of pretransplant diabetes mellitus of 10–15% [39–41] and new-onset posttransplant diabetes of <10% to up to 40% [14,24, 39–46] have been reported in liver transplant recipients. The wide range of values reported, particularly with the latter, is in part due to differences in the definition of diabetes. Even the largest study reporting a prevalence rate of new-onset posttransplant diabetes of 37.7% (28.3% transient and 9.4% persistent) in 555 liver transplant recipients followed for a median of 5 years at three American centers likely underestimated the true prevalence, since it defined diabetes as the use of antidiabetic medication [46].

The high prevalence of diabetes in liver transplant recipients may, in part, be explained by the association of hepatitis C virus (HCV) infection with insulin resistance/type II diabetes [41,45–49] and by HCV-related end-stage liver disease (ESLD) being the single most common indication for liver transplantation in the West. Thus, the relative risk of pretransplant diabetes has been reported to be increased more than threefold (adjusted odds ratio (OR) 3.77, 95% CI 1.80–7.87) [47] and that of new-onset posttransplant diabetes 2.5- to 5-fold in HCV-infected compared with non-HCV-infected patients, respectively [41,45]. While the exact mechanism(s) for this association of HCV infection and insulin resistance/type II diabetes remain(s) to be defined, HCV-induced TNF-alpha production might be involved (for review cf. [49]).

Moreover, an increasing number of liver transplants are performed for ESLD due to nonalcoholic steatohepatitis, the underlying insulin resistance likely persisting after transplantation.

Risk factors for developing/aggravating insulin resistance and type II diabetes are prevalent post liver transplant and include weight gain, as discussed earlier, but also immunosuppressive therapy with corticosteroids and calcineurin inhibitors, in particular tacrolimus. Thus, corticosteroid dose has been linked to posttransplant diabetes [24,39,41,45], and posttransplant diabetes was found to be around two times more frequent with tacrolimus-based than with cyclosporine-based regimens [14,41].

As in the nontransplant population, diabetes in liver transplant recipients is associated with significant morbidity and mortality. Thus, in a case control study, pretransplant diabetes was found to significantly increase posttransplant morbidity, in particular from cardiovascular, infectious, and renal diseases, and to decrease 5-year survival after liver transplantation from 67.7% to 34.5% [50]. Similarly, new-onset posttransplant diabetes was found to be associated with significantly increased morbidity, in particular from cardiovascular, infectious, and neurologic/neuropsychiatric diseases [51], and with a significantly decreased 2- to 5-year survival in most [24,39,43,45], but not all studies [51].

Precise diagnostic criteria and terminology is a prerequisite for classification of dysglycemic disorders. Table 23.5 summarizes the respective criteria according to the Canadian Diabetes Association [52]. The newest guidelines of the American Diabetes Association differ in that a fasting plasma glucose of <5.6 mmol/L (instead of <6.1 mmol/L) is defined as the upper limit of normal [53].

Impaired fasting glucose and impaired glucose tolerance are often termed "prediabetes"; they are per se not disease entities, but carry the risk of progressing to overt diabetes with time. Impaired fasting glucose and impaired glucose tolerance (insulin resistance) are associated with the metabolic syndrome and through that with increased cardiovascular risk [53].

Table 23.5 *Terminology and Diagnostic Criteria of Diabetes and Dysglycemic Disorders*

	Fasting Plasma Glucose (mmol/L)		2 h Plasma Glucose in a 75 g Oral Glucose Tolerance Test (mmol/L)
Impaired fasting glucose	6.1–6.9		NA
Impaired fasting glucose (isolated)	6.1–6.9	and	<7.8
Impaired glucose tolerance (isolated)	<6.1	and	7.8–11.0
Impaired fasting glucose and impaired glucose tolerance	6.1–6.9	and	7.8–11.0
Diabetes	≥7.0	or	≥11.1

New-onset posttransplant diabetes has been recently reviewed by an international expert panel; the resulting consensus guidelines have been published [54]. New-onset posttransplant diabetes was felt to resemble type II diabetes and the management aspects and differences given in Table 23.6 were emphasized.

■ METABOLIC SYNDROME AND CARDIOVASCULAR RISK

The metabolic syndrome is a clustering of cardiovascular risk factors, including overweight/obesity, dyslipidemia, insulin resistance, and arterial hypertension. Table 23.7 depicts the operational diagnostic criteria for the metabolic syndrome according to Ref. [55]. Other panels/organizations have used similar definitions/diagnostic criteria (for review cf. Ref. [56]).

The diagnosis of the metabolic syndrome is made if ≥3 of the abovementioned risk factors are present.

Many of the aforementioned studies in liver transplant recipients focused on some component(s) of the metabolic syndrome, but did not employ strict criteria for diagnosing the syndrome itself. Thus, exact prevalence rates of the metabolic syndrome in liver transplant recipients are lacking. However, from all the aforementioned studies, it seems clearly conceivable that the metabolic syndrome is highly prevalent among liver transplant recipients. Intuitively, it seems also to make sense that the clustering of cardiovascular risk factors within the metabolic syndrome should carry an increased risk for developing cardiovascular events, i.e. for cardiovascular morbidity and mortality. This is corroborated by an, albeit nontransplant, population-based study from Finland [57] and by the fact that the Framingham equation for estimating cardiovascular risk [58] contains with high-density lipid (HDL)–cholesterol and blood pressure two components of the metabolic syndrome (for discussion cf. Ref. [56]).

Thus, using the Framingham equation and comparing with an age- and sex-matched normal population, a recent study from a single center predicted an almost twofold increased 10-year risk for coronary events in 181 consecutive liver transplantation recipients at a median of 54 months after grafting [59]. While the observed cardiovascular event rate in the latter study did not differ from that in the normal population, another study clearly demonstrated a 3.07-fold (95% CI: 1.98–4.43) and 2.56-fold (1.52–4.05) increased risk for ischemic cardiac events and for cardiovascular death, respectively, in 100 consecutive liver transplant recipients followed for median 3.9 years after grafting [60]. Thus with long-term survival becoming routine after liver transplantation, cardiovascular morbidity and mortality will likely become increasingly

Table 23.6 *Selected Aspects of the Management of New-Onset Posttransplant Diabetes and Differences/Similarities to that of Type II Diabetes[a]*

Management Aspect	Recommendation/Frequency of Testing	Comments
Fasting plasma glucose (FPG) testing	• Weekly for first posttransplant month • At 2, 6, and 12 months • Annually thereafter	Identify patients with dysglycemia
Oral glucose tolerance test (OGTT)	Consider in patients with normal FPG or those with impaired glucose tolerance	Utility not validated in this population
Tailoring immunosuppressive therapy	• Decrease/withdraw corticosteroids as soon as possible • Consider switching to cyclosporine in poorly controlled tacrolimus-treated patients	Consider switching to calcineurin inhibitor-free regimen in poorly controlled cyclosporine-treated patients
Lifestyle modification	Council all patients with elevated FPG and/or abnormal OGTT regarding dietary measures, weight reduction, and exercise	
Oral agent pharmacotherapy		
• Monotherapy	Base choice of agent mainly on safety[b]	Comparative efficacy/tolerability not formally explored in this population
	Consider potential of serious adverse events in patients with renal impairment	
• Combination	Use same combinations as in nontransplant type II diabetics[b]	Efficacy/tolerability not formally explored in this population
Insulin + oral agent pharmacotherapy	Consider in patients poorly controlled on oral agent combination pharmacotherapy alone	Efficacy/tolerability not formally explored in this population

Self-monitoring of blood glucose	Essential component of management of patients receiving oral agent pharma-cotherapy/insulin	Similar to recommendation for patients with type II diabetes[c]
HbA1C	In patients with diabetes: • Measure every 3 months • Intervention if HbA1C $\geq 6.5\%$	Interpret with care in patients with anemia/renal impairment
Microalbuminuria	In patients with diabetes: consider annual screening	Not validated in this population
Diabetic complications	In patients with diabetes: screen annually	Similar to recommendation for patients with type II diabetes[c]
Lipid levels	In patients with diabetes: evaluate annually	Similar to recommendation for patients with type II diabetes[c]
Dyslipidemia	In patients with diabetes: aggressive lipid-lowering therapy according to NCEP[d]	All patients considered at high risk of coronary heart disease (CHD)
Hypertension	In patients with diabetes: keep blood pressure <130/80	Value of blood pressure lowering not tested in this population

[a]Modified for liver transplant setting from Ref. [54].
[b]For review cf. Ref. [57].
[c]cf. Ref. [57].
[d]cf. Ref. [16].

Table 23.7 *Clinical Identification of the Metabolic Syndrome using NCEP ATP III Criteria*[a]

Risk Factor	Defining Level[b]
Fasting plasma glucose	≥6.1
Arterial blood pressure	≥130/85 mmHg
Fasting triglycerides	≥1.7 mmol/L
• HDL–cholesterol	
Men	<1.0 mmol/L
Women	<1.3 mmol/L
• Abdominal obesity	Waist circumference
Men	>102 cm
Women	>88 cm

[a]cf. Refs [55,56].
[b]The diagnosis of metabolic syndrome is made when ≥3 of the risk factors are present.

relevant also in liver transplant recipients, just as it is well known for recipients of other solid organ transplants such as the kidney.

The therapy of the metabolic syndrome consists of lifestyle modifications, i.e. reduction of overweight/obesity by dietary measures and exercise, and, if this alone is insufficient in eliminating cardiovascular risk factors, of pharmacotherapy aimed at controlling dyslipidemia, insulin resistance, and blood pressure, as outlined above and recently summarized [61].

■ HYPERURICEMIA AND GOUT

Hyperuricemia is common in liver transplant recipients and was observed on average in 47% and 86% of patients 40 and 98 months after transplantation in two recent single center series ($n = 134$ and 75, respectively) [62,63]. The prevalence of hyperuricemia did not differ in cyclosporine- and tacrolimus-treated patients [62] and led to the clinical manifestation of gout in 6% and 2.6%, respectively [62,63].

Hyperuricemia in liver transplant recipients is attributable to decreased renal uric acid clearance, rather than increased uric acid production [64]. This seems largely due to a calcineurin inhibitor-induced decrease in glomerular filtration rate [65], but calcineurin inhibitor-induced decreased tubular uric acid secretion may contribute [66]. Additional factors predisposing to hyperuricemia in post-liver-transplant patients include obesity and diuretic therapy, in particular with thiazides.

Hyperuricemia may further impair an already decreased renal function (glomerular filtration rate), thus leading to more uric acid retention, increased hyperuricemia, and, thus, establishing a vicious cycle for renal function in liver transplant recipients. Indeed, allopurinol treatment of hyperuricemic liver transplant recipients with increased serum creatinin has been shown to improve renal function in a retrospective analysis [62].

Colchicin is the treatment of choice for acute gout attacks in the liver transplant recipient. Nonsteroidal anti-inflammatory drugs should be used with caution, since they bear the risk of further decreasing glomerular filtration rate, and thus uric acid clearance, by inhibiting renal prostaglandin synthesis. Allopurinol should be used as maintenance therapy to decrease uric acid blood levels and to secondarily prevent subsequent attacks in all patients with a history of gout. In addition, diuretic use should be critically reevaluated in these patients and, in particular, thiazides discontinued, if possible. In the absence of manifest gout, allopurinol maintenance therapy may be considered in hyperuricemic patients with impaired glomerular filtration rate (elevated serum creatinin) in an attempt to improve renal function [62]. Allopurinol by inhibiting xanthine oxidase interferes with azathioprine metabolism. This may lead to cumulation of a myelotoxic azathioprine metabolite and potentially life-threatening bone marrow suppression. For safety reasons, azathioprine should therefore not be used concomitantly with allopurinol.

■ OSTEOPOROSIS

Osteoporosis is a common finding in liver transplant recipients. Pooling results from cross-sectional studies and osteoporosis of the lumbar spine and hip (*T*-score in dual X-ray absorptiometry (DEXA) less than −2.5, i.e. bone mineral density more than 2.5 standard deviations below the mean for young healthy adults) was found in 32% and 27% of liver transplant recipients in a recent comprehensive review [67]. An additional proportion of post-liver-transplant patients have severely reduced bone mineral density (osteopenia with *Z*-scores between −1 and −2.5).

Longitudinal studies demonstrate that bone mineral density decreases rapidly in the initial 3–6 months posttransplant and subsequently stabilizes or improves again and reaches pretransplant levels in many patients at 1 year following grafting (for review cf. Ref. [67]).

Factors affecting osteopenia/osteoporosis in post-liver-transplant patients include pretransplant osteopenia/osteoporosis attributable to chronic ESLD (not only the cholestatic entities; for review cf. Refs [67–69]), perioperative immobilization, and immunosuppression with corticosteroids and calcineurin inhibitors. Corticosteroids inhibit intestinal calcium absorption and have in part cytokine-mediated, direct effects on bone metabolism [68]. The calcineurin inhibitors cyclosporine and tacrolimus have both been shown to cause bone loss (high-turnover osteoporosis) in animal models [70–73]. In addition, all other recognized risk factors for bone loss, including gender, hypogonadism/postmenopausal state, age, and smoking, pertain also to liver transplant recipients.

Based on the aforementioned it is not surprising that osteoporotic fractures, in particular of trabecular bone such as the vertebrae of the lumbar spine, occur in up to 30% of liver transplant recipients, typically within the first 3–6 months posttransplant (for review cf. Ref. [67]). Compression fractures of the lumbar spine early posttransplant impact on quality of life and mobilization, and often delay full rehabilitation with reintegration into daily life and professional activities.

It is therefore recommended that patients with chronic ESLD undergo a bone density measurement at the lumbar spine and at the femoral neck (DEXA) at least during evaluation for liver transplantation [63,65]. All cirrhotic patients including liver transplant candidates should get counseling regarding lifestyle measures (exercise and smoking cessation) and vitamin D (400–800 IU daily) and calcium (1–1.5 g daily) supplements. Biphosphonates should be started in patients with bone density measurements falling into the osteoporotic range and/or with a history of osteoporotic fractures. Hormone replacement therapy should be considered in appropriate patients [67]. This is aimed at preserving as much bone mass as possible up to transplant. After liver transplantation, corticosteroids should be tapered and withdrawn as soon as possible. Liver transplant recipients may profit from continuing vitamin D and calcium supplements, which are approved for prevention of corticosteroid-induced bone loss and have been shown to inhibit posttransplant bone loss in kidney and kidney/pancreas transplant recipients [74]. Continuing hormone replacement therapy should be considered in appropriate patients. In patients with pretransplant osteoporosis/osteoporotic fractures, it seems also reasonable to continue posttransplant with biphosponates. It seems reasonable to repeat bone density determination at 1 year after transplantation (or, as a baseline, if osteoporotic fractures occur) and adjust therapy accordingly.

■ SKIN DISORDERS

The skin of liver transplant recipients requires special attention. The mucocutaneous lesions associated with specific hepatic diseases and the dermatologic manifestations of ESLD usually improve or disappear after liver transplantation [75]. The skin of the liver transplant patient may, however, provide crucial diagnostic clues such as maculopapular lesions of the extremities, potentially heralding graft versus host disease [76]. In addition, liver transplant recipients are at risk of developing a number of skin disorders including infections with rare organisms alone or in combination, and nonmelanoma skin cancer, in particular squamous cell carcinoma [76–79]. Thus, the relative risk of developing squamous cell carcinoma has been found to be 70- to 100-fold higher after liver transplantation than in the general population [79,80] and to increase with the frequency and extent of lifetime sun exposure [77].

Liver transplant recipients should therefore be advised to protect their skin from intense exposure to sunlight, the best protection being to wear dark clothes. When exposure is unavoidable, sun blocker should be applied 30 min before exposure and reapplied frequently. They should be counseled to periodically check their integument themselves and to have less accessible regions such as the back checked by a partner. In addition, the transplant physician or a dermatologist should annually examine the entire integument of every liver transplant recipient including the oral cavity and the perianal area. A dermatologist should be consulted for evaluation of any suspicious lesion. Such systematic examination permits acting on early precancerous lesions such as actinic keratosis, oral leukoplakia, and verrucae and prevents their progression to stages requiring extensive (plastic) surgery.

■ FAMILY PLANNING

Secondary amenorrhea is frequent in premenopausal women suffering from ESLD. Within months of successful liver transplantation menses and libido return in approximately 90% of these women [81]. Obviously, genetic counseling should be offered to patients who were transplanted for an inheritable disease. Numerous successful deliveries in liver graft recipients have been reported [82]. Any pregnancy in a liver transplant recipient should, however, be regarded as a high-risk pregnancy, hypertension, preeclampsia, intrauterine growth retardation, and prematurity being more frequent than in the general population [83–87]. Respective close monitoring is therefore mandatory. It seems advisable for women to wait at least 1 year after transplantation before planning to conceive [82]. This allows the mother to recover from transplant surgery and any potential early complication, as well as to reach a stable allograft function with low-level maintenance immunosuppression. Calcineurin-inhibitors and azathioprine can be maintained during the pregnancy [83,86,87]; sirolimus, mycophenolate, and other newer immunosuppressive drugs should be stopped and replaced due to the lack of sufficient safety data [87]. Contraception with intrauterine devices is generally discouraged in liver transplant recipients because of the risk of pelvic infectious complications.

■ REFERENCES

1. Everhart JE, Lombardero M, Lake JR, et al. Weight change and obesity after liver transplantation: incidence and risk factors. Liver Transpl Surg 1998;4:285–296.

2. Guckelberger O, Bechstein WO, Neuhaus R, et al. Cardiovascular risk factors in long-term follow-up after orthotopic liver transplantation. Clin Transpl 1997;11:60–65.

3. Mazuelos F, Abril J, Zaragoza C, et al. Cardiovascular morbidity and obesity in adult liver transplant recipients. Transplant Proc 2003;35:1909–1910.

4. Sheiner PA, Magliocca JF, Bodian CA, et al. Long-term medical complications in patients surviving > or = 5 years after liver transplant. Transplantation 2000;15: 781–789.

5. Burke A, Lucey MR. Non-alcoholic fatty liver disease, non-alcoholic steatohepatitis and orthotopic liver transplantation. Am J Transplant 2004;4:686–693.

6. Health Canada. Canadian guidelines for body weight classification in adults. Ottawa, ON: Health Canada 2003. Publication H49-179/2003E. Available at: http://www.hc-sc.gc.ca/hpfb-dgpsa/onpp-bppn/weight_book_tc_e.html.

7. Krauss RM, Winston M, Fletscher BJ, Grundy SM. Obesity – impact on cardiovascular disease. Circulation 1998;98:1472–1476.

8. American Heart Association guidelines for weight management programs for healthy adults. AHA Nutrition Committee. Heart Dis Stroke 1994;3:221–228.

9. Thomson PD, Buchner D, Pina IL, et al. Exercise and physical activity in the prevention and treatment of atherosclerotic cardiovascular disease. A statement from the Council on Clinical Cardiology (subcommittee on exercise, rehabilitation and prevention) and the Council on Nutrition, Physical Activity, and Metabolism (subcommittee on physical activity). Circulation 2003;107:3109–3116.

10. Fletcher GF, Balady GJ, Amsterdam EA, et al. Exercise standards for testing and training. A statement for healthcare professionals from the American Heart Association. Circulation 2001;104:1694–1740.

11. Fernandez-Miranda C, Sanz M, dela Calle A, et al. Cardiovascular risk factors in 116 patients 5 years or more after liver transplantation. Transpl Int 2002;15:556–562.

12. Fernandez-Miranda C, dela Calle A, Morales JM, et al. Lipoprotein abnormalities in long-term stable liver and renal transplant patients. A comparative study. Clin Transpl 1998;12:136–141.

13. Reuben A. Long-term management of the liver transplant patient: diabetes, hyperlipidemia, and obesity. Liver Transpl 2001;7:S13–S21.

14. Levy G, Villamil F, Samuel D, et al. Results of lis2t, a multicenter, randomized study comparing cyclosporine microemulsion with C2 monitoring and tacrolimus with C0 monitoring in de novo liver transplantation. Transplantation 2004;77:1632–1639.

15. Neff GW, Montalbano M, Tzakis AG. Ten years of sirolimus therapy in orthotopic liver transplant recipients. Transplant Proc 2003;35(suppl 3A):209S–216S.

16. Grundy SM, Cleeman JI, Merz NB, et al., for the Coordinating Committee of the National Cholesterol Education Program. Implications of recent trials for the National Cholesterol Education Program Adult Treatment Panel III Guidelines. Circulation 2004;110:227–239.

17. Imagawa DK, Dawson S, 3rd, Holt CD, et al. Hyperlipidemia after liver transplantation: natural history and treatment with the hydroxy-methylglutaryl-coenzyme A reductase inhibitor pravastatin. Transplantation 1996;62:934–942.

18. Zachoval R, Gerbes AL, Schwandt P, et al. Short-term effects of statin therapy in patients with hyperlipoproteinemia after liver transplantation: results of a randomized cross-over trial. J Hepatol 2001;35:86–91.

19. Anfossi G, Masucco P, Bonomo K, et al. Prescription of statins to dyslipidemic patients affected by liver disease: a subtle balance between risks and benefits. Nutr Metab Cardiovasc Dis 2004;14:215–224.

20. Neal DA, Alexander GJ. Can the potential benefits of statins in general medical practice be extrapolated to liver transplantation? Liver Transpl 2001;7:1009–1014.

21. Edwards CJ, Hart DJ, Spector TD. Oral statins and increased bone-mineral density in postmenopausal women. Lancet 2000;355:2218–2219.

22. Meier CR, Schlienger RG, Kraenzlin ME, et al. HMG-CoA reductase inhibitors and the risk of fractures. JAMA 2000;283:3205–3210.

23. Chan KA, Andrade SE, Boles M, et al. Inhibitors of hydroxymethylglutaryl-coenzyme A reductase and risk of fracture among older women. Lancet 2000;355:2185–2188.

24. Stegall MD, Everson G, Schroter G, et al. Metabolic complications after liver transplantation. Diabetes, hypercholesterolemia, hypertension, and obesity. Transplantation 1995;15:1057–1060.

25. Canzanello VJ, Schwartz L, Taler SJ, et al. Evolution of cardiovascular risk after liver transplantation: a comparison of cyclosporine A and tacrolimus (FK 506). Liver Transpl 1997;3:1–9.

26. Johnston SD, Morris JK, Cramb R, et al. Cardiovascular morbidity and mortality after orthotopic liver transplantation. Transplantation 2002;73:901–906.

27. Rabkin JM, Corless CL, Rosen HR, et al. Immunosuppression impact on long-term cardiovascular complications after liver transplantation. Am J Surg 2002;183:595–596.

28. Gonwa TA. Hypertension and renal dysfunction in long-term liver transplant recipients. Liver Transpl 2001;7:S22–S26.

29. Hricik DE, Lautman J, Bartucci MR, et al. Variable effects of steroid withdrawal on blood pressure reduction in cyclosporine-treated renal transplant recipients. Transplantation 1992;53:1232–1236.

30. Chobanian AV, Bakris GL, Black HR, et al. Seventh report of the Joint National Committee on Prevention, Detection, Evaluation, and Treatment of High Blood Pressure. Hypertension 2003;42:1206–1252.

31. Moss NG, Powell SL, Falk RJ. Intravenous cyclosporine activates afferent and efferent renal nerves and causes sodium retention in innervated kidney in rat. Proc Natl Acad Sci USA 1985;822:8222–8226.

32. Scherrer U, Vissing SF, Morgan BJ, et al. Cyclosporine-induced sympathetic activation and hypertension after heart transplantation. New Engl J Med 1990;323:693–699.

33. Avdonin PV, Cottet-Maire F, Afanasjeva GV, et al. Cyclosporine A up-regulates angiotensin II receptors and calcium responses in human vascular smooth muscle cells. Kidney Int 1999;55:2407–2414.

34. Krauskopf A. Vasopressin type 1A receptor up-regulation by cyclosporin A in vascular smooth muscle cells is mediated by superoxide. J Biol Chem 2003;278:41685–41690.

35. Punch JD, Shieck VL, Campbell DA, et al. Corticosteroid withdrawal after liver transplantation. Surgery 1995;118:783–786.

36. Gomez R, Moreno E, Colina F, et al. Steroid withdrawal is safe and beneficial in stable cyclosporine-treated liver transplant patients. J Hepatol 1998;28:150–156.

37. Kuypers DR, Neumayer HH, Fritsche L, et al., on behalf of the Lacidipine Study Group. Calcium channel blockade and preservation of renal graft function in cyclosporine-treated recipients: a prospective randomized placebo-controlled 2-year study. Transplantation 2004;78:1204–1211.

38. Chanard J, Toupance O, Lavaud S, et al. Amlodipine reduces cyclosporin-induced hyperuricaemia in hypertensive renal transplant recipients. Nephrol Dial Transpl 2003;18:2147–2153.

39. Navasa M, Bustamante J, Marroni C, et al. Diabetes mellitus after liver transplantation: prevalence and predictive factors. J Hepatol 1996;25:64–71.

40. Knobler H, Stagnaro-Green A, Wallenstein S, et al. High incidence of diabetes in liver transplant recipients with hepatitis C. J Clin Gastroenterol 1998;26:30–33.

41. Aedosary AA, Ramji AS, Elliott TG, et al. Post-liver transplantation diabetes mellitus: an association with hepatitis C. Liver Transpl 2002;8:356–361.

42. Trail KC, McCashland TM, Larsen JL, et al. Morbidity in patients with posttransplant diabetes mellitus following orthotopic liver transplantation. Liver Transpl Surg 1996;2:276–283.

43. Steinmuller TH, Stockmann M, Bechstein WO, et al. Liver transplantation and diabetes mellitus. Exp Clin Endocrinol Diabetes 2001;108:401–405.

44. Jain A, Reyes J, Kashyap R, et al. What have we learned about primary liver transplantation under tacrolimus immunosuppression? Long-term follow-up of the first 1000 patients. Ann Surg 1999;230:441–448.

45. Baid S, Cosimi AB, Farrell ML, et al. Posttransplant diabetes mellitus in liver transplant recipients: risk factors, temporal relationship with hepatitis C virus allograft hepatitis, and impact on mortality. Transplantation 2001;72:1066–1072.

46. Khalili M, Lim JW, Bass N, et al. New onset diabetes mellitus after liver transplantation: the critical role of hepatitis C infection. Liver Transpl 2004;10:349–355.

47. Mehta SH, Brancati FL, Sulkowski MS, et al. Prevalence of type 2 diabetes mellitus among persons with hepatitis C virus infection in the United States. Ann Int Med 2000;133:592–599.

48. Bigam DL, Pennington JJ, Carpentier A, et al. Hepatitis C-related cirrhosis: a predictor of diabetes after liver transplantation. Hepatology 2000;32:87–90.

49. Knobler H, Schattner A. TNF-(alpha), chronic hepatitis C and diabetes: a novel triad. Q J Med 2005;98:1–6.

50. John RR, Thuluvath PJ. Outcome of liver transplantation in patients with diabetes mellitus: a case control study. Hepatology 2001;34:889–895.

51. John RR, Thuluvath PJ. Outcome of patients with new-onset diabetes mellitus after liver transplantation compared with those without diabetes mellitus. Liver Transpl 2002;8:708–713.

52. Canadian Diabetes Association. Clinical Practice Guidelines Expert Committee. Pharmacologic management of type II diabetes http://www.diabetes.ca/cpg 2003/downloads/defclassdiag.pdf.

53. American Diabetes Association. Diagnosis and classification of diabetes mellitus. Diabetes Care 2005; 28(suppl 1):S37–S42.

54. Davidson JA, Wilson A, on behalf of the International Expert Panel on New-Onset Diabetes after Transplantation. New-onset diabetes after transplantation 2003 International Consensus Guidelines. Diabetes Care 2004;27:805–812.

55. Third Report of the National Cholesterol Education Program (NCEP) Expert Panel. Expert Panel on detection, elevation and treatment of high blood cholesterol in adults (Adult Treatment Panel III). Final report. Circulation 2002;106:3143–3421.

56. Grundy SM, Brewer B, Cleeman JI, et al., for the conference participants. Definition of the metabolic syndrome. Report of the National Heart, Lung, and Blood Institute/American Heart Association Conference on scientific issues related to definition. Circulation 2004;109:433–438.

57. Lakka HM, Laaksonen DE, Lakka TA, et al. The metabolic syndrome and total and cardiovascular disease mortality in middle-aged men. JAMA 2002;288:237–252.

58. http://hin.nhlbi.nih.gov/atpiii/calculator.asp?usertype=prof#moreinfo.

59. Neal DA, Tom BD, Luan J, et al. Is there disparity between risk and incidence of cardiovascular disease after liver transplant? Transplantation 2004;77:93–99.

60. Johnston SD, Morris JK, Cramb R, et al. Cardiovascular morbidity and mortality after orthotopic liver transplantation. Transplantation 2002;73:901–906.

61. Grundy SM, Hansen B, Smith SC, et al., for the conference participants. Clinical management of metabolic syndrome. Report of the American Heart Association/ National Heart, Lung, and Blood Institute/American Diabetes Association conference on scientific issues related to management. Circulation 2004;109:551–556.

62. Neal DAJ, Tom BDM, Gimson AES, et al. Hyperuricemia, gout, and renal function after liver transplantation. Transplantation 2001;72:1689–1691.

63. Shibolet O, Elinav E, Ilan Y, et al. Reduced incidence of hyperuricemia, gout, and renal failure following liver transplantation in comparison to heart transplantation: a long-term follow-up study. Transplantation 2004;77:1576–1580.

64. Lin HY, Rocher LL, McQuillan MA, et al. Cyclosporin-induced hyperuricemia and gout. N Engl J Med 1989;321:287.

65. Zurcher R, Bock HA, Thiel G. Hyperuricemia in cyclosporin-treated patients: GFR-related effect. Nephrol Dial Transpl 1996;11:153–158.

66. Marcen R, Gallego N, Orofino L, et al. Impairment of tubular secretion of urate in renal transplant patients on cyclosporin. Nephron 1995;70:307–313.

67. Leslie WD, Bernstein CN, Leboff MS. AGA technical review on osteoporosis in hepatic disorders. Gastroenterology 2003;125:941–966.

68. Crippin JS. Bone disease after liver transplantation. Liver Transpl 2001;7:S27–S35.

69. Collier JD, Ninkovic M, Compston JE. Guidelines on the management of osteoporosis associated with chronic liver disease. Gut 50 (suppl 1):i1–i9.

70. Movsowitz C, Epstein S, Fallon M, et al. Cyclosporin-A in vivo produces severe osteopenia in the rat: effect of dose and duration of administration. Endocrinology 1988;123:2571–2577.

71. Schlosberg M, Movsowitz C, Epstein S, et al. The effect of cyclosporin A administration and its withdrawal on bone mineral metabolism in the rat. Endocrinology 1989;124:2179–2184.

72. Bowman AR, Sass DA, Dissanayake IR, et al. The role of testosterone in cyclosporin-induced osteopenia. J Bone Miner Res 1997;12:607–615.

73. Cvetkovic M, Mann GN, Romero DF, et al. The deleterious effects of long-term cyclosporin A, cyclosporin G, and FK 506 on bone mineral metabolism in vivo. Transplantation 1994;57:1231–1237.

74. Josephson MA, Schumm LP, Chiu MY, et al. Calcium and calcitriol prophylaxis attenuates posttransplant bone loss. Transplantation 2004;78:1233–1236.

75. Dufour JF, Schmied E. Dermatologic problems in patients who have undergone liver transplantation. In UpToDate, Rose, BD, ed., UpToDate, Wellesley, MA 2003.

76. Schmied E, Dufour JF, Euvrard S. Nontumoral dermatologic problems after liver transplantation. Liver Transpl 2004;10:331–229.

77. Mithoefer AB, Supran S, Freeman RB. Risk factors associated with the development of skin cancer after liver transplantation. Liver Transpl 2002;8:939–944.

78. Otley CC, Pittelkow MR. Skin cancer in liver transplant recipients. Liver Transpl 2000;6:253–262.

79. Haagsma EB, Hagens VE, Schaapveld M, et al. Increased cancer risk after liver transplantation: a population-based study. J Hepatol 2001;34:161–164.

80. Lindelof B, Sigurgeirsson B, Gabel H, et al. Incidence of skin cancer in 5356 patients following organ transplantation. Br J Dermatol 2000;143:513–519.

81. Parolin MB, Rabinovitch I, Urbanetz AA, et al. Impact of successful liver transplantation on reproductive function and sexuality in women with advanced liver disease. Transplant Proc 2004;36:943–944.

82. Nagy S, Bush MC, Berkowitz R, et al. Pregnancy outcome in liver transplant recipients. Obstet Gynecol 2003;102:121–128.

83. Scantlebury V, Gordon R, Tzakis A, et al. Childbearing after liver transplantation. Transplantation 2000;49:317–321.

84. Radomski JS, Moritz MJ, Munoz SJ, et al. National Transplantation Pregnancy Registry: analysis of pregnancy outcomes in female liver transplant recipients. Liver Transpl Surg 1995;1:281–284.

85. Tiely C. Contraception and pregnancy after liver transplantation. Liver Transpl 2001;7:S74–S76.

86. Jain AB, Reyes J, Marcos A, et al. Pregnancy after liver transplantation with tacrolimus immunosuppression: a single center's experience update at 13 years. Transplantation 2003;15:827–832.

87. Sivaraman P. Management of pregnancy in transplant recipient. Transplant Proc 2004;36:1999–2000.

88. Van de Borne P, Gelin M, Van de Stadt J, et al. Circadian rhythms of blood pressure after liver transplantation. Hypertension 1993;21:398–405.

89. Taler SJ, Textor SC, Canzanello VJ, et al. Loss of nocturnal blood pressure fall after liver transplantation during immunosuppressive therapy. Am J Hypertens 1995;8:598–605.

Recurrence of the Original Liver Disease

▼　▼　▼　▼　▼　▼　▼　▼　▼

Alastair D. Smith

24

■ INTRODUCTION

Despite many advances in orthotopic liver transplantation (OLT) during the past 40 years – more appropriate patient selection; improvements in surgical technique, anesthetic, and intensive care unit management; and more sophisticated immunosuppressive therapy, to name but a few – the issue of recurrent primary liver disease remains a problem for both transplant community members and patients alike. In contrast to chronic hepatitis C virus (HCV) liver disease, which recurs in almost all cases, other forms of acute and chronic liver disease have not been demonstrated to recur following OLT, e.g. Wilson's disease (Table 24.1). Somewhere between these two poles lies the future for patients in whom the prospect of disease recurrence is a distinct possibility. To what extent then are patients able to be advised that they have been "cured" of their original disease as a result of OLT?

In this chapter we review the frequency of and basis for diagnosis of recurrent primary liver disease, the recommended management thereof, and the implications that disease recurrence has upon medium- to long-term allograft function and patient outcome. Lastly, we assess the impact of recurrent primary liver disease upon the potential requirement for retransplantation within the context of scarce resource availability and organ allocation decision making.

■ VIRAL LIVER DISEASE

Hepatitis C

Decompensated chronic HCV liver disease is the commonest indication for OLT in the USA and the second most common indication in Europe [1,2]. Among patients infected with HCV at the time of OLT, reinfection of the

Table 24.1a *Diseases that do not recur after liver transplantation*

Fulminant hepatitis A

Fulminant hepatitis of unknown etiology

Extrahepatic biliary atresia

Benign tumours

Alpha-1-antitrypsin deficiency

Wilson's disease

Glycogen storage disease

Familial amyloid polyneuropathy

Primary hyperoxaluria

Tyrosinemia

Table 24.1b *Diseases that do recur after liver transplantation*

Hepatitis B virus liver disease

Hepatitis C virus liver disease

Alcoholic liver disease

Autoimmune hepatitis

Primary biliary cirrhosis

Primary sclerosing cholangitis

Malignant tumours

Haemochromatosis

Non-alcoholic fatty liver disease

Budd-Chiari syndrome

transplanted allograft is universal and occurs within a matter of days or weeks following surgery [3]. Thereafter, acute and chronic HCV liver disease ensue. Studies in which protocol liver biopsies were undertaken at least annually and with adequate years of patient follow-up demonstrated recurrent chronic liver disease rates ranging from 70% to 90% at 1 year, and 90% to 95% at 5 years. Moreover, cirrhosis was evident in 20–40% of patients at 5 years [4]. The accelerated clinical course of HCV liver disease after OLT is reflected by increased rates of fibrosis progression [5]. Clinical decompensation of cirrhosis heralds an inexorable downhill course and carries with it a poor medium-term prognosis [6]. These data are in contrast to earlier reports that suggested recurrent chronic HCV liver disease was less common, did not occur until the second year following OLT, and typically ran a more benign clinical course [7,8]. Analysis of the United Network for Organ Sharing (UNOS) database revealed that 5-year graft and patient survival rates (57% and 70%, respectively) among patients with chronic HCV liver disease undergoing OLT between 1992 and 1998 were poorer than among patients grafted for all other indications (68% and 77%, respectively) [9]. These data are similar to outcomes from a single-center Spanish study [10]. However, results of a recent multi-center study have challenged these findings: no appreciable patient and graft survival differences were evident between subjects undergoing OLT for HCV liver disease and those undergoing OLT for indications other than HCV [11]. Thus, there is continuing controversy about this issue.

Donor, recipient, and other variables that are important in the timing and extent of recurrent HCV liver disease include donor age and degree of steatosis, integrity of the host immune system, obesity, diabetes mellitus, alcohol consumption, prolonged cold- and warm-ischemia times, and both the extent of change of immunosuppressive therapy dosing and its nature [12,13]. As in the non-OLT population it appears that viral genotype may be important also; the role of gender and race on outcome after OLT is less clear.

Diagnosis

The diagnosis of recurrent viral disease rests squarely upon the presence of HCV ribonucleic acid (RNA) in serum, and demonstration of histological abnormalities referable to such infection. It is not sufficient to base the diagnosis of recurrent chronic HCV liver disease upon elevated serum aminotransferase concentrations in conjunction with a positive HCV RNA titer, especially during the weeks and months that follow soon after OLT, i.e. when the chances of acute cellular allograft rejection are greatest (Chapter 19). Histological features that favor the diagnosis of recurrent chronic HCV liver disease include lobular acidophil necrosis, absence of bile duct injury, mononuclear cell portal tract inflammation, interface hepatitis, and portal-based fibrosis, with or without the presence of steatosis and lymphoid aggregates (Chapter 22). Widespread endothelialitis and lymphocytic bile duct injury suggest that allograft rejection is the predominant problem. The presence of very considerable periportal and bridging fibrosis, centrilobular cholestasis, portal inflammation with interface hepatitis, and hepatocyte injury in a patient with jaundice and other features of graft dysfunction is of concern for fibrosing cholestatic hepatitis (FCH). Such features portend a poor outcome.

Management

Most experts would agree that antiviral therapy (AVT) should be recommended to patients with recurrent HCV liver disease. Indeed, if patients listed for or being evaluated for OLT are unsuitable recipients of interferon (IFN)-

based therapy (e.g. depression, complications of diabetes mellitus), or demonstrate unreasonable objections to the likelihood of such treatment following OLT then their candidacy should probably be reconsidered. That said, a number of key issues regarding AVT for patients with recurrent HCV liver disease remain unclear: first, the optimal timing of AVT following OLT; second, the duration of therapy (6 or 12 months as a minimum); third, whether pegylated interferon (peg-IFN)-based therapy is more efficacious than standard IFN, and last, the optimal dose of ribavirin (RBV) [14].

Detailed discussion of prophylactic therapy for prevention of recurrent chronic HCV liver disease is beyond the scope of this chapter (see Chapter 7). Several pilot studies have examined the impact of anti-HCV antibody preparations among patients undergoing OLT for HCV liver disease: the final results are awaited with considerable interest [15]. Deployment of AVT during the first few weeks after OLT, i.e. preemptively, in the hope of achieving sustained virologic response (SVR) is based on the following observations [16,17]. First, HCV-RNA titers are generally lower at this stage of the post-OLT course, and among pre-OLT patients with compensated chronic HCV liver disease, lower HCV-RNA titers predict a greater likelihood of success to AVT and attainment of SVR. Second, nontransplant patients infected acutely with HCV and treated soon thereafter have a much greater likelihood of achieving SVR. However, these theoretical advantages of AVT for recently transplanted patients are offset by the requirement for concomitant immunosuppressive therapy in which setting SVR occurs rarely, if at all; the possibility that acute cellular rejection may be precipitated; and the distinct possibility that AVT will not be well tolerated so soon after an heroic surgical procedure.

The efficacy and tolerability of preemptive AVT has been examined in a number of studies [16–19]. It is clear that only a proportion of patients are eligible for AVT under such circumstances and that limitations of therapy are significant, e.g. RBV-induced hemolytic anemia. In a multicenter study, Chalasani et al. randomized two groups of patients to receive either AVT (peg-IFN monotherapy: 48 weeks) or no treatment. In the first group, therapy was commenced within 3 weeks of OLT, and in the second it was started between 6 and 60 months of undergoing OLT [19]. Treatment was well tolerated for the most part in both groups; 8% in the first group and 12% in the second group achieved SVR, in contrast to untreated patients (no SVR). Moreover, AVT was associated with regression of fibrosis, especially among patients in the second group.

AVT for established recurrent chronic HCV liver disease is a common therapeutic strategy. It has the potential advantages that patients are further from surgery when treatment begins, and thus may have better conditioning, and they may be taking lower doses of immunosuppressive therapy so will be less likely to experience infective complications or reduced renal clearance of RBV. As Neuberger suggests, combination antiviral therapy (CAVT) may represent the best treatment approach currently for patients with recurrent histological disease [20]. The likelihood of achieving SVR appears greater with peg-IFN, and a realistic anticipated SVR rate is probably of the order of 25–30% based on data from recently reported studies [21–26]. The impact of CAVT upon hepatic fibrosis among patients achieving SVR is encouraging [27].

Just as CAVT prior to OLT for patients who have had clinical complications of cirrhosis and portal hypertension represents a major therapeutic challenge, so does treatment of recurrent disease. Patients may retain negative experiences of CAVT prior to OLT; may continue to exhibit thrombocytopenia, thus limiting the scope of treatment; and are at increased risk of infection by virtue of concomitant immunosuppressive therapy. Moreover, recent reports of acute and/or ductopenic allograft rejection during CAVT for recurrent HCV liver disease have given rise to the concern that CAVT may not be appropriate for every patient [28] (Chapter 19).

Nevertheless, in the face of early and aggressive recurrent chronic HCV liver disease, patients and physicians may have little or no alternative but to embark upon CAVT in the hope of attenuating subsequent allograft injury at the very least, thereby delaying the onset of advanced fibrosis, risk of graft failure, and premature death. Once significant graft fibrosis is established it would seem reasonable to restart screening for development of hepatocellular carcinoma (HCC).

Hepatitis B

Until the emergence of both hepatitis B virus immunoglobulin (HBIG) and antiviral agents such as lamivudine (LAM) and adefovir (ADV), the outcome for patients with chronic hepatitis B virus (HBV) liver disease undergoing OLT was invariably poor [29]. Allograft reinfection rates were at least 80% either as a result of direct infection from circulating HBV during transplant surgery or by infection with HBV from extrahepatic sites following OLT, or both. The likelihood of reinfection was related directly to the degree of viral replication occurring at the time of, or immediately before, OLT. Aggressive clinical disease was the hallmark with mortality rates of least 50% [30]. Indeed, when it became clear that the outlook for patients with HBV liver disease who underwent OLT was so bleak, third-party payers ceased underwriting OLT [31]. Now, with better anti-HBV therapy, patients undergoing OLT for HBV-related liver disease may anticipate outcomes that are similar to those who have HBV surface antigen (HBsAg)-negative disease [29].

Diagnosis

Elevated serum aminotransferase concentrations are accompanied by reemergence of HBsAg and HBV deoxyribonucleic acid (DNA) in serum. Depending on the time relationship between onset of these abnormalities and OLT, liver biopsy findings may demonstrate acute hepatitis, chronic hepatitis, or more advanced disease, similar to changes observed during the pretransplant disease course (Chapter 22). Immunohistochemical stains for both HBsAg and HBV core antigens are usually positive also. As with recurrent HCV liver disease histological findings representative of FCH may be evident.

Management

This may be considered in distinct, but complementary, phases. Prior to OLT, patients with active viral replication require AVT; following OLT, all patients should receive HBIG or HBIG in combination with AVT (evidence for sustained efficacy of LAM without HBIG post-OLT is lacking [32]). The principal objective of AVT before OLT is suppression of HBV replication so as to diminish the likelihood of graft reinfection thereafter (Chapter 7). Among patients with advanced fibrosis or cirrhosis, LAM is effective in achieving HBV-DNA loss from serum and delaying clinical decompensation and the emergence of HCC [33]. Moreover, LAM is well tolerated even in patients with decompensated disease, unlike IFN. However, its overall effectiveness is limited by three factors: recurrent viremia after treatment cessation, emergence of drug-resistant mutations in the YMDD component of the HBV-DNA polymerase gene (incidence of such mutations is estimated at 15–20% per year of treatment), and uncertainty as to the most appropriate time to initiate LAM in patients with advanced liver disease who are listed for OLT. ADV may be more efficacious in this setting than LAM, thereby leading to increased survival pre-OLT and even obviation of the need for OLT in some patients [34]. However, great care must be exercised among patients who have established renal insufficiency, and possibly in some patients with advanced portal hypertension also. Reduced dosing frequency of ADV may be required.

During the anhepatic phase of OLT and for 6 succeeding days HBIG (10 000 IU) is given intravenously to all patients. Thereafter, HBIG should be administered sufficiently frequently to maintain trough serum anti-HBsAB levels of 100–150 IU/L among patients who were HBV-DNA-negative, and >500 IU/L in those who demonstrated active viral replication prior to OLT [29]. The costs of these approaches, not to mention the demands of time and side-effects associated with intravenous HBIG administration, e.g. myalgia, facial flushing, and the potential risk of mercury poisoning, are considerable. Some units have transitioned patients who lacked evidence of viral replication prior to OLT to intramuscular (IM) HBIG in the interests of cost savings and the relative convenience for the patient, and in the knowledge that graft reinfection and disease recurrence are less likely in this setting. However, long-term outcome data to support this practice are limited.

Collated evidence from studies in which a combination of HBIG and LAM post-OLT was employed revealed an encouragingly low rate of recurrent HBV liver disease (<10% at 2 years), and negative HBV-DNA levels for the most part after further follow-up [29]. Moreover, IM HBIG was used in several of these studies, and it may be that this combination – AVT and lower-dose IM HBIG – represents the best approach for patients post-OLT, when cost and overall effectiveness are taken into consideration. However, severe recurrent HBV liver disease resulting in death has been reported among three patients receiving both HBIG and LAM. Two different mutations were demonstrated in elegant transfection studies: this combination and the ensuing viral replication were enhanced by the presence of LAM in vitro [35].

It is beyond the scope of this chapter to discuss the appropriateness and timing of HBIG withdrawal in detail. Both HBV vaccination and/or AVT may be possible in carefully selected patients. Further study is required to identify those patients in whom this strategy would be safest and most effective.

■ ALCOHOLIC LIVER DISEASE

Not unlike patients with chronic HBV liver disease, there was a period when the prospect of OLT for patients with alcoholic liver disease (ALD) was considered inappropriate. A belief prevailed that ALD was the predictable consequence of an individual's chosen behavior, thereby avoidable and not a justifiable indication for OLT [36]. However, presently, patients with ALD constitute approximately 20% of those undergoing OLT in both USA and Europe. Furthermore, 1-year and 5-year graft and patient survival rates for ALD are comparable with those for patients undergoing transplantation for indications other than ALD (Chapter 9) [1,2].

Some alcohol use following OLT appears to be relatively common, and duration of abstinence prior to OLT has little discriminatory ability to predict continuing abstinence thereafter [37]. A clear distinction needs to be drawn between consumption that may be of little consequence, and drinking behavior that may result directly in allograft injury or genuine risk of such poor adherence to clinical follow-up and immunosuppressive therapy that graft function and overall outcome are threatened. Despite these legitimate concerns, patients transplanted for ALD who then consumed significant amounts of alcohol following OLT fared no worse with respect to survival and episodes of graft rejection, compared with those who drank alcohol occasionally or not at all [38]. Factors that may help identify those patients who are more likely to return to heavy alcohol consumption post-OLT have been discussed in Chapter 4.

In contrast to recidivism, less is known about the true extent of recurrent ALD, i.e. heavy drinking with appropriate histological abnormalities in the allograft. Lee [39] examined a series of 29 liver biopsies from patients with "excessive" post-LT alcohol consumption and elevated liver test concentrations [39]. Although 83% of biopsy specimens demonstrated steatosis, only 28% revealed fibrosis; 23% (six patients) progressed to cirrhosis. However, five of the six patients with fibrosis had concurrent HCV infection, making it difficult to be certain whether cirrhosis was solely the result of alcohol. Nevertheless, when these findings are combined with rates of recidivism the extent of recurrent fibrotic ALD is probably less than 15%, a figure that is more encouraging than some other transplant indications, e.g. autoimmune hepatitis (AIH), primary biliary cirrhosis (PBC) (see later).

Diagnosis

Diagnosis should not be difficult: sustained, heavy alcohol consumption and manifestations of end-organ damage in the absence of other potential causes of liver disease are required. However, it is important to bear in mind that histological abnormalities of ALD are not specific and that widespread steatosis, associated lobular neutrophil inflammation, and centrilobular pericellular fibrosis may be a consequence of nonalcoholic steatohepatitis (NASH) primarily, rather than alcohol consumption (Chapter 22). A proportion of post-OLT candidates are at increased risk of developing NASH by virtue of obesity, further weight gain, type 2 diabetes mellitus, systemic hypertension, and other complications of immunosuppressive therapy, notably hyperlipidemia (Chapter 23).

Management

Abstinence is the key to success. If this can be achieved and maintained before bridging fibrosis or cirrhosis become established then the outcome should be favorable. However, once complications of portal hypertension have become evident the outlook is guarded.

■ AUTOIMMUNE LIVER DISEASE

Autoimmune Hepatitis

The first account of recurrent AIH was published in 1984 [40]. Further reports have followed, not least during the last 5 years [41–51]. These studies are primarily retrospective analyses of prospectively gathered data from single centers, with between 5, and in one case at least 10 years of patient follow-up [50]. The reported prevalence of recurrent AIH varies considerably: some authors described none or very few patients with compelling evidence of recurrent disease [41,42], whereas others reported recurrence rates approaching 20% and above – in two instances, 42% and 41%, respectively [46,50]. Reasons for these differences are unclear but small study numbers, limited periods of follow-up in some cases, and whether liver biopsies were performed according to protocol or only because of liver test abnormalities are all likely to be contributing factors. Moreover, the degree of graft dysfunction that arises following the diagnosis of recurrent AIH varies considerably from chronic hepatitis that can be controlled with increased levels of immunosuppressive therapy [47], to cirrhosis resulting in graft failure and the need for retransplantation, or death [46].

Factors that appear to be important in the development of recurrent AIH include positive HLA-DR3 status among recipients [47], a finding that has not been confirmed by other authors [45]. There is interest in whether mismatch of graft and recipient HLA-DR3 status (negative and positive, respectively) might contribute to disease recurrence, but this proposal has not been confirmed. Second, the degree to which immunosuppressive therapy has been tapered following OLT has been proposed as a contributing factor to the likelihood of disease recurrence; however, at least one group has been able to wean patients successfully from glucocorticoid therapy without compromise to graft or patient [52]. Although patients transplanted for AIH are at increased risk of allograft rejection compared with patients undergoing OLT for other indications [51], the incidence of rejection does not appear to be linked to the rates of recurrent AIH. Third, histological appearances of the explanted hepatectomy specimen have been reported by one group to be an important predictor of recurrent AIH, suggesting that in some patients certain histopathologic patterns identify patients with AIH who may be unresponsive or less responsive to immunosuppressive therapy [46].

De novo AIH is the development of clinical, serological, and histological features consistent with AIH [53], but among patients who underwent OLT for an indication other than AIH [54]. The first description of this phenomenon was among seven children [55]. Very similar findings have been reported in adult patients also: in one series, two patients had primary sclerosing cholangitis (PSC) and another had PBC prior to OLT [56]. Detailed consideration of the pathogenesis of de novo AIH is beyond the scope of this review, but possible mechanisms include autoantigen release from injured tissue and molecular mimicry, perhaps induced by an infectious agent [53,57].

Diagnosis

As with the other forms of autoimmune chronic liver disease (see later), establishing the diagnosis of recurrent AIH with confidence may be far from straightforward. First, increasing serum aminotransferase concentrations that follow dose reductions in immunosuppressive therapy may be a consequence of allograft rejection, emergence of recurrent disease, or some component of both. Second, circulating autoantibodies that are an integral component of the pre-OLT diagnosis persist in many cases (Chapter 10), albeit the titers may be less following OLT, and so cannot be relied upon as convincing evidence of recurrent disease. Third, some histological abnormalities of acute allograft rejection may be similar to and difficult to differentiate from those of recurrent AIH, e.g. mononuclear infiltrate of the portal tract with some disruption of the interface.

The median time from OLT to diagnosis of recurrent AIH is variable also. In at least one study, disease recurrence was evident in almost 50% of patients within 1 year of OLT [48], whereas in others this period was closer to 5 years [44,47,50]. In the only two studies in which protocol liver biopsies were performed, 28% (2/7) [47] and 56% (4/7) [50] of patients, respectively, were diagnosed with recurrent AIH in the absence of symptoms and/or elevated serum aminotransferase concentrations. However, no obvious link between protocol biopsies and earlier time to diagnosis of recurrent disease was observed, and it remains to be determined whether alteration of immunosuppressive therapy in light of such findings is important.

Management

Treatment of both recurrent and de novo AIH comprises prednisone alone, or in conjunction with azathioprine. In general, these agents would be added to the existing immunosuppressive regimen, and a successful response viewed as further indication of the correct diagnosis. The absence of a convincing response to therapy demands that the original diagnosis be reconsidered [57].

Primary Biliary Cirrhosis

Debate about the veracity of recurrent PBC has been considerable since the original report of three patients emerged more than 20 years ago [58,59]. At present, a diagnosis of recurrent PBC appears to have little meaningful impact on graft or patient survival, and of all the potential causes of primary disease recurrence would seem to carry the most favorable outlook. However, since long-term survival for patients undergoing OLT for PBC is as good, or better than for any other indication [60], increasing numbers of patients may develop recurrent disease, and in some cases, demonstrate significant progression and decompensation thereof. The implications this would have for possible retransplantation remain to be seen.

As with recurrent AIH (see earlier) reasons for uncertainty about the existence and extent of recurrent PBC include relatively small numbers of patients studied, short periods of patient follow-up, and lack of protocol biopsies in many instances. Several studies have demonstrated histological abnormalities consistent with recurrent PBC despite normal serum liver tests [61–63]. Furthermore, histological abnormalities may have a patchy distribution, as in the pre-OLT disease phase [59]. Results of studies based on protocol liver biopsies and with longer periods of follow-up suggest that the rate of recurrent PBC may be as high as 18% at 5 years, and up to 30% at 10 years [63].

There is agreement that risk factors for development of recurrent disease include recipient age (donor age, cold-, and warm-ischemia times may be important also), increasing duration from the time of OLT, and immunosuppressive drugs to which patients have been exposed. Patients transplanted under a tacrolimus rather than a cyclosporine-based regimen were more likely to develop recurrent PBC and to do so at an earlier stage [64]. Prolonged corticosteroid exposure after OLT may prevent or limit the emergence of findings consistent with recurrent PBC [59].

Diagnosis

There is currently a consensus that the diagnosis of recurrent PBC may be sustained in the presence of most or all of the following histological abnormalities: portal triad mononuclear cell inflammatory infiltrate, nonsuppurative bile duct injury, lymphoid aggregate formation, and epithelioid granulomata [65]. Moreover, the patient must have a definite pre-OLT diagnosis of PBC, and in most cases should demonstrate persistent circulating antimitochondrial antibodies (AMA) [65]. The diagnosis of recurrent PBC cannot be based on symptoms such as fatigue or pruritus, and/or the presence of cholestatic liver test abnormalities. The latter may exist for other reasons, e.g. chronic allograft rejection or biliary tract sepsis. Likewise, demonstration of circulating AMA post-OLT without appropriate histological abnormalities is insufficient evidence to confirm the diagnosis of recurrent PBC.

Management

There is no evidence that treatment of recurrent PBC with ursodeoxycholic acid (UDCA) alters the disease course; however, anecdotal improvement in liver test results may be achieved.

Primary Sclerosing Cholangitis

Single-center studies [66,67] have demonstrated allograft PSC recurrence rates of up to 37%. In one large study, recurrent PSC was documented in 24 of 120 patients (20%) based on radiographic evidence of multiple, nonanastomotic, and predominantly intrahepatic biliary strictures (22), or compatible histological abnormalities in those patients whose cholangiogram was normal (2)

[66]. In the large control group (415 patients without PSC who had undergone OLT) only one subject had histological findings suggestive of recurrent PSC (fibrous cholangitis following a Roux-en-Y anastamosis). Although no risk factors predictive of recurrent PSC were identified from this study, another study demonstrated associations between male sex and the presence of an intact colon prior to OLT, with recurrent PSC [67]. In a further study, patients administered OKT3 for steroid-resistant acute cellular rejection had greater likelihood of developing recurrent PSC. However, no link between primary immunosuppressive therapy (CyA or Tac) and the risk of recurrent PSC was established; and patients who could be weaned from corticosteroid therapy within 3 months of OLT exhibited a trend toward less recurrent PSC [68]. Review of the UNOS database revealed that patient and graft survival rates for subjects transplanted for PSC were significantly less good at 7 years and beyond than for a cohort with PBC who underwent OLT during the same period [69]. In addition, patients with PSC were significantly more likely to undergo retransplantation than patients who had PBC. Being a database analysis, the precise reasons for this are not clear, but it is reasonable to infer that disease recurrence was applicable in a significant proportion of cases.

Diagnosis

Like AIH and PBC, recurrent PSC may be very difficult to establish with certainty because laboratory, radiographic, and histological features upon which the diagnosis is based pre-OLT may arise in the post-OLT setting for wholly different reasons. Evidence of isolated anastomotic stricture formation, hepatic artery stenosis or thrombosis, established chronic allograft rejection, or ABO incompatibility between recipient and donor are circumstances in which the diagnosis of recurrent PSC would be difficult to sustain [70].

The pretransplant diagnosis must be secure (careful assessment of the explanted liver may be necessary); nonanastomotic intrahepatic and/or extrahepatic biliary strictures with beading and irregular narrowing should be evident on cholangiography at least 90 days post-OLT; and liver histology should reveal fibrous cholangitis, fibro-obliterative abnormalities, ductopenia, biliary cirrhosis, or some combination thereof.

Management

There is no compelling evidence that UDCA affords any lasting benefit to patients with recurrent PSC other than the hope of ameliorating pruritus should it exist. Once recurrent disease is established it would seem reasonable to restart periodic surveillance for cholangiocarcinoma (CCA) and hepatocellular cancer: one patient with recurrent PSC confirmed 7 years after OLT developed de novo CCA 2 years later [71]. Patients with coexisting inflammatory bowel disease (IBD) who undergo OLT for PSC and whose colon remains intact have significantly greater risk of developing advanced colorectal cancer (CRC) within 2–5 years of OLT [72]. Therefore, annual colonoscopy with multiple biopsies, in conjunction with a low threshold for colectomy in cases of dysplasia, is recommended. In contrast, no patient undergoing OLT for PSC, who did not have IBD prior to OLT, developed CRC thereafter.

■ MISCELLANEOUS LIVER DISEASES

Hepatocellular Carcinoma and Cholangiocarcinoma

Patients in the USA with end-stage liver disease (ESLD) and known, rather than incidental (i.e. tumor identified during examination of the explanted liver), HCC have enjoyed considerably greater access to OLT since February 2002 (Chapters 6 and 8). Therefore, it is conceivable that the rate of recurrent HCC may be greater during the next few years compared with the rates of tumor recurrence prior to introduction of the model for end-stage liver disease (MELD) scoring system [73]. In the face of recurrent HCC levels, immunosuppressive therapy should be reduced as far as is safely possible without precipitating allograft rejection. Even with neoadjuvant chemotherapy, the prognosis is not good.

Until development of specific protocols for pre-OLT management of patients with CCA in the setting of PSC by workers at the University of Nebraska and the Mayo Clinic, Minnesota, OLT was beset by the problem of recurrent cancer, premature death, and the sense that a donor organ might have been utilized better [74]. The prime function of these protocols is to weed out patients in whom locally invasive primary disease or metastases preclude OLT. As with recurrent HCC, reemergence of CCA in the post-OLT period carries a dismal prognosis. Effective treatment strategies for recurrent disease are lacking.

Nonalcoholic Steatohepatitis (NASH)

Several studies have demonstrated that nonalcoholic fatty liver disease (NAFLD) recurs in the majority of patients following OLT. In one study 30 patients transplanted either for NASH or for cryptogenic cirrhosis (CC) with phenotypic features of NASH had a recurrence rate of NAFLD (steatosis) of 100% at 5 years, compared with only 25% among control subjects (they had PBC, PSC, or ALD) [75]. Three patients (10%) developed steatohepatitis, with progression to fibrosis in one case, although increased rates of chronic rejection, graft failure, and/or mortality were not observed. The time to development of steatosis correlated directly with the cumulative steroid dose to which patients had been exposed. In another retrospective study of 71 patients who were transplanted for CC, NASH recurred in eight patients and CC in four, one of whom required retransplantation [76]. The 5-year cumulative incidence of graft failure was 7%. However, it is not known what proportion of patients undergoing OLT in this study may have had CC for reasons other than NAFLD. Recurrent NASH has been observed in a patient who underwent living donor liver transplantation [77].

Given that the burden upon OLT from NASH appears set to increase significantly during the next three decades it is safe to assume that the issue of recurrent disease will become an important consideration [78]. If recurrent steatosis is universal, not unlike HCV allograft reinfection and progression to NASH occurs in at least 10–20% of patients, then demands on services and donor organs will continue to outstrip supply.

Budd–Chiari Syndrome

Reports of recurrent Budd–Chiari syndrome (BCS) exist [79,80]. Lifelong anticoagulation with warfarin is recommended for most if not all patients following OLT, even in circumstances where the underlying cause of, or associated thrombotic disorder, has not been characterized completely. It may be the case that instances of recurrent BCS were linked to insufficient anticoagulation after OLT. However, in other cases, recurrent thrombosis developed in spite of adequate anticoagulation, e.g. in the face of recurrence of the underlying condition associated with BCS.

Hemochromatosis

Although overt clinical disease recurrence appears to be rare, accumulation of iron stores has been demonstrated after successful OLT for hemochromatosis. Therefore, it is reasonable to recommend that body iron stores be assessed annually and to institute phlebotomy as indicated. The impact of donor organs from patients who were heterozygous for the C282Y mutation on recipient is discussed in Chapter 11.

■ RETRANSPLANTATION

Given circumstances of very limited deceased donor organ availability in contrast to the number of patients listed for OLT, this is a difficult issue. As recurrent chronic HCV liver disease assumes greater significance with each passing year, members of the liver transplant community must exercise even greater responsibility toward appropriate organ allocation.

Our ability to make informed decisions regarding the utility (and appropriateness) of retransplantation is hampered somewhat by a lack of robust outcomes data. Analysis of the UNOS database has revealed similar survival rates for patients retransplanted for chronic HCV liver disease compared with other etiologies of cirrhosis, and for controlling for degree of illness at the time of retransplantation [81]. However, this database is unable to identify properly specific reason(s) for retransplantation, and some critical clinical and laboratory variables are missing. By contrast, two large single-center studies have reported much poorer survival among patients undergoing retransplantation for chronic HCV liver disease than for other indications [82,83].

Further analysis of the UNOS database, this time using graft and patient half-lives as end points rather than graft and patient survival rates, found that the median graft half-life for retransplantation taking all indications into consideration was only 1.5 years. By contrast, the median graft half-life for all first OLT was 12 years [84]. These data suggest that there may be no case to answer for retransplantation given the disparity between numbers of patients waiting and available deceased donor organs, with the possible exception of patients who develop primary allograft nonfunction. Conversely, if patients have very good functional status consideration of retransplantation may be appropriate (Chapter 1). However, if functional status is good, the MELD score may not especially high, thereby limiting priority. Therefore, adaptation of the MELD scoring system for patients being considered for retransplantation may be required. A retrospective, multicenter American study currently in progress may be able to provide answers for some of these key questions.

■ REFERENCES

1. Scientific Registry of Transplant Recipients. Transplant statistics: center-specific reports. Available at http://www.ustransplant.org/center-adv.html. Accessed January 2005.

2. Adam R, McMaster P, O'Grady JG, et al. Evolution of liver transplantation in Europe: report of the European Liver Transplant Registry. Liver Transpl 2003;9:1231–1243.

3. Garcia-Retortillo M, Forns X, Feliu A, et al. Hepatitis C virus kinetics during and immediately after liver transplantation. Hepatology 2002;35:680–687.

4. Gane E. The natural history and outcome of liver transplantation in hepatitis C virus-infected recipients. Liver Transpl 2003;9:S28–S34.

5. Berenguer M, Ferrell L, Watson J, et al. HCV-related fibrosis progression following liver transplantation: increase in recent years. J Hepatol 2000;32:673–684.

6. Berenguer M, Prieto M, Rayon J, et al. Natural history of clinically compensated hepatitis C virus-related graft cirrhosis after liver transplantation. Hepatology 2000;32:852–858.

7. Ferrell LD, Wright TL, Roberts J, et al. Hepatitis C viral infection in liver transplant recipients. Hepatology 1992;16:865–876.

8. Feray C, Gigou M, Samuel D, et al. The course of hepatitis C infection after liver transplantation. Hepatology 1994;20:1137–1143.

9. Forman LM, Lewis JD, Berlin JA, et al. Association between hepatitis C infection and survival after orthotopic liver transplantation. Gastroenterology 2002;122:889–896.

10. Berenguer M, Prieto M, San Juan F, et al. Contribution of donor age to the recent decrease in patient survival among HCV-infected liver transplant recipients. Hepatology 2002;36:202–210.

11. Charlton M, Ruppert K, Belle SH, et al. Long-term results and modeling to predict outcomes in recipients with HCV infection: results of the NIDDK liver transplantation database. Liver Transpl 2004;10(9):1120–1130.

12. Berenguer M. Host and donor risk factors before and after liver transplantation that impact HCV recurrence. Liver Transpl 2003;9:S44–S47.

13. Lake JR. The role of immunosuppressive in recurrence of hepatitis C. Liver Transpl 2003;9:S63–S66.

14. Samuel D. Hepatitis C, interferon and risk of rejection after liver transplantation (editorial; 26 references). Liver Transpl 2004;10:868–871.

15. Terrault NA. Prophylactic and preemptive therapies for hepatitis C virus-infected patients undergoing liver transplantation. Liver Transpl 2003;9:S95–S100.

16. Garcia-Retortillo M, Forns X. Prevention and treatment of hepatitis C virus recurrence after liver transplantation (review; 65 references). J Hepatol 2004;41:2–10.

17. Shergill AK, Khalili M, Straley S, et al. Applicability, tolerability, and efficacy of preemptive antiviral therapy in hepatitis C-infected patients undergoing liver transplantation. Am J Transplant, 2005; 5: 118-124.

18. Mazzaferro V, Sciavo M, Caccamo L, et al. Prospective randomized trial on early treatment of HCV infection after liver transplantation in HCV-RNA positive patients (abstract). Liver Transpl 2003;9:C-36.

19. Chalasani NP, Manzarbeitia C, Ferenci P, et al. Peginterferon alfa-2a (40 kD) as prophylaxis for recurrent hepatitis C virus infection (HCV) after orthotopic liver transplantation. Hepatology 2005;41:289–298.

20. Neuberger J. Treatment of hepatitis C virus infection in the allograft. Liver Transpl 2003;9:S101–S108.

21. Abdelmalek MF, Firpi RJ, Soldevila-Pico C, et al. Sustained viral response to interferon and ribavirin in liver transplant recipients with recurrent hepatitis C. Liver Transpl 2004;10:199–207.

22. Samuel D, Bizollon T, Feray C, et al. Interferon-alpha 2b plus ribavirin in patients with chronic hepatitis C after liver transplantation: a randomized study. Gastroenterology 2003;124:642–650.

23. Dumortier J, Scoazec JY, Chevallier P, et al. Treatment of recurrent hepatitis C after liver transplantation: a pilot study of peginterferon alfa-2b and ribavirin combination. J Hepatol 2004;40:669–674.

24. Rodriguez-Luna H, Khatib A, Sharma P, et al. Treatment of recurrent hepatitis C infection after liver transplantation with combination of pegylated interferon alpha 2b and ribavirin: an open label series. Transplantation 2004;77:190–194.

25. Ross AS, Bhan AK, Pascual M, et al. Pegylated interferon alpha-2b plus ribavirin in the treatment of post-liver transplant recurrent hepatitis C. Clin Transplant 2004;18:166–173.

26. Smith AD, Muir AJ, Heneghan MA, et al. What is the course of patients undergoing anti-viral therapy for recurrent hepatitis C virus liver disease? (Abstract) Am J Gastroenterol 2004;99:S85.

27. Bizollon T, Ahmed SNS, Radenne S, et al. Long term histological improvement and clearance of intrahepatic hepatitis C virus RNA following sustained response to interferon–ribavirin combination therapy in liver transplanted patients with hepatitis C virus recurrence. Gut 2003;52:283–287.

28. Kugelmas M, Osgood MJ, Trotter JF, et al. Hepatitis C virus therapy, hepatocyte drug metabolism, and risk for acute cellular rejection. Liver Transpl 2003;9:1159–1165.

29. Roche B, Samuel D. Evolving strategies to prevent HBV recurrence. Liver Transpl 2004;10:S74–S85.

30. O'Grady JG, Smith HM, Davies SE, et al. Hepatitis B virus re-infection after orthotopic liver transplantation. Serological and clinical implications. J Hepatol 1992;14:104–111.

31. Jury of the International Consensus Conference on Indications of Liver Transplantation. Consensus statement on indications for liver transplantation: Paris, June 22–23, 1993. Hepatology 1994;20:63S–68S.

32. Mutimer D, Dusheiko G, Barrett C, et al. Lamivudine without HBIG for prevention of graft reinfection with hepatitis B: long-term follow-up. Transplantation 2000;70:809–815.

33. Law YF, Sung JJ, Chow WC, et al. Lamivudine for patients with chronic hepatitis B and advanced liver disease. N Engl J Med 2004;351:1521–1531.

34. Schiff ER, Lai CL, Hadziyannis S, et al. Adefovir dipivoxil alone or in combination with lamivudine in patients with lamivudine-resistant hepatitis B in pre- and post-liver transplantation patients. Hepatology 2003;38:1419–1427.

35. Bock C-T, Tillmann HL, Torressi J, et al. Selection of hepatitis B virus polymerase mutants with enhanced replication by lamivudine treatment after liver transplantation. Gastroenterology 2002;122:264–273.

36. Lim JK, Keefe EB. Liver transplantation for alcoholic liver disease: current concepts and length of sobriety. Liver Transpl 2004;10:S31–S38.

37. Webb K, Neuberger J. Transplantation for alcoholic liver disease (editorial; 10 references). BMJ 2004;329:63–64.

38. Pageaux GP, Bismuth M, Perney P, et al. Alcohol relapse after liver transplantation for alcoholic liver disease: does it matter? J Hepatol 2003;38:629–634.

39. Lee RG. Recurrence of alcoholic liver disease after transplantation. Liver Transpl Surg 1997;3:292–295.

40. Neuberger J, Portmann B, Calne R, et al. Recurrence of autoimmune chronic active hepatitis following orthotopic grafting. Transplantation 1984;37:363–365.

41. Cattan P, Berney T, Conti F, et al. Outcome of orthotopic liver transplantation in autoimmune hepatitis according to subtypes. Transpl Int 2002;15:34–38.

42. Nunez-Martinez O, De la Cruz G, Salcedo M, et al. Liver transplantation for autoimmune hepatitis: fulminant versus chronic hepatitis presentation. Transplant Proc 2003;35:1857–1858.

43. Narumi S, Hakamada K, Saaki M, et al. Liver transplantation for autoimmune hepatitis: rejection and recurrence. Transplant Proc 1999;31:1955–1956.

44. Ratziu V, Samuel D, Sebagh M, et al. Long-term follow-up after liver transplantation for autoimmune hepatitis: evidence of recurrence of primary disease. J Hepatol 1999;30:131–141.

45. Reich DJ, Fiel I, Guarrera JV, et al. Liver transplantation for autoimmune hepatitis. Hepatology 2000;32:693–700.

46. Ayata G, Gordon FD, Lewis WD, et al. Liver transplantation for autoimmune hepatitis: a long-term pathologic study. Hepatology 2000;32:185–192.

47. Gonzalez-Koch A, Czaja AJ, Carpenter HA, et al. Recurrent autoimmune hepatitis after orthotopic liver transplantation. Liver Transpl 2001;7:302–310.

48. Molmenti EP, Netto GJ, Murray NG, et al. Incidence and recurrence of autoimmune/alloimmune hepatitis in liver transplant recipients. Liver Transpl 2002;8:519–526.

49. Heffron TG, Smallwood GA, Oakley B, et al. Autoimmune hepatitis following liver transplantation: relationship to recurrent disease and steroid weaning. Transplant Proc 2002;34:3311–3312.

50. Duclos-Vallee J-C, Sebagh M, Rifai K, et al. A 10 year follow up study of patients transplanted for autoimmune hepatitis: histological recurrence precedes clinical and biochemical recurrence. Gut 2003;52:893–898.

51. Vogel A, Heinrich E, Bahr MJ, et al. Long-term outcome of liver transplantation for autoimmune hepatitis. Clin Transplant 2004;18:62–69.

52. Trouillot TE, Shrestha R, Kam I, et al. Successful withdrawal of prednisone after adult liver transplantation for autoimmune hepatitis. Liver Transpl Surg 1999;5:375–380.

53. Mieli-Vergani G, Vergani D. De novo autoimmune hepatitis after liver transplantation (review; 34 references). J Hepatol 2004;40:3–7.

54. Alvarez F, Berg PA, Bianchi FB, et al. International autoimmune hepatitis group report: review of criteria for diagnosis of autoimmune hepatitis. J Hepatol 1999;31:929–938.

55. Kerkar N, Hadzic N, Davies ET, et al. De-novo autoimmune hepatitis after liver transplantation. Lancet 1998;351:409–413.

56. Heneghan MA, Portmann BC, Norris SM, et al. Graft dysfunction mimicking autoimmune hepatitis following liver transplantation in adults. Hepatology 2001;34:464–470.

57. Czaja AJ. Autoimmune hepatitis after liver transplantation and other lessons of self-intolerance (review; 92 references). Liver Transpl 2002;8:505–513.

58. Neuberger J, Portmann B, MacDougall B, et al. Recurrence of primary biliary cirrhosis after liver transplantation. N Engl J Med 1982;306:1–4.

59. Neuberger J. Recurrent primary biliary cirrhosis (review; 40 references). Liver Transpl 2003;9:539–546.

60. Roberts MS, Angus DC, Bryce CL, et al. Survival after liver transplantation in the United States: a disease-specific analysis of the UNOS database. Liver Transpl 2004;10:886–897.

61. Slapak GI, Saxena R, Portmann B, et al. Graft and systemic disease in long-term survivors of liver transplantation. Hepatology 1997;25:195–202.

62. Neuberger J, Wilson P, Adams D. Protocol liver biopsies: the case in favour. Transplant Proc 1998;30:1497–1499.

63. Garcia R, Garcia C, McMaster P, et al. Transplantation for primary biliary cirrhosis: retrospective analysis of 400 patients in a single center. Hepatology 2001;33:22–27.

64. Neuberger J, Gunson B, Hubscher S, et al. Immunosuppression affects the rate of recurrent primary biliary cirrhosis after liver transplantation. Liver Transpl 2004;10:488–491.

65. Hubscher S, Elias E, Buckels J, et al. Primary biliary cirrhosis. Histological evidence of disease recurrence after liver transplantation. J Hepatol 1993;18:173–184.

66. Graziadei IW, Wiesner RH, Batts KP, et al. Recurrence of primary sclerosing cholangitis following liver transplantation. Hepatology 1999;29:1050–1056.

67. Vera A, Moledina S, Gunson B, et al. Risk factors for recurrence of primary sclerosing cholangitis of liver allograft. Lancet 2002;360:1943–1944.

68. Kugelmas M, Spiegelman P, Osgood MO, et al. Different immunosuppressive regimens and recurrence of primary sclerosing cholangitis after liver transplantation. Liver Transpl 2003;9:727–732.

69. Maheshwari A, Yoo HY, Thuluvath PJ. Long-term outcome of liver transplantation in patients with PSC: a comparative analysis with PBC. Am J Gastroenterol 2004;99:538–542.

70. Graziadei IW. Recurrence of primary sclerosing cholangitis after liver transplantation (review; 25 references). Liver Transpl 2002;8:575–581.

71. Heneghan MA, Tuttle-Newhall JE, Suhocki PV, et al. De-novo cholangiocarcinoma in the setting of recurrent primary sclerosing cholangitis following liver transplantation. Am J Transplant 2003;3:634–638.

72. Vera A, Gunson BK, Ussatoff V, et al. Colorectal cancer in patients with inflammatory bowel disease after liver transplantation for primary sclerosing cholangitis. Transplantation 2003;75:1983–1988.

73. Wiesner RH, Freeman RB, Mulligan DC. Liver transplantation for hepatocellular cancer: the impact of the MELD allocation policy. Gastroenterology 2004;127:S261–S267.

74. Heimbach JK, Haddock MG, Alberts SR, et al. Transplantation for perihilar cholangiocarcinoma. Liver Transpl 2004;10:S65–S68.

75. Contos MJ, Cales W, Sterling RK, et al. Development of nonalcoholic fatty liver disease after orthotopic liver transplantation for cryptogenic cirrhosis. Liver Transpl 2001;7:363–373.

76. Sanjeevi A, Lyden E, Sunderman B, et al. Outcomes of liver transplantation for cryptogenic cirrhosis: a single-center study of 71 patients. Transplant Proc 2003;35:2977–2980.

77. Saab S, Cho D, Lassman RC, et al. Recurrent non-alcoholic steatohepatitis in a living related liver transplant recipient. J Hepatol 2005;42:148–149.

78. Charlton M. Nonalcohlic fatty liver disease: a review of current understanding and future impact (review; 117 references). Clin Gastroenterol Hepatol 2004;2:1048–1059.

79. Ruckert J, Ruckert R, Rudolph B, et al. Recurrence of the Budd–Chiari syndrome after orthotopic liver transplantation. Hepatogastroenterology 1999;46:867–871.

80. Renz JF, Ascher NL. Liver transplantation for nonviral, nonmalignant diseases: problem of recurrence. World J Surg 2002;26:247–256.

81. Watt KDS, Lyden ER, McCashland TM. Poor survival after liver re-transplantation: is hepatitis C to blame? Liver Transpl 2003;9:1019–1024.

82. Roayaie S, Schiano TD, Thung SN, et al. Results of re-transplantation for recurrent hepatitis C. Hepatology 2003;38:1428–1436.

83. Yao FY, Saab S, Bass NM, et al. Prediction of survival after liver re-transplantation for late graft failure based on preoperative prognostic scores. Hepatology 2004;39:230–238.

84. Smith AD, Marroquin CE, Edwards EB, et al. What is the anticipated half-life of a liver allograft? (Abstract) Gastroenterology 2004;126:A-665.

Infections in the Transplant Recipient

▼　▼　▼　▼　▼　▼　▼　▼　▼

**Barbara D. Alexander and
Kimberly Hanson**

25

INFECTION remains an important complication after solid organ transplantation (SOT). Despite advances in immunosuppressive regimens and surgical techniques, more than half of liver transplant recipients present with an infectious disease in the early posttransplant period [1]. The goal in the solid organ transplant recipient is to prevent infection and to recognize its presence early when it occurs.

The risk of infection is related to the balance between the patients' net state of immunosuppression and their epidemiological exposures [2]. The patient's level of immunosuppression is influenced by several factors including underlying disease, metabolic conditions (diabetes, malnutrition), immunosuppressive drugs, infection with immunomodulating viruses, and the presence of devitalized tissues, foreign bodies, or fluid collections from the surgical procedure.

Immunosuppression increases the risk of tissue invasion, dissemination, and superinfection once exposure to a potential pathogen occurs. Immunosuppression also blunts the typical inflammatory responses that clinicians and patients have come to recognize as markers of infection, thereby resulting in delayed therapeutic intervention. Epidemiological exposures encompass those occurring in the hospital as well as recent and remote exposures in the community. The clinician must take a detailed history of potential exposure to a variety of pathogens, realizing that the importance of environmental exposures will vary based on each individual's immune status. For example, bacterial and fungal pathogens may be more prominent in the setting of significant neutropenia while cytomegalovirus (CMV) and intracellular organisms may be more important with impaired T cell function.

■ TIMING OF INFECTION

Similar immunosuppressive regimens are used in all forms of SOT, and predictable patterns of infection have emerged. Based on these patterns, a timetable for infection in transplant recipients was developed by Fishman and Rubin [2]. The timetable is organized into three segments: the first month, 2–6 months, and more than 6 months posttransplant. The infections commonly encountered in the first month are caused by the same nosocomial pathogens that infect other postoperative patients with similar lengths of stay in the intensive care unit (ICU). The majority of these infections are due to bacterial and fungal agents. During the second to sixth months following transplantation, patients are at risk for opportunistic pathogens, most notably CMV and *Pneumocystis jiroveci* (formerly *Pneumocystis carinii*). Six months after transplantation, the etiology of infection depends on the function of the graft and the types of immunosuppressive regimens that have been employed. More than 80% of patients will have good graft function and can be maintained on minimal immunosuppressive regimens. Their infectious complications are few and typically related to pulmonary exposures. Ten percent of recipients will develop chronic viral infections and are at risk for developing late complications from these infections (e.g. Epstein–Barr virus (EBV) and posttransplant lymphoproliferative disorder (PTLD)). Another 10% of patients will be at high risk for life-threatening infections with opportunistic pathogens owing to their requirement for immunosuppressive antirejection therapy [2]. A timetable for infections commonly seen after SOT, adapted from Fishman and Rubin's work, is shown in Fig. 25.1.

■ INFECTION BY ORGAN

Blood

Several studies have shown that liver transplant recipients have a bacteremia rate ranging from 19% to 28%. This is higher than rates seen in other types of organ transplantation. The source of bloodstream infections in liver recipients appears to have shifted over the past several years from those related to intra-abdominal and/or wound infections to those associated with intravascular lines. Improved surgical techniques have resulted in a declining incidence of intra-abdominal infections at many transplant centers, and the organisms isolated from blood have reflected this change. Currently, Gram-positive cocci (e.g. *Staphylococcus aureus*, enterococci, and coagulase-negative staphylococci) cause 40–59% of all bacteremias in liver recipients. Diabetes mellitus, creatinine greater than 2.0 mg/dL, prolonged ICU stay, and higher APACHE II scores at the time of fever onset are significant predictors of bacteremia in this population [3].

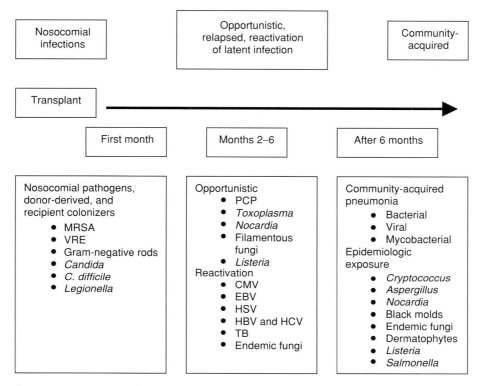

Fig. 25.1 *Sequence of posttransplant infections.*

Abdomen

Although a trend toward fewer intra-abdominal infections has been noted over the past several years, infections occurring in the abdomen remain a significant complication of liver transplantation. These infections are likely related to the complexity of the surgical procedure as well as its performance in a potentially contaminated environment. Breaches of bowel integrity and sacrifice of the sphincter of Oddi during Roux-en-Y biliary anastomosis may facilitate the reflux of enteric bacteria into the hepatobiliary system. Intrahepatic abscesses may also result from technical problems involving the implanted allograft such as hepatic artery thrombosis, biliary leak, or tear of the donor liver. Extrahepatic abscesses and peritonitis are typically related to biliary anastomotic leaks or bowel perforation, while cholangitis may be associated with biliary strictures.

An imaging study of the abdomen is often required to investigate the possibility of intra-abdominal infection after liver transplant, and any suggestion of biliary tract problems should lead to a cholangiogram. All fluid collections should be aspirated, examined for white blood cells, and evaluated with appropriate microbiologic staining and culture. Enteric Gram-negative bacteria, enterococci, anaerobes, and *Candida* species are the most likely pathogens involved in intra-abdominal infections.

Lung

Pneumonia is the second most common infection following liver transplantation [4]. It is reported in 13–34% of liver transplant recipients and accounts for 16–49% of all major infections in these patients. Even in the era of effective antimicrobial therapy, pneumonia is associated with a mortality rate up to 53% following liver transplant [5]. New pulmonary infiltrates in a liver recipient should be evaluated aggressively so that targeted antimicrobials can be utilized. Chest radiography is used to confirm the presence of pneumonia, but interpretation of the findings may be hampered by the presence of right-sided pleural effusion (infection in the pleural space is rare) or atelectasis immediately after surgery. In addition, the depressed inflammatory response of the immunocompromised host may modify or delay the appearance of abnormalities on chest X-ray (CXR). Chest computed tomogram (CT) should be considered when the CXR is negative or when the findings are subtle or nonspecific. Chest CT can help to define the extent of the disease and delineate the optimal diagnostic approach such as needle aspiration, bronchoscopy, or open lung biopsy.

Pneumonia may occur at any time during the posttransplant period, and the etiologic spectrum of pathogens is broad. Pneumonia occurring in the first month posttransplant is typically nosocomial and associated with the need for mechanical ventilation or intensive care. The most frequent cause of pneumonia during this period is aerobic Gram-negative rods including enterobacteriaceae and *Pseudomonas aeruginosa*. *S. aureus* is becoming recognized as a cause of hospital-acquired pneumonia in this population as well. Although pulmonary infections occurring after discharge may be due to common community-acquired pathogens such as *Streptococcus pneumoniae*, *Hemophilus influenzae*, and respiratory viruses, liver transplant recipients are also at high risk for infection with opportunistic pulmonary pathogens like *Legionella*, *Nocardia*, and *P. jiroveci*.

Central Nervous System

The presentation of central nervous system (CNS) infection in transplant recipients can be very different than that in normal hosts. The anti-inflammatory effects of immunosuppressive therapy may obscure signs of meningeal inflammation associated with meningitis. The most reliable constellation of symptoms suggestive of CNS infection includes unexplained fever and headache, which necessitates a complete and urgent neurological assessment with contrasted imaging of the head and lumbar puncture.

The majority of focal CNS lesions in liver transplant recipients arising within the first 30 days posttransplantation are the result of vascular events. However, up to 18% of these patients will have an infectious process. In a retrospective study by Selby et al., brain abscesses occurred in 0.63% of 2380 liver recipients and were associated with an overall mortality of 86%[6]. Those abscesses occurring acutely posttransplant were more likely to be fungal in origin while those manifesting long after transplantation, in otherwise healthy graft recipients, were typically nonfungal (i.e. *Nocardia or Toxoplasma*) [6]-[7].

Meningitis and encephalitis are also important infectious complications after SOT. The usual community-acquired bacterial and viral pathogens, in addition to more unusual organisms such as *Listeria*, are causes of acute meningitis. Subacute or chronic meningitis is more likely due to *Cryptococcus neoformans*, *Coccidioides immitus* (in areas of high endemicity), or *Mycobacterium tuberculosis*. Encephalitis may be caused by a number of viral pathogens including CMV, human herpesvirus (HHV-6), and such emerging pathogens as West Nile virus. Finally, progressive dementia, with or without focal neurological deficits, may occur as a result of infection with various viral pathogens.

■ SPECIFIC PATHOGENS

Bacteria

Bacteria are the most common cause of infection in liver transplant recipients, with a reported incidence ranging from 35% to 70%. Prolonged duration of surgery, large intraoperative transfusion requirements, additional immunosuppression, repeat abdominal surgery, use of Roux-en-Y rather than duct-to-duct biliary anastomosis, prolonged ICU stay, and CMV infection are factors associated with an increased risk of bacterial infection. Most bacterial infections occur in the first 8 weeks posttransplant and the infecting organism depends, to some degree, on the type of antimicrobial prophylaxis given [8]. Patients who receive broad-spectrum antibiotics are susceptible to aerobic Gram-negative infections and enteroccoci. Those who receive an oral antibiotic regimen for small bowel decontamination prior to surgery are susceptible to infections caused by Gram-positive organisms. Patients who receive any antibiotics, particularly β-lactam antibiotics or clindamycin, have increased risk for developing *Clostridium difficile* colitis.

Legionella species

Legionella is now recognized as a major opportunistic pathogen in SOT recipients. At certain institutions, up to 38% of bacterial pneumonias in liver recipients have been caused by *Legionella* species [9]. *Legionella pneumophila* serogroup 1 is estimated to cause 70% of reported human legionellosis. *Legionella micdadei* is also a documented pathogen in the immunosuppressed host [10]. Pneumonia is the predominant clinical syndrome and 25–50% of cases will be accompanied by watery diarrhea. In addition, transplant recipients seem to be at especially high risk for lung cavitation with this organism.

Outbreaks of *Legionella* have resulted from contaminated hospital water. As a result, some experts recommend routine culture of the water supply for this organism in all centers caring for transplant patients [11]. *Legionella* are fastidious organisms and do not grow on standard bacteriologic media. The clinical microbiology laboratory must be notified when *Legionella* is suspected so that special isolation media can be used. The *Legionella* urinary antigen test is also a useful adjunct to culture. It has a sensitivity of 70–80% and specificity of greater than 95% for the *Legionella pneumophila* serogroup [1].

Listeria monocytogenes

Listeria monocytogenes is a well-recognized cause of bacteremia and meningitis in immunocompromised individuals. It has been reported in patients with liver transplants [12,13], is life-threatening, and requires prompt diagnosis so that treatment with high-dose ampicillin can be initiated. Infection with *Listeria* typically occurs after the first month and is classically transmitted through contaminated food such as milk products, meat, and uncooked vegetables.

Nocardia Species

Another opportunistic bacterial pathogen in SOT recipients is *Nocardia*. *Nocardia* species are ubiquitous environmental saprophytes that infect humans either through direct inoculation or by inhalation of the organism. In one study from the UK, nocardiosis arose in 3.7% of liver transplant recipients over a 3.5-year period [14]. Pulmonary disease is the predominant clinical manifestation with seeding of the CNS via hematogenous spread in up to a quarter of all cases. Tropism for cerebral tissue has been confirmed experimentally and should prompt imaging studies of the CNS when pulmonary infection is diagnosed. Again, the laboratory should be notified when nocardiosis is suspected so that cultures may be held longer and appropriate media used. Sulfonamides, together with surgical drainage as clinically appropriate, are the mainstays of therapy. Prolonged therapy and monitoring is required for treatment in the nonimmunosuppressed host (6 months for pulmonary lesions and 12 months in CNS lesions). In organ transplant recipients, some experts recommend indefinite low-dose suppressive therapy after completion of the primary course of treatment [15]. Favorable therapeutic outcome may be anticipated if the diagnosis is made early and appropriate anitimicrobial therapy instituted.

■ MYCOBACTERIA

Mycobacterium tuberculosis

Tuberculosis (TB) occurs in 0.9–2.3% of liver transplant recipients, depending on the location of the center reporting. Reactivation of dormant disease is thought to be the most frequent mode of acquisition; however, transmission with the allograft, nosocomial spread, and community-acquired TB have also been documented in liver transplant recipients. Disease with TB typically occurs after the first month. During the first year posttransplant, TB is more likely to be disseminated at the time of diagnosis in the solid organ recipient as compared with the nonimmunocompromised host. In liver recipients, TB commonly involves the hepatic allograft and is associated with an overall mortality rate near 30% [16]. Treatment is complicated by the need to use drugs, such as rifampin, that can accelerate the metabolism of immuno-suppressive drugs and thereby place the patient at increased risk for rejection. All patients should undergo careful screening for TB, with a skin test and a CXR, with treatment for latent infection administered prior to transplant as indicated.

Fungi

The incidence of invasive fungal infections (IFIs) in liver transplant recipients is higher than that seen in most other types of solid organ transplants. The incidence has been reported to be as high as 42% [17]. More recent analysis, however, suggests that the overall rate of IFI is declining [18]. This shift may be a result of changing transplant practices in conjunction with effective antifungal prophylaxis targeting high-risk patients.

Specific risk factors predisposing liver recipients to fungal infection have been identified. Retransplantation, large intraoperative transfusion requirements, preoperative creatinine greater than 2 mg/dL, preoperative bilirubin greater than 10 mg/dL, choledochojejunostomy, and colonization by *Candida* species within 3 days of transplant are factors associated with a high risk for IFI [19–22]. CMV has also been shown to independently influence the risk for IFI after liver transplantation. A prospective analysis of 146 liver transplant recipients from four transplant centers in Boston demonstrated that 36% of patients with CMV disease developed an IFI within the first year posttransplant compared with 8% of those without CMV disease [23].

Singh et al. [24] evaluated the incidence of IFI in 190 consecutive liver transplant recipients over a 10-year period at a single institution. Infection rates were correlated with the evolution of transplant practices and patient characteristics. A statistically significant decrease in the duration of operation, intraoperative transfusion requirements, cold-ischemic time, use of Roux-en-Y biliary anastomosis, rate of biopsy-proven rejection, and retransplantation was documented over successive years. In addition, a significant decline in the Child–Pugh score at the time of transplantation was observed. The investigators found a significant decrease in invasive candidiasis, with an increase in invasive aspergillosis, despite little change in immunosuppressive regimens, no change in CMV infections, and no antifungal prophylaxis.

Candida and Aspergillus

Candida species remain the leading cause of fungal infection after liver transplantation, accounting for 77–83% of all IFIs. *Candida albicans* is the most frequently isolated species, followed by *Candida glabrata* and *Candida tropicalis* [17]. The abdomen continues to be the most likely site of infection.

Aspergillus species now account for 15–20% of all IFIs. The lungs are the most frequently involved site and dissemination to the brain may occur in patients with pulmonary aspergillosis. Singh et al. compared the characteristics of invasive Aspergillus (IA) infection among 26 liver recipients who underwent transplantation between 1990 and 1995 with 20 patients transplanted between 1998 and 2001 [25]. Significantly later infection (≥90 days after transplant) was seen in the 1998–2001 cohort while the earlier group was more likely to have dissemination and CNS involvement. In addition, the mortality rate appeared higher in the early cohort as compared with the later group (92% vs. 60%).

Cryptococcus, dematiaceous fungi, *Zygomycetes*, and the geographically restricted endemic fungi are also important causes of IFIs after liver transplantation. *Scedosporium apiospermum*, an asexual form of *Pseudallescheria boydii*, and *Scedosporium prolificans* have also been increasingly recognized as significant pathogens after transplant. Infection with these fungal pathogens tends to occur later in the posttransplant period.

Anitfungal Therapeutics

The number of antifungal therapeutic agents has greatly expanded in recent years. The three major classes of currently available drugs are the azoles, the enchinocandins, and the polyenes. The azole class, including fluconazole, itraconazole, ketoconazole, and the newer agents, voriconazole and posaconazole, are fungistatic drugs. Compared with fluconazole and itraconazole, voriconazole and posaconazole have a broadened spectrum of antifungal activity including activity against most yeast as well as *Aspergillus, Fusarium, Scedosporium*, and the dematiaceous fungi. Owing to its favorable therapeutic index and in vivo activity, voriconazole has become the treatment of choice for IA [26].

The echinocandins are cyclic hexapeptides that inhibit the biosynthesis of 1,3-β-glucan. These compounds function as noncompetitive inhibitors of 1,3-β-D-glucan synthase, an enzyme involved in the production of glucan polymers in the fungal cell wall [27,28]. The current generation of echinocandins includes caspofungin and micafungin (Food and Drug Administration (FDA)-approved in the USA) as well as, anidulafungin. These agents have fungicidal activity against *Candida* species and are fungistatic against *Aspergillus* species and *P. jiroveci*. The echinocandins have limited activity against *C. neoformans* and no activity against the *Zygomycetes*.

Amphotericin B, a polyene antifungal, remains the drug of choice for cryptococcal meningitis and zygomycoses. The polyenes are fungicidal drugs; however, achieving effective serum concentrations of amphotericin B is often limited by infusion-related side-effects and nephrotoxicity. The newer lipid formulations of amphotericin B have an improved safety/tolerability profile, and appear to be as effective as amphotericin B for the treatment of IFIs [29].

Diagnostic Testing

Despite improved recognition of risk factors for IFI and the availability of effective antifungal drugs, the mortality associated with invasive fungal disease remains high. This observation serves to highlight the need for aggressive diagnostic workup and treatment. In May 2003, a novel serologic assay designed to detect an antigen of *Aspergillus* was cleared by the FDA for diagnostic use. The assay is a sandwich enzyme immunoassay (EIA) using rat monoclonal antibody directed against the galactomannan epitope of *Aspergillus fumigatus*. The antibody reacts with several *Aspergillus* species as well as with exoantigens from several other molds [30]. In studies leading to FDA clearance, the galactomannan antigenemia EIA was shown to have a sensitivity of 81% and a specificity of 89% for the diagnosis of IA [30].

The utility of the galactomannan assay after liver transplant has been evaluated [31]. A study population comprising 154 liver transplant recipients was monitored twice weekly during posttransplant and subsequent hospitalizations. A total of 1594 serum samples were analyzed, and only one case of IA was documented during the study period. The patient with probable IA had a positive EIA result in three samples on initial testing, but not on repeat analysis. A total of 20 patients without IA had 23 false-positive tests (13% of patients). Patients undergoing transplant for autoimmune liver disease and those requiring dialysis were statistically more likely to have a false-positive test. In addition, 7 of the 20 patients with a false-positive test were receiving piperacillin–tazobactam (35% of patients). Even though a low incidence of IA precluded meaningful assessment of the sensitivity of the test for monitoring liver transplant recipients, it is clear that physicians must be aware of the potential for false-positive test results. The galactomannan antigenemia assay should not replace a careful microbiologic and clinical evaluation.

Cryptococcus

C. neoformans is a cause of subacute meningitis and pneumonia in SOT recipients. Its portal of entry is the lung, where it can cause local disease prior to dissemination. The clinical presentation can be subtle and often without CNS manifestations. Cyclosporine A, tacrolimus, and sirolimus are known to possess activity against *C. neoformans* [32–35]. Husain et al. [36] recently observed that SOT recipients who developed cryptococcosis while receiving tacrolimus were statistically less likely to have CNS involvement compared with other transplant recipients not receiving this drug [36].

The diagnosis of cryptococcal infection may be made through recovery of the organism from clinical specimens or with the cryptococcal antigen test on serum and/or spinal fluid. These tests are highly sensitive and specific for disease. Treatment of cryptococcal meningitis includes induction therapy with an amphotericin B product plus flucytosine followed by a switch to fluconazole for a minimum of 10 weeks to complete therapy. Treatment recommendations have been extrapolated from the guidelines for human immunodeficiency virus (HIV)-negative patients set forth by the Infectious Diseases Society of America [37].

Endemic Myscoses

Blastomyces dermatitidis, Coccidioides immitis, and *Histoplasma capsulatum* are geographically restricted fungi that cause disease in liver recipients. Three patterns of disease are observed with these organisms and include progressive primary infection, reactivation of latent infection, and reinfection. Systemic dissemination is common with all three pathogens. Clinical presentation may include fever of unexplained origin, pneumonitis unresponsive to antibiotics, or metastatic infection to skin, joints, bone, the genitourinary tract, and/or the CNS. Treatment varies based on infecting agent and site of infection.

Dematiaceous Fungi

Dematiaceous fungi, those with melanin in their cell walls, are becoming increasingly recognized as pathogens in the late posttransplant period. Average time to onset of infection with these organisms is 22 months. The majority of infections involve skin, joint, or soft tissue. Several of the organisms (*Cladophialophora bantiana* and *Dactylaria gallopava*) are neurotropic and have a tendency to cause CNS disease. The treatment of choice for these organisms is a third-generation triazole, with surgical excision if possible [38].

Pneumocystis jiroveci

P. jiroveci, previously thought to be a protozoan, has been reclassified as a fungus. *Pneumocystis pneumonia* (PCP) occurs during the second to sixth month following transplantation and has been reported to occur in 3–10% of liver recipients in the absence of prophylaxis. PCP usually presents with fever, cough, shortness of breath, and hypoxemia. CXR findings may be subtle and are characteristically interstitial and diffuse in nature. The treatment of choice is high-dose trimethopirm/sulfamethoxazole (TMP/SMX) with or without steroids, depending on the severity of the presenting illness.

■ VIRUSES

Cytomegalovirus

CMV is the most common opportunistic pathogen following liver transplantation. In one study, development of CMV disease was associated with an almost fourfold increase in the relative risk for death within 1 year following transplantation [39]. Three potential sources for CMV after liver transplantation have been identified: the donated allograft, blood products transfused from a seropositive donor, and reactivation of endogenous virus.

CMV is a herpesvirus that remains latent in cells of the myeloid lineage. Tumor necrosis factor-α (TNF-α) plays a key role in regulating the balance between latency and reactivation of CMV. Any physiological stimulus for TNF-α release has the potential to reactivate latent CMV. Unfortunately, triggers for TNF-α release include factors that occur frequently in SOT recipients such as: systemic infection, rejection, and therapy with antilymphocyte antibodies. Additionally, the main host defense against CMV is cytotoxic T-cell immunity, which is impaired in the transplant population [5].

Most CMV disease occurs between 1 and 4 months after transplantation. Patients at highest risk for CMV disease are CMV seronegative recipients of organs from seropositive donors and seropositive patients who require treatment with antilymphocyte antibodies for rejection. Without prophylaxis, attack rates for symptomatic disease of up to 64% have been described. Clinical manifestations range from a febrile viral syndrome (typically associated with leukopenia) to tissue-invasive disease. The allograft is the most frequent site of CMV-invasive disease and CMV hepatitis may occur in 4–25% of liver transplant patients [5]. Other commonly involved organs include the lungs and the gastrointestinal tract.

In the past, the diagnosis of CMV infection was typically accomplished by rapid shell vial antigen detection or by culturing the organism from clinical specimens. Care should be taken when interpreting culture results, as asymptomatic shedding is known to occur. Correlation must be made with histopathologic and immunohistochemical stains of tissue if possible. Newer, more rapid methods for diagnosing CMV infection include detection of the pp65 antigen, the CMV DNA hybrid capture test, and polymerase chain reaction (PCR) assays targeting CMV DNA. All of these methods have improved sensitivity and specificity as compared with culture. The choice of the diagnostic assay employed is typically based on the needs and resources of each individual transplant center.

Antiviral therapy with either intravenous (IV) or oral ganciclovir has been proven effective for the prevention of CMV disease in SOT recipients, but no consensus exists regarding the optimal treatment for CMV disease. Some basic principles should be followed however. Initial therapy for disease should include IV ganciclovir for 2–4 weeks, with clearance of viremia documented prior to stopping therapy. This strategy helps to prevent disease relapse as well as the development of ganciclovir resistance. Some experts add anti-CMV hyperimmune globulin for the treatment of severe or relapsing disease while others follow the IV course with 2–3 months of oral ganciclovir. Leukopenia is a common side-effect of ganciclovir, and granulocyte colony-stimulating factor (G-CSF) can be safely used as support [40]. The dose of ganciclovir should be adjusted for renal function.

Epstein–Barr Virus

EBV is a herpesvirus that has been associated with the development of PTLD. PTLD occurs in up to 2.7% of all liver recipients. As with CMV, infection with EBV may be a result of exposure to the virus in the community or from the receipt of an infected graft. Risk factors for PTLD are primary EBV infection (patients seronegative for EBV pretransplant who develop infection posttransplant), CMV disease, and treatment with antilymphocyte antibodies. Unchecked viral replication can occur in the setting of defective cytotoxic T-cell immunity, and EBV-infected B lymphocytes may undergo uncontrolled expansion leading to lymphoproliferative disease. Not all PTLD is of B cell origin however. Up to 2% of PTLD may be T-cell derived [41].

PTLD usually occurs 6 or more months after transplantation and typically involves the transplanted graft. Extranodal presentations with invasion of the brain, bone marrow, gastrointestinal tract, or lung are seen as well. Mortality rates range from 69% to 81%. Older age, longer interval to onset after transplantation, and monoclonality of the lymphoma are associated with poor outcomes [42]. Tissue biopsy with histologic classification is the mainstay of diagnosis.

Treatment of PTLD remains controversial. Initial intervention should be a reduction in immunosuppression, but there are no established guidelines regarding "how much" to reduce or "how long" to maintain the reduction. Additionally, the effectiveness of antiviral therapy (such as acyclovir) in this setting has not been established. Chemotherapy, immunotherapy, radiation, and surgical excision have also been used to treat PTLD. Clinical trials comparing the various treatment regimens are just beginning. Future strategies will likely involve PCR testing to detect replicating EBV in blood as a marker of risk for developing PTLD. Such surveillance could allow a targeted decrease in immunosuppression to help control expansion of proliferating lymphocyte clones and, in theory, prevent the development of PTLD [43].

Human Herpesvirus-6

HHV-6 is a recognized pathogen in transplant recipients, but the precise epidemiological and clinical aspects of infection with this virus remain to be resolved. The primary target of HHV-6 is the CD4+ lymphocyte, a characteristic shared with HIV. Primary infection with HHV-6 is a significant risk factor for CMV disease in liver transplant recipients. Similarly, CMV infection is associated with concurrent HHV-6 antigenemia in liver transplant patients [44]. The usual timing of infection is 2–4 weeks after transplantation. Bone marrow suppression, pneumonitis, and encephalopathy are the most commonly reported clinical manifestations. Cell culture remains the gold standard for the diagnosis. A shell vial assay, antigenemia assay, and PCR test are also available and may expedite viral detection. The organism's susceptibility profile echoes that of CMV; it is resistant to acyclovir but sensitive to ganciclovir and foscarnet [45,46].

Varicella–Zoster Virus

Varicella–zoster virus (VZV) reactivates as dermatomal zoster in 3–7% of liver recipients. Reactivation occurs approximately 3 months after transplantation. As with the other herpesviruses, use of antilymphocyte antibodies confers a risk for VZV reactivation. Occasionally zoster, and in patients without prior infection or vaccination, primary varicella, can be disseminated and associated with a high mortality. Acyclovir is the drug of choice for these infections.

Respiratory Viruses

The respiratory viruses include influenza A and B; respiratory syncytial virus (RSV); parainfluenza 1, 2, and 3; and adenovirus. The clinical importance of infection with these viruses in the SOT population is not well defined. However, immunosuppressed patients may have more severe infection and/or have symptoms that persist longer than those occurring in normal hosts. Infections with these agents are likely underreported given their wide range of clinical manifestations and the poor availability of adequate diagnostic laboratory tests. Similarities amongst the respiratory viruses include seasonality, person-to-person transmission, relatively short incubation periods, acquisition in the community or nosocomially, and use of the respiratory tract as the portal of entry and site of disease expression.

Although these pathogens often produce similar symptoms, the risk of complications varies considerably by virus and transplant type [47]. Hierholzer et al. performed a comprehensive review of over 300 cases of adenoviral infection in immunocompromised patients [48]. The study revealed that 11% of the transplant recipients evaluated became infected with adenoviruses, and the infection frequently involved the organ system transplanted. The level of immunosuppression, patient age, and serotype of the infecting virus were all associated with mortality. Most of the adenovirus infections observed in renal transplant patients were caused by subgenus B, and these infections had a fatality rate of 17%. In comparison, subgenus C serotypes were more common in liver recipients and had an overall fatality rate of 53%.

Direct antigen detection is the most rapid means for diagnosing respiratory viral infections. Antigen detection can be performed in a matter of hours on clinical specimens with relatively good sensitivity and specificity. In addition, these viruses often grow well in cell culture, and standard culture should be a part of the routine laboratory evaluation for respiratory viruses.

The mainstay of treatment for viral respiratory infection is supportive care. Unfortunately, there are no well-defined treatment options for adenovirus infections. Amantidine and rimantidine were the first licensed antiviral agents for the treatment of influenza A in adults in the USA. The neuraminidase inhibitors zanamavir (inhaled) and oseltamivir (oral) are now FDA-cleared for the treatment of both influenza A and B. All of these agents must be started within the first 48 hours of symptoms. Treatment benefit is typically a modest decrease in the duration of symptoms. Possible benefits in the prevention of complications or the treatment of influenza pneumonia are unproven, and trials in the transplant population have not been conducted. Nevertheless, most authorities support the use of these agents in the treatment of complicated influenza infection. Precaution should be taken when prescribing zanamivir to patients with underlying asthma or chronic obstructive pulmonary disease due to its risk of bronchospasm. Ribavirin, a synthetic nucleoside, is approved (by aerosol delivery) for the treatment of RSV pneumonia and bronchiolitis in hospitalized infants and children. Studies of ribavirin in the transplant population have not been performed. In addition to being expensive, administration of the drug requires special precaution owing to its toxicity in people wearing contacts or who are pregnant. Although ribavirin may be used in severe cases of RSV pneumonia, routine use of this medication is not recommended.

■ PROTOZOA/PARASITES

Toxoplasma gondii

Toxoplasmosis, caused by the protozoan *Toxoplasma gondii*, is an important disease in immunocompromised hosts. Although heart recipients have the highest incidence of disease among SOT recipients, toxoplasmosis has been described in recipients of liver transplants as well. The disease results from transmission in an infected organ or due to reactivation of latent infection. Clinical findings range from headaches associated with ring-enhancing lesions in the brain to multiorgan failure from disseminated disease. A review of the literature reported six cases of disseminated disease in liver recipients with a mortality rate of 83% [49]. The disease occurred within the first 3 months after transplant and initial manifestations of dissemination were fever and pneumonia. Treatment of disease is with high-dose TMP/SMX.

Strongyloides stercoralis

Strongyloidiasis is a potentially lethal nematode infection in transplant patients. One-third of infected individuals are asymptomatic, and patients may not be aware of their colonization prior to transplant. The typical route of infection is through skin contact with contaminated soil. Following immunosuppression, patients carrying the parasite may develop a hyperinfection syndrome as the worms migrate from the intestine to the lung by way of the blood. Severe abdominal pain, diffuse pulmonary infiltrates, ileus, shock, meningitis, and sepsis with multiple Gram-negative rods may occur. Treatment includes thiabendazole or albendazole. The mortality rate is high despite therapy.

Prevention/Prophylaxis

One double-strength TMP/SMX tablet taken once a day or three times a week helps to prevent infection with PCP, *Listeria monocytogenes*, and *T. gondii*. Prophylaxis should be continued for 6 months after transplantation or longer in patients receiving continued heavy immunosuppression. Patients allergic to sulfa-containing medications may be given dapsone or inhaled pentamidine as alternatives for PCP prophylaxis.

Antifungal Prophylaxis

Studies evaluating the efficacy of fluconazole as prophylaxis during the peri-transplant period have shown a decrease in the overall incidence of IFI from 23% to 5.6% [17]. Interestingly, two randomized controlled trials demonstrating the efficacy of prophylactic fluconazole did not document an increase in azole-resistant *Candida* species compared with the control groups [50,51]. As expected, fluconazole was not effective in preventing *Candida krusei* and *C. glabrata* infection. Liposomal amphotericin B has also been shown to effectively reduce candidal infection during the first months after liver transplant [52], but no multicenter trials have been performed. Whether the preemptive use of antifungal therapy improves overall clinical outcome remains to be proven and additional clinical trials are required to delineate the optimal prophylaxis against molds.

Antiviral Prophylaxis

Antiviral prophylaxis should begin with assessment of donor and recipient CMV serostatus. Two therapeutic strategies have been evaluated for the prevention of CMV disease after SOT. These strategies include universal prophylaxis, in which all patients at risk for CMV infection/disease receive antiviral therapy, and preemptive therapy that is guided by the results of frequent laboratory surveillance. In terms of CMV-related mortality, the two strategies appear to be equivalent [53]. Most experts agree that patients at high risk for CMV disease (donor seropositive and recipient seronegative) should receive ganciclovir prophylaxis immediately posttransplant for up to 90 days. Patients requiring treatment with antilymphocyte antibodies should receive ganciclovir prophylaxis as well. Patients with an intermediate risk for CMV (seropositive recipients) may do equally well with a preemptive approach. Patients at low risk for CMV disease (seronegative donor and seronegative recipient) but with positive serology for HSV can be prophylaxed with oral acyclovir [54].

The efficacy and safety of once-daily valganciclovir, a valine ester prodrug of ganciclovir, was compared with oral ganciclovir for the prevention of CMV disease in 364 high-risk SOT recipients [55]. In an intention-to-treat analysis,

12% of valganciclovir recipients and 15.2% of ganciclovir recipients developed CMV disease by the 6-month analysis. At 12 months, the incidence of CMV disease in the valganciclovir and ganciclovir groups was 17.2% and 18.4%, respectively. The differences between groups were not statistically significant, and the study established the overall noninferiority of valganciclovir as compared with oral ganciclovir. Time to onset of CMV disease and viremia was delayed in the valganciclovir group, and a higher incidence of neutropenia was noted. In subgroup analysis, a statistically significant interaction between treatment and organ type was observed. The 6-month incidence of CMV disease in liver recipients ($n = 118$) receiving valganciclovir was 19% as compared with 12% in the ganciclovir group. As a result, valganciclovir was not approved by the FDA for prophylaxis in liver transplant recipients. Further studies are needed to better understand whether the efficacy of valganciclovir might be different than oral ganciclovir after liver transplantation.

Vaccination

Vaccination status should be reviewed and updated prior to transplantation. Although vaccine immune responses may be less robust in transplant recipients, studies have demonstrated clinical benefit from incomplete responses. In general, live vaccines should be avoided due to the risk of viral dissemination in the transplanted population. Hepatitis A, hepatitis B, and varicella immune status should be determined and vaccines administered as appropriate [56, 57]. Patients born before 1957 and those without written documentation of having received the measles–mumps–rubella (MMR) vaccine should receive the MMR vaccine. Pneumococcal vaccine should be administered pretransplant and every 5 years thereafter. Yearly administration of the influenza vaccine is recommended for all transplant recipients and a booster for tetanus toxoid should be given every 5 years as well.

■ REFERENCES

1. Paya CV, Hermans PE, Washington JA, et al. Incidence, distribution, and outcome of episodes of infection in 100 orthotopic liver transplantations. Mayo Clin Proc 1989;64(5):555–564.

2. Fishman JA, Rubin RH. Infection in organ-transplant recipients. N Engl J Med 1998;338(24):1741–1751.

3. Chang FY, Singh N, Gayowski T, et al. Fever in liver transplant recipients: changing spectrum of etiologic agents. Clin Infect Dis 1998;26(1):59–65.

4. Kusne S, Dummer JS, Singh N, et al. Infections after liver transplantation. An analysis of 101 consecutive cases. Medicine 1988;67(2):132–143.

5. Singh N. Infectious diseases in the liver transplant recipient. Semin Gastrointest Dis 1998;9(3):136–146.

6. Selby R, Ramirez CB, Singh R, et al. Brain abscess in solid organ transplant recipients receiving cyclosporine-based immunosuppression. Arch Surg 1997;132(3):304–310.

7. Bonham CA, Dominguez EA, Fukui MB, et al. Central nervous system lesions in liver transplant recipients: prospective assessment of indications for biopsy and implications for management. Transplantation 1998;66(12):1596–1604.

8. Winston DJ, Emmanouilides C, Busuttil RW. Infections in liver transplant recipients. Clin Infect Dis 1995;21(5):1077–1089.

9. Chow JW, Yu VL. Legionella: a major opportunistic pathogen in transplant recipients. Semin Resp Infect 1998;13(2):132–139.

10. Knirsch CA, Jakob K, Schoonmaker D, et al. An outbreak of *Legionella micdadei* pneumonia in transplant patients: evaluation, molecular epidemiology, and control (see comment). Am J Med 2000;108(4):290–295.

11. Singh N, Gayowski T, Wagener M, et al. Pulmonary infections in liver transplant recipients receiving tacrolimus. Changing pattern of microbial etiologies. Transplantation 1996;61(3):396–401.

12. Limaye AP, Perkins JD, Kowdley KV. Listeria infection after liver transplantation: report of a case and review of the literature. Am J Gastroenterol 1998;93(10):1942–1944.

13. Bourgeois N, Jacobs F, Tavares ML, et al. *Listeria monocytogenes* hepatitis in a liver transplant recipient: a case report and review of the literature. J Hepatol 1993;18(3):284–289.

14. Forbes GM, Harvey FA, Philpott-Howard JN, et al. Nocardiosis in liver transplantation: variation in presentation, diagnosis and therapy. J Infect 1990;20(1):11–19.

15. Sorrell TC, Iredell JR, Mitchell DH. Nocardia species. In Mandell GL, Bennett JE, Dolin R, eds., Principles and practice of infectious diseases. Philadelphia, PA: Churchill Livingstone, 2000:2637–2645.

16. Nishizaki T, Yanaga K, Soejima Y, et al. Tuberculosis following liver transplantation: report of a case and review of the literature. Transpl Int 1996;9(6):589–592.

17. Paya CV. Fungal infections in solid-organ transplantation. Clin Infect Dis 1993;16(5):677–688.

18. Pappas PG, ABMKKDH Seal. Invasive fungal infections (IFIs) in hematopoietic stem cell (HSCTs) and organ transplant recipients (ORTs): overview of the TRANSNET database. 42nd Annual Meeting of the Infectious Diseases Society of America 42 (abstract number 682), 2004;174.

19. Castaldo P, Stratta RJ, Wood RP, et al. Clinical spectrum of fungal infections after orthotopic liver transplantation. Arch Surg 1991;126(2):149–156.

20. Collins LA, Samore MH, Roberts MS, et al. Risk factors for invasive fungal infections complicating orthotopic liver transplantation. J Infect Dis 1994;170(3):644–652.

21. Hadley S, Samore MH, Lewis WD, et al. Major infectious complications after orthotopic liver transplantation and comparison of outcomes in patients receiving cyclosporine or FK506 as primary immunosuppression. Transplantation 1995;59(6):851–859.

22. Karchmer AW, Samore MH, Hadley S, et al. Fungal infections complicating orthotopic liver transplantation. Trans Am Clin Climatol Assoc 1994;106:38–47.

23. George MD, Snydman MD, Werner P, et al. The independent role of cytomegalovirus as a risk factor for invasive fungal disease in orthotopic liver transplant recipients. Am J Med 1997;103(2):106–113.

24. Singh N, Wagener MM, Marino IR, et al. Trends in invasive fungal infections in liver transplant recipients: correlation with evolution in transplantation practices. Transplantation 2002;73(1):63–67.

25. Singh N, Avery RK, Munoz P, et al. Trends in risk profiles for and mortality associated with invasive aspergillosis among liver transplant recipients. Clin Infect Dis 2003;36(1):46–52.

26. Herbrecht R, Denning DW, Patterson TF, et al. Voriconazole versus amphotericin B for primary therapy of invasive aspergillosis. N Engl J Med 2002;347(6):408–415.

27. Denning DW. Echinocandins: a new class of antifungal. J Antimicrob Chemother 2002;49(6):889–891.

28. Walsh TJ. Echinocandins – an advance in the primary treatment of invasive candidiasis. N Engl J Med 2002;347(25):2070–2072.

29. Dupont B. Overview of the lipid formulations of amphotericin B. J Antimicrob Chemother 2002;49(90001):31–36.

30. Wheat LJ. Rapid diagnosis of invasive aspergillosis by antigen detection. Transpl Infect Dis 2003;5(4):158–166.

31. Kwak EJ, Husain S, Obman A, et al. Efficacy of galactomannan antigen in the *Platelia aspergillus* enzyme immunoassay for diagnosis of invasive aspergillosis in liver transplant recipients. J Clin Microbiol 2004;42(1):435–438.

32. Odom A, Del Poeta M, Perfect J, et al. The immunosuppressant FK506 and its nonimmunosuppressive analog L-685,818 are toxic to *Cryptococcus neoformans* by inhibition of a common target protein. Antimicrob Agents Chemother 1997;41(1):156–161.

33. Cruz MC, Cavallo LM, Gorlach JM, et al. Rapamycin antifungal action is mediated via conserved complexes with FKBP12 and TOR kinase homologs in *Cryptococcus neoformans*. Mol Cell Biol 1999;19(6):4101–4112.

34. Cruz MC, Del Poeta M, Wang P, et al. Immunosuppressive and nonimmunosuppressive cyclosporine analogs are toxic to the opportunistic fungal pathogen

Cryptococcus neoformans via cyclophilin-dependent inhibition of calcineurin. Antimicrob Agents Chemother 2000;44(1):143–149.

35. Odom A, Muir S, Lim E, et al. Calcineurin is required for virulence of *Cryptococcus neoformans*. EMBO J 1997;16(10):2576–2589.

36. Husain S, Wagener MM, Singh N. *Cryptococcus neoformans* infection in organ transplant recipients: variables influencing clinical characteristics and outcome. Emerg Infect Dis 2001;7(3):375–381.

37. Saag MS, Graybill RJ, Larsen RA, et al. Practice guidelines for the management of cryptococcal disease. Infectious Diseases Society of America. Clin Infect Dis 2000;30(4):710–718.

38. Singh N, Chang FY, Gayowski T, et al. Infections due to dematiaceous fungi in organ transplant recipients: case report and review. Clin Infect Dis 1997;24(3):369–374.

39. Falagas ME, Snydman DR, Griffith J, et al. Effect of cytomegalovirus infection status on first-year mortality rates among orthotopic liver transplant recipients. The Boston Center for Liver Transplantation CMVIG Study Group. Ann Intern Med 1997;126(4):275–279.

40. Winston DJ, Foster PF, Somberg KA, et al. Randomized, placebo-controlled, double-blind, multicenter trial of efficacy and safety of granulocyte colony-stimulating factor in liver transplant recipients. Transplantation 1999;68(9):1298–1304.

41. Paya CV, Fung JJ, Nalesnik MA, et al. Epstein–Barr virus-induced posttransplant lymphoproliferative disorders. ASTS/ASTP EBV–PTLD Task Force and the Mayo Clinic Organized International Consensus Development Meeting. Transplantation 1999;68(10):1517–1525.

42. Manez R, Breinig MC, Linden P, et al. Posttransplant lymphoproliferative disease in primary Epstein–Barr virus infection after liver transplantation: the role of cytomegalovirus disease. J Infect Dis 1997;176(6):1462–1467.

43. Scheenstra R, Verschuuren EAM, de Haan A, et al. The value of prospective monitoring of Epstein–Barr virus DNA in blood samples of pediatric liver transplant recipients. Transpl Infect Dis 2004;6(1):15–22.

44. Lautenschlager I, Lappalainen M, Linnavuori K, et al. CMV infection is usually associated with concurrent HHV-6 and HHV-7 antigenemia in liver transplant patients. J Clin Virol 2002;25(suppl 2):S57–S61.

45. Dockrell DH, Smith TF, Paya CV. Human herpesvirus 6. Mayo Clin Proc 1999;74(2):163–170.

46. Singh N, Carrigan DR. Human herpesvirus-6 in transplantation: an emerging pathogen. Ann Intern Med 1996;124(12):1065–1071.

47. Sable CA, Hayden FG. Orthomyxoviral and paramyxoviral infections in transplant patients. Infect Dis Clin North Am 1995;9(4):987–1003.

48. Hierholzer JC. Adenoviruses in the immunocompromised host. Clin Microbiol Rev 1992;5(3):262–274.

49. Lappalainen M, Jokiranta TS, Halme L, et al. Disseminated toxoplasmosis after liver transplantation: case report and review. Clin Infect Dis 1998;27(5):1327–1328.

50. Lumbreras C, Cuervas-Mons V, Jara P, et al. Randomized trial of fluconazole versus nystatin for the prophylaxis of Candida infection following liver transplantation. J Infect Dis 1996;174(3):583–588.

51. Winston DJ, Pakrasi A, Busuttil RW. Prophylactic fluconazole in liver transplant recipients. A randomized, double-blind, placebo-controlled trial. Ann Intern Med 1999;131(10):729–737.

52. Tollemar J, Hockerstedt K, Ericzon BG, et al. Prophylaxis with liposomal amphotericin B (AmBisome) prevents fungal infections in liver transplant recipients: long-term results of a randomized, placebo-controlled trial. Transplant Proc 1995;27(1):1195–1198.

53. Singh N. Preemptive therapy versus universal prophylaxis with ganciclovir for cytomegalovirus in solid organ transplant recipients. Clin Infect Dis 2001;32(5):742–751.

54. Patel R, Snydman DR, Rubin RH, et al. Cytomegalovirus prophylaxis in solid organ transplant recipients (review; 58 references). Transplantation 1996;61(9):1279–1289.

55. Paya C, Humar A, Dominguez E, et al. Efficacy and safety of valganciclovir vs. oral ganciclovir for prevention of cytomegalovirus disease in solid organ transplant recipients. Am J Transplant 2004;4(4):611–620.

56. Cohen JI, Brunell PA, Straus SE, et al. Recent advances in varicella–zoster virus infection. Ann Intern Med 1999;130(11):922–932.

57. White CJ. Varicella–zoster virus vaccine. Clin Infect Dis 1997;24(5):753–761.

Renal Function Posttransplant

▼ ▼ ▼ ▼ ▼ ▼ ▼ ▼ ▼

Stephen R. Smith

WITH BROADENING of the inclusion criteria for liver transplantation, the majority of liver transplant recipients have some impairment of renal function prior to transplantation and most have clinically apparent renal insufficiency at some time in the posttransplant period [1–3]. Among those with renal impairment at the time of transplant are patients whose renal failure comes from the same underlying process that caused the liver disease (hepatitis B, hepatitis C, analgesic overdose, amyloidosis, auto-immune disease), patients with underlying parenchymal renal disease from diseases such as diabetes and hypertension, and other patients in whom the functional renal impairment is caused by the liver failure itself and its complications. The latter group may have manifestations ranging from mild sodium retention to oliguric renal failure termed hepatorenal syndrome (HRS).

For both prognostic and therapeutic reasons it is important to assess the level of renal function in patients being considered for liver transplantation and to determine if there is any reversible component. A general approach to the patient with liver disease and renal insufficiency is presented below, followed by discussion of specific causes of renal dysfunction in the posttransplant period, including calcineurin inhibitor (cyclosporine and tacrolimus) toxicity and virus-associated glomerulonephritis.

■ MEASUREMENT OF RENAL FUNCTION

The most commonly used markers of glomerular filtration rate (GFR), blood urea nitrogen (BUN) and serum creatinine, have limitations that should be kept in mind, especially in the setting of liver transplantation.

Because urea is generated by the liver from the metabolism of protein and ammonia, both malnutrition and poor hepatic function may cause a "falsely" low BUN that can lead to an overestimation of GFR. Conversely, corticosteroids, bleeding (particularly in the gastrointestinal tract), and renal hypoperfusion cause BUN levels higher than one would expect for a given level of GFR. Furthermore, because urea is reabsorbed by the nephron (to a varying degree dependent on urine flow), urea clearance underestimates GFR.

Creatinine is generated predominantly in the skeletal muscle. Thus, patients with decreased muscle mass (most cirrhotic patients) may have a misleadingly low serum creatinine. Furthermore, creatinine is both filtered and secreted by the nephron, so that the clearance of creatinine is an overestimate of GFR. In addition, a number of medications (including trimethoprim, cimetidine, and cefazolin) inhibit the secretion of creatinine, so that when these medications are used the serum creatinine may rise without any true change in GFR. It should also be noted that the relationship between the serum creatinine and GFR is not linear; at high levels of GFR, the serum creatinine is insensitive to large changes in GFR, while at low levels of GFR, small changes in GFR cause large changes in serum creatinine [4].

Despite these limitations, the endogenous creatinine clearance from a timed urine collection or as calculated from the Cockcroft–Gault formula [5] $\{(140-\text{age})/\text{Cr} \times (\text{wt. in kg}/72) \ (\times \ 0.85 \text{ for females})\}$ remains the most common measure of GFR. The accuracy of this calculation can be enhanced by pretreatment with cimetidine to block the tubular secretion of creatinine. If a timed urine collection is performed, the amount of creatinine excreted in 24 h should be 12–25 mg/kg body weight as a crude test for completeness of the collection. Because of the variability in the accuracy of timed collections performed by outpatients, and the excellent correlation of the Cockcroft–Gault calculation with timed creatinine clearance measurements under controlled conditions, a timed collection may be necessary only for a baseline creatinine clearance and to measure protein excretion. It can then be repeated only as necessary to confirm abrupt or unexpected changes in the serum creatinine. There are numerous other methods to estimate GFR from demographic and laboratory variables such as the modification of diet in renal disease (MDRD) and the modified MDRD formulas [6] and there are now online calculators that provide a convenient way to estimate GFR (e.g. http://nephron.com/gi-bin/MDRDSIdefault.cgi). However, in liver transplant recipients, even the best performing equation, the six-variable MDRD equation, provides an estimate that is within 30% of the actual GFR only two-thirds of the time [7].

Where available, the measurement of GFR using an exogenous substance such as ethylenediaminetetraacetic acid (EDTA), diethylenetriamine pentaacetic acid (DTPA), iothalamate, or iohexol is preferred. Like inulin, these substances are filtered, but neither secreted nor reabsorbed, and are easier to use than inulin [8]. The cost of the radiolabeled GFR markers and the precautions needed in handling them make these tests expensive. Many nuclear medicine departments now perform isotopic GFR measurements based on the decay of the plasma level of an injected radiolabeled GFR marker over a few hours.

■ GENERAL APPROACH TO ACUTE DECREASES IN RENAL FUNCTION

As in all patients with a decline in renal function, the initial efforts should be directed toward eliminating urinary tract obstruction and poor renal perfusion as causes. Ultrasound examination of the kidneys is a highly sensitive screen for obstruction of the collecting systems. Marked volume depletion and retroperitoneal fibrosis can rarely lead to a false-negative ultrasound in patients with obstruction. Furthermore, not all dilated collecting systems are obstructed. Congenital abnormalities are the most common cause of false-positive ultrasounds. Nuclear medicine scans performed before and after the administration of furosemide can often differentiate between a congenitally dilated collecting system and an obstructed one. At the time of ultrasonography, the renal vascular resistance can be assessed. Hepatorenal syndrome (and to a lesser extent prerenal azotemia) is characterized by intense renal vascular constriction measurable by Doppler techniques as high renal vascular resistance.

The determination of the patient's volume status can be particularly difficult in the setting of liver disease. In addition to orthostatic changes in blood pressure and heart rate and inspection of the jugular venous contour, the spot urine sodium concentration and urine to plasma ratio of creatinine can be helpful in the differential diagnosis if diuretics have not been given recently (see Table 26.1) [2]. In a patient taking diuretics, a fractional excretion of urea ([(urine urea nitrogen/BUN)/(urine creatinine/plasma creatinine)] $\times 100$) less than 35% is a better indicator of reduced renal perfusion than indices based on the urine sodium concentration [9]. Volume depletion, hypotension, low car-

Table 26.1 *Differential Diagnosis of Renal Failure in Advanced Liver Disease (adapted from Eckardt [2])*

	Prerenal Azotemia	Acute Tubular Necrosis	Hepatorenal Syndrome	Primary Nephropathy
Urine sodium	<10 meq/L	>30 mmol/L	<10 mmol/L	>30 mmol/L
Urine to plasma creatinine ratio	>30:1	<20:1	>30:1	<20:1
Proteinuria	<100 mg	<500 mg	<500 mg	Variable

diac output, and sepsis are common causes of poor renal perfusion. In addition, HRS and intravenous administration of contrast material are both associated with renal vasoconstriction and avid sodium retention by the kidneys. Renal artery stenosis should be considered in the presence of new or worsening hypertension associated with a decline in GFR. Magnetic resonance angiography provides a sensitive, noninvasive, and nonnephrotoxic way to diagnose renovascular disease. If there is uncertainty with regard to the possible presence of intravascular volume depletion, a therapeutic trial of 1.5 L of isotonic saline intravenously should be considered.

Having ruled out pre- and postrenal causes of renal insufficiency, attention can be turned to parenchymal renal disease. The evaluation should include a urinalysis, and especially if qualitative proteinuria is present, a 24-h collection of urine for protein and creatinine. Serologic studies for complement components, antinuclear antibodies, hepatitis B surface antigen, hepatitis C antibody, cryoglobulins, and rheumatoid factor may be indicated. In patients with a history of glucose intolerance, formal ophthalmologic evaluation for diabetic retinopathy may be useful. Renal biopsy is occasionally required for clarification of the diagnosis and for renal prognosis.

■ RENAL DISEASE ASSOCIATED WITH VIRAL HEPATITIS

Both hepatitis B and hepatitis C have been associated with glomerular disease. The data that hepatitis B virus (HBV) and hepatitis C virus (HCV) cause glomerulonephritis in some patients are indirect, but compelling. The most common clinical presentation in both cases is the nephrotic syndrome with a slowly progressive decline in renal function [10,11]. The proteinuria remits spontaneously in a minority of patients, but may also recur. The degree of proteinuria appears to correlate with viremia as spontaneous remission of the glomerulopathy is usually associated with clearance of viral antigens from the blood. End-stage renal disease may result from the glomerulonephritis induced by either hepatitis B or C.

The renal histology in HBV-associated renal disease is that of membranous glomerulonephritis in most cases, but membranoproliferative glomerulonephritis, mesangial proliferative glomerulonephritis, focal segmental glomerulosclerosis, and minimal change disease have all been described. In addition, in patients with HBV-associated polyarteritis nodosa, a variety of histologic patterns have been documented. HBV antigens have been localized in the glomeruli using immunofluorescent antibodies, electron microscopy, and molecular techniques. HBeAg has been consistently associated with capillary basement membrane deposits (membranous form of glomerulopathy), while HBsAG is more closely associated with deposits in the mesangium [10,12].

Hepatitis C has been associated most closely with membranoproliferative glomerulonephritis [13–15]. Many of the patients with chronic HCV and membranoproliferative glomerulonephritis also have hypocomplementemia, cryoglobulinemia (the cryoprecipitates contain HCV-RNA), and rheumatoid factors (IgM antibodies directed against anti-HCV antibodies) [13–15]. Other symptoms and signs of mixed cryoglobulinemia such as skin lesions, arthritis, and neuropathy may not be present. Indeed, even the hepatitis associated with the renal disease may be asymptomatic and the transaminases may be normal [14]. A purely membranous glomerulonephritis has also been reported in patients with HCV, and may have a different pathogenesis [16]. Whether the natural history of virus-associated glomerulonephritis is different in transplanted patients taking immunosuppressive agents is not known, but these entities do occur in transplanted patients [13].

Therapy in patients with glomerulonephritis associated with chronic viral hepatitis should be aimed at clearing the viremia. Corticosteroids have not been shown to be of benefit. For patients with hepatitis C, treatment with α-interferon may result in clearance of the viral antigenemia and decrease in proteinuria in some cases. Unfortunately, cessation of therapy is often associated with recurrent viremia and increased proteinuria [14]. Combination therapy with α-interferon and ribavirin provides a sustained virological remission in some patients [17]. However, ribavirin is contraindicated in patients with kidney disease. Treatment with pegylated interferon α2b alone is successful in clearing the virus in a minority of treated patients with kidney disease, but is poorly tolerated [18]. Likewise, in patients with hepatitis B, lamivudine [19], α-interferon, and hepatitis B immune globulin have been used to render patients free of hepatitis B DNA. The optimal timing and combination of agents for the treatment of viral hepatitis continues to evolve. It is clear that it is much more difficult to achieve sustained virological remission in patients being treated with immunosuppressant agents after transplantation.

Nonspecific therapy for the nephrotic syndrome should include diuretics, and, if hyperkalemia can be managed, the use of an angiotensin-converting enzyme inhibitor or angiotensin receptor blocker. Control of hyperlipidemia is also important, but can be complicated by the presence of impaired liver transplant function.

■ RENAL DISEASE ASSOCIATED WITH POOR HEPATIC FUNCTION

Patients with poor hepatic function of any cause may develop parenchymal renal disease manifested by nonnephrotic proteinuria, microscopic hematuria, and reduced GFR. The most common histologic picture is a mesangiopathic glomerulonephritis with deposition of IgM and often IgA, perhaps because of impaired clearance by the liver. It has not been proved that these immune complexes are the cause of the renal disease.

Hepatorenal Syndrome

Patients with end-stage liver disease may exhibit a spectrum of functional renal impairment from mild sodium retention and clinically unapparent reduction in GFR, to an oliguric state with severe intrarenal vasoconstriction, avid sodium conservation, and very low GFR referred to as hepatorenal syndrome [2]. HRS is a diagnosis of exclusion, requiring the absence of sepsis and nephrotoxic agents, less than 500 mg/day of protein excretion, an ultrasound showing no evidence of obstruction or parenchymal renal disease, and a lack of improvement with cessation of diuretic therapy and plasma volume expansion [20]. If the syndrome persists, acute tubular necrosis may result. Thus, the urine sodium concentration is less than 10 meq/L early in the process, but as tubular ischemia occurs, the urine sodium rises, clouding the diagnostic issue (see Table 26.1) [2,21]. The mechanisms underlying the development of HRS, reviewed in detail elsewhere [22], have not been fully elucidated but are likely in part on the basis of splanchnic vasodilatation as well as abnormalities in autoregulation of renal blood flow due to changes in sympathetic nervous system output, levels of endothelins, vasoconstrictor prostaglandins, the renin/angiotensin system, and nitric oxide metabolism.

Transjugular intrahepatic portosystemic shunt (TIPS) placement ameliorates the tendency toward sodium retention and improves GFR in the majority of patients with HRS, in addition to lowering portal pressures [23]. The procedure has significant risks including precipitation of hepatic encephalopathy and, in the patient with poor left ventricular function, pulmonary edema.

■ SURVIVAL AFTER LIVER TRANSPLANTATION IN PATIENTS WITH RENAL DISEASE

Retrospective studies indicate that patient survival after liver transplantation is reduced in patients with HRS pretransplant versus patients without HRS, but the majority have improvement in renal function after liver transplantation [24]. HRS is thus not a contraindication to liver transplantation.

Although improvement in renal function often occurs in the first 6 weeks after successful liver transplantation, approximately 7–10% of patients with HRS develop end-stage renal disease in the posttransplant period.

Renal replacement therapy is required in the first month in approximately 10% of patients with renal insufficiency pretransplant versus 2% of those with normal renal function prior to transplant [25]. Approximately 35% of patients experience a permanent decline in GFR of $30 \, \text{mL/min/1.73 m}^2$ after transplantation, with the rate of decline maximal at 1 month posttransplant [26]. Registry data indicate that the pretransplant level of renal function is also predictive of graft and patient survival after transplantation. For instance, the adjusted odds ratio for death within 30 days of transplantation is 1.5 for patients with creatinine clearance 40–70 mL/min, 2.9 for creatinine clearance 20–40 mL/min. and 3.4 for creatinine clearance <20 mL/min, compared with a reference group with creatinine clearance > 70 mL/min. With the adoption of allocation of organs based on model for end-stage liver disease (MELD) score, more patients with renal disease are likely to receive a liver transplant, and lower than expected outcomes may be observed [27].

The indications for combined liver/kidney transplantation are continuing to evolve. It is clear that patients with functional renal insufficiency including those with HRS should not receive a simultaneous kidney transplant because of the high likelihood of improvement in native renal function post liver transplant. The combined procedure should probably be reserved for a subset of those patients with end-stage renal disease due to genetic disease that can be functionally cured by transplantation of a liver (e.g. primary oxalosis), and those with end-stage liver disease and biopsy-proved parenchymal renal disease.

Calcineurin Inhibitor Nephrotoxicity

Cyclosporine and tacrolimus are common causes of reduced GFR in liver transplant recipients. The adverse renal effects of these drugs take several forms [28–30]. Almost all patients taking cyclosporine or tacrolimus in therapeutic dosages experience a dose-related decrease in renal blood flow and GFR. This reduction in GFR is largely due to renal vasoconstriction, with both the afferent and the efferent arterioles affected. In its most extreme form, there is tubular damage and a clinical picture of acute tubular necrosis, perhaps on the basis of ischemia. Calcineurin inhibitors appear to be direct proximal tubule toxins only at blood levels an order of magnitude higher than therapeutic levels. The mechanism of the renal hemodynamic effects of calcineurin inhibitor toxicity involves increased production of thromboxane A_2 and perhaps endothelin, another potent vasoconstrictor. In addition, there is evidence for contraction of mesangial cells, the specialized pericytes that modulate the glomerular capillary surface area [28].

These effects occur with acute infusion and persist with maintenance oral dosing. They are completely reversible early on, but may play a role in some of the chronic effects discussed below. Calcium channel blockers attenuate the vasoconstriction caused by calcineurin inhibitors. Some of the calcium channel blockers also slow the hepatic metabolism of these agents (nicardipine, diltiazem, verapamil), and are used in some centers to reduce the doses required to achieve the target trough blood level. Other agents of this class have little if any effect on cyclosporine and tacrolimus metabolism (nifedipine, felodipine, amlodipine).

Calcineurin inhibitors can also cause an acute form of nephrotoxicity manifested by acute renal failure in the early posttransplant period. Renal biopsy in these patients shows endothelial damage, formation of fibrin thrombi in capillary loops (Fig. 26.1), eosinophilic material in the walls of arterioles and small arteries, with patchy necrosis of smooth muscle cells (Fig. 26.2). This lesion is histologically similar to that seen in malignant hypertension and thrombotic thrombocytopenic purpura. Indeed, thrombocytopenia sometimes accompanies this syndrome in transplanted patients and responds to plasmapheresis and withdrawal of the calcineurin inhibitor [28]. Fortunately, this form of nephrotoxicity is uncommon.

The most important adverse effect of calcineurin inhibitor is chronic nephrotoxicity. This is manifested clinically by slowly deteriorating renal function over months to years, usually without heavy proteinuria. Histologic examination shows interstitial fibrosis, sometimes in a striped pattern (Fig. 26.3), and tubular atrophy in the regions of fibrosis. Arteriolar walls contain degenerative hyaline changes, although the glomeruli are initially

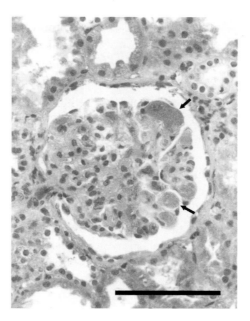

Fig. 26.1 *Thrombotic angiopathy of cyclosporine toxicity. The arrowheads point to fibrin thrombi in the capillary loops of a glomerulus from a patient with acute cyclosporine toxicity. Bar indicates 100 μm. (Photomicrograph courtesy of David Howell, M.D., Ph.D.)*

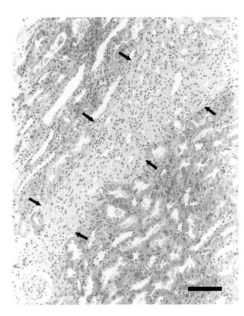

Fig. 26.2 *Cyclosporine-associated arteriolopathy. The arrowheads indicate a markedly thickened arteriole in a patient with acute cyclosporine toxicity. G, glomerulus; A, artery. Bar indicates* 100 μm. *(Photomicrograph courtesy of David Howell, M.D., Ph.D.)*

well preserved [28–30]. The pathogenesis of this lesion has been reviewed elsewhere [30].

It has become increasingly clear from the accumulated experience in solid organ transplantation and from the use of low-dose cyclosporine in autoimmune disease that although many patients can tolerate cyclosporine in a dose of 3–5 mg/kg/day without progressive loss of GFR, there is a subgroup of patients who develop chronic cyclosporine toxicity and eventual end-stage renal disease with this treatment, even in the absence of blood levels above the usual therapeutic range. Treatment includes decreasing the dose or discontinuing the agent altogether if possible. Other agents such as fish oil, the prostaglandin E_1 analog misoprostol, and calcium channel blockers have not been of demonstrated benefit in halting the progression of renal failure. When unexplained progressive decrease in renal function occurs in a patient taking cyclosporine, renal biopsy should be considered in order to identify the problem while it is early enough that an alternative immunosuppressive strategy might halt the decrease in renal function. There are no data to suggest that switching from one calcineurin inhibitor to another at equipotent doses will result in less nephrotoxicity [31]. However, as trough tacrolimus levels correlate more closely with the area under the curve of drug exposure than do trough cyclosporine levels, it may be easier to avoid calcineurin inhibitor

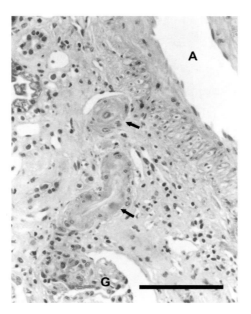

Fig. 26.3 *Chronic cyclosporine toxicity. A stripe of interstitial fibrosis is shown by the arrowheads in a patient with chronic cyclosporine toxicity. Bar indicates 100 μm. (Photomicrograph courtesy of David Howell, M.D., Ph.D.)*

toxicity using tacrolimus. If cyclosporine is used, the blood level drawn 2 h post dose (C_2 level) should be used to monitor therapy.

Several small studies have reported on switching from a calcineurin inhibitor to mycophenolate mofetil when renal function is worsening [32–36]. In the aggregate it appears that calcineurin reduction or withdrawal after introduction of mycophenolate has beneficial effects on the progression of renal disease and blood pressure at the cost of a slightly increased risk of rejection. Substitution of sirolimus for the calcineurin inhibitor has also been reported with or without concomitant use of mycophenolate with favorable effect on renal function in three series with small numbers of patients [36–38].

■ DIALYSIS IN THE LIVER TRANSPLANT PATIENT

Dialytic therapy in the immediate postoperative period requires close attention to hemodynamics and coagulation parameters. In the hypotensive patient, the most appropriate means of renal replacement therapy is continuous venovenous hemofiltration dialysis (CVVHD), while conventional hemodialysis can be used in the more stable patient. In the liver transplant patient with impaired hepatic clearance and renal failure, attention should be paid to the route of excretion of all pharmacologic agents given and doses adjusted accordingly.

Cyclosporine, tacrolimus, prednisone, and mycophenolate mofetil are not removed by hemodialysis to any significant extent, while methylprednisolone and azathioprine (and its active metabolite mercaptopurine) are cleared partially during dialysis. Most angiotensin-converting enzyme inhibitors are dialyzable, with benazepril and quinapril being exceptions. Calcium channel blockers are generally not cleared by hemodialysis, while many of the beta-blockers are (atenolol, acebutalol, metoprolol, nadalol, sotalol). Because atenolol is primarily cleared by the kidneys, the dose to achieve a desired effect is much lower in patients with poor renal function. Metoprolol on the other hand is primarily metabolized by the liver. Metabolites of verapamil with atrioventricular (AV) node-blocking properties, but little antihypertensive effect can accumulate in patients on hemodialysis. This agent is thus best avoided in end-stage renal disease.

■ REFERENCES

1. Distant DA, Gonwa TA. The kidney in liver transplantation. J Am Soc Nephrol 1993;4:129–136.

2. Eckardt KM. Renal failure in liver disease. Intensive Care Med 1999;25:5–14.

3. Fisher NC, Nightingale PG, Gunson BK, et al. Chronic renal failure following liver transplantation. Transplantation 1998;66:59–66.

4. Shemesh O, Golbetz H, Kriss JP, et al. Limitations of creatinine as a filtration marker in glomerulopathic patients. Kidney Int 1985;28:830–838.

5. Cockcroft SW, Gault HM. Prediction of creatinine clearances from serum creatinine. Nephron 1986;16:31–41.

6. Levey AS, Coresh J, Balk E, et al. National Kidney Foundation practice guidelines for chronic kidney disease: evaluation, classification, and stratification. Ann Intern Med 2003;139:137–147.

7. Gonwa TA, Jennings L, Mai ML, et al. Estimation of glomerular filtration rates before and after orthotopic liver transplantation: evaluation of current equations. Liver Transpl 2004;10:301–309.

8. Perrone RD, Steinman TI, Beck GJ, et al. Utility of radioisotopic filtration markers in chronic renal insufficiency: simultaneous comparison of ^{125}I-iothalamate, [169]Yb-DTPA, ^{99m}Tc-DTPA, and inulin. Am J Kidney Dis 1990;16:224–235.

9. Carvounis CP, Nisar S, Guro-Razuman S. Significance of the fractional excretion of urea in the differential diagnosis of acute renal failure. Kidney Int 2002;62:2223–2229.

10. Lai KN, Lai FM. Clinical features and the natural course of hepatitis B virus-related glomerulopathy in adults. Kidney Int 1991;40(suppl 35):S40–S45.

11. Johnson RJ, Willson R, Yamabe H, et al. Renal manifestations of hepatitis C virus infection. Kidney Int 1994;46:1255–1263.

12. Takekoshi Y, Tochimaru H, Nagata Y, et al. Immunopathogenetic mechanisms of hepatitis B virus-related glomerulopathy. Kidney Int 1991;40(suppl 35):S34–S39.

13. Johnson RJ, Gretch DR, Yamabe H, et al. Membranoproliferative glomerulonephritis associated with hepatitis C virus infection. N Engl J Med 1993;328:465–470.

14. Johnson RJ, Gretch DR, Couser WG, et al. Hepatitis C virus-associated glomerulonephritis. Effect of α-interferon therapy. Kidney Int 1994;46:1700–1704.

15. Bursten DM, Rodby RA. Membranoproliferative glomerulonephritis associated with hepatitis C virus infection. J Am Soc Nephrol 1993;4:1288–1293.

16. Stehman-Breen C, Alpers CE, Couser WG, et al. Hepatitis C virus associated membranous glomerulonephritis. Clin Nephrol 1995;44:141–147.

17. Younossi ZM, Singer ME, McHutchison JG, et al. Cost effectiveness of interferon α2b combined with ribavirin for the treatment of hepatitis C. Hepatology 1999;30:1318–1324.

18. Mukherjee S, Gilroy RK, McCashland TM, et al. Pegylated interferon for recurrent hepatitis C in liver transplant recipients with renal failure: a prospective cohort study. Transplant Proc 2003;35:1478–1479.

19. Jarvis B, Faulds D. Lamivudine. A review of its therapeutic potential in chronic hepatitis B. Drugs 1999;58:101–141.

20. Arroyo V, Gines P, Gerbes AL, et al. Definition and diagnostic criteria of refractory ascites and hepatorenal syndrome in cirrhosis. Hepatology 1996;23:164–176.

21. Epstein M. Hepatorenal syndrome: emerging perspectives of pathophysiology and therapy. J Am Soc Nephrol 1994;4:1735–1753.

22. Arroyo V, Gines P, Rhodes J, et al., eds. Ascites and renal dysfunction in liver disease, diagnosis and treatment. Malden, MA: Blackwell Science, 1999:175–303.

23. Brensing KA, Textor J, Strunck H, et al. Transjugular intrahepatic portosystemic stent-shunt for hepatorenal syndrome. Lancet 1997;349:697–698.

24. Gonwa TA, Klintmalm GB, Levy M, et al. Impact of pretransplant renal function on survival after liver transplantation. Transplantation 1995;59:361–365.

25. Brown RS, Lombardero M, Lake JR. Outcome of patients with renal insufficiency undergoing liver or liver–kidney transplantation. Transplantation 1996;62:1788–1793.

26. Pawarode A, Fine DM, Thuluvath PJ. Independent risk factors and natural history of renal dysfunction in liver transplant recipients. Liver Transpl 2003;9:741–747.

27. Nair S, Verma S, Thuluvath PJ. Pretransplant renal function predicts survival in patients undergoing orthotopic liver transplantation. Hepatology 2002;35:1179–1185.

28. Remuzzi G, Bertani T. Renal vascular and thrombotic effects of cyclosporine. Am J Kidney Dis 1989;13:261–272.

29. Kopp JB, Klotman PE. Cellular and molecular mechanisms of cyclosporin nephrotoxicity. J Am Soc Nephrol 1990;1:162–179.

30. Bennett WM, DeMattos A, Meyer MM, et al. Chronic cyclosporine nephropathy: the Achilles' heel of immunosuppressive therapy. Kidney Int 1996;50:1089–1100.

31. Henry ML. Cyclosporine and tacrolimus (FK506): a comparison of efficacy and safety profiles. Clin Transplant 1999;13:209–220.

32. Schlitt HJ, Barkmann A, Boker KHW, et al. Replacement of calcineurin inhibitors with mycophenolate mofetil in liver-transplant patients with renal dysfunction: a randomized controlled trial. Lancet 2001;357(9256):587–591.

33. Stewart SF, Hudson M, Talbot D, et al. Mycophenolate mofetil monotherapy in liver transplantation. Lancet 2001;357:609–610.

34. Raimondo ML, Dagher L, Papatheodoridis GV, et al. Long-term mycophenolate mofetil monotherapy in combination with calcineurin inhibitors for chronic renal dysfunction after liver transplantation. Transplantation 2003;75:186–190.

35. Cantarovich M, Tzimas GN, Barkun K, et al. Efficacy of mycophenolate mofetil with very low-dose cyclosporine microemulsion in long-term liver-transplant patients with renal dysfunction. Transplantation 2003;76:98–102.

36. Ziolkowski J, Paczek L, Senatorski G, et al. Renal function after liver transplantation: calcineurin inhibitor toxicity. Transplant Proc 2003;35:S2307–S2309.

37. Kniepass D, Iberer F, Grasser B, et al. Sirolimus and mycophenolate mofetil after liver transplantation. Transpl Int 2003;16:504–509.

38. Fairbanks KD, Eustace JA, Fine D, et al. Renal function improves in liver transplant recipients when switched from a calcineurin inhibitor to sirolimus. Liver Transpl 2003;10:1079–1085.

Cutaneous Diseases in the Transplant Recipient

27

**Sarah A. Myers and
Juan-Carlos Martinez**

C UTANEOUS DISEASE is a significant cause of morbidity in organ transplant recipients (OTRs). Due to chronic posttransplant immunosuppression, this population is at increased risk for inflammatory cutaneous conditions, cutaneous and systemic infections, lymphoproliferative disease, and cutaneous malignancy. Routine dermatologic follow-up is important in the management of both acute and chronic skin problems associated with the long-term immunosuppression of transplantation.

■ INFLAMMATORY CONDITIONS

Hepatitis C Virus-Associated Mixed Cryoglobulinemia

Hepatitis C virus (HCV)-related cirrhosis is a major cause of liver failure leading to transplantation. Unfortunately, HCV almost uniformly recurs after transplantation. Accordingly, several HCV-related cutaneous conditions can be seen in this cohort of liver transplant recipients. These include porphyria cutanea tarda (PCT), lichen planus (LP), and, most importantly, HCV-associated mixed cryoglobulinemia (MC), which can lead to systemic vasculitis. In recent studies, MC has been documented in up to 20–30% of HCV-positive liver transplant patients [1,2]. Cutaneous lesions consist primarily of nonblanching palpable purpura, which can be either acrally or diffuse distributed. Its recognition should prompt evaluation of a liver transplant patient's HCV status and treatment with antiviral therapy if indicated.

Graft-versus-Host Disease

Although rarely seen after solid organ transplantation, graft-versus-host disease (GVHD) has been reported in liver transplant patients. Extracutaneous manifestations such as fever, elevated transaminases, and bile duct injury leading to cholestasis are more common, but cutaneous manifestations have been reported in liver transplant patients. Often, these cutaneous lesions are the presenting sign of GVHD [3,4]. Both acute and chronic forms can be seen and have very different cutaneous presentations.

Acute GVHD usually develops in the third week following transplantation and manifests as burning or pruritic erythematous papules and macules that may coalesce into a more diffuse morbilliform eruption. In severe cases, bullae or generalized erythroderma can occur. Acute GVHD must be considered in patients presenting with fever, skin rash, gastrointestinal (GI) symptoms, and panyctopenia following solid organ transplantation. Diagnosis of acute GVHD is suggested by histological findings on biopsy. This can be confirmed by the presence of donor lymphocytes in the affected tissues. Because profound immunosuppression is the treatment of GVHD, the mortality rate due to infection is high.

Chronic cutaneous GVHD has been described but is exceedingly rare in liver transplant patients. It can present as lichenoid or sclerodermoid types. Lichenoid GVHD resembles LP and can present as pruritic purple papules. It differs from classic LP in that it initially often involves the palms and soles, then generalizes. Individual lesions of lichenoid GVHD may be less angular and geometric than the polygonal papules seen in classic LP. Sclerodermoid GVHD presents as indolent sclerotic, indurated plaques on the trunk and extremities of affected individuals. Chronic GVHD is most often treated with the lowest effective dose of systemic steroids.

■ INFECTIONS

There are two primary factors that determine the risk of infection in OTRs. The first is the overall degree of immunosuppression, including potency and duration, and the other is the amount of exposure to potential pathogenic organisms. Specific, consistent, and recognizable patterns of postoperative and opportunistic infections arise in transplant recipients because the immunosuppresive regimens are fairly similar in all forms of solid organ transplantation [5].

The vast majority of infections occurring in the first month after transplantation are caused by the same pathogens that afflict immunocompetent surgical patients, namely, nosocomial bacteria and Candida. After the first month, the immunomodulating viruses – cytomegalovirus (CMV), Epstein–Barr virus (EBV), other human herpesviruses, hepatitis B virus (HBV), and HCV – as well as other infections become more problematic. In particular, infection by opportunistic pathogens such as *Pneumocystis carinii*, Aspergillus, and Listeria monocytogenes may occur. More than 6 months after transplantation, infections can develop from conventional or community-acquired pathogens, chronic viruses including human papillomaviruses (HPV), or opportunistic organisms such as Pneumocystis and endemic fungi [5,6] (see Chapter 25).

Cutaneous lesions may be important and early manifestations of systemic infection in OTRs [7]. Table 27.1 lists opportunistic and primary pathogens that can lead to disseminated disease. Unfortunately, the majority of these infections do not cause specific skin lesions, and skin biopsy specimens in this setting must be processed with both special stains and various culturing techniques to evaluate all the possible culprits.

■ BACTERIAL INFECTIONS

The majority of cutaneous bacterial infections in OTRs, as in the general population, are due to *Staphylococcus aureus* and *Streptococcus pyogenes*. Superficial bacterial infections, folliculitis, abscesses, furuncles, wound infections, cellulitis, and bacteremia with septic skin emboli all occur with increased frequency. Ecthyma gangrenosum due to *Pseudomonas aeruginosa* is also a potential complication in OTRs. Ecthyma patients develop tense, grouped vesicles surrounded by pink or violaceous halos. The lesions secondarily ulcerate and develop necrotic black eschars.

Skin infections due to opportunistic organisms such as Nocardia and mycobacteria also have been reported in transplant patients. Nocardiosis may present as subcutaneous nodules at sites of primary inoculation, though these are more commonly due to hematogenous dissemination from a pulmonary focus. Mycobacterial infection, caused by both *Mycobacterium tuberculosis* and atypical mycobacterial organisms, occurs with increased incidence in transplant patients. Cutaneous lesions are present in approximately 10% of patients with disseminated *Mycobacterium tuberculosis*.

Atypical mycobacterial infection may present as erythematous, indurated, and sometimes fluctuant nodules, papules, or vesicles, usually on the extremities. Atypical mycobacterium known to cause infection in immunosuppressed patients includes *Mycobacterium kansasii*, *Mycobacterium haemophilum*, *Mycobacterium fortuitum*, *Mycobacterium chelonei*, *Mycobacterium marimun*, and *Mycobacterium scrofulaceum*.

All the preceding infections are diagnosed based on tissue gram stain or acid-fast stain and tissue culture.

■ FUNGAL INFECTIONS

Superficial Mycosis

Superficial fungal infections, including dermatophytosis, tinea versicolor, Malassezia furfur folliculitis, and widespread cutaneous candidiasis, are com-

Table 27.1 *Processing of Skin Specimens to Establish Cause of Infection*

───

I. Laboratory identification of causative infectious agents from skin specimens (biopsy, curettage, wound drainage)

   A. Direct preparations for microscopic examination

      1. Wet mount for fungal elements

         a. KOH

         b. Saline solution

         c. India ink

      2. Stained smears

         a. Gram stain

         b. Acid-fast stain

   B. Organisms

      1. Actinomycetes: delicate filaments $<1\,\mu m$; with or without granules (Nocardia Actinomyces)

      2. Spherules: thick-walled cells with endospores (*Coccidioides immitis*)

      3. Zygomycetes: Aseptate hyphae; $10\text{--}15\,\mu m$ (Rhizopus, Mucor)

      4. Septate hyphae: $2.5\text{--}4\,\mu m$ (*Aspergillus fumigatus, Pseudallescheria boydii*)

      5. Pseudohyphae: hyphae with indentations at septa (Candida)

      6. Yeasts

         a. Small: $1\text{--}3\,\mu m$ (*Histoplasma capsulatum*)

         b. Medium: $2\text{--}5\,\mu m$ (*Candida albicans*)

         c. Large

            1) $8\text{--}20\,\mu m$ (*Blastomyces dermatitidis*)

            2) $8\text{--}40\,\mu m$ (*Paracoccidioides brasiliensis*)

            3) $5\text{--}30\,\mu m$ (*Cryptococcus neoformans*)

II. Isolation of causative agents: cultures of skin specimens for laboratory examination

   A. Aerobic and anaerobic bacteria

      1. Thioglycollate broth

      2. Sheep blood agar

   B. Atypical mycobacteria (25–37°C)

      1. Löwenstein–Jensen culture medium

      2. Middlebrook 7H10 agar

   C. Fungal

      1. Sabouraud's dextrose agar

      2. Mycosel agar (Becton–Dickinson)

   D. Viral: obtain appropriate holding media (e.g. sterile veal heart infusion broth)

───

mon in OTRs. Dermatophyte infection may present as widespread or refractory to treatment of epidermal scaly patches with an annular border or deeper dermal involvement such as dermal nodules or Majocchi's granuloma (granulomatous folliculitis). Although dermatophytes typically do not invade living tissue, disseminated dermatophyte infection with spread to viscera may occur as a result of immunosuppressive drug therapy [8,9].

Deep Mycosis

Systemic fungal infections are fairly common in OTRs and are frequently fatal [10]. The most common deep fungal infections are caused by the Candida and Aspergillus species, but rarer organisms, previously considered to be "contaminants" or saprophytes, are increasingly pathogenic in immunocompromised patients. Cutaneous involvement suggests hematogenous spread and disseminated infection but can rarely represent sites of primary inoculation.

Disseminated candidiasis is particularly common in liver transplant patients; 62–91% of fungal infections are attributed to Candida species in this patient population [11]. It is often fatal and can be difficult to diagnose as blood cultures are positive for Candida organisms in only 25% of cases [12]. Skin lesions are present in 10–15% of patients and can be extremely helpful in establishing the diagnosis. The cutaneous lesions include erythematous macules that become purpuric; pustular papules; nodules with pale centers; and subcutaneous nodules. Histologic examination of tissue reveals aggregates of hyphae and spores within the dermis or at the site of vascular damage. Culture of a cutaneous lesion is positive in 60% of cases.

Aspergillosis is a common systemic mycosis but skin lesions associated with disseminated disease occur in only 10% of patients. Lesions are multiple scattered papules or hemorrhagic vesicles or bullae that rapidly progress into necrotic ulcers covered by a heavy black eschar. Primary cutaneous aspergillosis has also been described in immunosuppressed patients as a single or multiple painful erythematous indurated plaques usually at sites of occlusion of intravenous access [13]. Histologic examination of skin biopsies from both forms of cutaneous aspergillosis reveals an absence of spores and numerous septate hyphae with acute angle branching in the dermis.

The importance of non-Aspergillus hyalohyphomycotic fungi has been increasing in recent years. These organisms are much more likely than Aspergillus to lead to disseminated infections and infection has a poor prognosis. Both localized and disseminated Fusarium infection can occur. Disseminated Fusarium infection occurs almost exclusively in immunocompromised individuals, particularly in neutropenic patients [14]. Lesions usually present as multiple painful red macules and papules, often with some central necrosis. Paecilomyces organisms have been reported to cause primary cutaneous mycosis (usually a focal nodule or cellulitic plaque) and are emerging as a significant pathogen in the immunosuppressed population. Pseudallescheria is a soil fungus that has been reported to cause disseminated disease in immuno-compromised patients as well.

Zygomycosis organisms are common opportunistic pathogens that infect immunosuppressed patients. Rhizopus is the most common pathogen, followed by Basidiobolus, Mucor, Cunninghamella, Saksenaea, and Absidia. There are different clinical forms of Zygomycete infection including rhinocer-ebral, pulmonary, GI, cutaneous, central nervous system (CNS), and renal disease. Cutaneous disease often begins with plaque-like or pustular lesions that progress to black necrotic plaques and ulcers. The histopathologic hall-marks are invasion of blood vessel walls by broad, nonseptate hyphae, with branching at right angles, thrombus formation, and infarction of surrounding tissue. Disseminated disease occurs in severely immunocompromised patients with mortality rates of nearly 100% in some studies [15].

The dematiaceous fungi have brown hyphae and pseudohyphae and yeast-like cells in tissue; they produce dark colonies on culture. Alternaria, Curvularia, Phialophora, and Scytalidium species all can produce soft tissue infection. These organisms are becoming more frequent pathogens in immuno-compromised hosts. Cutaneous lesions from primary inoculation are charac-terized by pigmented firm nodules and papules that evolve into ulcerated plaques [16]. Skin lesions can also be seen in disseminated disease and al-though dissemination is very rare, mortality rates approach 80%.

Cryptococcus neoformans is a relatively common pathogen in immunocom-promised patients. While primary cutaneous cryptococcosis can occur in trans-plant patients, involvement of the skin in cryptococcosis is usually indicative of disseminated disease. Approximately 15% of patients with disseminated cryptococcosis have cutaneous involvement presenting as papules, molluscum contagiosum-like lesions, nodules, plaques, tumors, abscesses, and occasion-ally lesions that resemble bacterial cellulitis. Biopsy of involved skin reveals encapsulated spores.

Dimorphic fungi constitute a significant risk for disseminated infections in immunocompromised patients and include histoplasmosis, coccidioidomyco-sis, blastomycosis, and sporotrichosis. Transplant patients may develop di-morphic infections from three possible sources: reactivation of prior infection, the organ itself (also reactivation), or as a newly acquired infection. As with cryptococcosis, cutaneous lesions are variable. Organisms are often apparent on skin biopsy and their identification can aid in early initiation of antifungal therapy.

■ VIRAL INFECTIONS

Viral infections of the skin are common in immunocompromised hosts. Reactivation of latent viral infections caused by herpes simplex, varicella–zoster, and CMV is a frequent and troublesome problem in OTRs.

Herpes Simplex Virus

Herpes simplex infection occurs most commonly during the first 3 weeks after transplantation. Most infections represent reactivation of latent infection, although there have been several case reports of herpes simplex virus (HSV) transmission through transplantation. Typical mucocutaneous lesions are grouped vesicles on an erythematous base. Systemic disease with scattered cutaneous lesions may also occur. The diagnosis can be made by demonstration of multinucleated giant cells on a Tzanck preparation, although this does not distinguish between HSV and varicella–zoster virus (VZV) infections, and/or by culture, polymerase chain reaction (PCR), or direct immunofluorescence. Treatment with acyclovir or its derivatives results in healing of lesions. Prolonged courses may be required for complete healing in the immunosuppressed host.

Varicella–Zoster Virus

Herpes zoster is common in transplant recipients. Clinical disease is characterized by unilateral grouped vesicles on an erythematous base localized to one or few dermatomes. As with herpes simplex infection, varicella–zoster infections may be associated with prolonged viral shedding, a decreased healing time, and an increased incidence of viral dissemination in the immunocompromised patient. Postherpetic neuralgia also occurs at an increased incidence. Manifestations of herpes zoster may be prolonged for up to several months in immunosuppressed patients, and the disease has been found to clear after immune suppressants are decreased. Acyclovir is the treatment of choice.

Cytomegalovirus

CMV is one of the most common opportunistic infections in transplant recipients. CMV infection may represent new infection introduced by the donor organ or the reactivation of prior infection in the recipient. Cutaneous involvement is present in 10–20% of patients with systemic CMV infection and is a sign of poor prognosis [17]. Ulcerations on the perianal and rectal mucosa and the buttocks and thighs may occur. Other skin lesions include morbilliform eruptions, indurated hyperpigmented nodules or plaques, vesiculobullous eruptions, and petechial and purpuric eruptions indicative of a vasculitis. Localized CMV disease can occur in wounds or other sites of trauma without systemic involvement. Skin lesions in both primary and disseminated disease are characterized by the presence of large intranuclear inclusions with a surrounding halo in endothelial cells. Ganciclovir is effective for the treatment of CMV infections.

Epstein–Barr Virus

Epstein–Barr virus has been implicated in posttransplant lymphoproliferative disorder (see later) [18]. This disorder is usually a B cell lymphoproliferative process ranging in severity from a benign polyclonal process that wanes when immunosuppressive therapy is decreased to a highly malignant monoclonal lymphoma that is resistant to all forms of treatment.

Molluscum Contagiosum

Molluscum contagiosum is a DNA-containing pox virus that appears commonly on the face or genital areas as umbilicated skin-colored to erythematous papules. These lesions have been observed in large numbers in patients after transplantation. Because lesions resembling molluscum occur in patients with cryptococcal (and some of the dimorphic fungal) infections, a skin biopsy is recommended when the diagnosis is uncertain.

Human Papillomavirus

There is an increased incidence of common warts in OTRs, and the prevalence increases with duration of immunosuppression. These warts are frequently multiple and may be recalcitrant to treatment. In addition, common verrucae or condyloma acuminata may present as scaly, verrucous, keratotic papules or fleshy, pedunculated papules and may be difficult to distinguish from squamous cell carcinoma (SCC) in transplant patients. The threshold for biopsy in these patients should be low, and aggressive treatment is important, as verrucae in OTRs have an increased rate of malignant degeneration when compared with the general population. Treatment for verrucae includes topical therapies such as imiquimod 5% cream, topical 5-FU, or locally destructive methods such as curettage, laser, surgical removal, and/or cryotherapy. In addition, regular gynecologic and rectal/anal examination is especially important in the transplant population due to the association of certain HPV types (HPV-16, -18, -31, and -33) with cervical dysplasia, cervical carcinoma, and SCC of the anus.

Kaposi's Sarcoma

Like other variants of Kaposi's Sarcoma, transplant assaciated KS is cansed by human he, pesvilus 8 (HHV-8). The risk of Kaposi's sarcoma (KS) is greatly increased in transplant recipients compared with a control population of the same ethnic origin [19–21]. Although it may develop as early as 6 months after transplantation, KS appears an average of 21 months after transplantation and is directly related to the amount of immunosuppression. Presumably, because liver transplant recipients require relatively less immunosuppression than other OTRs, the incidence of KS in the former population is significantly lower.

Cutaneous manifestations include violaceous plaques or nodules on the skin and mucous membranes. If present, these findings provide an opportunity for early diagnosis. Patients who do not develop skin lesions and have isolated visceral disease often go undiagnosed and untreated, leading to a much higher mortality rate. Internal KS should be suspected in patients with allograft dysfunction of unknown etiology, pleural effusions, or recalcitrant ascites [22]. KS in liver transplant recipients is not as aggressive as in the human immunodeficiency virus (HIV)-infected population, and partial or complete remission has been reported with lowering of immunosuppressive medications.

Posttransplantation Lymphoproliferative Disorder

There is a well-established correlation between immunosuppression and lymphoproliferative disorders. This group of diseases ranges in spectrum from mild polyclonal proliferations and infectious mononucleosis-like symptoms to life-threatening lymphomas. The incidence of posttransplantation lymphoproliferative disorder (PTLD) in OTRs is approximately 2% and associated mortality can range from 50% to 80% [18]. Usually, PTLDs are EBV-induced B cell proliferations, although EBV-negative PTLD has been described. Identified risk factors for development of PTLD include type and amount of immunosuppressive medications, younger age at time of transplant, and primary EBV infection after transplantation [23]. Type of organ transplanted has been linked to incidence as well; renal and liver transplant patients have a relatively lower risk compared with heart, lung, and bone marrow transplant recipients [24].

PTLD most often presents nodally or extranodally in the GI tract, CNS, lungs, and transplanted allograft. PTLD confined to the skin, although quite rare, has been described. These patients have been reported to present with subcutaneous nodules on the trunk and extremities, erythematous plaques on the face, and reticulate erythematous plaques on the thighs [23,25]. These respond to treatment more favorably than do PTLDs with extracutaneous involvement. It is unknown whether this more favorable outcome pertains to the specific biology of the process or to earlier diagnosis because of cutaneous, and therefore easily visible, manifestations.

Treatment of PTLD usually consists of reductions in immunosuppression, which can lead to cure rates of 25–50%. Few alternatives exist beyond this, although new treatments, including antiviral agents, passive antibody therapy, surgical resection, local irradiation, anti-B cell monoclonal antibody therapy, and interferon-alpha, are being investigated [26].

■ CUTANEOUS MALIGNANCY

Background

Data pertaining specifically to skin cancer in liver transplant recipients are lacking. However OTRs have a well-documented, increased risk for development of cutaneous malignancy [27–30]. In addition, the skin cancers that afflict these patients tend to be both more numerous and more aggressive, with higher rates of local invasion, recurrence, and both nodal and distant metastases. Not surprisingly, these confer higher rates of morbidity and mortality when compared with those found in the general population.

Epidemiology and Risk Factors

Perhaps the best epidemiological data defining the increased risk post solid organ transplantation can be found in two large population-based studies performed in Holland and Norway. These found the overall incidence of SCC to be from 65 to 250 times higher than in the general population [31,32]. Several recently published studies monitoring de novo malignancies after liver transplantation have demonstrated variable rates of SCC development in liver transplant recipients ranging from 1.1% to almost 23%. Generalizations may be difficult to make from these data, as the studies have different monitoring methodologies, and there may be a tendency to underestimate the actual number of skin cancers [33–37]. Of note, relatively less immunosuppression is required to prevent allograft rejection in liver transplant recipients. Accordingly, although liver transplant recipients have increased rates of posttransplantation cutaneous malignancy, these rates are lower than those found in renal or cardiac transplant recipients [38,39].

In the general population, the ratio of incidence of basal cell carcinoma (BCC) to SCC is approximately 4:1. This ratio is reversed in OTRs, with SCC being the most common skin cancer. Identified risk factors for development of skin cancer in OTRs include increased age, duration and intensity of immunosuppression, extensive ultraviolet radiation exposure, low CD4 counts, HPV infection, and fair complexion [40,41]. Cadaveric versus live donor transplantation, treatment with antithymocyte globulin or OKT3, and sex of the recipient does not appear to increase risk of posttransplant skin cancer.

The pathogenesis of skin cancer in these patients has not been fully elucidated, but it is felt that immunosuppressive medication regimens play a role in the increased incidence of SCC. Proposed mechanisms include direct carcinogenic effects of some medications, such as azathioprine and cyclosporine, and decreased host immunosurveillance, which creates a carcinopermissive environment [28,42–45]. The role of specific immunosuppressives in the development of skin cancer is difficult to ascertain because many patients are treated with multiple agents. New immunosuppressive medication regimens with less carcinogenic potential and even antitumoral effects, such as sirolimus, are being developed and actively investigated [43].

Although the role of HPV infection in the pathogenesis of epithelial lining of the genital tract is well established, its role in transplant-associated cutaneous malignancy remains unclear. OTRs have increased rate of HPV infection, and verrucae in this population have increased rates of malignant degeneration. It has been postulated that infection with HPV types 5 and 8 may be associated with increased risk of development of SCC in OTRs [40,46,47].

Management

Ideal management of any transplant recipient requires a multidisciplinary approach. The role of the dermatologist in the management of posttransplant skin cancer is essential. Prevention is perhaps the most elemental tool. Because transplant recipients can develop premalignant and malignant lesions at an alarming rate, close and frequent observation is critical. Early visits should include proper education regarding behavioral modifications and instruction in the proper, daily use of high sun protection factor (SPF) sunscreen and protective clothing. Patients who have extensive actinic damage or history of skin cancer prior to transplantation are especially at risk, and OTRs should be made aware of their increased risk for skin cancer. Websites and informational brochures should be provided to the patients. The International Transplant Skin Cancer Collaborative (ITSCC), an organization founded in part to educate transplant recipients and their physicians, has a website at www.itscc.org with available educational material.

In addition to sun protection and close follow-up, management of skin lesion requires biopsy of any suspicious lesions and treatment of premalignant lesions. Early and aggressive treatment of premalignancies such as actinic keratoses and verrucae can be of great benefit. These lesions can be treated with local destruction such as cryotherapy or curettage. In addition, some topical treatments have been found to be chemopreventive in the development of skin cancers in OTRs. Topical agents such as 5-fluorouracil and topical retinoids have been found to reduce the numbers of both malignant and premalignant lesions [48,49]. Prevention of premalignant lesions not only decreases the risk of new malignancies but also serves to facilitate clinical detection of malignant lesions.

Patients who develop new premalignant and malignant lesions despite topical therapy may require more aggressive chemoprevention. Systemic retinoids such as acitretin and isotretinoin have been shown to be effective in prevention of keratotic neoplasms in OTRs [50]. These can be used in combination with topical retinoids to decrease the risk of systemic side-effects. Benefit from systemic retinoids is seen only as long as the drug is continued, and, as such, long-term use is usually required. Close observation of laboratory values, particularly in liver transplant patients, is necessary in these patients; common side-effects of systemic retinoid therapy include increased triglycerides and elevation of liver function tests. Due to the risk of systemic side-effects as well as reports of poor tolerance in OTRs with advanced SCC, it is recommended that systemic retinoids be started at a low dose (10–25 mg/day) and slowly increased as patient tolerance allows.

Recent guidelines have been set forth for the management of SCC in OTRs [51]. As with premalignant lesions, tumors should be treated early and aggressively. Specific tumors in any given patient may be classified as low- or high-risk using specific criteria. High-risk features include tumor size greater than 2 cm on the trunk or extremities, greater than 1 cm on the cheeks, forehead, neck, and scalp, or greater than 0.6 cm on the "mask" areas of the face. In addition, aggressive histologic subtype, presence of ulceration, rapid rate of development or growth, occurrence in a scar, and recurrence after previous treatment are all features of a high-risk tumor. Low-risk tumors can be treated with electrodesiccation and curettage, cryosurgery, curettage and cryotherapy, and excisional modalities such as Mohs' micrographic surgery (MMS) or surgical excision with postoperative histological margin assessment. High-risk tumors should be treated with aggressive surgical excision or with radiation therapy in inoperable tumors or in patients either unwilling or unable to undergo surgical excision. However, for some 10% of OTRs, multiple and severe SCC detrimentally affects quality of life and carries a significant risk of nodal and systemic metastases. This population underscores the need for prevention and early treatment, as metastatic SCC in OTRs causes significant morbidity and carries a 3-year survival rate of only 56% [52].

Management of these challenging patients may require reduction in immunosuppressant medications as cutaneous carcinogenesis begins to develop. As previously mentioned, liver transplant patients require less immunosuppression than most other OTRs, and accordingly, the problem of posttransplantation skin cancer is fortunately not as severe. Regardless, cutaneous malignancy in liver transplant recipients is a problem, and close collaboration between the dermatologist and the transplant team is essential.

■ REFERENCES

1. Abrahamian GA, Cosimi AB, Farrell ML, et al. Prevalence of hepatitis C virus-associated mixed cryoglobulinemia after liver transplantation. Liver Transpl 2000;6(2):185–190.

2. Duvoux C, Tran Ngoc A, Intrator L, et al. Hepatitis C virus (HCV)-related cryoglobulinemia after liver transplantation for HCV cirrhosis. Transpl Int 2002;15(1):3–9.

3. Schmuth M, Vogel W, Weinlich G, et al. Cutaneous lesions as the presenting sign of acute graft-versus-host disease following liver transplantation. Br J Dermatol 1999;141(5):901–904.

4. Walling HW, Voigt MD, Stone MS. Lichenoid graft vs. host disease following liver transplantation. J Cutan Pathol 2004;31(2):179–184.

5. Fishman JA, Rubin RH. Infection in organ-transplant recipients. N Engl J Med 1998;338(24):1741–1751.

6. Hogewoning AA, Goettsch W, van Loveren H, et al. Skin infections in renal transplant recipients. Clin Transplant 2001;15(1):32–38.

7. Abel EA. Cutaneous manifestations of immunosuppression in organ transplant recipients (Part 1). J Am Acad Dermatol 1989;21(2):167–179.

8. Demidovich CW, Kornfeld BW, Gentry RH, et al. Deep dermatophyte infection with chronic draining nodules in an immunocompromised patient. Cutis 1995;55(4):237–240.

9. Squeo RF, Beer R, Silvers D, et al. Invasive *Trichophyton rubrum* resembling blastomycosis infection in the immunocompromised host (Part 2). J Am Acad Dermatol 1998;39(2):379–380.

10. Radentz WH. Opportunistic fungal infections in immunocompromised hosts. J Am Acad Dermatol 1989;20(6):989–1003.

11. Husain S, Tollemar J, Dominguez EA, et al. Changes in the spectrum and risk factors for invasive candidiasis in liver transplant recipients: prospective, multi-center, case-controlled study. Transplantation 2003;75(12):2023–2029.

12. Bodey GP, Luna M. Skin lesions associated with disseminated candidiasis. JAMA 1974;229(11):1466–1468.

13. Allo MD, Miller J, Townsend T, et al. Primary cutaneous aspergillosis associated with Hickman intravenous catheters. N Engl J Med 1987;317(18):1105–1108.

14. Martino P, Gastaldi R, Raccah R, et al. Clinical patterns of Fusarium infections in immunocompromised patients. J Infect 1994;28(suppl 1):7–15.

15. Jimenez C, Lumbreras C, Aguado JM, et al. Successful treatment of mucor infection after liver or pancreas–kidney transplantation. Transplantation 2002;73(3):476–480.

16. Merino E, Banuls J, Boix V, et al. Relapsing cutaneous alternariosis in a kidney transplant recipient cured with liposomal amphotericin B. Eur J Clin Microbiol Infect Dis 2003;22(1):51–53.

17. Lesher JL, Jr. Cytomegalovirus infections and the skin. Am Acad Dermatol 1988;18(6):1333–1338.

18. Paya CV, Fung JJ, Nalesnik MA, et al. Epstein–Barr virus-induced posttransplant lymphoproliferative disorders. ASTS/ASTP EBV–PTLD Task Force and the Mayo Clinic Organized International Consensus Development Meeting. Transplantation 1999;68(10):1517–1525.

19. Penn I. Cancers in renal transplant recipients. Adv Ren Replace Ther 2000;7(2):147–156.

20. Berg D, Otley CC. Skin cancer in organ transplant recipients: epidemiology, pathogenesis, and management. J Am Acad Dermatol 2002;47(1):1–17.

21. Andreoni M, Goletti D, Pezzotti P, et al. Prevalence, incidence and correlates of HHV-8/KSHV infection and Kaposi's sarcoma in renal and liver transplant recipients. J Infect 2001;43(3):195–199.

22. Marcelin AG, Roque-Afonso AM, Hurtova M, et al. Fatal disseminated Kaposi's sarcoma following human herpesvirus 8 primary infections in liver-transplant recipients. Liver Transpl 2004;10(2):295–300.

23. Beynet DP, Wee SA, Horwitz SS, et al. Clinical and pathological features of posttransplantation lymphoproliferative disorders presenting with skin involvement in 4 patients. Arch Dermatol 2004;140(9):1140–1146.

24. Green M, Webber S. Posttransplantation lymphoproliferative disorders. Pediatr Clin North Am 2003;50(6):1471–1491.

25. Schumann KW, Oriba HA, Bergfeld WF, et al. Cutaneous presentation of posttransplant lymphoproliferative disorder (Part 2). J Am Acad Dermatol 2000;42(5):923–926.

26. Preiksaitis JK. New developments in the diagnosis and management of posttransplantation lymphoproliferative disorders in solid organ transplant recipients. Clin Infect Dis 2004;39(7):1016–1023.

27. Sheil AG. Organ transplantation and malignancy: inevitable linkage. Transplant Proc 2002;34(6):2436–2437.

28. Berg D, Otley CC. Skin cancer in organ transplant recipients: epidemiology, pathogenesis, and management. J Am Acad Dermatol 2002;47(1):1–17.

29. Euvrard S, Kanitakis J, Claudy A. Skin cancers after organ transplantation. N Engl J Med 2003;348(17):1681–1691.

30. Ong CS, Keogh AM, Kossard S, et al. Skin cancer in Australian heart transplant recipients. J Am Acad Dermatol 1999;40(1):27–34.

31. Jensen P, Hansen S, Moller B, et al. Skin cancer in kidney and heart transplant recipients and different long-term immunosuppressive therapy regimens (Part 1). J Am Acad Dermatol 1999;40(2):177–186.

32. Hartevelt MM, Bavinck JN, Kootte AM, et al. Incidence of skin cancer after renal transplantation in the Netherlands. Transplantation 1990;49(3):506–509.

33. Haagsma EB, Hagens VE, Schaapveld M, et al. Increased cancer risk after liver transplantation: a population-based study. J Hepatol 2001;34(1):84–91.

34. Xiol X, Guardiola J, Menendez S, et al. Risk factors for development of de novo neoplasia after liver transplantation. Liver Transpl 2001;7(11):971–975.

35. Saigal S, Norris S, Muiesan P, et al. Evidence of differential risk for posttransplantation malignancy based on pretransplantation cause in patients undergoing liver transplantation. Liver Transpl 2002;8(5):482–487.

36. Sanchez EQ, Marubashi S, Jung G, et al. De novo tumors after liver transplantation: a single-institution experience. Liver Transpl 2002;8(3):285–291.

37. Mithoefer AB, Supran S, Freeman RB. Risk factors associated with the development of skin cancer after liver transplantation. Liver Transpl 2002;8(10):939–944.

38. Penn I. Posttransplantation de novo tumors in liver allograft recipients. Liver Transpl Surg 1996;2(1):52–59.

39. Frezza EE, Fung JJ, van Thiel DH. Non-lymphoid cancer after liver transplantation. Hepatogastroenterology 1997;44(16):1172–1181.

40. Ulrich C, Schmook T, Sachse MM, et al. Comparative epidemiology and pathogenic factors for nonmelanoma skin cancer in organ transplant patients (Part 2). Dermatol Surg 2004;30(4):622–627.

41. Fortina AB, Piaserico S, Caforio AL, et al. Immunosuppressive level and other risk factors for basal cell carcinoma and squamous cell carcinoma in heart transplant recipients. Arch Dermatol 2004;140(9):1079–1085.

42. Tremblay F, Fernandes M, Habbab F, et al. Malignancy after renal transplantation: incidence and role of type of immunosuppression. Ann Surg Oncol 2002;9(8):785–788.

43. Euvrard S, Ulrich C, Lefrancois N. Immunosuppressants and skin cancer in transplant patients: focus on rapamycin (Part 2). Dermatol Surg 2004;30(4):628–633.

44. Servilla KS, Burnham DK, Daynes RA. Ability of cyclosporine to promote the growth of transplanted ultraviolet radiation-induced tumors in mice. Transplantation 1987;44(2):291–295.

45. Ryffel B. The carcinogenicity of cyclosporin. Toxicology 1992;73(1):1–22.

46. Bouwes Bavinck JN, Feltkamp M, Struijk L, et al. Human papillomavirus infection and skin cancer risk in organ transplant recipients. J Investig Dermatol Symp Proc 2001;6(3):207–211.

47. Stockfleth E, Nindl I, Sterry W, et al. Human papillomaviruses in transplant-associated skin cancers (Part 2). Dermatol Surg 2004;30(4):604–609.

48. Euvrard S, Verschoore M, Touraine JL, et al. Topical retinoids for warts and keratoses in transplant recipients. Lancet 1992;340(8810):48–49.

49. Kanitakis J, Euvrard S, Faure M, et al. Porokeratosis and immunosuppression. Eur J Dermatol 1998;8(7):459–465.

50. De Graaf YG, Euvrard S, Bouwes Bavinck JN. Systemic and topical retinoids in the management of skin cancer in organ transplant recipients (Part 2). Dermatol Surg 2004;30(4):656–661.

51. Stasko T, Brown MD, Carucci JA, et al. Guidelines for the management of squamous cell carcinoma in organ transplant recipients (Part 2). Dermatol Surg 2004;30(4):642–650.

52. Martinez JC, Otley CC, Stasko T, et al. Defining the clinical course of metastatic skin cancer in organ transplant recipients: a multicenter collaborative study. Arch Dermatol 2003;139(3):301–306.

Productivity and Social Rehabilitation of the Transplant Recipient

▼　　▼　　▼　　▼　　▼　　▼　　▼　　▼　　▼

28

Karli S. Pontillo

■ INTRODUCTION

Ethical allocation of scarce donor organs requires assessing the likelihood that a person undergoing liver transplantation will experience a successful outcome. Zilberfein et al. [1] observed that effective and ethical decision making in the transplant evaluation process requires fulfillment of both medical and psychosocial criteria. As medical and psychosocial variables continue to be assessed throughout the transplant process, the common goal remains the achievement of maximal productivity and social rehabilitation of liver transplant recipients.

Liver transplant programs employ an interdisciplinary team approach in the evaluation of potential recipients. The core team of hepatologists, surgeons, nurse coordinators, licensed clinical social workers (LCSWs), psychologists, and financial coordinators each has a unique role to perform, striving to be supportive, yet as objective as possible and providing continuity of care. The LCSW has a crucial role to play during every phase of liver transplantation: from evaluating psychosocial factors that determine whether the patient is prepared for the procedure to helping patients and their families adjust to life afterward. The degree to which a successful outcome can be achieved depends significantly upon the LCSW's effectiveness at patient assessment, psychological care, and adherence to the transplant regimen.

■ PSYCHOSOCIAL ASSESSMENT

Liver transplantation is adversely influenced by donor organ scarcity and extended waiting times [2]. The psychosocial assessment is designed to identify patients at high risk of experiencing negative transplant outcomes, and therefore more likely to require a greater amount of mental health, behavioral, and/or social support services and interventions before and after transplantation [3]. One tool commonly used during this process is the Psychosocial Assessment of Candidates for Transplantation (PACT), developed by Olbrisch et al. [4], with the view that reliability and validity of psychosocial criteria used to predict transplant outcome are limited. The PACT scales measure quantity and quality of social supports, psychological health, lifestyle factors, substance abuse, compliance with and knowledge regarding the transplant process. It has been demonstrated to be a useful and reliable tool for studying clinical decision making. Olbrisch et al. [4] reported that 96% of those who use the tool agree to accept or deny patients based on their PACT score. For example, a good transplant candidate would have stable, committed support networks, no major psychopathology, good coping skills; be willing and able to make lifestyle changes, e.g. substance abstinence; and display a realistic understanding and expectation of transplantation. As PACT is used to assess patients' readiness for transplantation, LCSWs are better able to recognize their ability to achieve the best possible outcome and rehabilitation posttransplant.

Zilberfein et al. state that clinical social work and psychiatric support services are often critical in achieving adherence to transplant process requirements. In a study of psychosocial risk factors, interventions, and medical outcomes at one transplant center, they reported a need for ongoing individual counseling by 42% of pretransplant patients, compared with 70% after orthotopic liver transplantation (OLT) [1]. At most transplant centers, both a LCSW and a medical psychologist evaluate potential transplant candidates. Substance abuse screening and psychological assessments are two integral and overlapping aspects of this process. This is particularly helpful and important when inconsistencies are discovered in histories reported to different providers. Patients with a substance abuse history require ongoing assessment for and compliance with substance abstinence. Identification of psychological risk factors, such as recurrent depression or anxiety for patient or caregiver, will require counseling and/or psychotropic medications. The LCSW and the medical psychologist work collaboratively to monitor progress and continue interventions, which include counseling, support, advocacy, and availability of resources. The most valuable resource for transplant patients and families, however, is the relationship with the transplant team.

■ SOCIAL SUPPORT

Patients undergoing liver transplantation experience multiple physical and emotional changes, e.g. depression and anxiety. Therefore, it is critical that they have committed caregivers and a robust support network throughout the process, consisting of family, friends, neighbors, and groups. Dobbels et al. [5] demonstrated that social support helps reduce stressors associated with patients' illnesses.

The evaluation assesses each patient's and caregiver's level of understanding, functional ability, and commitment. The LCSW evaluates the quality of support and family interactions to help clarify roles and responsibilities. Some of the post-OLT responsibilities include monitoring medications, awareness of physical symptoms of infection or rejection, driving the patient to and from clinic appointments, staying locally with the patient in a furnished apartment or hotel, as well as providing both general physical and emotional support. Research suggests that both transplant and nontransplant patients with inadequate support are more likely to develop an affective psychiatric disorder [5], the corollary being that patients who have a strong support network have better overall outcomes. The transplant team, in turn, commits itself not only to the patient but also to his or her caregivers. The support plan is reviewed continually for major life changes, particularly if the patient has a considerable period of time on the waiting list prior to OLT. Dew et al. [6] reported that patients and families often identify the wait as the "most psychologically stressful part of the transplant experience."

Most transplant programs provide pre- and posttransplant support groups for patients and their families. This sharing of common experiences and concerns, particularly when offered by posttransplant patients, has been shown to reduce both anxiety and isolation [7]. Some of these stressors include anxiety about loss of income, increasingly high health care costs, feelings of uselessness and loss of control, and fear of dying without undergoing liver transplantation, including how death would affect the family [7]. Addressing such issues with patients and caregivers in a confidential group setting is the responsibility of a LCSW or equivalent mental health professional.

◼ PSYCHOLOGICAL HEALTH

Most, if not all, liver transplant candidates undergoing evaluation have already experienced life-threatening complications of end-stage liver disease (ESLD) and will experience typical adjustment reactions, e.g. anxiety, depression, anger, fear, loss of independence, and frustration. The prevalence of anxiety and depression is 4–20 times more common among pre-solid organ transplant recipients than in the general population [5]. Patients and families must learn to be prepared for and cope with many potential stressors that surface during the transplant process, as well as the effects of illness on health-related quality of life and family function. In addition, O'Carroll et al. [8] suggest, "highly neurotic or anxious individuals may have unrealistic expectations regarding liver transplantation and may be more likely to be disappointed with the eventual outcome."

Emotional stability is a significant factor in determining a patient's readiness for transplantation. The psychosocial assessment also involves identifying personality disorders, organic brain disorders, and suicidal ideation. The prevalence of personality disorders in transplant candidates ranges between 11% and 35%, comparable with the general population [5]. Personality disorders may result in nonadherence with diet, appointments, medications, and the requirement for smoking cessation. By using PACT, a patient's psychological health is rated, from severe ongoing psychopathology such as personality disorders to stable personality factors [4]. Individuals with stable personality factors tend to accept their illness and their need for transplantation better and adjust more readily during all phases of the process.

In addition to psychological factors, it is important to recognize biological factors such as hepatic encephalopathy, since it may contribute to mood and personality changes [5]. Lack of energy, loss of appetite, and sleep problems may be symptoms of depression and/or effects of liver disease and require consideration of pharmacotherapy [3].

Liver transplant support groups provide a forum where patients and caregivers can discuss the many challenges of mood and personality changes and their impact upon family relationships. For instance, those with no history of alcohol abuse may feel a stigma associated with a diagnosis of cirrhosis. Baker and McWilliam [7] suggest that stigmatization generates negative feelings, isolating patients within their social environment. Some patients with ESLD even choose not to reach out to support networks for fear of being labeled an alcoholic. However, transplant candidates with determination and a positive mindset tend to cope better with these challenges, especially when discussed within a support group forum.

It is an integral part of the evaluation process that caregivers are also assessed for mental health issues that could affect the patient's care and subsequent outcome. Dew et al. discuss how "family members' own mental health history and social functioning are relevant in understanding the psychosocial environment of the patient." These mental health issues can be significant sources of stress for the patient and may rob the patient of needed support [3].

■ LIFESTYLE FACTORS

Assessment of the ability and willingness of a potential transplant candidate and their support network to adhere to the medical regimen is a fundamental concern, and one that is discussed in detail at the outset of the evaluation process (Chapter 4). Pretransplant nonadherence is a risk factor for negative results following transplantation [5]. In order to address this issue, patients sign a behavioral contract, which assists them in understanding requirements for listing as a transplant candidate. These requirements include attending regular clinic visits; taking medications as prescribed; maintaining a healthy weight; securing the commitment of family and friends; abstaining from alcohol, tobacco, and other nonprescription drugs; and communicating physical and/or emotional problems to transplant team members in a timely manner. Such a contract promotes and models a healthy lifestyle before transplant occurs. As noted by Nelson et al. [9], behavioral contracting encourages patients to alter behavior as the transplant team monitors adherence, and it provides a reward: being approved for transplantation. Behavioral contracting is not used as a treatment but as a tactic to address nonadherence among liver transplant candidates.

One major necessity for success is the lifelong requirement for and necessary commitment to costly immunosuppressive drug therapy (Chapter 29). As noted by Bunzel and Laederach-Hofmann [10], poor adherence with this regimen impairs both quality of life and life span among transplant recipients, being a "major risk factor for graft rejection," and is responsible for up to 25% of deaths after transplant. Medical adherence is one area in which patients can have some sense of control in their recovery and quality of life. However, Bunzel and Laederach-Hofmann [10] conclude that overall nonadherence ranges between 20% and 50% and continues to persist posttransplant.

Alcohol remains a common cause of ESLD (Chapter 10) [11], and is a significant lifestyle factor that must be addressed. Since denial is a cardinal feature of alcohol dependence, it should not be surprising that some patients deny alcohol use was a contributing factor to their disease. Alcohol abuse and dependence can also lead to problems at work, in relationships, and with the legal system. The psychological and social problems that arise from alcohol dependence may compromise adherence and thus, transplant outcome, with data showing 15–25% of pretransplant alcoholic patients relapsing episodically or drinking continuously after transplantation [5]. Dobbels et al. demonstrated that longer periods of sobriety before transplantation have been associated with a decrease in relapse rate after transplantation. Of course, this is dependent on other factors: the number of years of drinking, number of alcoholic drinks consumed daily, and previous alcohol treatment programs [5]. It is commonplace amongst liver transplant programs that patients demonstrate at least 6 months of abstinence from alcohol and other substances and, if applicable, provide documentation of their substance abuse treatment. This may comprise inpatient rehabilitation, outpatient counseling programs, and attendance at Alcoholics Anonymous. As noted earlier, both the LCSW and the medical psychologist monitor the patient's treatment and progress.

Addictive behavior patterns may limit a patient's ability to care for himself or herself post-OLT, which then interferes with rehabilitation goals. Research studies have shown that 11–48% of liver transplant recipients return to some level of alcohol use during the first year after OLT, and an additional 5–10% return to drinking 2 and 3 years thereafter. The substance use component in the evaluation should consider patients' "personal triggers for renewed substance use," their desire to use the substance, and what coping mechanisms are in place to help prevent relapse [3]. Substance abuse and nonadherent behavior in other areas adversely affect transplant rehabilitation and success, and these issues need to be identified at an early stage and addressed where possible.

■ TRANSPLANT EDUCATION

A major objective of psychosocial evaluation is to determine the patient's and family's understanding of the illness and necessity for transplant. PACT is useful, to assess both relevant knowledge and receptiveness to this type of education [4], and has been shown to be important for maximizing psychosocial and medical adherence [6]. Liver transplantation is a lifetime commitment, and many patients have unrealistic expectations about recovery and posttransplant quality of life. Despite extensive discussion about the risks and benefits of OLT, psychological defense mechanisms, e.g. denial and avoidance, may lead to an exaggerated positive interpretation of such information. This positive outlook regarding posttransplant life can actually be helpful as a coping mechanism within the context of surgery and recovery, but result in disappointment thereafter. In one study of 55 liver transplant patients Holzner et al. [12] found that 60% expected to lead a normal life posttransplant, but only 40% of the group felt as though their expectations had been fulfilled. This sense of normality is dependent on both physical and emotional factors, as each patient's functional level may continue to be impaired, and overall quality of life improved.

Education is also essential for helping patients and families cope with the financial considerations of transplantation. The financial coordinator should meet with transplant candidates and their supporters to discuss insurance coverage and out-of-pocket costs liable to patients and family members. In many cases, patients are required to raise funds when finances are limited. The LCSW can assist to identify financial resources for posttransplant care issues, e.g. accommodation, subsistence, temporary loss of income, and immunosuppressive drugs, in particular. Having realistic expectations decreases anxiety over these transplant-associated costs. Once the financial aspect of transplantation has been addressed, patients can focus more energy on the physical and emotional aspects thereof.

■ QUALITY OF LIFE PRETRANSPLANT

Bravata and Keeffe state, "health-related quality of life is a multidimensional construct, reflecting an individual's global physical and psychosocial well-being." This includes not only physical and psychological health, but also social and sexual functioning, ability to perform regular daily activities, and overall well-being [13]. Some transplant programs use the Medical Outcomes Survey Short Form (SF-36), a generic tool that is well validated to assess health-related quality of life. It includes 36 items divided into eight scales: physical functioning, role-physical, bodily pain, general health, vitality, social functioning, role-emotional, and mental health. In one particular study using this tool, Younossi et al. [14] concluded that the quality of life among patients awaiting liver transplantation was severely impaired when compared with that reported by the general population.

Many lifestyle adjustments are necessary before transplantation occurs. When patients present for evaluation, they may exhibit many physical symptoms of liver disease that can prevent participation in regular daily activities. Lack of energy and fatigue are commonplace. Since diet and exercise may be significant contributing factors and both are critical to recovery, patients are often advised to maintain dietary and exercise programs pretransplant. A transplant dietician is available to assist with individualized dietary plans.

A major adjustment for patients is when they are required to quit work or interrupt their education as the result of illness. Unemployment places a financial burden on the family, with the spouse or partner often having to assume responsibility for providing and managing finances. Such a role reversal may be difficult to endure; work and education give a sense of purpose and accomplishment. When they are interrupted, patients need to find new ways to give their lives meaning.

As a result of their illness, many patients must apply for Social Security Disability. This can be a frustrating process, especially when there is an extended waiting period between their application and receipt of first disability check. In addition, some patients' insurance coverage may change. Patients must remain aware of transplant and immunosuppressive drug coverage under any new policies.

Social activities with family and friends are altered as patients deal with increased physical limitations. Baker and McWilliam concluded that while waiting to undergo transplantation, patients often withdrew from activities that they perceived defined who they were. Thus, as their physical and emotional health declined, so participation in social activities became more limited [7]. During this difficult waiting period, the transplant team plays an important role in helping patients set and achieve reasonable goals to achieve a more satisfying quality of life.

■ QUALITY OF LIFE POSTTRANSPLANT

Quality of life has been shown to increase in both physical and psychological domains within 6 months of undergoing liver transplantation. DeBona et al. [15] suggest that in these first few months patients feel a sense of "rebirth," positively influencing their overall outlook. However, recovery rates vary and it is not uncommon for patients to require hospital admission with acute rejection or other complications of OLT. The average recovery time for a liver transplant recipient is 6–12 months, and the 1-year anniversary of surgery marks an important time for patients and families. Relative stability in their lives is usually achieved once this critical milestone is passed [6], thereby allowing patients to change their focus and priorities with this new lease on life.

Immediately after transplant surgery, patients and their families experience a period of relief and euphoria [16]; this psychological boost often aids the recovery process. However, happiness may be tempered by the knowledge that another family has lost a loved one, and feelings of remorse and grief are prevalent during the postoperative period. Zilberfein et al. [1] discuss how patients may preoccupy themselves with the donor, wanting to know personal information such as age, gender, and cause of death: these feelings are a "common emotional burden [1]." It is suggested that patients wait until after their initial recovery, when a sense of normality has been restored, before making a decision to contact the donor family or not. One potential drawback, however, is that patients and families may be less able to focus on and accept information about potential complications [6]. DeBona et al. [15] state, "quality of life and psychological distress after OLT may be influenced by complications following surgery, by the effect of immunosuppressive therapy, and by recurrence of liver disease, particularly HCV." As a result, education, supportive counseling, and other resources remain as important post-OLT as they were pretransplant.

■ PRODUCTIVITY AND SOCIAL REHABILITATION

During the early postoperative period, liver transplant recipients continue to experience and demonstrate both physical and social limitations. They are advised to regain physical strength by walking once they are moved from the intensive care unit (ICU), where a physical therapist works extensively with them. After discharge from hospital, patients are expected to continue ambulating on their own, with assistance and supervision from caregivers, and to maintain an exercise and dietary regimen. As with the pretransplant phase, it is often difficult for patients to accept continued physical limitations. The stability and availability of support networks is critical as patients become dependent on them during the postoperative phase. As they slowly begin to feel more independent in their recovery, patients will involve themselves in more social activities. The ability to adjust to the many physical and social changes improves adherence with posttransplant regimens.

Body and self-image changes also occur that can precipitate negative feelings. The most significant bodily change is the extensive scarring from transplant surgery. Other body changes result from side-effects of medications, including steroids. Patients, both male and female, may gain weight, grow excessive body and facial hair, and suffer from mood changes. Sexual activity is affected during the recovery process, which can influence relationships. The social worker can help patients and families reprioritize their lives and achieve new goals, as they are sometimes not mentally ready to take on new responsibilities.

■ RETURNING TO WORK

Returning to work should be an important rehabilitation goal for most liver transplant recipients. However, after OLT a patient may not view it as important, especially if his or her life priorities have been altered. Potential barriers that may limit transplant recipients' ability and willingness to return to work include discrimination by potential employers, economic conditions, availability of health insurance, limited education and/or work skills, and the belief that some obstacles are "insurmountable [17]." Depression is an important predictor of posttransplant patients' capacity to return to work: 60% of depressed recipients who were at least 6 months posttransplant were not working [18]. Some patients are able to return to work at their former jobs, whereas others may have to reduce their hours or change careers in order to adjust to physical limitations. A recent study following patients returning to work 5 years after liver transplantation observed that before liver transplant, 44% of study patients were employed, in contrast to only 22% employed 6.4 years posttransplant [19]. This finding is significant, since returning to work is an important rehabilitation goal for many patients and also can be used as an index of transplant success. As reported by Carter et al. [17], those patients who are able to return to work reported "less depression, higher self-esteem, improved relationships, and an increased motivation to stay as healthy as possible."

■ EMOTIONAL CHANGES

Patients are confronted with varying degrees of emotional stress throughout the transplant process. The extent to which counseling is utilized before transplantation is contingent on the severity of depression, anxiety, or other mood changes identified during the assessment. The medical psychologist and/or the LCSW would have followed-up with these patients more frequently, to offer appropriate psychosocial recommendations. Once transplant surgery and the immediate postoperative period are completed, it is expected that some patients will develop some depressive symptoms as a result of their experience, and the effects of immunosuppressive drug therapy. This can occur even if they did not display symptoms before surgery. Forsberg et al. reported that coping mechanisms change over time and are affected by situational contexts. Antonovsky's theory of coping states, "a person who finds that there is meaning in daily existence will also be determined to make sense of difficult situations [20]." As patients and caregivers experience more physical and emotional adjustments during the first year posttransplant, they will most likely experience increased stress. Therefore, as patients continue to adjust during the recovery process, they learn to accept their situation with more patience and enthusiasm.

As the transplant experience can have an emotional impact on recipients and caregivers, the social worker can be a valuable resource. In our program, a psychosocial assessment of liver recipients and families is completed within 72 h posttransplant. A study by Nickel et al. concluded that coping, anxiety, and depression, in addition to social factors, determine overall well-being and health-related quality of life after liver transplantation. Using SF-36, they found that depression was the strongest factor in both physical and mental quality of life [21]. If patients and/or their families display signs of depression or anxiety, they may require more counseling and support services. Some patients are also prescribed antidepressants or other mood-adjusting medications to help them recover, especially when they are hospitalized repeatedly for complications. Repeated hospitalization delays the transplant patient's ability to reach his or her goals, which may, in turn, affect his or her emotional health.

Anxiety, anger, and denial are all important factors in patients' adherence with the medical regimen [10]. Posttransplant depression can also trigger noncompliance, a significant risk factor for negative outcome [5]. Encouragement and motivation from support systems during times of depression are necessary to keep the patient equally motivated. The clinical social worker and other mental health professional team members are responsible for providing necessary interventions for these patients to facilitate their reintegration into their personal and professional lives. As declared by Jones and Egan [22], social work has an ethical obligation to patients during the initial recovery period and throughout the transplant process.

■ RESOURCES

There are many resources available to patients and families that focus on specific liver diseases, the transplantation process at each stage, related information and support services (Table 28.1).

Table 28.1 *Resources for Liver Transplant Patients*

Organization	Description
Alcoholics Anonymous www.alcoholics-anonymous.org 212-870-3400	Fellowship of men and women who share their experience, strength, and hope with each other in order to solve their common problems and help others recover from alcoholism
American Liver Foundation www.liverfoundation.org 1-800-223-719	National, voluntary nonprofit health agency dedicated to preventing, treating, and curing hepatitis and other liver diseases through research, education, and advocacy
American Liver Society www.liversociety.org	Provides information and resources on various liver diseases and transplantation through research, advocacy, awareness, and support
Centers for Medicare and Medicaid Services (CMS) www.cms.hhs.gov www.medicare.gov	CMS is a Federal agency within the U.S. Department of Health and Human Services responsible for both Medicare and Medicaid services
National Clearing House for Alcohol and Drug Information www.health.org 1-800-729-6686	Information provided on alcohol, tobacco, and mental health services including local mental health centers
National Foundation for Transplant (NFT) www.transplants.org 1-800-489-3863	Provides information for fundraising to help patients overcome financial hurdles in receiving a life-saving transplant, the follow-up treatment, and medications essential to their continued health
Organ Procurement and Transplantation Network (OPTN) www.optn.org	The OPTN is a unique public/private partnership that links all of the professionals involved in the donation and transplantation system
Pharmaceutical Research and Manufacturers Association of America (PhRMA) www.phrma.org 1-800-762-4636	The PhRMA represents the leading research-based pharmaceutical and biotechnology companies in the USA offering information on patient assistance programs

Table 28.1 *Continued*

Social Security Administration www.socialsecurity.gov 1-800-772-1213	Information and applications provided for retirement and disability including supplemental security income (SSI) and Medicare benefits
Substance Abuse and Mental Health Services Administration www.samhsa.gov	Provides information on substance abuse and mental health services including local mental health centers
United Network for Organ Sharing (UNOS) www.unos.org 1-800-292-9548	UNOS provides transplant publications, reports, and resources specifically of interest to patients. UNOS brings together medicine, science, public policy, and technology to facilitate every organ transplant performed in the USA

Vocational Rehabilitation is one such resource available to patients who have been out of work. This state-funded agency assists individuals with physical, sensory, or mental disabilities to undergo training or gain employment. Patients may decide to return to school to complete or start a new education program, or may involve themselves in volunteer work if they are unable to return to employment. The Ticket to Work and Self-Sufficiency Program for people with disabilities increases opportunities and choices for Social Security beneficiaries.

Liver transplant support groups continue to be available to patients and families post-OLT as well. As time goes on, however, patients return to clinic less frequently and others live far from the hospital, making such a group less accessible. If there are support groups in their own area, they are encouraged to participate. Transplant patients able to attend a support group regularly have the opportunity of meeting other transplant recipients and form connections that go well beyond the counseling and support undertaken in an individual or group setting.

■ SUMMARY

Psychosocial status before transplantation has the potential to influence medical outcomes post-OLT [3]. Rehabilitation of patients with ESLD who become liver transplant recipients begins when they arrive for their initial transplant evaluation. Psychosocial assessments are essential tools, with all team members playing fundamental roles in this process. Once a patient is listed for transplantation, psychosocial adjustments continue throughout the waiting period, transplant, and recovery. The transplant team must identify high-risk patients in the early stages of their evaluation and provide appropriate interventions and referrals. Although a liver transplant recipient is never fully prepared for what lies ahead, professional relationships with the transplant team facilitate the ability to understand, accept, and cope with an intense and grueling process. If patients are to obtain the best possible quality of life posttransplant, committed care must begin with the transplant evaluation and continue throughout their lives.

■ REFERENCES

1. Zilberfein F, Hutson C, Snyder S, et al. Social work practice with pre- and post-liver transplant patients: a retrospective self study. Soc Work Health Care 2001;33:91–104.

2. Wang VS, Saab S. Liver transplantation in the era of model for end-stage liver disease. Liver Int 2004;24:1–8.

3. Dew MA, Switzer G, DiMartini A. Psychosocial assessments and outcomes in organ transplantation. Prog Transplant 2000;10(4):239–259.

4. Olbrisch ME, Levenson JL, Hamer R. The PACT: a rating scale for the study of clinical decision-making in psychosocial screening of organ transplant candidates. Clin Transplant 1989;3:164–169.

5. Dobbels F, De Geest S, Cleemput I, et al. Psychosocial and behavioral selection criteria for solid organ transplantation (review; 120 references). Prog Transplant 2001;11:121–130.

6. Dew MA, Manzetti J, Goycoolea J, et al. Psychosocial aspects of transplantation. In Smith S, ed., Organ transplantation: concepts, issues, practice, and outcomes 2002; Chapter 8. Available at http://www.medscape.com.

7. Baker MS, McWilliam C. How patients manage life and health while waiting for a liver transplant. Prog Transplant 2003;13:47–60.

8. O'Carroll RE, Couston M, Cossar J, et al. Psychological outcome and quality of life following liver transplantation: a prospective, national, single-center study. Liver Transpl 2003;9:712–720.

9. Nelson MK, Presberg BA, Olbrisch ME, et al. Behavioral contingency contracting to reduce substance abuse and other high-risk health behaviors in organ transplant patients. J Transpl Coord 1995;5:35–40.

10. Bunzel B, Laederach-Hofmann K. Solid organ transplantation: are there predictors for posttransplant noncompliance? A literature overview. Transplantation 2000;70: 711–716.

11. DiMartini A, Day N, Dew MA, et al. Alcohol use following liver transplantation: a comparison of follow-up methods. Psychosomatics 2001;42:55–62.

12. Holzner B, Kemmler G, Kopp M, et al. Preoperative expectations and postoperative quality of life in liver transplant survivors. Arch Phys Med Rehabil 2001;82:73–79.

13. Bravata D, Keeffe E. Quality of life and employment after liver transplantation. Liver Transpl 2001;7:S119–S123.

14. Younossi Z, McCormick M, Price LL, et al. Impact of liver transplantation on health-related quality of life. Liver Transpl 2000;6:779–783.

15. DeBona M, Ponton P, Ermani M, et al. The impact of liver disease and medical complications on quality of life and psychological distress before and after liver transplantation. J Hepatol 2000;33:609–615.

16. Dew MA. Quality of life studies: organ transplantation research as an exemplar of past progress and future directions. J Psychosom Res 1998;44:189–195.

17. Carter J, Winsett R, Rager D, et al. A center-based approach to a transplant employment program. Prog Transplant 2000;10:204–208.

18. Newton S. Relationship between depression and work outcomes following liver transplantation: the nursing perspective. Gastroenterol Nurs 2002;26:68–72.

19. Moyzes D, Walter M, Rose M, et al. Return to work 5 years after liver transplantation. Transplant Proc 2001;33:2878–2880.

20. Forsberg A, Backman L, Svensson E. Liver transplant recipients' ability to cope during the first 12 months after transplantation – a prospective study. Scand J Caring Sci 2002;16:345–352.

21. Nickel R, Wunsch A, Egle UT, et al. The relevance of anxiety, depression, and coping in patients after liver transplantation. Liver Transpl 2002;8:63–71.

22. Jones J, Egan M. The transplant experience of liver recipients: ethical issues and practice implications. Soc Work Health Care 2000;31:65–88.

▼   ▼   ▼   ▼   ▼   ▼   ▼   ▼   ▼   ▼

Medications

Immunosuppressive Medications

▾ ▾ ▾ ▾ ▾ ▾ ▾ ▾ ▾

Andrew J. Muir

29

A LTHOUGH other advances have made contributions, developments in immunosuppressive therapy have had significant impact on both graft and patient survival. The introduction of cyclosporine was a landmark event that made transplantation a reasonable clinical option [1]. Even with current therapies, clinically significant acute cellular rejection occurs in 24–80% of patients [2,3]. In addition, 5–10% ultimately develop chronic rejection, and repeated episodes of acute cellular rejection may increase the risk of chronic rejection [4]. The dominant cells in most rejection episodes are T cells, and successful transplantation requires blunting this response.

Immunosuppressive strategies vary from center to center in the selection of specific agents, number of agents, and the duration of use of each agent. A common theme among these diverse approaches is to combine agents with different mechanisms. This approach leads to additive immuno-suppression while minimizing adverse effects from any individual drug. In spite of this approach, management of adverse effects remains a significant component of immunosuppressive therapy. The current range of available agents does allow some flexibility for individualization as side-effects occur. To that end, this chapter addresses some of the agents in current practice.

■ CORTICOSTEROIDS

Despite the development of other agents, corticosteroids remain a key component of immunosuppression, both for initial therapy and for acute cellular rejection. The side-effects of corticosteroids have led to the pursuit of other regimens that eliminate the need for long-term steroid therapy.

Mechanism

Corticosteroids exert their anti-inflammatory activities through a variety of mechanisms. Within several hours after a dose, there is a significant reduction in the number of lymphocytes as a result of redistribution into lymphoid tissues. More importantly, corticosteroids also inhibit cytokine expression, including interleukin-1 (IL-1), IL-2, IL-6, and tumor necrosis factor (TNF) alpha gene transcription and secretion [5,6]. Corticosteroids also block the ability of macrophages to respond to lymphocyte-derived signals. Receptors are also present on monocytes, neutrophils, and eosinophils.

Administration

The use of corticosteroids varies widely among transplant programs. Most groups, however, give large doses of an intravenous form (usually methylprednisolone) at the time of transplantation and then quickly move to prednisone. For patients who are unable to take or absorb the oral preparation, the conversion from oral to parenteral dosing is provided in Table 29.1. The rate and duration of the prednisone taper are the major areas of variation and may depend not only on the center but also on the indication for transplantation. Due to the increased viral loads in the setting of immunosuppression and hepatitis C virus infection [7], these patients may expect more rapid tapering. There has been limited experience with steroid-free immunosuppression; a pilot study of 21 transplants demonstrated acute rejection requiring steroids in 23.5% and 3-year graft survival of 95% [8].

Management of acute cellular rejection also involves corticosteroids. Patients typically receive several days of high-dose intravenous methylprednisolone and then resume prednisone. The first controlled trial comparing different regimens for liver allograft rejection found that a starting dose of methylprednisolone of 1000 mg followed by a taper over 6 days was superior to 3 consecutive days of methylprednisolone 1000 mg [9].

Table 29.2 provides a summary of the administration characteristics of prednisone and the other immunosuppressive agents discussed in this chapter.

Table 29.1 *Equivalent Dosing of Common Corticosteroids*

Corticosteroid	Equivalent Dose (mg)
Hydrocortisone	20
Prednisolone	5
Prednisone	5
Methylprednisolone	4

Table 29.2 *Dose Administration*

Drug	Maintenance Dose	Tablets/ Capsule	Oral Suspension	Parenteral	Monthly Monitoring
Prednisone	5–20 mg/day	✓	✓		Glucose
Cyclosporine	8 ± 4 mg/kg/day in 2 doses	✓	✓	✓	Drug level, Crt, K, lipids
Tacrolimus in 2 doses	0.10–0.30 mg/kg/day	✓	✓	✓	Drug level, Crt, K, lipids
Mycophenolate mofetil	500–1000 mg bid	✓	✓	✓	CBC
Azathioprine	1–2 mg/kg/day	✓	a	✓	CBC, AST, ALT, alk phos, bilirubin
Sirolimus	2 mg/day	✓	✓		CBC, Crt, K, lipids

(Formulations spans the Tablets/Capsule, Oral Suspension, and Parenteral columns.)

Note: ALT, alanine aminotransferase; AST, aspartate aminotransferase; alk phos, alkaline phosphatase; bili, total bilirubin; CBC, complete blood count; Crt, creatinine; K, potassium.
[a]Not commercially available but can be prepared with tablets by a pharmacist.

Pharmacokinetics

After oral administration, prednisone is rapidly absorbed, and peak levels can be observed in 1–2 h. Prednisone undergoes metabolism by the liver to the active metabolite prednisolone, which is then further metabolized to inactive compounds. Increased levels may therefore occur with hepatic insufficiency. The major route of excretion is renal, and dialysis does not substantially affect clearance. Prednisone does cross the placenta and is also found in breast milk.

Table 29.3 *Pregnancy and Lactation Risk*

Medication	Pregnancy Classification[a]	Found In Breast Milk?
Cyclosporine	C	Yes
Tacrolimus	C	Yes
Mycophenolate mofetil	C	b
Azathioprine	D	Yes
Sirolimus	C	b

[a]Classification: C, lack of human studies and results of animal studies positive or lacking; D, positive evidence of risk in humans.
[b]Positive results of animal studies, unknown in humans.

Table 29.4 *Pharmacokinetics of Immunosuppressive Agents*

Medication	Metabolism	Excretion	Dose Adjustment In Renal Failure	In Hepatic Failure	Dialyzable?
Prednisone	Metabolism	Excretion	None	None	No
Cyclosporine	Hepatic	Renal	↓[a]	↓	No
Tacrolimus	Hepatic	Bile	↓[a]	↓	No
Mycophenolate mofetil	Hepatic	Renal	↓	None	No
Azathioprine	Hepatic	Renal	↓	None	Partially
Sirolimus	Hepatic	Bile	None	↓	No

[a]Related to toxicity, not drug accumulation.

Table 29.3 summarizes the pregnancy and lactation risk with the common immunosuppressive agents. Table 29.4 provides a summary of the pharmacokinetics of corticosteroids and the other immunosuppressive agents discussed later in this chapter.

Adverse Effects

The many side-effects related to corticosteroids have led to attempts to decrease or eliminate their use in immunosuppressive regimens. In the acute setting, hyperglycemia and neurological impairment may occur. The neurological findings can range from insomnia to overt psychosis. Appetite stimulation is quite common and often leads to considerable weight gain after transplant. Problems associated with long-term steroid use also include cushingoid appearance, osteoporosis, cataracts, and myopathy. Rapid tapers or sudden discontinuation of corticosteroids may result in acute adrenal insufficiency. A summary of the common adverse effects is given in Table 29.5.

■ CYCLOSPORINE

Neoral® and Sandimmune®

The modern era of liver transplantation began with the introduction of cyclosporine. In 1976, Borel et al. [10] reported the discovery of the immunosuppressive properties of this fungal metabolite extracted from *Cylindrocarson lucidum*. After an initial successful series [1], the University of Pittsburgh group reported their first 1000 patients treated with cyclosporine and steroids and found that the survival rate was three times greater than in the precyclosporine era [11]. Most transplant centers select either cyclosporine or tacrolimus as a component of their initial immunosuppressive regimen. Studies comparing these two agents are discussed in the section about tacrolimus.

Table 29.5 *Adverse Effects*

	Prednisone	Cyclosporine	Tacrolimus	Azathioprine	Mycophenolate Mofetil	Sirolimus
Leukopenia				✓	✓	✓
Anemia				✓	✓	✓
Thrombocytopenia				✓	✓	✓
Nephrotoxicity		✓	✓			
Hypertension	✓	✓	✓			
Hyperkalemia		✓	✓			
Hypomagnesemia		✓	✓			
Neurotoxicity	✓	✓	✓			
Gastrointestinal					✓	
Pancreatitis				✓		
Hepatoxicity				✓		
Hyperlipidemia	✓	✓	✓			✓
Hyperglycemia	✓	✓	✓			
Gingival hyperplasia		✓	✓			

Mechanism

Cyclosporine binds to cyclophilin, a cytoplasmic receptor protein, and creates an active complex. This complex then binds to calcineurin, a calcium-activated serine–threonine phosphatase, and inhibits the expression of several critical T cell activation transcription factors. Cyclosporine's regulation of IL-2 gene transcription appears to be especially important [12]. The inhibition of IL-2 activity is associated with a decreased response to class I and II antigens, which are critical for the rejection cascade. The inhibition of these transcription factors limits the activation and proliferation of lymphocytes.

Administration

Neoral has largely replaced Sandimmune as the dominant preparation of cyclosporine. Sandimmune has pharmacokinetic properties that have presented problems for many patients. Cyclosporine is quite hydrophobic, and absorption of Sandimmune requires good motility and emulsification by luminal bile salts. Consequently, higher doses are required immediately after surgery if bile output is being diverted to external drainage by a T-tube. Neoral is prepared as a microemulsion of cyclosporine and therefore mixes well with intestinal contents [13]. T-tube drainage therefore does not impact its dosing. Neoral also has increased bioavailability and decreased intrapatient and interpatient variability. The correlation between cyclosporine trough blood concentrations and total systemic exposure measured by the area under the curve is also greater with Neoral [14]. As a result, Neoral and Sandimmune cannot be used interchangeably.

The initial doses of cyclosporine may be delivered intravenously, but the patient is soon converted to the oral route. Doses may vary widely, but the typical dose is 8 ± 4 mg/kg in two doses. If the patient is unable to take oral medication, the dose can be given parenterally but at approximately one-third of the daily oral dose. When given parentally, the drug should be mixed in a glass container (its lipophilic properties cause it to bind to plastics) in a dedicated line. When the patient is taking oral cyclosporine, food may impact the absorption [15], and this effect may be less common with Neoral [16]. However, to prevent alterations in drug levels, patients should take the medicine at the same interval after each meal. The oral solution is not palatable and can be mixed in orange or apple juice. Grapefruit juice should be avoided because of reports of significant increases in cyclosporine levels [17].

Despite the improvements with Neoral, the variability associated with cyclosporine requires frequent monitoring of drug trough levels. Patients need to be reminded to hold their medications on the morning that a cyclosporine level is going to be measured; unexpected high levels warrant clarification of the timing of the last dose of medication. Multiple assays are now available to measure drug levels, and the particular assay used may impact the drug level. Both immunoassays and a high-pressure liquid chromatograph (HPLC) assay are available [18]. The immunoassays use antibodies directed against cyclosporine, but the antibodies may also cross-react with inactive metabolites of cyclosporine. The HPLC technique separates cyclosporine from its metabolites by liquid chromatography. This method therefore reports the level of the parent drug only. The immunoassay may therefore overestimate the cyclosporine concentration by approximately 40%. The goal for levels may vary with the overall immunosuppressive regimen and may also vary from center to center. Our center's guidelines for cyclosporine levels with the HPLC assay are described in Table 29.6.

Pharmacokinetics

The bioavailability of oral cyclosporine varies between 20% and 50%. Cyclosporine is metabolized primarily by the cytochrome P450 system of the liver, generating more than 17 metabolites. Although several metabolites show detectable immunosuppressant activity, the contribution of active metabolites to immunosuppression is minimal [19]. The half-life is approximately 15 h (range 10–40 h). Excretion in the urine is minimal, and neither renal failure nor dialysis alters clearance. Renal failure does not warrant dose reduction to

Table 29.6 *Cyclosporine Levels After Transplantation*

Months After Transplantation	Level (ng/ml)
0–3	200–250
3–6	150–200
6–12	120–150
>12	80–120

prevent high-drug levels, but dose reduction may be necessary if nephrotoxicity caused by cyclosporine is a concern. Given cyclosporine's hepatic metabolism, significant hepatic insufficiency may warrant dose monitoring. Cyclosporine does cross the placenta and is present in breast milk.

Adverse Effects

When cyclosporine was introduced, the absence of significant myelosuppression was an important advantage over other available immunosuppressive agents. However, experience with cyclosporine has revealed a number of other side-effects. Nephrotoxicity often develops with cyclosporine use and may require dose reduction or conversion to another agent. Other potentially nephrotoxic agents should be cautiously used, including amphotericin B, acyclovir, aminoglycosides, and nonsteroidal anti-inflammatory drugs (NSAIDs). Hypertension and hypomagnesaemia may also occur. Because of the risk of hyperkalemia, potassium-sparing diuretics should be avoided.

Neurotoxicity is another common finding with cyclosporine, affecting as many as a third of patients [20]. Findings have included altered mental status, motor polyneuropathy, dysarthria, myoclonus, seizures, hallucinations, and cortical blindness. Other common problems include hyperlipidemia, gingival hyperplasia, and hirsutism. Hepatotoxicity has been reported but was associated with high drug levels [21].

■ TACROLIMUS

Prograf®

With a similar action to cyclosporine, tacrolimus has emerged as another option for immunosuppression. Tacrolimus is a macrolide antibiotic that was isolated from the soil fungus *Streptomyces tsukubaensis*. Like cyclosporine, tacrolimus blocks the activation of calcineurin and inhibits the expression of critical T cell activation gene transcription factors. Tacrolimus, however, binds to a highly conserved cytosolic protein (FK-506 binding protein (FKBP)) [22]. In this manner, it limits the activation and proliferation of lymphocytes.

Although initially used for rescue therapy in acute rejection, tacrolimus has also become a first-line agent. Two randomized, controlled trials from the 1990s compared cyclosporine and tacrolimus and found similar patient and graft survival rates [23,24]. Although fewer rejection episodes occurred with tacrolimus, there were also more side-effects. Since that time, the microemulsified preparation of cyclosporine (Neoral) with increased bioavailability emerged. As a result, a randomized controlled trial was conducted in patients undergoing liver transplantation [25]. The patients received either open-label tacrolimus or microemulsified cyclosporine in combination with prednisolone and azathioprine. The primary end points were death, retransplantation, or treatment failure due to immunological reasons. Twelve months after transplantation, the primary end points were reached in 62 (21%) of 301 patients receiving tacrolimus versus 99 (32%) of 305 patients receiving cyclosporine ($P = 0.001$). Rates of renal dysfunction and need for antihypertensives were similar. Diabetes was more frequent with tacrolimus.

Administration

Tacrolimus is available in oral and parenteral forms. Even in the early postoperative setting, absorption through gastrointestinal tract is adequate, and the parenteral form is rarely necessary. The typical maintenance dose is 0.10–0.30 mg/kg/day divided into two doses. Bioavailability with the oral formulation is variable, however, and close monitoring of drug trough levels remains necessary. Our center's recommended trough levels are included in Table 29.7. More than 1 year after transplantation, lower levels are acceptable if liver enzymes remain normal. Food recommendations are similar to those for cyclosporine. Food may reduce bioavailability, and patients need to be consistent in timing of food intake and dose. In addition, patients taking tacrolimus should avoid grapefruit juice because of potential for increased levels.

Pharmacokinetics

The metabolism of tacrolimus occurs mainly through the hepatic cytochrome P450 system. As a result, hepatic dysfunction may be associated with increased plasma concentrations and reduced clearance. Renal insufficiency does not

Table 29.7 *Tacrolimus Levels After Transplantation*

Months After Transplantation	Level (ng/ml)
0–6	7–10
>6	5–7

lead to elevated drug levels, but dose reduction may be necessary if nephrotoxicity is a concern. The elimination half-life of tacrolimus in liver transplant patients is about 12 h [26]. Tacrolimus does cross the placenta and is present in breast milk.

Adverse Effects

Like cyclosporine, nephrotoxicity and neurotoxicity have been reported with tacrolimus. However, nephrotoxicity caused by cyclosporine is not necessarily a contraindication to the use of tacrolimus. In a series of 19 patients with cyclosporine nephrotoxicity converted to tacrolimus, 13 patients had a decrease in serum creatinine and stable graft function [27].

Diabetes has also been reported with tacrolimus. Other side-effects are similar to those of cyclosporine, including hyperkalemia, hypomagnesemia, and hyperlipidemia. In addition, cardiomyopathy has been reported in children [28]. Side-effects seen less frequently with tacrolimus include gingival hyperplasia, hirsutism, and hypertension.

■ AZATHROPRINE

Imuran®

Azathroprine remains a common component of initial regimens for liver transplantation, although mycophenolate mofetil has emerged as another option. Azathroprine interferes with purine synthesis via the "salvage" pathway and, therefore, complements the activity of corticosteroids and the calcineurin inhibitors.

Mechanism

Azathroprine is a purine analog that is metabolized in the liver to 6-mercaptopurine (6-MP). Further conversion of 6-MP results in a series of MP-containing nucleotides that interfere with de novo purine synthesis and therefore both deoxyribonucleic acid (DNA) and ribonucleic acid (RNA) synthesis. These effects result in decreased production of T and B lymphocytes, reduced immunoglobulin secretion, and decreased IL-2 secretion.

Administration

Azathioprine is available in both oral and parenteral forms. Although not available commercially, an oral solution can be prepared from the tablets by a pharmacist. When parenteral dosing is required, the dose is equivalent to the oral dose. The typical dose is 1–2 mg/kg daily.

One component of 6-MP metabolism is methylation of both 6-MP and the initial MP nucleotide by the enzyme thiopurine methyltransferase (TPMT). Considerable genetic polymorphism exists with this enzyme. Within the general population, approximately 11% of individuals may have intermediate (heterozygote) activity, and 1 in 300 may have no TPMT activity [29]. TPMT activity correlates with the response to azathroprine or 6-MP, and lack of TPMT activity is associated with myelosuppression [30]. Although not commonly used in transplantation, the assays for TPMT activity and genotypes are commercially available and may assist in management.

Pharmacokinetics

Azathroprine is metabolized by the liver with renal clearance. Renal insufficiency may therefore necessitate dose reduction. The half-life ranges from 0.7 to 3 h. Azathroprine is partially removed with dialysis, and doses should therefore be given after dialysis on these days. In addition, azathroprine does cross the placenta and is present in breast milk.

Adverse Effects

The most common and dose-limiting side-effect of azathiopurine is bone marrow suppression. As a result, routine monitoring is necessary. Typically, bone marrow suppression is reversible with a decreased dose or discontinuation. Pancreatitis is another common side-effect. In addition, liver enzyme abnormalities may occur in as many as 5% of patients. Venoocclusive disease has also rarely occurred with long-term treatment.

■ MYCOPHENOLATE MOFETIL

Cellcept®

Mycophenolate mofetil inhibits de novo purine biosynthesis and has become more common in liver transplantation as an alternative to azathroprine. The major advantage over azathroprine is its more selective inhibition of lymphocytes. Mycophenolate mofetil is used by many centers as a component of the initial immunosuppression regimen in combination with corticosteroids and a calcineurin inhibitor. Other indications have included rescue therapy for steroid-resistant rejection and also as an alternative if intolerance develops with other agents. Mycophenolate mofetil has been used as a first-line agent and allowed early cessation of prednisone [31]. The active drug, mycophenolic acid (MPA), is produced by Penicillium fungus.

Mechanism

After oral administration, mycophenolate mofetil is rapidly and completely converted to MPA. MPA then inhibits inosine monophosphate dehydrogenase, thus preventing the formation of guanosine monophosphate (GMP) and therefore guanine triphosphate and deoxyguanine triphosphate. These substrates are necessary for DNA and RNA synthesis. Unlike other cells, lymphocytes cannot synthesize GMP sufficiently through the salvage pathway that involves the enzyme hypoxanthine–guanine phosphoribosyltransferase. MPA acid therefore selectively inhibits the proliferation of both T and B lymphocytes.

Administration

Mycophenolate mofetil is available in both oral and parenteral forms. After oral administration, mycophenolate mofetil is rapidly and extensively absorbed. The typical dose is 1 g twice per day. Administration with food may decrease peak levels, and patients should therefore take the dose 1 h before or 2 h after a meal.

Pharmacokinetics

MPA is poorly absorbed after oral administration, and the semisynthetic prodrug mycophenolate mofetil improves the bioavailability. MPA is metabolized principally by glucuronyl transferase; the glucuronide metabolite is not pharmacologically active. About 90% of the administered drug is eliminated in the urine as MPA glucuronide. The elimination half-life is approximately 18 h. Renal impairment leads to accumulation of the MPA glucuronide metabolite, and dose reduction is necessary with renal insufficiency. Hemodialysis does not allow the clearance of MPA. MPA does cross the placenta and is found in breast milk.

Adverse Effects

Mycophenolate mofetil may have significant gastrointestinal side-effects, including nausea, anorexia, and diarrhea. Gastritis may develop, and the drug should be avoided in the setting of active peptic ulcer disease. Other side-effects include leukopenia, anemia, and thrombocytopenia.

■ SIROLIMUS

Rapamune®

Sirolimus is a macrolide antibiotic produced by *Streptomyces hygriscopicus* that has demonstrated potent immunosuppressive activity in a number of studies. In 1999, the U.S. Food and Drug Administration approved sirolimus for the prevention of acute transplant rejection. Soon after introduction, sirolimus emerged as an effective alternative for patients with renal insufficiency related to calcineurin inhibitor toxicity [32]. More recently, sirolimus has been increasingly used for initial immunosuppression in liver transplantation [33–35]. Three case series have now reported decreased incidence of rejection compared with historic controls. A pilot study randomized patients to tacrolimus and corticosteroids or sirolimus and low-dose tacrolimus with corticosteroids. The sirolimus group had lower graft and patient survival, and there was also increased wound infection and hepatic artery thrombosis [36]. A large international liver transplant trial was also halted due to increased incidence of hepatic artery thrombosis in patients receiving sirolimus. The manufacturer ultimately issued a letter warning physicians of this risk, and sirolimus now carries a "black box" warning in its package insert [37]. The warning notes that most cases of hepatic artery thrombosis occurred within 30 days of transplantation. These study findings continue to be debated. Sirolimus continues to be used later in the posttransplantation course; its role in initial immunosuppression remains controversial.

Mechanism

Sirolimus is structurally related to tacrolimus and shares the same binding site. However, sirolimus possesses a distinct mechanism of action [38]. The sirolimus–FKBP complex does not affect calcineurin activity. Instead, sirolimus blocks signals transduced from IL-2 receptors and other growth factors to the nucleus, thus inhibiting T and B cell proliferation.

Administration

Sirolimus is administered orally, and the typical maintenance dose is 2 mg/day. Food may alter the bioavailability of sirolimus, and the dose should be taken consistently in relation to eating.

Pharmacokinetics

Sirolimus is rapidly absorbed in 1–2 h. The bioavailability is approximately 14%. The major route of excretion appears to be the feces, with only 2.2% excreted in the urine. The half-life increased from 79 h in normal patients to 113 h in those with hepatic dysfunction. Dosage adjustments may therefore be necessary in patients with mild to moderate liver dysfunction.

Adverse Effects

Common adverse effects with sirolimus include anemia, leukopenia, and thrombocytopenia. Headache, hypertension, hyperlipidemia, and hypokalemia have also been reported. Hepatic artery thromosis has previously been discussed. Increased incidence of wound dehiscence was reported in a pilot study of sirolimus in liver transplant patients [36]. This complication was not increased in other reports and may be associated with the use of higher doses of sirolimus [33].

■ ANTIBODY THERAPY

Antibody therapy has been used for treatment of steroid-resistant rejection and induction therapy. The development of monoclonal technology has provided a more specific and consistent response. At this time, these agents do not have a routine role in maintenance immune suppression, but they have been utilized in isolated circumstances. Regimens examining a variety of strategies and combinations are currently under investigation.

■ ANTITHYMOCYTE GLOBULIN

Atgam® and Thymoglobulin®

Antithymocyte globulin is a purified immunoglobulin prepared from hyperimmune serum of horse, rabbit, sheep, or goat immunized with human thymic lymphocytes. Antithymocyte globulin binds to the surface of the T lymphocytes in the circulation, resulting in lymphopenia and impairment of T lymphocyte immune responses. Antithymocyte globulin is administered parentally at a daily dose of 10–30 mg/kg over several hours. Adverse effects include serum sickness, fever, chills, rash, leucopenia, thrombocytopenia, and nephritis.

■ MUROMONAB-CD3 MONOCLONAL ANTIBODY

Orthoclone OKT3®

OKT3 was the first monoclonal antibody approved by the Food and Drug Administration for use in humans. OKT3 is directed to the epsilon-chain of CD3, a three-chain molecule that is associated with T cell antigen receptor (TCR) [39]. CD3 is necessary for CD4+ T cell activation by alloantigen, and for CD8+ T cell direct cellular cytotoxicity. The main indication of OKT3 is for control of acute rejection [40]. OKT3 is administered intravenously. After administration, a cytokine-release syndrome with flu-like symptoms is evident within 30–60 min. OKT3 may also lead to pulmonary edema and exacerbate congestive heart failure or coronary artery disease.

■ DACLIZUMAB

Zenapax®

Daclizumab is a chimeric monoclonal antibody produced by recombinant DNA technology. The recombinant genes encoding daclizumab are a composite of human (90%) and murine (10%) antibody sequences. Daclizumab binds to the alpha subunit of the IL-2 receptor on lymphocytes, thus interfering with the signal that activates T cells. When used as part of induction therapy in combination with corticosteroids and cyclosporine, daclizumab reduced rejection episodes in renal transplantation [41]. It is administered intravenously 1 mg/kg every 14 days for five doses. Daclizumab is generally well tolerated with a side-effect profile comparable with that of placebo.

■ BASILIXIMAB

Simulect®

Basiliximab is also a chimeric (murine/human) monoclonal antibody that blocks the IL-2 receptor. When combined with standard immunotherapy in renal transplant recipients, basiliximab reduced acute rejection and graft loss at 3 years without increasing adverse events, including infection and malignancy [42]. The recommended dosing regimen is 20 mg intravenously within 6 h of reperfusion and also on day four posttransplantation. Basiliximab also has a benign side-effect profile, including lack of cytokine release syndrome.

■ CONCLUSION

The current range of available immunosuppressive agents allows some flexibility to tailor the regimen for the individual patient. At the same time, rejection and significant adverse effects continue to complicate the posttransplant period for many patients. Future work will include different combinations as well as development of new agents. Efforts will also focus on improving the balance of maximizing immunosuppression while minimizing adverse effects.

■ REFERENCES

1. Starzl TE, Klintmalm GB, Porter KA, et al. Liver transplantation with use of cyclosporin A and prednisone. N Engl J Med 1981;305:266–269.

2. Neuberger J. Incidence, timing, and risk factors for acute and chronic rejection. Liver Transpl Surg 1999;5(suppl 1):S30–S36.

3. Adams DH, Neuberger JM. Treatment of acute rejection. Semin Liver Dis 1992; 12:80–88.

4. Soin AS, Rasmussen A, Jamieson NV, et al. CsA levels in the early posttransplant period – predictive of chronic rejection in liver transplantation? Transplantation 1995;59:1119–1123.

5. Almawi WY, Lipman ML, Stevens AC, et al. Abrogation of glucocorticoid-mediated inhibition of T cell proliferation by the synergistic action of IL-1, IL-6, and IFN-gamma. J Immunol 1991;146:3523–3527.

6. Vacca A, Felli MP, Farina AR, et al. Glucocorticoid receptor-mediated suppression of the interleukin 2 gene expression through impairment of the cooperativity between nuclear factor of activated T cells and AP-1 enhancer elements. J Exp Med 1992;175:637–646.

7. Magy N, Cribier B, Schmitt C, et al. Effects of corticosteroids on HCV infection. Int J Immunopharmacol 1999;21:253–261.

8. Pirenne J, Aerts R, Koshiba T, et al. Steroid-free immunosuppression during and after liver transplantation – a 3-yr follow-up report. Clin Transplant 2003;17: 177–182.

9. Volpin R, Angeli P, Galioto A, et al. Comparison between two high-dose methyl-prednisolone schedules in the treatment of acute hepatic cellular rejection in liver transplant recipients: a controlled clinical trial [see comment]. [Clinical Trial. Journal Article. Randomized Controlled Trial] Liver Transpl 2002;8(6): 527–534.

10. Borel JF, Feurer C, Gubler HU, et al. Biological effects of cyclosporin A: a new antilymphocytic agent. Agents Actions 1976;6:468–475.

11. Iwatsuki S, Starzl TE, Todo S, et al. Experience in 1,000 liver transplants under cyclosporine-steroid therapy: a survival report. Transplant Proc 1988;20 (suppl 1):498–504.

12. Clipstone NA, Crabtree GR. Identification of calcineurin as a key signalling enzyme in T-lymphocyte activation. Nature 1992;357:695–697.

13. Levy G, Grant D. Potential for CsA–Neoral in organ transplantation. Transplant Proc 1994;26:2932–2934.

14. Mueller EA, Kovarik JM, van Bree JB, et al. Pharmacokinetics and tolerability of a microemulsion formulation of cyclosporine in renal allograft recipients – a concentration-controlled comparison with the commercial formulation. Transplantation 1994;57:1178–1182.

15. Keogh A, Day R, Critchley L, et al. The effect of food and cholestyramine on the absorption of cyclosporine in cardiac transplant recipients. Transplant Proc 1988;20:27–30.

16. Mueller EA, Kovarik JM, van Bree JB, et al. Influence of a fat-rich meal on the pharmacokinetics of a new oral formulation of cyclosporine in a crossover comparison with the market formulation. Pharm Res 1994;11:151–155.

17. Ku YM, Min DI, Flanigan M. Effect of grapefruit juice on the pharmacokinetics of microemulsion cyclosporine and its metabolite in healthy volunteers: does the formulation difference matter? J Clin Pharmacol 1998;38:959–965.

18. Hamwi A, Veitl M, Manner G, et al. Evaluation of four automated methods for determination of whole blood cyclosporine concentrations. Am J Clin Pathol 1999;112:358–365.

19. Schlitt HJ, Christians U, Bleck J, et al. Contribution of cyclosporin metabolites to immunosuppression in liver-transplanted patients with severe graft dysfunction. Transpl Int 1991;4:38–44.

20. Guarino M, Stracciari A, Pazzaglia P, et al. Neurological complications of liver transplantation. J Neurol 1996;243:137–142.

21. Yuan QS, Zheng FL, Sun Y, et al. Rescue therapy with tacrolimus in renal graft patients with cyclosporine A-induced hepatotoxicity: a preliminary study. Transplant Proc 2000;32:1694–1695.

22. Wiederrecht G, Lam E, Hung S, et al. The mechanism of action of FK-506 and cyclosporin A. Ann NY Acad Sci 1993;696:9–19.

23. The U.S. Multicenter FK506 Liver Study Group. A comparison of tacrolimus (FK 506) and cyclosporine for immunosuppression in liver transplantation. N Engl J Med 1994;331:1110–1115.

24. European FK506 Multicentre Liver Study Group. Randomised trial comparing tacrolimus (FK506) and cyclosporin in prevention of liver allograft rejection. Lancet 1994;344:423–428.

25. O'Grady JG, Burroughs A, Hardy P, et al. Tacrolimus versus microemulsified ciclosporin in liver transplantation: the TMC randomised controlled trial. Lancet 2002;360:1119–1125.

26. Hooks MA. Tacrolimus, a new immunosuppressant – a review of the literature. Ann Pharmacother 1994;28:501–511.

27. Pratschke J, Neuhaus R, Tullius SG, et al. Treatment of cyclosporine-related adverse effects by conversion to tacrolimus after liver transplantation. Transplantation 1997;64:938–940.

28. Nakata Y, Yoshibayashi M, Yonemura T, et al. Tacrolimus and myocardial hypertrophy. Transplantation 2000;69:1960–1962.

29. Vuchetich JP, Weinshilboum RM, Price RA. Segregation analysis of human red blood cell thiopurine methyltransferase activity. Genet Epidemiol 1995;12:1–11.

30. Lennard L, Van Loon JA, Weinshilboum RM. Pharmacogenetics of acute azathioprine toxicity: relationship to thiopurine methyltransferase genetic polymorphism. Clin Pharmacol Ther 1989;46:149–154.

31. Stegall MD, Wachs ME, Everson G, et al. Prednisone withdrawal 14 days after liver transplantation with mycophenolate: a prospective trial of cyclosporine and tacrolimus. Transplantation 1997;64:1755–1760.

32. Neff GW, Montalbano M, Slapak-Green G, et al. Sirolimus therapy in orthotopic liver transplant recipients with calcineurin inhibitor-related chronic renal insufficiency. Transplant Proc 2003;35:3029–3031.

33. Dunkelberg JC, Trotter JF, Wachs M, et al. Sirolimus as primary immunosuppression in liver transplantation is not associated with hepatic artery or wound complications. Liver Transpl 2003;9:463–468.

34. McAlister VC, Peltekian KM, Malatjalian DA, et al. Orthotopic liver transplantation using low-dose tacrolimus and sirolimus. Liver Transpl 2001;7:701–708.

35. Trotter JF, Wachs M, Bak T, et al. Liver transplantation using sirolimus and minimal corticosteroids (3-day taper). Liver Transpl 2001;7:343–351.

36. Wiesner R, Rapamune Liver Transplant Study Group. The safety and efficacy or sirolimus and low-dose tacrolimus versus tacrolimus in de novo orthotopic liver transplant patients: results from a pilot study (abstract). Hepatology 2002;36:208A.

37. Package insert. Rapamune (sirolimus). Philadelphia, PA: Wyeth Laboratories, September 2002.

38. Molnar-Kimber KL. Mechanism of action of rapamycin (sirolimus, Rapamune). Transplant Proc 1996;28:964–969.

39. Chang TW, Kung PC, Gingras SP, et al. Does OKT3 monoclonal antibody react with an antigen-recognition structure on human T cells? Proc Natl Acad Sci USA 1981;78:1805–1808.

40. Ortho Multicenter Transplant Study Group. A randomized clinical trial of OKT3 monoclonal antibody for acute rejection of cadaveric renal transplants. N Engl J Med 1985;313:337–342.

41. Vincenti F, Kirkman R, Light S, et al. Interleukin-2-receptor blockade with daclizumab to prevent acute rejection in renal transplantation. Daclizumab Triple Therapy Study Group. N Engl J Med 1998;338:161–165.

42. Chapman TM, Keating GM. Basiliximab: a review of its use as induction therapy in renal transplantation. Drugs 2003;63:2803–2835.

Drug Interactions with Commonly Used Immunosuppressive Agents

Paul G. Killenberg

▼ ▼ ▼ ▼ ▼ ▼ ▼ ▼ ▼

■ INTRODUCTION

Following liver transplantation (LT), patients characteristically receive several medications in addition to antirejection drugs. The opportunity for significant drug interactions is, therefore, great. Drug interactions are particularly frequent during the first 6 months after LT when the immunosuppressive dose is greater.

Drug interactions can be grouped into two types: pharmacokinetic interactions (where one drug alters the absorption, distribution, or elimination of another) and pharmacodynamic interactions (where a second drug potentiates or interferes with the action or side-effects of another).

This chapter focuses on drug interactions of both types that involve the commonly used immunosuppressive agents. Synergism in immunosuppressive effect between agents is not considered.

Certain drug interactions occur with sufficient frequency and uniformity within the patient population that the practicing physician can anticipate the interaction and make rational adjustments in the dose of the immunosuppressive agent, thus avoiding toxic or inadequate levels. In other instances, the literature reports a few cases of possible interaction. The latter reports may reflect genetic idiosyncrasies or other factors not substantiated by pharmacokinetic studies. Reports of infrequent drug interactions should not be dismissed as irrelevant; rather, they should prompt increased vigilance including frequent determinations of immunosuppressive drug levels or measurements related to potential toxicity. Drug interactions are not necessarily to be avoided; some drug interactions, once understood, can be used to the patient's benefit. Intentional coadministration of certain antifungal agents [1] or calcium channel blocking drugs [2] has permitted lower dosing of cyclosporine A while maintaining the target trough level. These interactions have resulted in financial savings without sacrificing immunosuppression. Intentional drug interactions, however, should always be followed by increased surveillance of relevant drug levels in order to avoid complications resulting from individual variations in response.

■ DRUGS THAT INTERACT WITH CYCLOSPORINE A, SIROLIMUS, AND TACROLIMUS

Cyclosporine A, sirolimus, and tacrolimus (FK506) share several features that enable them to be considered together with respect to drug interactions. In addition to a similar mechanism of action, all three drugs are biodegraded in the intestine and in the liver by the mixed function oxidase (p450) system, specifically by the CYP3A4 isoform. In addition, cyclosporine A and tacrolimus bind to the ATPase portion of the p-glycoprotein, multidrug resistance (MDR) gene. Any other drug that either binds to the CYP3A4 site or is transported by the p-glycoprotein has the potential to interact with all three drugs. Drugs that are avidly bound to CYP3A4 may inhibit these immunosuppressive agents, with the result that the levels of cyclosporine A, tacrolimus, or sirolimus will rise to potentially toxic levels unless the dose of the immunosuppressive is decreased. Similarly, in instances, where the binding of the immunosuppressive agents to CYP3A4 is stronger, toxic levels of other drugs may be reached. Finally, drugs that over time induce an increase in activity of CYP3A4 may be associated with increased rates of degradation of the immunosuppressive agents and result in lowering of the blood levels, potentially below effective immunosuppression.

The occurrence of genetic polymorphism in the mixed function oxidase system further adds to the complexity of these drug interactions. Since the therapeutic window for cyclosporine A, sirolimus, and tacrolimus is relatively narrow, minor changes in the blood levels can have significant, and at times, disastrous results.

Most of the known drug interactions were originally reported with cyclosporine A, fewer documented with tacrolimus, and even less with sirolimus. However, given the similar metabolism of these three drugs, it is reasonable to consider any demonstrated interaction with one as pertaining to all three. In the following sections, we assume similar interactions among the three drugs unless specifically noted.

Fortunately, the list of known, frequent, and significant drug interactions with cyclosporine A or tacrolimus is relatively small. The data in Tables 30.1 and 30.2 should be considered appropriate to all formulations of cyclosporine A, although most of the data were developed with Sandimmune® [3–8].

Table 30.1 *Anti-infection Drugs that Interact with Cyclosporine A, Tacrolimus, or Sirolimus*

Drug	Increases Immunosuppressant Levels	Decreases Immunosuppressant Levels	Increases Toxicity
Antibacterial agents			
Aminoglycosides			
(e.g. gentamicin, tobramycin, amikacin)			+++ (renal)
Chloramphenicol	+		
Ciprofloxacin	+		
Imipenem/cilastatin			++ (neuro)
Macrolides			
(e.g. erythromycin, azithromycin)	+++		
Penicillins (e.g. nafcillin)		?	
Quinupristin/dalfopristin	++		
Sulfa agents			+ (renal)
Vancomycin			+ (renal)
Antituberculosis agents			
Isoniazid		+	
Rifampicin, rifampin, rifabutin		+++	
Antifungal agents			
Amphotericin B			+++ (renal)
Azoles			
(e.g. ketoconazole, itraconazole, clotrimazole)	+++		
Antimalarial			
Chloroquine	++		
Antiviral agents			
Acyclovir, ganciclovir	+		+ (renal)
Protease inhibitors (HIV)			
(e.g. indinavir, ritonavir/lopinavir, saquinavir)	++		

+++, Well-established, significant; ++, probable, variable; +, possible, individual.

Table 30.2 *Other Drugs that Interact with Cyclosporine A, Tacrolimus, or Sirolimus*

Drug	Increases Immunosuppressant Levels	Decreases Immunosuppressant Levels	Increases Toxicity
Anticonvulsants			
Carbamazepine		+	
Phenobarbital		++	
Phenytoin		+++	
Primidone		+	
Antihypertensives			
ACE inhibitors			++ (hyperkalemia)
Calcium channel inhibitors			
(e.g. verapamil, diltiazem, amlodipine)	++		
(e.g. felodipine, nicardipine)	+++		
Anti-inflammatory agents			
Nonsteroidal, cyclooxygenase inhibitors			+ (renal)
Psychotropic agents			
Benzodiazepines	++		
(e.g. alprazolam, diazepam, midazolam, triazolam)			
Modafinil			++
Serotonin uptake inhibitors	+++		
(e.g. nefazodone, sertraline)			
Steroid hormones			
Miscellaneous agents			
Allopurinol	++		
Alendronate	+		
Danazol	++		
Grapefruit juice	++		
Orlistat		++	
St. John's wort		+++	
Ticlopidine		++	
Vinblastine	++		

+++, Well-established, significant; ++, probable, variable; +, possible, individual.

Antibacterials

The most significant and consistent interactions between antibacterial agents and cyclosporine A, sirolimus, or tacrolimus involve the aminoglycoside and macrolide antibiotics.

The nephrotoxicity of the commonly used aminoglycosides gentamycin, tobramycin, and amikacin is enhanced when these drugs are given to patients receiving cyclosporine A or tacrolimus. This interaction may require a reduction in the dose of the antibacterial as the creatinine clearance decreases. There usually is no effect on blood levels of the immunosuppressive drugs. When possible, an alternative antibacterial should be used.

Among the antibiotics, the natural and semisynthetic macrolide agents have the greatest potential for increasing immunosuppressive drug blood levels. Numerous reports in the literature attest to the potential that administration of erythromycin, by binding to the P-450 sites in the intestine and the liver results in significant elevations of the blood levels of the immunosuppressives. If an oral macrolide is the antibiotic agent of choice for a transplant patient on cyclosporine A, sirolimus, or tacrolimus, one should be prepared to effect up to a 50% reduction in the oral dose of the immunosuppressive drug. Blood levels of intravenous cyclosporine A, sirolimus, and tacrolimus are less affected by the macrolides [3,4,9].

A single report and occasional clinical observation suggest that the incidence of neurotoxicity may be increased when imipenem/cilastin and cyclosporine A are given together. Symptoms of confusion and headache occur without change in the cyclosporine A blood level; all symptoms abate when the antibiotic is discontinued.

An increase in rejection of renal grafts was reported in patients receiving both cyclosporine A and ciprofloxacin. Levofloxacin appears to be free of any interaction with cyclosporine A and may be the drug of choice in this setting [10]. A very significant increase in cyclosporine A levels has been reported in a group of patients receiving quinupristin/dalfopristin [11].

Report of an interaction with chloramphenicol resulting in toxic levels of tacrolimus suggests that patients receiving the drug should be monitored carefully [12].

Other reports of drug interactions between antibacterial agents and cyclosporine A or tacrolimus are less convincing.

Antituberculous Agents

Several studies indicate that rifampicin decreases cyclosporine A and tacrolimus blood levels, probably by inducing P-450 metabolism. It may take several days to 2 weeks to observe the maximum reduction in blood levels;

stepwise increments in cyclosporine A dose are necessary to prevent rejection. The literature suggests that an eventual two- to threefold increment in immunosuppressant dose may be required to maintain appropriate trough levels. CYP3A4 induction by rifampicin may persist for 2–3 weeks after discontinuation of rifampicin. Rifabutin has effects similar to rifampicin, but to a lesser degree; experience with this interaction is limited. Although there are reports in the literature that isoniazid may affect cyclosporine A metabolism, in all instances the isoniazid was given in conjunction with rifampicin.

Antifungal Agents [11–14]

The pharmacokinetic interaction between ketoconazole, itraconazole, and either cyclosporine A, sirolimus, or tacrolimus results in a significant increase in immunosuppressant blood levels. Within 2–3 days of starting either azole, the dose of these immunosuppressives must be reduced by at least 50% in order to avoid toxic blood levels. At usual therapeutic doses of ketoconazole or itraconazole, the cyclosporine A dose will eventually need to be reduced to about 25% of its original dose. This interaction may persist for several days after discontinuing the antifungal agent. The rate of return of cyclosporine A pharmacokinetics to baseline after stopping ketoconazole is subject to considerable interindividual variation. At usual therapeutic doses of ketoconazole, or itraconazole, the cyclosporine A dose will need to be reduced to about 25% of the original dose. The interaction may persist for several days after discontinuing the antifungal agent; the rate of return of cyclosporine A pharmacokinetics to baseline after stopping ketoconazole is subject to considerable individual variation.

Fluconazole is much less potent; significant interactions are rare unless the dose of fluconazole equals or exceeds 200 mg per day [15]. Miconazole is also an infrequent offender.

Clotrimazole is frequently employed as an oral troche for prevention of thrush. When used properly, most of the drug binds to the oral mucosa and is released into the mouth over several hours; there is no appreciable systemic absorption across the buccal mucosa. However, clotrimazole is well absorbed from the gastrointestinal tract. Patients who swallow all or a substantial part of the troche may exhibit increased cyclosporine A levels. Topical administration of clotrimazole to intact or inflamed skin does not result in significant systemic absorption of the drug.

Amphotericin B does not affect cyclosporine A blood levels but is more nephrotoxic in the presence of cyclosporine A. Hypomagnesemia also may be more pronounced when the two drugs are used together.

Antiviral Agents

Acyclovir and gancyclovir have been reported to increase cyclosporine A blood levels and enhance nephrotoxicity. However, this interaction is very infrequent. These agents are used regularly in patients receiving all three immunosuppressives without ill effects. Ritinavir is a potent inhibitor of CYP3A4 and can be expected to interact with cyclosporine A, sirolimus, or tacrolimus. Ritinavir and saquinavir bind to the p-glycoprotein and may affect cyclosporine A or tacrolimus blood levels [16,17].

Anticonvulsants

Patients treated with usual doses of oral or intravenous phenytoin will experience decreased levels of cyclosporine A or tacrolimus unless the dose of immunosuppressant is increased [4,18]. Two- to fourfold increases in the cyclosporine A dose may be necessary to maintain prephenytoin trough levels. Phenytoin probably induces the rate of cytochrome P-450 metabolism in both intestine and liver.

A similar mechanism is proposed for the interaction with phenobarbital. This effect of phenobarbital, however, appears to be dose-related and has been reported only in children receiving over 25 mg of the drug per day [19].

Since induction of CYP3A4 may require a few days to reach maximal rates of metabolism, lower immunosuppressant levels may not be immediately evident upon addition of either phenytoin or phenobarbital. Blood levels need to be checked repeatedly in the first week to 10 days of these anticonvulsants in order to establish the final dose adjustment. As noted earlier, the metabolic activity of CYP3A4 may not immediately revert to the basal state upon stopping either anticonvulsant.

Carbamazepine also has been reported to decrease trough levels of cyclosporine A in several patients; the mechanism is not known. There is a single report of primidone-associated low blood levels of cyclosporine A.

Antihypertensives

Among the antihypertensive agents, the most significant pharmacokinetic interactions occur with some of the calcium channel blockers [2,5,7,8]. These drugs decrease CYP3A4 metabolism of cyclosporine A, sirolimus, and tacrolimus; verapamil also competes by binding to the p-glycoprotein. Of the calcium channel blockers, nicardipine and mebefradil are particularly potent inhibitors; the others have the potential of interacting with the immunosuppressives, but are less potent. Given interindividual variation in drug metabolism, it is wise to follow cyclosporine A, sirolimus, or tacrolimus blood levels more closely for the first 2 months after starting any calcium channel blocker. The interaction may be delayed for several weeks after starting the drug.

The angiotensin-converting enzyme (ACE) inhibitor agents do not affect immunosuppressant blood levels. However, ACE inhibitors and the potassium-sparing diuretics such as spironolactone and amiloride exacerbate hyperkalemia, which is common in patients on cyclosporine A and tacrolimus.

With the exception of carvedilol, the alpha adrenergic agents and the beta-blockers do not interact with either cyclosporine A or tacrolimus. Although interindividual variation was observed, concomitant administration of cavedilol and cyclosporine A required an average reduction of 20% in the dose of the latter [20].

Adrenal and Gonadal Steroids

Although it has been reported that high doses of adrenal steroids (~1 g of methyl prednisolone a day) may raise cyclosporine A blood levels [21], in clinical practice this interaction is rarely appreciated. In most instances, doses of corticosteroids of this magnitude are employed for less than a week; in usual practice, the cyclosporine A dose is not reduced during this time.

The synthetic steroid danazol regularly causes a rise in trough levels of these immunosuppressant drugs. Other natural and synthetic estrogenic steroids including birth control pills have the potential to increase cyclosporine A levels through an interaction with CYP3A4; however, there are no convincing reports of this interaction. Women beginning birth control pills or receiving estrogen therapy for bone disease should be observed for a possible change in the steady-state level of cyclosporine A.

Nonsteroidal Anti-inflammatory Drugs

The effect of nonsteroidal anti-inflammatory drugs (NSAIDs) on intrarenal prostaglandin metabolism may exacerbate the nephrotoxicity of cyclosporine A and tacrolimus. However, careful studies in patients with rheumatoid arthritis failed to show any worsening of the creatinine clearance when several NSAIDs were added to patients already receiving 5 mg/kg cyclosporine A [22]. Addition of NSAIDs to the therapeutic regimen of liver transplant patients receiving either cyclosporine A or tacrolimus should be followed by close surveillance of the serum creatinine concentration.

Chemotherapeutic Agents

Cyclosporine A and tacrolimus bind to and inhibit the MDR gene p-glycoprotein on the cell membrane of hepatocytes and many other cells. This can result in a decreased rate of excretion of several chemotherapeutic agents, including vinblastine daunomycin and etoposide. This property of cyclosporine A has led to intentional addition of the drug to chemotherapy regimens in an attempt to overcome the effect of the MDR gene. Melphalan potentiates renal dysfunction when given to patients receiving cyclosporine A.

Agents Acting on the Gastrointestinal Tract

The somatostatin analog, octreotide, is reported to decrease cyclosporine A blood levels in patients receiving oral but not intravenous cyclosporine A. This suggests an effect on absorption, but the actual mechanism of this interaction is not known. Metoclopramide increases cyclosporine A blood levels by an as-yet-not-understood effect on absorption.

Cimetidine is known to inhibit a P-450 isoenzyme other than CYP3A4. Nevertheless, administration of cimetidine to patients receiving cyclosporine A has been shown to alter peak cyclosporine A blood levels [23].

Hypocholesterolemic Agents

An increased incidence of rhabdomyolysis-induced renal failure due to myoglobinuria is reported in patients receiving HMG-CoA reductase inhibitors and either tacrolimus or cyclosporine A [24]. Patients requiring these drugs for treatment of hypercholesterolemia posttransplantation should be treated with the lowest effective dose. Routine determination of serum creatine phosphokinase (CPK) is recommended while patients are on these immunosuppressives and any of the "statin" HMG-CoA inhibitors. Progressive elevation of the CPK or unexpected myalgia should lead to immediate discontinuation of the hypocholesterolemic drug until the patient is evaluated further.

Fluvistatin, simvistatin, and pravistatin are the least susceptible to inhibition and may be the drugs of choice in liver transplant patients [6].

Antihistamines

Terfenadine is metabolized by CYP3A4 in both intestine and liver. Its metabolism is therefore subject to inhibition by all three immunosuppressants.

Psychotropic Agents

Some benzodiazepines (e.g. midazolam, triazolam, alprazolam, and diazepam) are susceptible to drug interactions based on their metabolism by CYP3A4; midazolam has been associated with elevation of cyclosporine A levels in patients. Temazepam, nitrazepam, and lorazepam do not interact significantly and may be preferred [6].

Several of the selective serotonin reuptake inhibitors (SSRIs) are metabolized by and inhibit CYP3A4 [8,25]. Addition of nefazodone to one heart transplant patient resulted in an almost tenfold increase in the cyclosporine A blood level; interactions have been reported with sertraline and fluoxetine [26,27].

St. John's wort (*Hypericum perforatum*) can significantly reduce the bioavailability of oral cyclosporine A [28]. This interaction has resulted in acute cellular rejection.

Miscellaneous

Bromocriptine and chloroquine are known to increase blood levels of cyclosporine A. Ticlopidine may affect cyclosporine A bioavailability; reduction in the dose of ticlopidine in patients receiving both drugs does not change cyclosporine A pharmacokinetics and preserves the antiplatelet function of ticlopidine.

Grapefruit and grapefruit juice can enhance the bioavailability of oral cyclosporine A, with resulting toxic blood levels [29,30]. The extent of this interaction depends on variables such as the species of the grapefruit and the process used to prepare the juice. Although this interaction has been used to reduce the cost of cyclosporine A in some patients, constant vigilance is necessary to avoid clinically significant variations in blood levels of the drug.

■ DRUGS THAT INTERACT WITH AZATHIOPRINE

Drugs that Exacerbate Marrow Suppression (Table 30.3)

Allopurinol, sulfasalazine, and 5-amino salicylic acid inhibit enzymes that degrade purines; concomitant use of these drugs results in enhanced bone marrow toxicity [31–33]. When allopurinol is used, the dose of azathioprine should be reduced to 25–33% of the initial dose in order to avoid cytopenia. Sirolimus may also have a pharmacodynamic interaction with azathioprine and accentuate bone marrow inhibition [34].

The use of ACE inhibitors to control hypertension in patients receiving azathioprine can also lead to anemia and leukopenia [35]; the mechanism of this interaction is not known.

Miscellaneous

There are several case reports suggesting that azathioprine interacts with warfarin to reduce the dose-related anticoagulant effect [36,37]. Patients should be monitored at the start of concomitant therapy, with adjustments in the warfarin dose as necessary.

DRUGS THAT INTERACT WITH MYCOFENOLATE MOFETIL

Drugs interacting with mycofenolate mofetil (MMF) are few and fall into two categories: drugs that inhibit absorption and drugs that reduce renal excretion [38–40] (Table 30.4). Antacids and cholestyramine decrease the blood levels of mycophenolic acid (MPA), the active metabolite, by 30–40%, presumably by interfering with absorption. Acyclovir interacts with the inactive metabolite, mycofenolic acid glucuronide (MPAG), with the result that the blood levels of both MPAG and acyclovir rise by 11% and 22%, respectively. This interaction probably occurs because of competition for renal tubular secretion, which is necessary for the excretion of both agents. Similarly, animals given probenecid, a known inhibitor of renal tubular secretion, experienced a twofold increase in blood levels of MPA as well as a marked rise in MPAG. The increase in MPA that follows probenecid suggests that when other drugs that are dependent on renal tubular secretion for elimination (the penicillins, aspirin, etc.) are given to patients receiving MMF, careful monitoring for evidence of bone marrow suppression may be necessary. No pharmacokinetic drug interaction was noted when cyclosporine or sirolimus was given with MMF; however, in the presence of tacrolimus, blood levels of MPA increase. A review of renal transplant patients receiving MMF and allopurinol failed to reveal evidence to suggest an interaction.

Table 30.3 *Drugs Potentiating Marrow Toxicity When Given to Patients Receiving Azathioprine*

Allopurinol
Sulfasalazine
ACE inhibitors
5-Amino salicylate
Sirolimus

Table 30.4 *Drugs that Interact with Mycophenolate Mofetil*

Drug	Effect
Antacids, cholestyramine	Decreases absorption of mycophenolate mofetil
Acyclovir	Increases blood levels of acyclovir
Probenecid	Increases blood levels of mycophenolate[a]
Tacrolimus	Increases blood levels of mycophenolic acid[a]

[a]Demonstrated only in animals, but probable in humans.

■ OTHER IMMUNOSUPPRESSIVE DRUGS

Adrenal Steroids

With the exception of the interaction between high-dose methylprednisolone and cyclosporine A, as noted above, there is little clinical evidence that adrenal steroids exhibit any pharmacokinetic interactions in liver transplant patients. Pharmacodynamic interactions with hypoglycemic agents are well known and attributed to an increase in insulin resistance due to the steroids. Similarly, impairment of naturesis induced by diuretics occurs.

Immunoglobulins

Other than the elevation in cyclosporine A blood levels associated with concomitant administration of OKT3 (see above), there are no known drug–drug interactions with any of the other immunoglobulins [41].

■ REFERENCES

1. First M, Schroeder T, Weiskittel P, et al. Concomitant administration of cyclosporin and ketoconazole in renal transplant recipients. Lancet 1982;1(8673):1198–1201.

2. Duvoux C, Cherqul D, DiMartino V, et al. Nicardipine as antihypertensive therapy in liver transplant recipients: results of long-term use. Hepatology 1997;25:430–433.

3. Grebenau M. Sandimmune® (cyclosporine) drug interactions. East Hanover, NJ: Sandoz Pharmaceuticals, 1994.

4. Yee G, McGuire T. Pharmacokinetic drug interactions with cyclosporin (Part I). Clin Pharmacokinet 1990;19:319–332.

5. Yee G, McGuire T. Pharmacokinetic drug interactions with cyclosporin (Part II). Clin Pharmacokinet 1990;19:400–415.

6. Dresser G, Spence J, Bailey D. Pharmacokinetic–pharmacodynamic consequences and clinical relevance of cytochrome p450 3A4 inhibition. Clin Pharmacokinet 2000;38:41–57.

7. Ingle G, Sievers T, Holt C. Sirolimus: continuing the evolution of transplant immunosuppression. Ann Pharmacother 2000;34:1044–1045.

8. Fireman M, DiMartini A, Armstrong S, et al. Immunosuppressants. Psychsomatics 2004;45:354–360.

9. Gupta S, Bakran A, Johnson R, et al. Cyclosporin–erythromycin interaction in renal transplant patients. Br J Clin Pharmacol 1989;27:475–481.

10. Doose D, Walker S, Chien S, et al. Levofloxacin does not alter cyclosporine disposition. J Clin Pharmacol 1998;38:90–93.

11. Stamatakis M, Richards J. Interaction between quinupristin/dalfopristin and cyclosporine. Ann Pharmacother 1997;31:576–578.

12. Schulman S, Shaw L, Jabs K, et al. Interaction between tacrolimus and chloramphenicol in a renal transplant recipient. Transplantation 1998;65:1397–1398.

13. Albengres E, Le Louet H, Tillement J. Systemic antifungal agents. Drug interactions of clinical significance. Drug Saf 1998;18:83–97.

14. Katz H. Drug interactions of the newer oral antifungal agents. Br J Dermatol 1999;141(suppl 56):26–32.

15. Ventkatakrishnan K, von Moltke L, Greenblatt D. Effects of the antifungal agents on oxidative drug metabolism: clinical relevance. Clin Pharmacokinet 2000;38:111–180.

16. Lee C, Gottesman M, Cardarelli C, et al. HIV-1 protease inhibitors are substrates for the MDR1 multidrug transporter. Biochemistry 1998:37:3594–3601.

17. Gutmann H, Fricker G, Drewe J, et al. Interactions of HIV protease inhibitors with ATP-dependent drug export proteins. Mol Pharmacol 1999;56:383–389.

18. Keown P, Laupacis A, Carruthers G, et al. Interaction between phenytoin and cyclosporine following organ transplantation. Transplantation 1984;38:304–306.

19. Yee G, Lennon T, Gmur D, et al. Age-dependent cyclosporine pharmacokinetics in marrow transplant recipients. Clin Pharmacol Ther 1986;40:438–443.

20. Kaijser M, Johnsson C, Zezina L, et al. Elevation of cyclosporin A blood levels during carvedilol treatment in renal transplant patients. Clin Transpl 1997;11:577–581.

21. Klintmalm G, Sawe J. High dose methylprednisolone increases plasma cyclosporin levels in renal transplant recipients. Lancet 1984;1(8379):731.

22. Tugwell P, Ludwin D, Gent M, et al. Interaction between cyclosporin A and nonsteroidal antiinflammatory drugs. J Rheumatol 1997;24:1122–1125.

23. Lewis S, McCloskey W. Potentiation of nephrotoxicity by H2-antagonists in patients receiving cyclosporine. Ann Pharmacother 1997;31:363–365.

24. Cohen E, Kramer M, Maoz C, et al. Cyclosporine drug-interaction-induced rhabdomyolysis, a report of two cases in lung transplant recipients. Clin Transplant 200;70:119–122.

25. von Moltke L, Greenblatt D, Schmider J, et al. Metabolism of drugs by cytochrome p450 3A isoforms. Implications for drug interactions in psychopharmacology. Clin Pharmacokinet 1995;29(suppl 1):33–43.

26. Wright D, Lake K, Bruhn P, et al. Nefazodone and cyclosporine drug–drug interaction. J Heart Lung Transplant 1999;18:913–915.

27. Greene D, Barbhaiya R. Clinical pharmacokinetics of nefazodone. Clin Pharmacokinet 1997;33:260–275.

28. Fugh-Berman A. Herb–drug interactions. Lancet 2000;355:134–138.

29. Fuhr U. Drug interactions with grapefruit juice. Extent, probable mechanism and clinical relevance. Drug Saf 1998;18:251–272.

30. Bailey D, Malcolm J, Arnold O, et al. Grapefruit juice–drug interactions. Br J Clin Pharmacol 1998;46:101–110.

31. Rundles R, Wyngaarden J, Hitchings G, et al. Effects of a xanthine oxidase inhibitor on thiopurine metabolism, hyperuricemia and gout. Trans Assoc Am Physicians 1963;76:126–140.

32. Zimm S, Collins J, O'Neill D, et al. Inhibition of first-pass metabolism in cancer chemotherapy: interaction of 6-mercaptopurine and allopurinol. Clin Pharmacol Ther 1983;34:810–817.

33. Szumlanski C, Weinshilboum R. Sulphasalazine inhibition of thiopurine methyl-transferase: possible mechanism for interaction with 6-mercaptopurine and azathioprine. Br J Clin Pharmacol 1995;39:456–459.

34. Mignat C. Clinically significant drug interactions with new immunosuppressive agents. Drug Saf 1997;16:267–278.

35. Gossmann J, Kachel H-G, Schoeppe W, et al. Anemia in renal transplant recipients caused by concomitant therapy with azathioprine and angiotensin-converting enzyme inhibitors. Transplantation 1993;56:585–589.

36. Singleton J, Conyers L. Warfarin and azathioprine: an important drug interaction. Am J Med 1992;92:217.

37. Rivier G, Khamashta M, Hughes G. Warfarin and azathioprine: a drug interaction does exist. Am J Med 1992;95:342.

38. Hoffman-La Roche, Inc. CellCept (mycophenolate mofetil capsules). Package insert. 1995.

39. Bullingham R, Nicholls A, Kamm B. Clinical pharmacokinetics of mycophenolate mofetil. Clin Pharmacokinet 1998;34:429–455.

40. Hübner GI, Eismann R, Sziegoleit W. Drug interaction between mycophenolate mofetil and tacrolimus detectable within therapeutic mycophenolic acid monitoring in renal transplant patients. Ther Drug Monit 1999;21:536–539.

41. Vasquez E, Pollak R. OKT3 therapy increases cyclosporine blood levels. Clin Transplant 1997;11:38–41.

PART 5

Pediatric Liver Transplantation

Special Considerations for Liver Transplantation in Children

31

▼　▼　▼　▼　▼　▼　▼　▼　▼

Martin Burdelski and Xavier Rogiers

P EDIATRIC liver transplantations represent about 10% of all liver transplantations registered in the European Liver Transplantation Register (ELTR) [1]. This percentage has been stable over the last decades. The pediatric transplant population differs widely in many respects from the adult one. These differences refer to the natural course of the underlying diseases, indications, surgical techniques, posttransplant complications, and long-term results and are elucidated in this chapter.

■ INDICATIONS

The predominant indication for liver transplantation in children is extrahepatic biliary atresia, which represents more than 50% of all pediatric liver transplantations worldwide (Fig. 31.1) [2–5]. More than 80% of affected children are nonsymptomatic at birth. Thus the term "atresia" is misleading. Only in those patients with associated vascular malformations a developmental defect may be assumed. In the majority of patients, infections or infection-induced immunological or inflammatory processes must be regarded as responsible for the development of cholestatic cirrhosis. In general, first symptoms are detectable during the first weeks of life, with a rapid development of cholestatic liver cirrhosis that presents with clinical signs of decompensation at the age of 4–6 months [2]. The natural course of this disorder does not allow survival beyond the age of 2 years. If performed in time, i.e. before the development of cirrhosis, a hepatoportoenterostomy (Kasai operation) [2] can prevent this rapid deterioration. There is clear evidence that the Kasai procedure prevents fatal outcome of the affected children in up to 60% of cases if performed before the age of 60 days. In the long-term, follow-up centers with a long-standing experience

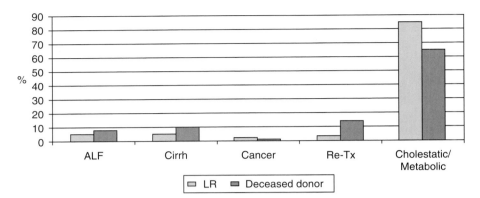

Fig. 31.1 *Indications in pediatric liver transplantation according to [1] (n = 4313, Oct 1991–Dec 2001). ALF, acute liver failure; Cirrh, cryptogenic cirrhosis, autoimmune cirrhosis; Re-Tx, retransplantation.*

in both diagnosing and treating these patients may have about 10% of children surviving longer than 10 years without transplantation. In general, patients without Kasai operation and patients with a failed Kasai operation will need liver transplantation within the first year of life [6]. This accounts for about 30% of affected children. Another 30% can survive with slower progress toward chronic end-stage liver disease (ESLD). These patients will need liver transplantation before 6 years of age. Only 30% of the operated children will have a chance to survive until adolescence without transplantation and only 10% of the initial cohort of patients will be cirrhosis-free longer than 10 years after operation [7].

In addition to biliary atresia there are another 20–25% of patients suffering from cholestatic liver disorders leading to chronic ESLD. In this group, there are patients with progressive familial intrahepatic cholestasis types 1, 2, and 3 (PFIC 1, 2, and 3) [2]. An underlying genetic defect is responsible for a defective bile salt export pump, which leads to bile salt-induced toxic hepatocyte damage with giant cell formation and rapid progress to cholestatic cirrhosis in patients with type 1 and 2 disease. The characteristic finding in these patients is normal γ-glutamyltransferase (γGT) in serum in combination with high serum bile acids [8]. In patients with type 3 disease, the genetic defect is responsible for a defect transporter of phospholipids. These patients do have increased serum catalytic concentrations of γGT [9]. The lack of phospholipids leads to destruction of the bile ducts by the toxic bile salts. Bile duct proliferation and cholestatic liver cirrhosis are the characteristic histopathological features of this disease. In all types of PFIC, life expectancy is less than 18 years of age, some patients deteriorating rapidly after viral infections and even vaccination with live vaccines. Other patients will have only mild hepatopathy until adolescence but a very fast decompensation at this age [8].

Among the patients with cholestatic liver disease there is another group suffering from neonatal hepatitis syndrome. Only a minority of these patients can be identified to suffer from cytomegalovirus (CMV), herpes simplex, parvo B19, or adenovirus infection [2]. The rest remains unclear with regard to the underlying infectious agent [10–13]. The differential diagnosis must include metabolic disorders, the characteristic histological feature of giant cell hepatitis just reflecting a nonspecific reaction of the neonatal hepatocyte to any kind of injury. In the later course, these patients will show the histological pattern of paucity of intrahepatic bile ducts. The fate of this nonsyndromatic paucity of intrahepatic bile ducts is comparable with that of extrahepatic biliary atresia although the percentage of affected children going to rapidly progressing liver cirrhosis is assumed to be about 25% [13].

Alagille syndrome is a syndromatic bile duct hypoplasia characterized by additional features such as facial stigmata, congenital heart defects with peripheral pulmonary artery stenosis, butterfly vertebrae, vascular and intracranial vascular malformations, and embryotoxon posterior [14]. It is an autosomal dominant inherited syndrome with a wide range of phenotypic expressions. It has been shown that the genetic background is a defect in the JAG 1 gene responsible for the formation of notch proteins, which are needed for specific differentiation of organs and tissues. Liver transplantation is needed in patients with severe cholestasis, which is characterized by high serum cholesterol and high serum bile acid concentration [15]. The majority of affected children, however, will experience complications of their congenital heart defect and pulmonary artery stenosis.

Inherited metabolic disorders account for up to 20% of liver transplantations in children [16]. Cystic fibrosis, α1-antitrypsin deficiency, tyrosinemia, urea cycle defects, Crigler–Najjar syndrome, respiratory chain disorders, and some patients with neonatal hemochromatosis are found in this group. Elaborating the diagnosis may be difficult since it is almost impossible to differentiate between primary and secondary findings in patients with advanced liver cirrhosis. Metabolic disorders should only be considered as indications for liver transplantation if the natural course of other affected organs is benign [17,18]. In cystic fibrosis for instance, the progress of pulmonary disease is stopped unexpectedly despite immunosuppression. In contrast, respiratory chain disorders and Niemann–Pick type C show rapid progress of the cerebral manifestation after transplantation. These disorders are therefore considered to be contraindicated in pediatric liver transplantation. The workup of these metabolic disorders being difficult and even time-consuming, it is mandatory to have a close cooperation between hepatologists and metabolists at the transplant center.

Acute liver failure is another important indication for liver transplantation in children (Fig. 31.1). The ELTR report 2004 counts 13.2% of transplantations in this category [1]. The causes of acute liver failure are metabolic disorders such as neonatal hemochromatosis, hereditary tyrosinemia, respiratory chain disorders, Wilson's disease, autoimmune hepatitis (AIH), viral hepatitis due to herpesvirus, parvo B19, and hepatitis B virus (HBV) infections [19–25]. About 16–26% of causes in pediatric acute liver failure remain unclear even if most sensitive methods such as polymerase chain reaction (PCR) techniques are used. Mushroom poisoning and drug toxicity account for another important group of patients [19]. The indication for liver transplantation is based in most centers on disturbances of the clotting system. International normalized ratio (INR) findings above 4 or Quick test below 20% or factor V below 20% of normal are considered as bad prognostic indicators [22]. Since increased intracranial pressure may induce irreversible brain damage the most important issue in treating these patients is to recognize when a patient has already passed the therapeutic window in which liver transplantation can be offered with good prognosis [26].

In contrast to the adult experience, chronic viral hepatitis due to HBV or hepatitis C virus (HCV) infection is a rare indication for liver transplantation in children. Cryptogenic cirrhosis is even more frequent than these viral hepatitis forms (Fig. 31.1). Another important issue in chronic ESLD may be autoimmune disorders (AIH). AIH types 1 and 2 normally respond to steroid- and azathioprine-based immunosuppression very well; only 5–10% of patients need liver transplantation, especially if the diagnosis is made late after cirrhosis has already been established [27]. Primary sclerosing cholangitis with or without active colitis is another indication for pediatric liver transplantation. In contrast to other cholestatic disorders mentioned earlier, the progress of this disease is comparable with the adult experience. The risk of experiencing a cholangiocarcinoma, however, must be taken into account if the course of the disease is longer than 10 years.

Malignant disorders such as hepatoblastoma and hepatocellular carcinoma are the smallest group among the indications for liver transplantation in children, ranging from 2% to 4% of all indications (Fig. 31.1). In hepatoblastoma, the orchestrated combination of chemotherapy and surgery with optional liver transplantation has been shown to be very effective [28,29], whereas in hepatocellular carcinoma results in pediatric liver transplantation are very disappointing [30].

Finally, secondary liver diseases such as posttraumatic or post-liver-resection in hepatic malignancies or short gut syndrome after multiple and extensive small bowel resection with less than 20 cm small bowel left and the need of total parenteral nutrition [31,32] and veno-occlusive disease after chemotherapy and/or bone marrow transplantation or Budd–Chiari syndrome in thrombocytosis [33] are considered as indications for liver transplantation. In total parenteral nutrition-associated secondary cholestatic liver cirrhosis, a combined liver and small bowel transplantation is needed.

■ PRETRANSPLANT CARE OF THE PEDIATRIC LIVER TRANSPLANT CANDIDATE

After the challenge of establishing a diagnosis in a given child with ESLD and after defining the individual prognosis, the optimized medical and nutritional therapy of a patient can help to avoid serious complications before transplantation. The real advances in pediatric liver transplantation compared with the experience in the 1980s are due to the fact that transplantation can be performed in an earlier state of the disease, since the major problem of children with chronic end-stage cholestatic liver disease is multimorbidity (Fig. 31.2). Malnutrition is one aspect of multimorbidity and is observed in 50–60% if defined as body weight below the third percentile. Recurrent infections including spontaneous bacterial peritonitis may occur in 30–50% of children; portal hypertension with bleeding from varices is seen in 20–50%. In addition there are complications such as renal insufficiency, including hepatorenal syndrome (HRS) in about 17–50%, osteopathy with pathological fractures in 18–50% of patients, abnormal vascular patterns leading to pre- and intrahepatic shunting in 3–50% of patients and hepatopulmonary syndrome finally, which is found in 1–5% of patients.

Malnutrition is pronounced in cholestatic liver disorders due to fat maldigestion, serious anorexia, and catabolic state [34–39] (Fig. 31.2). The management of this complication is difficult. In most patients, supplementation of fat-soluble vitamins and substitution of essential fatty acids by medium-chained fatty acids and intravenous (IV) fat infusions are necessary. It can be done via nasogastric tube, which may be difficult in patients with esophageal varices. In most patients, however, an IV supplementation in weekly intervals becomes

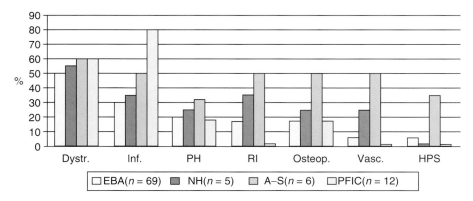

Fig. 31.2 *Multiorgan morbidity in pediatric transplant candidates (own data). Dystr., malnutrition, body weight < 3rd percentile; Inf., recurrent infections; PH, portal hypertension requiring medical/endoscopic therapy; RI, renal insufficiency; Osteop., osteopathy; Vasc., vascular complications due to either congenital or acquired abnormalities; HPS, hepatopulmonary syndrome defined as low oxygen saturation in cirrhotic patients.*

necessary. In encephalopathic patients, protein supplementation should include branched amino acids. The efficacy of lactulose or sodium benzoate therapy needs further evaluation. If a patient does not respond to nutritional support with high-energy intake with up to 120–180% of recommended daily intake, liver transplantation should be performed as soon as possible.

The risk of recurrent infections of the respiratory tract is explained by mechanical effects of pulmonary compression by ascites, increased size of liver and spleen, and by the fact that the macrophage system of the liver is destroyed (Fig. 31.2). Patients with chronic end-stage cholestatic liver disease are further bound to overwhelming Gram-negative septicemia, which can lead to acute multiorgan failure even within hours. Close monitoring of the patient and guided antibiotic therapy rather than prophylactic antibiotic therapy is recommended.

Portal hypertension is a major feature of chronic ESLD (Fig. 31.2). Esophageal and gastric varices need close monitoring. If ultrasound examinations reveal collaterals at the spleen, the risk of having esophageal varices is high. In children, primary and secondary prophylaxis are justified as soon as cherry red spots are detected on the varices [40]. It is recommended that esophageal varices be treated with rubber band ligation whereas gastric varices should be treated with cyanoacrylate [41,42]. Again, liver transplantation should be considered in these patients as soon as possible as a curative therapy in portal hypertension. With regard to supportive therapy, there are no evidence-based data available in children. Nonselective beta-blockers are reported to show frequent side-effects such as fatigue, nausea, and arterial hypotension and are even more pronounced than in adults where up to 30% of patients need either reduced dosages or even finishing treatment.

Renal insufficiency in chronic or acute ESLD must be seen as a serious problem in a transplant candidate (Fig. 31.2). The use of calcineurin inhibitors in the posttransplant phase will aggravate this problem further [43]. Renal insufficiency in the context of HRS has a bad prognosis, with less than 10% spontaneous recovery [44]. The pathophysiology is not well understood [45]. After exclusion of secondary renal failure due to shock, infection, and diuretics, true HRS is defined as occurring in chronic liver failure with portal hypertension if the glomerular filtration rate is less than $40\,\mathrm{mL/min/1.73\,m^2}$ body surface area in the absence of structural abnormalities of the kidneys investigated, for instance, by ultrasound. The urine output is less than 2 mL/kg/h, the sodium excretion is less than 10 mmol/L, the urine osmolality is lower than plasma osmolality, and the serum sodium concentration is less than 130 mmol/L. There should be no significant erythrocyturia. The prevalence of HRS in pediatric transplant candidates is low; most of the patients with renal function impairment suffer from preexisting disease due to either drug-related, dysplastic kidneys or renal vascular malformation. Renal insufficiency thus may vary between 2% and 50% according to the underlying disease (Fig. 31.2). The management of HRS includes control of electrolytes and water by restriction of fluid intake and hemofiltration or hemodialysis if necessary. In the future, a molecular adsorbent recycling system [46] may be applied since a pediatric size adaptation is now available. But still, no controlled pediatric trials using such a device were performed until recently. In general, renal insufficiency in a transplant recipient requires careful use of calcineurin inhibitors.

Osteopathy is a frequent comorbidity in cholestatic chronic ESLD (Fig. 31.2) [47]. It is observed in up to 50% of patients and characterized by pathological fractures, which may be seen in 16% of all patients (Fig. 31.2). The pathophysiology is complex, malabsorption of vitamin D, impaired bone repair, and disturbances in metabolism of parathormone [48]. Therapy is difficult, since treatment with calcium and 1-25-dihydroxycholecalciferol does not seem to be efficient and is even hazardous in the presence of hypercalciuria and may lead to renal calcinosis. Even worse, after transplantation the use of calcineurin inhibitors may interfere with a recovery of osteopathy [49]. As a consequence, early transplantation preventing the manifestation of osteopathy seems to be the best option.

Vascular abnormalities may be observed in children with symptomatic extrahepatic biliary atresia presenting with partial Ivemark syndrome (Fig. 31.2). The features of this entity are aplasia of the superrenal inferior vena cava, azygos or hemiazygos continuation, preduodenal portal vein, asplenia or polysplenia syndrome, and abdominal situs inversus with the risk of intestinal volvulus [50,51]. In children with nonsyndromatic extrahepatic biliary atresia, hypoplasia of the portal vein is frequently observed leading to extensive intra- and extra-abdominal collateral formation [52]. Sufficient portal flow may be difficult to obtain under this predisposition. In this case, careful ligation of these collaterals can become necessary during transplantation in order to enhance the portal flow. Reduced portal vein flow due to increased resistance in the cirrhotic liver may worsen and finally end up in oscillating or even reversing the hepatofugal portal vein flow. This situation can only be detected by Doppler ultrasound. The risk of this reversal of the portal vein flow is the manifestation of portal vein thrombosis [52]. Liver transplantation in this situation then is almost impossible. Thus, monitoring of the patient by Doppler ultrasound is the only way to recognize the development of this complication, with the chance of preventing real portal vein thrombosis by early transplantation.

The hepatopulmonary syndrome is a rare complication of chronic ESLD in children. It is observed in 1–30% of children with chronic ESLD (Fig. 31.2). It is important to know that the development of this complication is not in parallel with the progress of the liver disease. The first clinical symptoms are dyspnoe and oxygen desaturation not responding to increased oxygen supply. The diagnosis is established by bubble echocardiography and right heart catheter [53,54]. The cause of this complication is thought to be lack of NO inactivation in the liver or increased NO formation in the lungs [55]. Development of spider naevi and teleangiectasies is caused by the same pathophysiology. The right heart catheter is essential in order to exclude pulmonary hypertension, which means a clear contraindication for liver transplantation. The outcome of liver transplantation in hepatopulmonary syndrome is worse than in normal transplantation, the recovery of the patient may be very prolonged. The best option is to prevent the development of hepatopulmonary syndrome by early transplantation.

The last entity is acute-on-chronic liver failure [56,57]. Chronic ESLD aggravated by infection, toxins, or gastrointestinal bleeding may lead to further consumption of clotting factors with the risk of intracranial or gastrointestinal bleeding (Fig. 31.3). The metabolic balance may collapse by hypoglycemia and acidemia with lactate acidosis and ATP depletion. All factors may induce cerebral edema. In addition, shock may contribute to further deterioration with multiorgan failure with renal, intestinal, circulatory, and pulmonary impairment. It goes without saying that this combination of complication is difficult to manage. If any kind of artificial liver support, including molecular adsorbents recirculating system (MARS) [46], is able to reverse this, complication needs further randomized controlled studies in adult and pediatric patients.

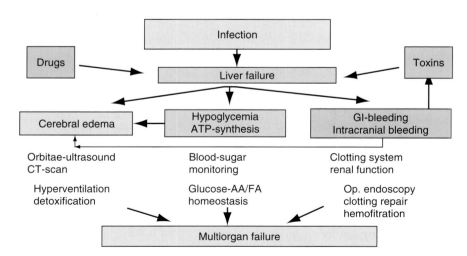

Fig. 31.3 *Development of acute-on-chronic liver failure and ways to prevent, diagnose, and treat this complication. Level 1, causes of liver failure; level 2, consequences of liver failure; level 3, diagnostic approach; level 4, interventions in order to prevent further progress to multiorgan failure.*

■ CONTRAINDICATIONS

In the beginning of liver transplantation up to 40% of patients on the waiting list experienced either primary or secondary contraindications. Body weight below 10 kg was one of the most frequent contraindications since it was most unlikely that a suitable donor was available in time [58]. Hypoplasia of the portal vein, advanced liver disease with more than one organ failure, and active infections were the other contraindications. Today, only active infection, extrahepatic spread of hepatic malignancy, and progressive involvement of other organs are still considered as contraindications [59]. This means that contraindications have almost been abolished.

■ TIMING OF TRANSPLANTATION

Timing of transplantation plays a role with regard to pre- and posttransplant survival (Fig. 31.3). Prediction of pretransplant survival is essential in order to allocate a donor organ in the sense of "sickest first" policy. This situation is applicable to adults, where waiting list mortality is essential, reaching up to 20%. In children, however, the use of all technical variants, i.e. full-size, reduced-size organs, split- and living-related segments has provided enough organs to cover the needs [60]. The only exception is the young adolescent who is competing with small adults with a long waiting time in the actual allocation prescription of Eurotransplant. If this is kept in mind, the pediatric end-stage liver disease (PELD) score makes no sense in Eurotransplant. This score has been established in the USA and in Canada in order to guarantee an easily obtainable, objective, and verifiable parameter for organ allocation. The PELD calculator uses serum albumin (g/dL), bilirubin (mg/dL), INR, growth failure based on gender, height, and weight, and age at listing (Fig. 31.4) [61]. Some 12 years ago, a similar score had been developed using serum bilirubin ($>300 \mu mol/L$), prothrombin time ($<50\%$ of normal), cholinesterase (<1.5 kU/ L), and weight ($<$3rd percentile) as prognostic parameters of a risk score [62]. Other prognostic indicators of pretransplant survival used the metabolizing capacity of the diseased liver after either lidocaine injection or oral applied caffeine. Indocyanine green had been used either alone or in combination with the Pugh score as a prognostic indicator of pretransplant survival reflecting the perfusion rather than the metabolic capacity of the liver. These systems can be used in order to identify the patients with a high risk of death while on the waiting list by significant deterioration of the PELD or any other score [63,64]. With regard to posttransplant survival, however, these scoring systems turned out to be less efficient. In the meantime, survival rates after pediatric liver transplantation have reached almost 97% [60]. This progress makes a prediction of the posttransplant survival almost unnecessary.

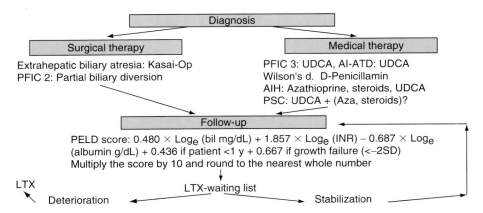

Fig. 31.4 *Follow-up algorithm of a potential transplant candidate in order to achieve appropriate timing of LTX.*

■ SURGICAL OPTIONS IN PEDIATRIC LIVER TRANSPLANTATION

The last 14 years have shown a significant change in the use of donor organs with regard to the use of technical variants. After living-related liver transplantation had been shown to be effective [65], the surgical experience derived from living donation was applied to split-liver transplantation, leading to a renaissance of this technique by avoiding nonacceptable risks for the recipient of the right part of the liver [66]. This technique helped to avoid wasting of organs, which had to be done in those patients who were transplanted with reduced-size organs. In general, reduced-size organs should no longer be used; splitting should be the first choice. However, the ELTR report including data until December 2002 shows a major role of reduced-size liver transplantation in the pediatric age group. In experienced centers, the outcome of pediatric liver transplantation is not influenced by the use of technical variants [67]. This is a strong argument for focusing pediatric liver transplantation to only a few centers as is done in the UK, where only three centers are allowed to perform pediatric liver transplantation [68].

■ IMMUNOSUPPRESSIVE THERAPY

Modern immunosuppression uses a triple therapy consisting of calcineurin inhibitors, interleukin-2 receptor antibodies, and steroids. There has only been one paper comparing both available calcineurin inhibitors in a prospective randomized controlled study [69]. The results showed no difference with regard to patient and graft survival and adverse events. However, there was a significant difference in corticosteroid-resistant acute rejection-free survival in favor of tacrolimus. Oversized immunosuppression exposes the pediatric recipient at risk of developing a posttransplant lymphoproliferative disease (PTLD) [70]. PTLD is reported to be seen in up to 20% of patients [69,71–73]. Since PTLD is EBV-driven, this high risk of PTLD in children is easily explained by the high prevalence of EBV in donors but almost zero prevalence in small children. Most immunosuppressive protocols aim to have a steroid-free therapy already 1 year after transplantation. Thus, catch-up growth in children as one essential aspect of quality of life after transplantation starts significantly at this time only [74]. Long-term side-effects of calcineurin inhibitors may contribute to cardiovascular complications such as arterial hypertension and coronary heart disease and to renal insufficiency [67]. Therefore close drug monitoring of cyclosporine and tacrolimus is essential (Tables 31.1 and 31.2). Whether C_2 rather than C_0 values give better information with regard to optimized immunosuppression in cyclosporine therapy is discussed at the moment [75,76]. Since more than 90% of children have a biliodigestive anastomosis instead of a choledochocholedochostomy, leading to significant delay or enhancement of transit, it is almost unlikely that the C_2 measurement grants an advantage over C_0 values.

There is some evidence that immunization in pediatric liver transplant candidates shifts the T-helper cell state 2 into T-helper cell state 1 with predominant interferon and interleukin-2 production. This state seems to predispose to rejection [77]. In addition, posttransplant vaccination seems not to show significant complications and good immunological response. Therefore it makes sense to perform only hepatitis B vaccination and to postpone the normal vaccination program to the second half-year after transplantation when immunosuppression is comparably low.

■ POSTTRANSPLANT COMPLICATIONS

In a systematic view, both medical and surgical complications may be encountered after transplantation (Fig. 31.5). The prevalence of medical complications is as high as 60–80% so that a single patient is at a high risk of experiencing one or even multiple complications [67]. In the immediate perioperative phase, bacterial infections may be encountered [78,79]. These may present as general, local, or organ-bound infections or abscesses. Septicemia, peritonitis, pneumonitis, or abscesses in kidney, brain, and osteomyelitis due to staphylococcus and *Enterococcus coli* infection are the most frequent agents. Unreflected pretransplant prophylaxis bears the risk of bacterial resistance. Perioperative antibiotic therapy is recommended as long as central venous lines or intra-abdominal drains are used. The antibiotics given should reflect the local commonest bacterial agents and should cover staphylococci. A daily swab from tracheal secretions as long as the patient is on the ventilator, from ascitic

Table 31.1 *Anti-infection Drugs that Interact with Cyclosporine A, Tacrolimus, or Sirolimus*

Drug	Increases Immunosuppressant Levels	Decreases Immunosuppressant Levels	Increases Toxicity
Antibacterial agents			
Aminoglycosides			+++ (renal)
(e.g. gentamicin, tobramycin, amikacin)			
Chloramphenicol	+		
Ciprofloxacin	+		
Imipenem/cilastatin			+ (neuro)
Macrolides	+++		
(e.g. erythromycin, azithromycin)			
Penicillins (e.g. nafcillin)	+	+++	
Quinupristin/dalfopristin	++		
Sulfa agents			+ (renal)
Vancomycin	+++		+ (renal)
Antituberculosis agents			
Isoniazid		+	
Rifampicin, rifampin, rifabutin		+++	
Antifungal agents			
Amphotericin B	+++		+++ (renal)
Azoles	+++		
(e.g. ketoconazole, itraconazole, clotrimazole)			
Antimalarial			
Chloroquine	++		
Antiviral agents			
Acyclovir, ganciclovir	+		+ (renal)
Protease inhibitors (HIV)	++		
(e.g. indinavir, ritonavir/lopinavir, saquinavir)			

+++, Well-established, significant; ++, probable, variable; +, possible, individual.

fluid as long as the patient has abdominal drains, and of blood samples drawn from central lines is recommended in order to achieve a guided antibiotic therapy. Acute rejection was observed in up to 60% of patients in the first week after transplantation. By using interleukin-2 receptor antibodies the

Table 31.2 *Other Drugs that Interact with Cyclosporine A, Tacrolimus, or Sirolimus*

Drug	Increases Immunosuppressant Levels	Decreases Immunosuppressant Levels	Increases Toxicity
Anticonvulsants			
Carbamazepine		+	
Phenobarbital		++	
Phenytoin		+++	
Primidone		+	
Antihypertensives			
ACE inhibitors			++ (hyperkalemia)
Calcium channel inhibitors			
(e.g. verapamil, diltiazem, amlodipine)	++		
(e.g. felodipine, nicardipine)	+++		
Anti-inflammatory agents			
Nonsteroidal cyclooxygenase inhibitors			+ (renal)
Psychotropic agents			
Benzodiazepines			
(e.g. alprazolam, diazepam, midazolam, triazolam)	++		
Modafinil		++	
Serotonin uptake inhibitors			
(e.g. nefazodone, sertraline)	+++		
Steroid hormones			
Danazol	++		
Miscellaneous agents			
Allopurinol	++		
Alendronate	+		
Grapefruit juice	++		
Orlistat		++	
St. John's wort		+++	
Ticlopidine		++	
Vinblastine	+		

+++, Well-established, significant; ++, probable, variable; +, possible, individual.

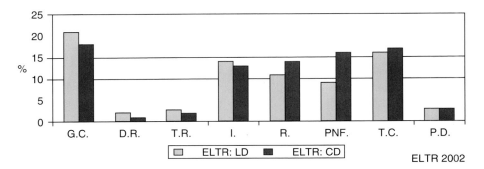

Fig. 31.5 *Causes of graft/patient loss in ELTR expressed as percent in pediatric liver transplantation (Oct 1991–Dec 2001). G.C., general complication; D.R., disease recurrence; T.R., tumor recurrence; I., infection; R., rejection; PNF, primary nonfunction; T.C., technical complication; P.D., perioperative death.*

prevalence of rejection has been lowered to about 20% [80–83]. However, there are two remarkable observations: (1) acute rejection in patients with IL2ra therapy is postponed to the third and fourth week after transplantation and does not present with clinical symptoms as has been common in the pre-IL2ra period. Thus the only way to detect these rejections is close monitoring [2]. The prevalence of steroid-resistant rejection has not been changed by IL2ra therapy. In the beginning of immunosuppression, absorption of calcineurin inhibitors may be varying very much. In some patients even toxic drug concentrations may be seen, leading to impaired renal, cerebral, and even hepatic function [82]. Using tacrolimus in normal dosage in organs with primary malfunction or nonfunction thus may be critical. In cyclosporine-based immunosuppression primary malfunction or nonfunction may lead to intoxication or to not achieving targeted trough levels. Primary nonfunction is defined as retransplantation within 10 days after transplantation or death resulting from a nonfunctioning graft, primary poor function as a Quick-test below 30% requiring substitution of fresh frozen plasma and AT III [60]. Especially at risk for this critical complication are patients with small-for-size transplants, which are defined as <0.8% of body weight. Other factors contributing to primary nonfunction or malfunction are fatty degeneration of the donor organ in combination with perfusion damage or cold- or warm-ischemic time beyond 12 and 60 min, respectively.

As far as surgical complications are concerned, bleeding from the cut surface in split-, living-related or reduced-size organs, biliary leakage from the cut surface or bile duct anastomosis and intestinal leakages from small bowel perforations after adhesiolysis or from anastomotic insufficiencies are best detected by controlling the drain fluids for blood, bilirubin, and amylase. In experienced centers using all surgical technical variants, i.e. full-size, reduced-size, split-, and living-related transplantations, however, there has been a steady improvement with regard to surgical complications. Biliary, arterial, portal, intestinal, and bleeding complications have reached a prevalence of less than 10% [60]. In addition, close monitoring with Doppler ultrasound starting already in the intraoperative phase and continued on a daily basis will show either fluid retention or portal venous, arterial, or venous flow impairment. The intraoperative Doppler ultrasound has been shown to be essential in preventing late sequelae from perfusion damage such as ischemic-type bile duct lesions, portal vein thrombosis, and hepatic venous outflow obstruction [60,67].

Bile duct and vascular obstructions are treated by either interventional radiography or surgery [84–86]. Portal vein obstruction after transplantation can be approached by performing a mesenteric-recessus umbilicalis shunt with vascular interposition (Mesorex shunt) [87,88].

Retransplantation results from either acute or chronic organ failure due to different causes: failed immunosuppression, viral infection, vascular, and bile duct complications. The ELTR report counts for the time period of 1991–2002 in 4313 pediatric recipients shows no statistical differences of causes of graft loss or death between living-related donation and organs from deceased donors with regard to general complications (21% vs. 18%), disease recurrence (2% vs. 1%), tumor recurrence (3% vs. 2%), infection (14% vs. 13%), rejection (11% vs. 14%), primary non- or dysfunction (9% vs. 16%), technical complications (16% vs. 17%) and preoperative death (3% vs. 3%) (Fig. 31.5) [1].

■ LONG-TERM RESULTS AFTER PEDIATRIC LIVER TRANSPLANTATION

Aspects of long-term results after pediatric liver transplantation are of increasing interest. The natural history of a long-term survivor after liver transplantation is characterized by viral infections due to CMV, Epstein–Barr virus (EBV), adenovirus, and herpes simplex virus infection [89–92] and by drug-related impairment of liver, kidney, and brain function and arterial hypertension [67]. There are additional complications because of vascular obstruction of the hepatic artery, the portal and the hepatic vein, and secondary lesions of the biliary tract. Due to the use of technical variants, the pediatric transplant recipient is at a high risk of experiencing biliary complications, since almost every patient is subjected to biliodigestive anastomosis.

Viral infections due to CMV, EBV, and herpes simplex virus infection are treatable by ganciclovir, cidofovir, and acyclovir. In case of drug-related impairment of renal or hepatic function, alternative immunosuppressants are available such as rapamune or mycofenolate mofetil [93–95]. Attention deficit syndromes and cerebral convulsions, however, are difficult to manage. Calcineurin inhibitors are associated with attention deficit syndrome and cerebral convulsion in children with preexisting brain damage and can contribute significantly to an impairment of posttransplant quality of life even in other children [96,97]. Very young infants and neonates have a higher risk of suffering from such complications [98]. However, it is difficult to asses any potential brain damage in this especial age group at the time of transplantation, so a "normal" neurological finding in such a patient cannot exclude such an important complication in the later course [99]. Arterial hypertension is observed in children after liver transplantation in about 30% of patients and is of great importance for the late outcome [69] (Fig. 31.1). Patients with preexisting renal damage are at high risk of developing renal dysfunction. As a consequence, intensive monitoring of renal function and blood pressure is essential in any patient after liver transplantation, and guided therapy is mandatory. Calcineurin inhibitor-free immunosuppression is recommended in these children [94].

Vascular complications may be prevented by intraoperative Doppler ultrasound examinations, which are often undetectable by just clinical means. In case of late manifestations of bile duct, hepatic artery, portal, and hepatic vein obstruction, the first attempt to correct is made by interventional radiology approach [67]. Only in those cases where these interventions are contraindicated or associated with a high risk for the patient, surgical interventions such as reanastomosing or extrahilar mesenterico left portal vein shunt are considered. Apart from mechanical portal vein complications due to anastomotic or inflammatory processes, effects of chronic rejection as a cause of arterial and portal vein obstruction are difficult to identify. Chronic rejection can only be identified after explantation.

There are new disorders observed after pediatric liver transplantation. The de novo hepatitis with autoimmune antibodies and atypical histology are such new detected disorders requiring additional azathioprine medication [100–102].

Quality of life measurements in recipients and their families are necessary to assess the quality of long-term survival. Patients estimate their all-day strength better than their parents and probably better than teachers and instructors. The integration of a transplant recipient into normal life is still suboptimal and needs to be improved.

◼ GENERAL ASPECTS OF PEDIATRIC CARE AFTER LIVER TRANSPLANTATION

Liver transplantation in children today covers all ages from newborns until late adolescence. It is performed in children who have no other option for survival or in children with poor quality of life. In newborns and infants, parents are responsible for the decision to undergo transplantation. The actual results of liver transplantation in children justify such a decision since they have reached an almost 95% survival for the first 6 postoperative months and an almost 80% survival for 10 years. These high standards expose transplanted children to everyday risks under immunosuppression.

Infections of the upper respiratory tract and gastroenteritis may influence absorption of immunosuppressants directly or by the use of antibiotics interfering with metabolism of calcineurin inhibitors. In general, however, normal immunosuppression does not expose children to a higher risk than nonimmunosuppressed siblings. Treatment with macrolides such as erythromycin, amphotericin B, and fluconazol, on the other hand, increases cyclosporine A and tacrolimus levels, so toxic liver, cerebral, and renal damage must be taken into consideration. On the contrary, phenobarbiton, carbamacepin, and rifampicin as an anti-itching agent will lower the trough levels of both calcineurin inhibitors and thus increase the risk of underimmunosuppression-caused rejection. Any therapy with the agents mentioned above must be balanced with regard to risks and benefits.

High immunosuppression in combination with primary EBV infection exposes the pediatric recipient to the risk of EBV-driven PTLD. Especially at risk are children with negative EBV status. Close monitoring of EBV serology and EBV PCR thus is essential in these children. Apart from typical EBV-related symptoms, anemia, gastrointestinal pain, and bleeding need thorough workup.

In adolescents, the acceptance of being transplanted turns out to be much more difficult [103]. Transplantation in an adolescent is really challenging with regard to acceptance of surgical and medical care. Children growing up after transplantation show a changing pattern of compliance once adolescence is reached [104]. Noncompliance with its risk of rejection and organ damage becomes an essential problem. Many efforts are needed to instruct children about the importance of compliance. Quality of life measurements have become an important measure of success of liver transplantation.

■ REFERENCES

1. ELTR report, 2004. Available at www.eurotransplant.org.

2. Suchy FJ, Burdelski M, Tomar BS, et al. Cholestatic liver disease: Working Group report of the first World Congress of Pediatric Gastroenterology, Hepatology and Nutrition. J Pediatr Gastroenterol Nutr 2002;34(suppl 2):S89–S97.

3. McDiarmid SV. Current status of liver transplantation in children. Pediatr Clin North Am 2003;50:1335–1374.

4. McDiarmid SV, Anand R, Lindblad AS, et al. Studies of pediatric liver transplant-ation: 2002 update. An overview of demographics, indications, timing and im-munosuppressive practices in pediatric liver transplantation in the United States and Canada. Pediatr Transplant 2004;8:284–294.

5. Diem HV, Evrard V, Vinh HT, et al. Pediatric liver transplantation for biliary atresia: results of primary grafts in 328 recipients. Transplantation 2002;75:1692–1697.

6. Wildhaber BE, Coran AG, Drongowski RA, et al. The Kasai portoenterostomy for biliary atresia: a review of a 27-year experience with 81 patients. J Pediatr Surg 2003;38:1480–1485.

7. Hadzic N, Davenport M, Tizzard S, et al. Long-term survival following Kasai portoenterostomy: is chronic liver disease inevitable? J Pediatr Gastroenterol Nutr 2003;37:430–433.

8. Knisely AS. Progressive familial intrahepatic cholestasis. Pediatr Dev Pathol 2004;7:309–314.

9. Baussan C, Cresteil D, Gonzales E, et al. Genetic cholestasis and related disorders. Acta Gastroenterol Belg 2002;67:179–183.

10. Kneepkens CM, Douwes AC. Idiopathic neonatal hepatitis. Tijdschr Kindergen-eeskd 1993;61:141–146.

11. Adrian-Casavilla F, Reyes J, Tzakis A, et al. Liver transplantation for neonatal hepatitis as compared to the other two leading indications for liver transplantation in children. J Hepatol 1994;21:1035–1039.

12. Patrinos ME, Hardman JM, Easa D, et al. Idiopathic neonatal hepatitis associated with a fatal coagulopathy. J Perinatol 1999;19:599–602.

13. Roberts EA. Neonatal hepatitis syndrome. Semin Neonatol 2003;7:357–374.

14. Hadchouel M. Alagille syndrome. Indian J Pediatr 2002;69:815–818.

15. Ganschow R, Grabhorn E, Helmke K, et al. Liver transplantation in children with Alagille syndrome. Transplant Proc 2001;33:3608–3609.

16. Burdelski M. Liver transplantation in metabolic diseases: current status. Pediatr Transplant 2002;6:361–363.

17. Kayler LK, Rasmussen CS, Dykstra DM, et al. Liver transplantation in children with metabolic disorders in the United States. Am J Transplant 2003;3:334–339.

18. Rodeck B, Melter M, Kardorrf R, et al. Liver transplantation in children with chronic end stage liver disease: factors influencing survival after transplantation. Trans-plantation 1996;62:1071–1076.

19. Mondragon R, Mieli-Vergani G, Heaton ND, et al. Liver transplantation for fulmin-ant liver failure in children. Transpl Int 1992;(5 suppl 1):S206–S208.

20. Kelly DA. Managing liver failure. Postgrad Med J 2002;78:660–667.

21. Durand P, Debray D, Mandel R, et al. Acute liver failure in infancy: a 14-year experience of a pediatric liver transplantation center. J Pediatr 2001;139:871–876.

22. Aw MM, Dhawan A. Acute liver failure. Indian J Pediatr 2002;69:87–91.

23. Ec LC, Shepherd RW, Cleghorn GJ, et al. Acute liver failure in children: a regional experience. J Pediatr Child Health 2003;39:107–110.

24. Tessier G, Villeneuve E, Villeneuve JP. Etiology and outcome of acute liver failure: experience from a transplant center in Montreal. Can J Gastroenterol 2002;16: 672–676.

25. Kelly DA. Acute liver failure. Indian J Pediatr 1999;66(suppl):104–109.

26. Helmke K, Burdelski M, Hansen HC. Detection and monitoring of intracranial pressure dysregulation in liver failure by ultrasound. Transplantation 2000;70: 392–395.

27. Vogel A, Heinrich E, Bahr MJ, et al. Long-term outcome of liver transplantation for autoimmune hepatitis. Clin Transplant 2004;18:62–69.

28. Haberle B, Bode U, von Schweinitz D. Differentiated treatment protocols for high- and standard-risk hepatoblastoma – an interim report of the German Liver Tumor Study HB99. Klin Padiatr 2003;215:159–165.

29. Perilongo G, Shafford E, Maibach R, et al. Risk-adapted treatment for childhood hepatoblastoma: final report of the second study of the International Society of Paediatric Oncology-SIOPEL 2. Eur J Cancer 2004;49:411–421.

30. Yoo HY, Patt CH, Geschwind JF, et al. The outcome of liver transplantation in patients with hepatocellular carcinoma in the United States between 1988 and 2001: 5-year survival has improved significantly with time. J Clin Oncol 2003;21:4329–4335.

31. Weber TR, Keller MS. Adverse effects of liver dysfunction and portal hypertension on intestinal adaptation in short bowel syndrome in children. Am J Surg 2002;184:582–586.

32. Forchielli ML, Walker WA. Nutritional factors contributing to the development of cholestasis during parenteral nutrition. Adv Pediatr 2003;50:245–267.

33. Cario H, Pahl HL, Schwarz K, et al. Familial polycythemia vera with Budd–Chiari syndrome in childhood. Br J Haematol 2003;123:346–352.

34. Pierro A, Koletzko B, Carnielle V, et al. Resting energy expenditure is increased in infants with extrahepatic biliary atresia. J Pediatr Surg 1989;24:534–538.

35. Ksiazyk J, Lyszkowska M, Kierkus J. Energy metabolism in portal hypertension in children. Nutrition 1996;12:469–474.

36. Greer R, Lehnert M, Lewindon P, et al. Body composition and components of energy expenditure in children with end-stage liver disease. J Pediatr Gastroenterol Nutr 2003;36:358–363.

37. Kelly DA. Nutritional factors affecting growth before and after liver transplantation. Pediatr Transplant 1997;1:80–84.

38. Burdelski M, Nolkemper D, Ganschow R, et al. Liver transplantation in children: long-term outcome and quality of life. Eur J Pediatr 1999;158(suppl 2): S34–S42.

39. Collemaes M, Sokal E, Otte JB. Growth factors in children with end-stage liver disease before and after liver transplantation: a review. Pediatr Transplant 1997;1:171–175.

40. Goncelves MEP, Cardoso SR, Maksoud JG. Prophylactic sclerotherapy in children with esophageal varices. Long-term results of a controlled prospective randomized trial. J Pediatr Surg 2000;35:401–405.

41. McKiernan PJ. Treatment of variceal bleeding. Gastrointest Endosc Clin North Am 2001;11:789–812.

42. Celinska-Cedro D, Teisseyre M, Woynarowski M. Endoscopic ligation of esophageal varices for prophylaxis of first bleeding in children with portal hypertension. Preliminary results of a prospective randomised study. J Pediatr Surg 2003;38:1008–1011.

43. Berg UB, Ericzon BG, Nemeth A. Renal function before and long after liver transplantation in children. Transplantation 2001;27:561–562.

44. McDiarmid SV. Renal function in pediatric liver transplant patients. Kidney Int 1996;53(suppl):S77–S84.

45. Gentilini P, Vizutti F, Gentilini A, et al. Update on ascites and hepatorenal syndrome. Dig Liver Dis 2002;34:592–605.

46. Mitzner SR, Klammt S, Peszynski P, et al. Improvement of multiple organ functions in hepatorenal syndrome during albumin dialysis with the molecular adsorbent recirculating system. Ther Apher 2001;5:417–422.

47. D'Antiga L, Dhawan A, Moniz C. Bone mineral density and height gain in children with chronic cholestatic liver disease undergoing transplantation. Transplantation 2002;73:1788–1793.

48. Rittinghaus EF, Jüppner H, Burdelski M, et al. Selective determination of C-terminal (70–84) hPTH: elevated concentrations in cholestatic liver disease. Acta Endocrinol 1986;111:62–68.

49. D'Antiga L, Ballan D, Luisetto G, et al. Long-term outcome of bone mineral density in children who underwent a successful liver transplantation. Transplantation 2004;78:899–903.

50. Chardot C, Carton M, Spire-Bendelac N, et al. Prognosis of biliary atresia in the era of liver transplantation: French national study from 1986 to 1996. Hepatology 1999;30:606–611.

51. Kataria R, Kataria A, Gupta DK. Spectrum of congenital anomalies associated with biliary atresia. Indian J Pediatr 1996;63:652–654.

52. Helmke K. Imaging of the pediatric transplant candidate. In Bücheler E, Nicolas V, Broelsch CE, et al., eds., Diagnostic and interventional radiology in liver transplantation. Berlin, Heidelberg, New York, Hong Kong, Paris: Springer, 2003:211–236.

53. Hoeper MM, Krowka MJ, Strassburg CP. Portopulmonary hypertension and hepatopulmonary syndrome. Lancet 2004;364:26–27.

54. Paramesh AS, Husain SZ, Shneider B, et al. Improvement of hepatopulmonary syndrome after transjugular portasystemic shunting. Case report and review of literature. Pediatr Transplant 2003;7:157–161.

55. Dinh-Xuan AT, Naeije R. The hepatopulmonary syndrome: NO way out? Eur Respir J 2004;23:661–662.

56. Sen S, Williams R, Jalan R. The pathophysiological basis of acute-on-chronic liver failure. Liver 2002;22(suppl 2):5–13.

57. Kelly DA. Managing liver failure. Postgrad Med J 2002;78:660–667.

58. Burdelski M, Pichlmayr R, Ringe B, et al. Pediatric liver transplantation – ten years experience in Hanover. Clin Transpl 1987;1:55–62.

59. Kelly DA. Current results and evolving indications for liver transplantation in children. J Pediatr Gastroenterol Nutr 1998;27:214–221.

60. Broering DC, Kim JS, Mueller T, et al. 132 consecutive pediatric liver transplantations without hospital mortality. Ann Surg 2004;240:1002–1012.

61. McDiarmid SV, Anand R, Lindblad AS. Principal Investigators and Institutions of the Studies of Pediatric Liver Transplantation (SPLIT) Research Group. Development of a pediatric end-stage liver disease score to predict poor outcome in children awaiting liver transplantation. Transplantation 2002;27:173–181.

62. Burdelski M, Oellerich M, Düwel J, et al. Pre- and posttransplant assessment of liver function in paediatric liver transplantation. Eur J Pediatr 1992;151(suppl):S39–S43.

63. Burdelski M, Schütz E, Nolte-Buchholtz S, et al. Prognostic value of the monoethylglycinexylidide test in pediatric liver transplant candidates. Ther Drug Monit 1996;18:378–382.

64. Oellerich M, Burdelski M, Lautz HU, et al. Assessment of pretransplant prognosis in patients with cirrhosis. Transplantation 1991;51:801–806.

65. Wadstrom J, Rogiers X, Malago M, et al. Experience from the first 30 living related liver transplant in Hamburg. Transplant Proc 1995;27:1173–1174.

66. Rogiers X, Malago M, Gawad K, et al. In situ splitting of cadaveric livers: the ultimate expansion of the limited donor pool. Ann Surg 1996;224:339–431.

67. Burdelski M, Rogiers X. What lessons have we learned in pediatric liver transplantation. J Hepatol 2005;42:28–33.

68. Davenport M, De Ville de Goyet J, Stringer MD, et al. Seamless management of biliary atresia in England and Wales. Lancet 2004;363:1354–1357.

69. Kelly DA, Jara P, Rodeck B, et al. Tacrolimus and steroids versus ciclosporin microemulsion, steroids and azathioprine in children undergoing liver transplantation: randomized European multicenter trial. Lancet 2004;364:1054–1061.

70. Ganschow R, Schulz A, Meyer T, et al. Low-dose immunosuppression reduces the incidence of post-transplant lymphoproliferative disease in pediatric liver graft recipients. J Pediatr Gastroenterol Nutr 2004;38:198–203.

71. Penn I. De novo malignancies in pediatric organ transplant recipients. Pediatr Transplant 1998;2:56–63.

72. Molmenti EP, Nagata DE, Roden JS, et al. Post-transplant lymphoproliferative syndrome in the pediatric liver transplant population. Am J Transplant 2001;1:356–359.

73. Koh BY, Rosenthal P, Medeiros LJ, et al. Posttransplantation lymphoproliferative disorders in pediatric patients undergoing liver transplantation. Arch Pathol Lab Med 2001;125:227–343.

74. Nemeth A, Berg B, Ericzon G. Height and growth in children following liver transplantation. Pediatr Transplant 2000;4(suppl):139–143.

75. Ganschow R, Richter A, Grabhorn E, et al. C2 blood concentrations of orally administered cyclosporine in pediatric liver graft recipients with a body weight below 10 kg. Pediatr Transplant 2004;8:185–188.

76. Burdelski M. The impact of cyclosporine on the development of immunosuppressive therapy for pediatric transplantation. Transplant Proc 2004;36(suppl 2):S295–S298.

77. Ganschow R, Broering DC, Nolkemper D, et al. Th2 cytokine profile in infants predisposes to improved graft acceptance after liver transplantation. Transplantation 2001;72:929–934.

78. Drews D, Sturm E, Latta A, et al. Complications following living-related and cadaveric transplantation in 100 children. Transplant Proc 1997;29:421–423.

79. Ganschow R, Nolkemper D, Helmke K, et al. Intensive care management after pediatric liver transplantation: a single center experience. Pediatr Transplant 2000;4:273–279.

80. Ganschow R, Grabhorn E, Burdelski M. Basiliximab in paediatric liver transplantat recipients. Lancet 2001;357:388.

81. Ganschow R, Broering DC, Stuerenburg I, et al. First experience with basiliximab in pediatric liver graft recipients. Pediatr Transplant 2001;5:353–358.

82. Arora N, McKiernan PJ, Beath SV, et al. Concomitant basiliximab with low-dose calcineurin inhibitors in children post-liver transplantation. Pediatr Transplant 2002;6:214–218.

83. Martin SR, Atkinson P, Anand R, et al. Studies of Pediatric Liver Transplantation 2002: patient and graft survival and rejection in pediatric recipients of a first liver transplant in the United States and Canada. Pediatr Transplant 2004;8: 273–283.

84. Chardot C, Evrard F. Liver transplantation in children. Soins Pediatr Pueric 2004;216:23–27.

85. Roberts JP, Hulbert-Shearon TE, Merion RM, et al. Influence of graft type on outcome after pediatric liver transplantation. Am J Transplant 2004;4:373–377.

86. Yersiz H, Renz JF, Farmer DG, et al. One hundred in situ split-liver transplantations: a single-center experience. Ann Surg 2003;238(4):496–505.

87. De Ville de Goyet J, Alberti D, Falchetti D, et al. Treatment of extrahepatic portal hypertension in children by mesenteric-to-left portal vein bypass: a new physiological procedure. Eur J Surg 1999;165:777–781.

88. Stenger AM, Broering DC, Gundlach M, et al. Extrahilar mesenterico-left portal vein shunt for portal vein thrombosis after liver transplantation. Transplant Proc 2001;33:1739–1741.

89. Feldstein AE, Razonable RR, Boyce TG, et al. Prevalence and clinical significance of human herpesviruses 6 and 7 active infection in pediatric liver transplant patients. Pediatr Transplant 2003;7:125–129.

90. McLaughlin GE, Delis S, Kashimawo L, et al. Adenovirus infection in pediatric liver and intestinal transplant recipients: utility of DNA detection by PCR. Am J Transplant 2003;3:224–228.

91. Vilchez RA, Fung J, Kusne S. The pathogenesis and management of influenza virus infection in organ transplant recipients. Transpl Infect Dis 2002;4:177–182.

92. Their M, Holmberg C, Lautenschlager I, et al. Infections in pediatric kidney and liver transplant patients after perioperative hospitalization. Transplantation 2000;69:1617–1623.

93. Jiminez-Rivera C, Avitzur Y, Fecteau AH, et al. Sirolimus for pediatric liver transplant recipients with post-transplant lymphoproliferative disease and hepatoblastoma. Pediatr Transplant 2004;8:243–248.

94. Nobili V, Comparcola D, Sartotelli MR, et al. Mycophenolate mofetil in pediatric transplant patients with renal dysfunction: preliminary data. Pediatr Transplant 2003;7:454–457; erratum in Pediatr Transplant 2004;8:94.

95. Markiewicz M, Karlicinski P, Teisseyre J, et al. Rapamycine in children after liver transplantation. Transplant Proc 2003;35:2284–2286.

96. Alonso EM, Neighbors K, Mattson C, et al. Functional outcomes of pediatric liver transplantation. J Pediatr Gastroenterol Nutr 2003;37:155–160.

97. Krull K, Fuchs C, Yurk H, et al. Neurocognitive outcome in pediatric liver transplant recipients. Pediatr Transplant 2003;7:111–118.

98. Schulz KH, Wein C, Boeck A, et al. Cognitive performance of children who have undergone liver transplantation. Transplantation 2003;75:1236–1240.

99. Grabhorn E, Schulz A, Helmke K, et al. Short- and long-term results of liver transplantation in infants aged less than 6 months. Transplantation 2004;78:235–241.

100. Czaja AJ. Autoimmune hepatitis after liver transplantation and other lessons of self-intolerance. Liver Transpl 2002;8:505–513.

101. Mieli-Vergani G, Vergani D. De novo autoimmune hepatitis after liver transplantation. J Hepatol 2004;40:3–7.

102. Gupta P, Hart J, Millis JM, et al. De novo hepatitis with autoimmune antibodies and atypical histology: a rare cause of late grafts dysfunction after pediatric liver transplantation. Transplantation 2001;71:664–668.

103. Kelly DA. Strategies for optimising immunosuppression in adolescent transplant recipients: a focus on liver transplantation. Pediatr Drugs 2003;5:177–183.

104. Shemesh E, Shneider BL, Savitzky JK, et al. Medication adherence in pediatric and adolescent liver transplant recipients. Pediatrics 2004;113:825–832.

Liver Transplantation in the Future

New Approaches

▼ ▼ ▼ ▼ ▼ ▼ ▼ ▼ ▼ ▼

Markus Selzner and Leo Bühler

TREATMENT of advanced acute or chronic liver failure generally remains supportive. Currently, liver transplantation is the only available therapy for end-stage liver disease (ESLD). However, the increasing shortage of cadaveric organ donors for transplantation motivates researchers to find methods to preserve damaged liver tissue or new sources for organs and tissues. Therefore developing alternative methods for liver transplantation is crucial. Among the new approaches that are under investigation in experimental settings, methods that protect against ischemic injury and improve liver regeneration, and the use of hepatocyte transplantation, liver xenotransplantation, and stem cell technology are discussed.

■ PROTECTIVE STRATEGIES AGAINST ISCHEMIC INJURY

During the past decade, the number of patients waiting for a liver transplantation has by far outnumbered the available grafts for liver transplantation. As a result of the current donor shortage the number of patients awaiting an organ has grown dramatically over the past decade, triggering interest to maximize and optimize the use of potential organs. For example, marginal organs (i.e. organs not used previously or expected to be associated with increased risk of malfunction) and partial liver transplantation such as living-related and split-liver transplantations are increasingly used in most transplant centers [1,2]. A common issue inherent to all strategies is the need to preserve the graft from the time of harvesting until implantation [3]. From cooling of the graft, initiated in the 1950s, and the introduction of the University of Wisconsin (UW) solution for cold preservation in the mid-1980s [4], many experimental studies have suggested novel protective strategies, although very few have yet reached clinical practice.

Reperfusion Injury

During liver transplantation the ischemic injury can be divided into warm- and cold-ischemic injury. Cold-ischemic injury occurs during the preservation period until implantation of the graft. Cold ischemia is mainly associated with injury to the sinusoidal endothelial cells (SECs) [5]. During cold preservation the cytoskeleton of the endothelial cells develops structural changes, inducing cell rounding and detachment from the basal membrane. Despite rounding and detachment the SECs stay alive until reperfusion, when rapid cell death is induced in the presence of oxygen. It has been demonstrated that the injury to the endothelial cells is synergistically enhanced in the presence of leukocytes and platelets [6].

In contrast, warm ischemia is only tolerated poorly by the liver, resulting in rapid hepatocyte death. The detachment of SECs during cold preservation allows leukocyte and thrombocyte adhesion during reperfusion, inducing disturbance of the microcirculation. At the time of reperfusion free oxygen radicals are formed and Kupffer cells are activated, resulting in tumor necrosis factor-α (TNFα) release. Leukocyte and thrombocyte recruitment further aggravates the injury, inducing parenchymal cell death.

Organ Cooling

Reduction of the organ temperature to 1–4°C was the first strategy applied to protect the liver against ischemic injury, allowing a preservation of up to 8 h. In the mid-1980s, a specific preservation solution was developed by Belzer and Southerland to counteract the known and suspected effects of hyperthermia [4]; these effects included cell swelling due to inhibition of the Na+/K+ pump, intracellular acidosis, and disturbance of the cytosolic Ca++ homeostasis [7] and with this preservation solution (UW solution), the limit of liver preservation could be extended up to 24 h. Since the UW solution mainly protects SECs it has been speculated that prevention of cytoskeleton changes by inhibition of matrix metallo-protease (MMP) is of importance. One of the main ingredients of the UW solution (lactobionic acid) is a potent inhibitor of metallo-proteases. Recently Bretschneider's solution, also known as histidine/tryptophan/keto-glutarate solution or HTK solution, has been shown to be as effective as the UW solution at the usual periods of cold preservation used in human transplantation [8]. This is a surprising outcome, because the compositions of these two solutions are very different, and, seemingly, the only property shared by these solutions is buffering capacity and MMP inhibition. However, buffering capacity alone cannot explain their effectiveness, because solutions with excellent buffering capacity, such as Krebs–Henseleit solution and Eurocollins solution, are poor preservation solutions. These results underline the lack of understanding of protective mechanisms of preservation solutions.

Ischemic Preconditioning

Many protective strategies have been developed during the past decade, which rarely reached the clinical practice. A novel approach to protect the liver against reperfusion injury is ischemic preconditioning (i.e. a short period of ischemia followed by a short period of reperfusion prior to a prolonged ischemic insult) (Fig. 32.1). Ischemic preconditioning was first described in 1986 in the heart in a canine model by Murry et al. [9]. The authors found that a short period of ischemia protects the heart against a sustained ischemic injury. Subsequently, the protective effect of ischemic preconditioning has been described in most other organ systems including the brain [10], skeletal muscle [11], kidney [12], intestine [13], retina [14], and the liver [15].

In a recent large randomized trial the protective effect of ischemic preconditioning was determined in human liver resection [16]. In the setting of rat liver transplantation several groups demonstrated protection of the graft by ischemic preconditioning of the donor [17,18]. Arai et al. [18] showed in a model of rat liver transplantation decreased SEC death and diminished Kupffer cell activation if ischemic preconditioning was applied prior to harvesting. Others [17] found in a model of 30 h preservation of rat livers in UW solution that ischemic preconditioning decreases sinusoidal cell detachment and reduces the activity of MMPs. Furthermore, endothelial cell apoptosis was prevented if preconditioning was used prior to harvesting. Interestingly, it was shown recently that ischemic preconditioning can be performed only on one hepatic lobe, resulting in protection of the ipsilateral and the contralateral side [19]. This offers new options for living-related liver transplantation when the transplant surgeon hesitates to apply ischemia to the transplanted lobe.

Although the effects of preconditioning are well documented the mechanisms of protection remain unclear. Various potential mediators have been proposed but the interaction of the different pathways is only poorly understood to date. It has been proposed recently that ischemic preconditioning provides a sublethal oxidative stress, inducing protection against the sustained ischemia and reperfusion [20]. Ischemia and reperfusion are associated with large oxidative stress-inducing injury in hepatocytes and nonparenchymal cells. The authors demonstrated that ischemic preconditioning provides a small sublethal oxidative stress, which prevents the larger oxidative stress at

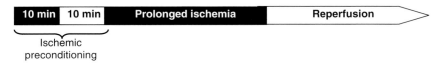

Fig. 32.1 *Ischemic preconditioning represents a short time of ischemia followed by a short time of reperfusion prior to a prolonged ischemic insult.*

the time of reperfusion. Preventing the small oxidative stress during preconditioning with antioxidants resulted in loss of the preconditioning effect and increased hepatocyte injury. In contrast, providing a small oxidative stress pharmacologically with hydrogen peroxide (H_2O_2) imitated the effect of ischemic preconditioning and protected the liver against ischemia and reperfusion injury.

Studies in the myocardium indicated that the protective effect of preconditioning is mediated by a receptor-dependent mechanism [21]. In the case of liver, one of the most studied candidates of receptor-mediated preconditioning is adenosine. Adenosine is an extracellular molecule, which is generated during ischemia by the degradation of ATP into adenosine and phosphate. Ischemic preconditioning resulted in a threefold increase of adenosine in the liver [22]. Arai et al. [18] demonstrated that the protective effect of preconditioning is associated with the activation of adenosine 2 receptors. In this study, ischemic preconditioning of 5 min ischemia followed by 5 min of reperfusion prior to harvesting of the rat liver resulted in a decrease in SEC death. Blocking the adenosine 2 receptor resulted in loss of the preconditioning effect, while blockage of the adenosine 1 receptor did not alter protection of preconditioning. Pharmacologic stimulation of the adenosine 2 receptor provided protection against ischemic injury similar to ischemic preconditioning. The authors proposed that the protective effect of adenosine is mediated by the increase of cAMP levels in SECs. Several other effects of adenosine might be associated with protection. Adenosine inhibits leukocyte adhesion and decreases the expression of adhesion molecules. Kupffer cell activation is decreased by adenosine. Furthermore, it is a potent vasodilatator and adenosine inhibits the formation of free oxygen radicals.

NO has been described as an important signaling molecule in most organ systems. It is produced from L-arginine by nitric oxide synthase. Peralta et al. [22,23] have proposed that the protective effect of adenosine 2 receptor activation is mediated by the intracellular formation of NO. The authors described that the activation of adenosine 2 receptors was associated with an induction of nitric oxide synthesis in rat livers. Inhibition of NO production results in a loss of the preconditioning effect. In contrast, NO donor pretreatment prior to harvesting protected the rat liver against reperfusion injury similar to ischemic preconditioning. Interestingly, NO pretreatment provided also protective effects against ischemic injury with simultaneous inhibition of adenosine. This indicates that NO is downstream of adenosine in the protective cascade. In the study by Peralta et al. the effect of preconditioning was associated with improved hepatic microcirculation, decreased lipid peroxidation, and diminished leukocyte accumulation.

This pathway offers the possibility for a pharmacological intervention, including agents such as adenosine receptor (A2) agonists and nitric oxide precursors ('NO donors'). Several studies in animal models indicate that synthetic adenosine receptor agonists (e.g. CGS-21680) may confer protection to the liver against cold-ischemic injury [18]. Alternatively, administration of NO donors such as L-arginine [24], NONOate [22], FK409 [25] and others induced protection against warm-ischemic hepatic insults in rat models.

Heat Shock Preconditioning

Several studies have indicated that livers can be protected against ischemic injury by exposing the whole body to hyperthermia of 42°C. The heat exposure triggers the induction of several stress proteins (heat shock proteins (HSPs)), such as HSP72, HSP90, and heme oxygenase-1 (HO-1). They belong to a class of proteins called chaperones that are involved in protein folding [26] during synthesis and represent cellular mechanisms of protection from protein degradation. In particular, HO-1 or Hsp32 [27] contributes to the protective mechanism of hyperthermic preconditioning, based on the finding that overexpression of these two molecules increases the resistance of the liver and other organs to ischemic injury. HO-1 catalyzes the breakdown of heme into biliverdin, carbon monoxide, and iron. Biliverdin is further converted into bilirubin, which is a potent antioxidant.

Redaelli et al. [28] performed heat shock preconditioning by placing rats for 20 min in a 42°C water bath. Afterwards, the liver was harvested and orthotopic liver transplantation was performed after 44 h preservation in UW solution. While all control animals without heat shock preconditioning died within 3 days, 89% of the rats in the heat shock preconditioning group survived permanently. Heat shock preconditioning was associated with decreased transaminases, improved bile flow, and decreased necrosis. Pharmacological blockage of HO-1 resulted in loss of the protective effect of heat shock preconditioning. In contrast, induction of HO-1 with cobalt protoporphyrin protected the liver against reperfusion injury similar to heat shock preconditioning. Similar results were obtained from Mokuno et al. [29]. The authors placed rats for 10 min in a 43°C water bath and found an induction of HSP72, HSP90, and HO-1. Heat shock preconditioning reduced transaminases and significantly improved survival after liver transplantation. In addition, TNFα and IL-10 were decreased in the heat shock preconditioning group in comparison with animals with transplantation without heat shock exposure. The maximum effect of heat shock preconditioning was observed by the authors if liver transplantation was performed 6–48 h after preconditioning, indicating a delayed protective effect in comparison with ischemic preconditioning, which is present immediately. Matsumoto et al. [30] performed heat shock preconditioning in rats and found HSP70 as late as 48 h after preconditioning in hepatocytes as well as in SECs. Heat shock preconditioning reduced transaminases and improved survival of the rats. In addition, the authors reported that heat shock preconditioning particularly protected the SECs with significant reduction of apoptosis.

Since HO-1 catalyzes the reaction of heme in biliverdin and carbon monoxide, Kato et al. [31] compared heat shock preconditioning with carbon monoxide or bilirubin rinse of rat livers prior to transplantation. The authors demonstrated the protective effect of heat shock preconditioning on hepatocyte injury and bile flow in comparison with rats receiving liver transplantation without heat shock preconditioning. Pharmacologic inhibition of HO-1 resulted in a loss of the preconditioning effect. Bilirubin but not carbon monoxide administration provided a protective effect against ischemic injury. The authors concluded that the protective effect of HO-1 could be mediated by an increase of bilirubin.

■ THE FATTY LIVER

Steatosis is an increasing problem in liver transplantation, affecting currently about 26% of all donors. In the USA 20% of the population has a body mass index above 30%, and obesity is currently regarded as the leading health problem in the USA. Several groups have described the increased frequency of primary graft dysfunction or nonfunction after liver transplantation with steatotic organs. In a multivariate analysis including 227 patients, severe steatosis was identified as an important significant risk factor for primary graft nonfunction or dysfunction [32]. Currently, severe steatosis (>60%) is considered a contraindication for liver transplantation by most transplant centers while organs with moderate steatosis (30–60%) are marginal. Since a large percentage of the donor livers are steatotic, research has focused on improving the function of these marginal grafts.

Several hypotheses have been developed to explain the decreased tolerance of fatty livers against ischemia/reperfusion injury. These include decreased energy content, increased lipid peroxidation, and decreased microcirculation in fatty livers [33,34]. We investigated the energy content in lean and fatty livers prior and after hepatic ischemia and reperfusion [33]. Steatosis was associated with significantly decreased intrahepatic ATP content before ischemia, but also after 4 h of 24 h of reperfusion. While lean hepatocytes after warm ischemia develop a predominant ATP-dependent apoptotic cell death, fatty livers undergo necrosis. Ischemic preconditioning improved the intrahepatic ATP content and resulted in a significant reduction of postreperfusion aspartate transaminase (AST) levels and decreased necrosis. Similarly, Serafin et al. [35] reported that ischemic preconditioning enhances the ATP content of the lean liver and reduces reperfusion injury.

Lipid peroxidation has been discussed as a second important mechanism of injury in fatty livers. During reperfusion, oxygen-free radicals are formed, resulting in peroxydation of the cell membranes and other lipids. Gao et al. [36] suggested that after rat liver transplantation of fatty liver, the increased lipid peroxydation resulted in cell death. Serafin et al. [35] investigated lipid peroxidation in a model of warm ischemia and reperfusion in fatty and lean rats. Steatosis was associated with significantly increased reperfusion injury and reduced survival. The authors found an eightfold increase of lipid peroxidation in steatotic livers, when compared with the lean control group. Ischemic preconditioning decreased reperfusion injury and improved survival. In addition, ischemic preconditioning was associated with a threefold decrease of lipid peroxidation in the steatotic livers. Inhibition of NO production resulted in a loss of the preconditioning effect with high levels of lipid peroxidation. In contrast, administration of NO prior to the ischemic injury resulted in effects similar to ischemic preconditioning. With NO injection the fatty livers were protected against ischemic injury, with a threefold reduction of lipid peroxidation. These findings indicate that lipid peroxidation is one mechanism of injury in fatty livers and that ischemic preconditioning protects fatty livers by reducing lipid peroxidation.

Finally, disturbance of the sinusoidal microcirculation has been proposed by us and others as a mechanism of reperfusion injury in fatty livers. We determined that ischemic injury decreases the hepatic microcirculation in lean and fatty livers. However, in lean livers, the sinusoidal perfusion is rapidly restored within 4 h of reperfusion, while steatosis is associated with a prolonged period of low sinusoidal microcirculation up to 24 h after reperfusion. Ischemic preconditioning resulted in an improvement of sinusoidal perfusion in lean and fatty livers. While lean livers demonstrated a normal microcirculation despite ischemic injury the sinusoidal perfusion in fatty livers was significantly improved.

■ HEPATOCYTE TRANSPLANTATION

Over the last three decades, transplantation of isolated liver cells has been used by several investigators either as a "bridge" for patients awaiting liver transplantation or as metabolic replacement therapy. The main advantages of cell transplantation over whole organ transplantation are: (1) cell transplantation has been shown to be minimally invasive, with decreased morbidity, mortality, and costs; (2) cells can be stored by cryopreservation for immediate availability in emergencies; (3) the recipient liver remains intact, subsequent orthotopic liver transplantation remains open; and (4) isolated hepatocytes can be modified by gene therapy and allow metabolic corrections. We here present the basic methods for hepatocyte isolation and review experimental and clinical data of hepatocyte transplantation.

Tissue Procurement and Isolation of Hepatocytes

Mouse and rat hepatocytes are obtained from whole livers according to the technique developed by Seglen [37]. The portal vein is used to perfuse the liver with the collagenase solution. Porcine and human hepatocytes are obtained from surgical liver biopsies and are perfused by a system of multiperfusion through several portal veinules (Fig. 32.2). Human liver biopsies are taken from patients undergoing segmental hepatectomies for liver tumors. At the start of the intervention, a wedge of macroscopically normal tissue (15–30 g) located within the part of the liver to be resected is excised, immersed in ice-cold buffered medium, and carried to the laboratory. Rodent, porcine, and human hepatocyte isolations are performed in two steps. The first step is the perfusion of the liver with a buffer solution. This perfusion is used to wash out the vascular network and to keep the cells in a physiological environment. The second step is the perfusion of the liver with a buffer solution containing collagenase and constitutes the digestion phase. The digested liver breaks up and the hepatocytes sediment in a dense fluid (Fig. 32.3).

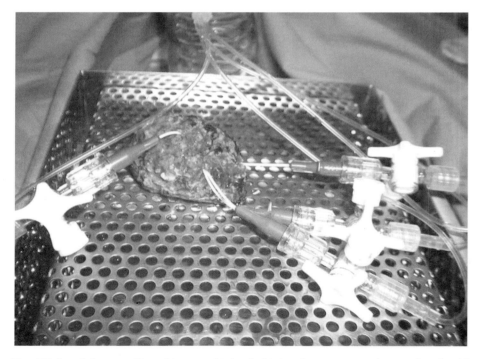

Fig. 32.2 *A human liver biopsy, obtained during hepatectomy, is canulated with three venous catheters and perfused with an enzymatic solution.*

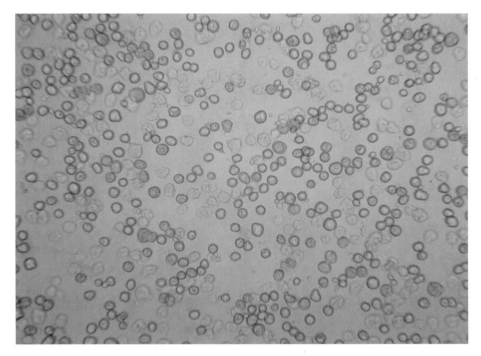

Fig. 32.3 *Human hepatocytes after isolation in culture. (Light microscopy ×40.)*

Sites of Hepatocyte Transplantation

The liver and spleen are the optimal sites for hepatocyte engraftment and function [38,39]. The peritoneal cavity has also been used for transplantation of encapsulated hepatocytes [38,39], but ectopic sites appear to be less favorable for hepatocyte engraftment. Hepatocytes are transplanted into the liver by portal vein injection, or by injection into the spleen from which cells migrate to the liver through the splenic vein. After implantation into the liver, hepatocytes integrate the liver parenchyma, leaving the hepatic architecture intact. These engrafted cells benefit from exposure to portal nutrients and growth factors and contact with other hepatocytes and nonparenchymal cells, and have the capability to secrete bile into the native biliary system.

Hepatocyte Transplantation in Animal Models

Hepatocyte transplantation has been used in rodent [40–42] and large animal models [43,44] for rescue therapy of liver failure and support of liver-based metabolic diseases.

Hepatocyte transplantation has been studied in animal models of liver failure since the 1970s and has been shown to improve the survival of animals with both chemically and surgically induced acute liver failure [45].

Hepatocyte transplantation prevented the development of intracranial hypertension in pigs with acute ischemic liver failure [46]. Several animal models of human metabolic liver diseases are available and allow testing the use of hepatocyte transplantation for these indications. Transplantation of hepatocytes, equivalent to 1–5% of the total hepatic mass, resulted in partial correction of hyperbilirubinemia in uridine diphosphate (UDP)–glucuronyl-transferase-deficient Gunn rats, an animal model of Crigler–Najjar syndrome type 1 [47], or increased serum albumin levels in Nagase analbuminemic rats [48]. Furthermore, hepatocyte transplantation allowed partial metabolic improvement in the Long-Evans Cinnamon rat model that presents a copper metabolism defect similar to Wilson's disease [49], or in the Watanabe hyperlipidemic rabbit model that presents a low-density lipoprotein (LDL) receptor deficiency similar to familial hypercholesterolemia [50].

Laboratory studies clearly indicate that hepatocyte transplantation can be an effective alternative to whole liver transplantation for the treatment of a variety of liver disorders. However, translation of these strategies into clinical practice requires further intense research.

Hepatocyte Transplantation in Clinical Trials

Following the encouraging laboratory results, several centers have initiated clinical hepatocyte transplantation trials. First, hepatocyte transplantation has been used to "bridge" patients with acute liver failure to liver transplantation [51,52]. Patients were transplanted with 10^7 to 10^{10} allogeneic hepatocytes, injected into the splenic artery or the portal vein, corresponding to 1–4% of the native hepatocyte mass. Transplanted cells were found in the liver and the spleen and anecdotal improvements of encephalopathy, ammonia, prothrombin time, and cerebral perfusion pressure were reported. Complications were rare and included transient hemodynamic instability, sepsis, and embolization of hepatocytes into the pulmonary circulation [51,52]. Although transplanted cells may have provided clinical benefits, convincing evidence of engraftment and function of transplanted hepatocytes has been difficult to prove. Treatment of chronic liver failure by hepatocyte transplantation has also been studied in a few centers. In Japan, ten cirrhotic patients were treated with hepatocytes recovered from their own left lateral liver segments [53]. Hepatocytes were transplanted into the spleen by direct splenic puncture, or by infusion into the splenic artery of the portal vein. Modest improvement of encephalopathy, synthetic liver, and renal functions was observed, but overall no significant prolongation of survival was obtained.

Several liver-based metabolic diseases have been treated by hepatocyte transplantation. Allogeneic hepatocytes were transplanted for correction of ornithine transcarbamylase (OTC) deficiency [54], glycogen storage disease type Ia [55], and Crigler–Najjar syndrome type 1 [56]. Hepatocyte transplantation resulted in transient improvement of hepatic OTC deficiency, but hepatocyte long-term function was assessed in a patient with glycogen storage disease type Ia [55] and in a 10-year-old patient with Crigler–Najjar syndrome [56]. Posttransplant, this patient showed a 50% decrease of bilirubin levels compared with pretransplant, and 5% of the deficient hepatic enzymatic function was restored. However, the metabolic correction was not sufficient to eliminate the need for phototherapy. Therefore, the patient ultimately underwent successful auxiliary liver transplantation [56].

Both experimental and clinical studies of hepatocyte transplantation indicate great potential of this approach; however, adequate supply of donor hepatocytes remains a serious barrier to wide clinical application and other sources of cells must be identified.

■ LIVER XENOTRANSPLANTATION

Xenotransplantation, the use of animals for transplantation into humans, represents a potentially unlimited source of organs that would solve the current shortage of human organs that limits clinical allotransplantation worldwide.

Largely for logistic reasons, the pig has been identified as the most suitable donor animal. When transplanted into untreated humans or nonhuman primates, pig organs are rejected hyperacutely within minutes by antibody-mediated complement activation. Hyperacute rejection is the result of this incompatibility between donor and recipient encountered in vascularized organ xenotransplantation [57,58]. Hyperacute rejection is characterized by the destruction of the xenograft parenchyma and vasculature immediately after reperfusion, resulting in widespread interstitial hemorrhage and thrombosis [57]. Hyperacute rejection is induced by naturally occurring antibodies reactive against donor antigens [57,59,60]. The major target antigen of human natural xenogeneic antibodies is the galactoseα1,3galactose (Gal) sugar residue present on the cell surface of lower mammals and New World monkeys [57]. The presence of natural antibodies against Gal in human and Old World monkeys and humans relates to evolutionary differences among species in the basic immune defense against bacterial pathogens [61]. The main components implicated in hyperacute rejection are xenoreactive antibodies and complement and endothelial cells. It has been shown that removal of xenoreactive antibodies can prevent hyperacute rejection [57,59,62]. Complement also plays a crucial role in hyperacute rejection, mainly through activation of the classical pathway by xenoreactive antibodies and directly through the alternative pathway without antibody binding. Complement depletion can be achieved by administration of various agents, e.g. cobra venom factor or soluble complement receptor-1, and allows prevention of hyperacute rejection [63].

The birth of the first homozygous galactosyltransferase-knockout (GT-KO) pigs, not expressing the major xenoantigen recognized by human natural anti-Gal antibodies, was reported by PPL Therapeutics and the Pittsburgh team in 2003 [64]. Immerge Biotherapeutics also announced the production of GT-KO pigs and, in collaboration with the Massachusetts General Hospital group, recently published first in vivo results following the transplantation of these pig organs into baboons [65]. GT-KO pig hearts were transplanted heterotopically in immunosuppressed baboons. The immunosuppression consisted of antihuman thymocyte globulin as induction, followed by maintenance therapy combining a human anti-CD154 monoclonal antibody, mycophenolate mofetil, and methylprednisolone. The mean organ xenograft survival was around 80 days, but some hearts survived up to 180 days, demonstrating clearly that these newly modified pig organs offer a significant progress in term of graft survival. Thrombotic microangiopathy occurred in several xenografted hearts, indicating that remaining coagulation disturbances have to be solved to allow long-term survival. Further genetic modifications allowing control of coagulopathy should further improve results and new clinical trials could be initiated again in the near future.

A number of molecular incompatibilities have been identified between pigs and humans. The physiological and biochemical variations that exist between these species include blood viscosity, enzymes, hormones, and liver metabolism. Of particular concern has been the incompatibility of coagulation factors that are produced by the liver and might lead to the development of a procoagulant state in the graft with subsequent thrombosis. Genetic engineering approaches might be considered to overcome these barriers.

Experimental Liver Xenotransplantation

Only a few studies performing pig-to-nonhuman primate liver transplantation have been reported [66–68]. The initial studies reported recipient survival of maximum 3 days with features of hyperacute rejection, despite strong immunosuppression [66,67]. More recently, Ramirez et al. [68] reported transplantation of livers obtained from transgenic pigs for human decay accelerating factor (hDAF) into baboons. Baboons were extubated at postoperative day 1 and were awake and able to eat and drink. Clotting parameters, including porcine fibrinogen, reached nearly normal levels at postoperative day 2 and remained detectable up to the end of the experiments. Maximum recipient survival was 8 days. Histopathological examination of livers revealed absence of hyperacute rejection. These results indicate that porcine livers are able to maintain sufficient coagulation and protein levels in primates up to 8 days after transplantation [68].

Clinical Trials of Liver Xenotransplantation

Only one clinical pig-to-human liver transplantation was reported in 1994, in a patient with fulminant hepatitis [69]. The patient underwent preoperative plasmapheresis to remove circulating xenoantibodies and the porcine liver graft was placed in a heterotopic position. The liver did not show any signs of metabolic function and the patient died 30 h after transplantation [69]. This case confirms that major immunological hurdles still prevent xenotransplantation to enter clinical application and emphasize the importance of preclinical experiments that must be performed prior to initiation of new clinical trials.

Xenogeneic Hepatocyte Transplantation

Transplantation of xenogeneic primary or immortalized hepatocytes instead of whole liver has been considered as a possibility, allowing unlimited availability of liver cells to treat liver diseases. Hepatocyte xenotransplantation is progressing, and recent experiments in small animal models used porcine hepatocytes transplanted into spleens of cirrhotic rats without immunosuppression and allowed restoration of metabolic functions and prolonged recipient survival [70]. These results demonstrate the feasibility of this approach to support liver failure by xenogeneic cells, but they need to be validated in large preclinical animal models.

■ STEM CELL TECHNOLOGY

Controlled differentiation of stem cells to obtain specialized cells for treatment of various diseases is another approach to find new sources of tissues for transplantation or to regenerate diseased organs. Stem cells are self-renewing progenitor cells that can differentiate into one or more specialized cell types. Traditionally, pluripotent stem cells were thought to be found only in embryos. Recently, several studies have shown that adult organ-specific stem cells can differentiate into cells of other organs. For example, it has been shown that bone marrow-derived cells can differentiate into muscle [71], cartilage [72], fat tissue [72], neural tissue [73], or liver [74]. The enormous potential of adult stem cell technology would be to provide a source of functional hepatocytes without the need of fetal, allogeneic, or xenogeneic tissues.

Adult bone marrow contains two types of multipotential stem cells – the hematopoietic stem cell and the mesenchymal stem cell. Each of them is capable of producing progeny that differentiate to several cell types.

Hematopoietic Stem Cells

Lagasse et al. [74] have demonstrated that hematopoietic stem cells can differentiate into hepatocytes in a mouse model of chronic liver failure [74]. They transplanted adult bone marrow cells into fumarylacetoacetate hydrolase (FAH)-deficient mice, an animal model of fatal hereditary tyrosinemia type I. The recipient mice were preconditioned by receiving lethal whole body irradiation, followed by injection of purified wild-type adult hematopoietic bone marrow cells. The transplanted mice restored deficient liver biochemical functions and showed long-term survival, whereas all control mice died within 2 months. Liver histology of transplanted mice revealed extensive liver repopulation by hepatocytes of donor-type origin, indicating that hematopoietic stem cells can differentiate into liver cells and could be used as regenerative therapy of various liver diseases.

So far, no clinical trial has been initiated using hematopoietic stem cells for treatment of liver diseases, but Körbling et al. [75] have analyzed in patient recipients of bone marrow cells for treatment of malignant hematopoietic diseases if cells of donor-type origin were detectable in various tissues [75]. Biopsy specimens from the liver, gastrointestinal tract, and skin were obtained from female patients who had undergone transplantation of hematopoietic stem cells from peripheral blood or bone marrow from a male donor. The biopsies were studied for the presence of donor-derived epithelial cells or hepatocytes with the use of fluorescence in situ hybridization of interphase nuclei and immunohistochemical staining for cytokeratin, CD45 (leukocyte common antigen), and a hepatocyte-specific antigen. All recipients of sex-mismatched transplants showed evidence of complete hematopoietic donor chimerism. XY-positive epithelial cells or hepatocytes accounted for 0–7% of the cells in histologic sections of the biopsy specimens. These cells were detected in liver tissue as early as day 13 and in skin tissue as late as day 354 after the transplantation of peripheral blood stem cells. These data confirm that circulating stem cells can differentiate into mature hepatocytes and epithelial cells of the skin and gastrointestinal tract [75].

Mesenchymal Stem Cells

Mesenchymal cells represent the second stem cell population within the bone marrow. Among the mesenchymal cells, a less differentiated cell type has been described and isolated: the multipotent adult progenitor cells. These cells can be cultured and expanded for more than 80 divisions and are able to differentiate under specific in vitro conditions into specialized cell types of mesodermal as well as endodermal origin, such as pulmonary epithelium and hepatocytes [76,77]. Lee et al. have recently published a cell culture protocol using specific hepatic growth factors (e.g. hepatocyte growth factor, oncostatin) and showed that after 4 weeks of culture, mesenchymal stem cells not only expressed marker genes specific of liver cells, but were also capable of albumin production, glycogen storage, urea secretion, uptake of LDL, and phenobarbital-inducible cytochrome P450 activity [78]. These in vitro results are very encouraging and show that adult-derived bone marrow cells are self-renewing progenitor cells that can differentiate into different specialized cell types, including hepatocyte-like cells. Further studies will test their potential engraftment and regeneration of damaged liver tissue in vivo.

■ REFERENCES

1. Loinaz C, Gonzalez EM. Marginal donors in liver transplantation. Hepatogastroenterology 2000;47(31):256–263.

2. Marcos A. Right-lobe living donor liver transplantation. Liver Transpl 2000;6(6 suppl 2):S59–S63.

3. Clavien PA, Harvey PR, Strasberg SM. Preservation and reperfusion injuries in liver allografts. An overview and synthesis of current studies. Transplantation 1992;53(5):957–978.

4. Belzer FO, Southard JH. Principles of solid-organ preservation by cold storage. Transplantation 1988;45(4):673–676.

5. Clavien PA. Sinusoidal endothelial cell injury during hepatic preservation and reperfusion. Hepatology 1998;28(2):281–285.

6. Sindram D, Porte RJ, Hoffman MR, et al. Platelets induce sinusoidal endothelial cell apoptosis upon reperfusion of the cold ischemic rat liver. Gastroenterology 2000;118(1):183–191.

7. Marsh DC, Belzer FO, Southard JH. Hypothermic preservation of hepatocytes. II. Importance of Ca2 and amino acids. Cryobiology 1990;27(1):1–8.

8. Hatano E, Kiuchi T, Tanaka A, et al. Hepatic preservation with histidine–tryptophan–ketoglutarate solution in living-related and cadaveric liver transplantation. Clin Sci (Lond) 1997;93(1):81–88.

9. Murry CE, Jennings RB, Reimer KA. Preconditioning with ischemia: a delay of lethal cell injury in ischemic myocardium. Circulation 1986;74(5):1124–1136.

10. Glazier SS, O'Rourke DM, Graham DI, et al. Induction of ischemic tolerance following brief focal ischemia in rat brain. J Cereb Blood Flow Metab 1994;14(4):545–553.

11. Pang CY, Yang RZ, Zhong A, et al. Acute ischemic preconditioning protects against skeletal muscle infarction in the pig. Cardiovasc Res 1995;29(6):782–788.

12. Turman MA, Bates CM. Susceptibility of human proximal tubular cells to hypoxia: effect of hypoxic preconditioning and comparison to glomerular cells. Ren Fail 1997;19(1):47–60.

13. Hotter G, Closa D, Prados M, et al. Intestinal preconditioning is mediated by a transient increase in nitric oxide. Biochem Biophys Res Commun 1996;222(1):27–32.

14. Roth S, Li B, Rosenbaum PS, et al. Preconditioning provides complete protection against retinal ischemic injury in rats. Invest Ophthalmol Vis Sci 1998;39(5):777–785.

15. Peralta C, Closa D, Hotter G, et al. Liver ischemic preconditioning is mediated by the inhibitory action of nitric oxide on endothelin. Biochem Biophys Res Commun 1996;229(1):264–270.

16. Clavien PA, Selzner M, Rudiger HA, et al. A prospective randomized study in 100 consecutive patients undergoing major liver resection with versus without ischemic preconditioning. Ann Surg 2003;238(6):843–850; discussion 851–852.

17. Sindram D, Rudiger HA, Upadhya AG, et al. Ischemic preconditioning protects against cold ischemic injury through an oxidative stress dependent mechanism. J Hepatol 2002;36(1):78–84.

18. Arai M, Thurman RG, Lemasters JJ. Contribution of adenosine A(2) receptors and cyclic adenosine monophosphate to protective ischemic preconditioning of sinusoidal endothelial cells against storage/reperfusion injury in rat livers. Hepatology 2000;32(2):297–302.

19. Arai M, Thurman RG, Lemasters JJ. Ischemic preconditioning of rat livers against cold storage–reperfusion injury: role of nonparenchymal cells and the phenomenon of heterologous preconditioning. Liver Transpl 2001;7(4):292–299.

20. Rudiger HA, Graf R, Clavien PA. Sub-lethal oxidative stress triggers the protective effects of ischemic preconditioning in the mouse liver. J Hepatol 2003;39(6):972–977.

21. Nakano A, Cohen MV, Downey JM. Ischemic preconditioning: from basic mechanisms to clinical applications. Pharmacol Ther 2000;86(3):263–275.

22. Peralta C, Hotter G, Closa D, et al. The protective role of adenosine in inducing nitric oxide synthesis in rat liver ischemia preconditioning is mediated by activation of adenosine A2 receptors. Hepatology 1999;29(1):126–132.

23. Peralta C, Hotter G, Closa D, et al. Protective effect of preconditioning on the injury associated to hepatic ischemia–reperfusion in the rat: role of nitric oxide and adenosine. Hepatology 1997;25(4):934–937.

24. Cottart CH, Do L, Blanc MC, et al. Hepatoprotective effect of endogenous nitric oxide during ischemia–reperfusion in the rat. Hepatology 1999;29(3):809–813.

25. Dhar DK, Yamanoi A, Ohmori H, et al. Modulation of endothelin and nitric oxide: a rational approach to improve canine hepatic microcirculation. Hepatology 1998;28(3):782–788.

26. Gething MJ, Sambrook J. Protein folding in the cell. Nature 1992;355(6355):33–45.

27. Coito AJ, Buelow R, Shen XD, et al. Heme oxygenase-1 gene transfer inhibits inducible nitric oxide synthase expression and protects genetically fat Zucker rat livers from ischemia–reperfusion injury. Transplantation 2002;74(1):96–102.

28. Redaelli CA, Tian YH, Schaffner T, et al. Extended preservation of rat liver graft by induction of heme oxygenase-1. Hepatology 2002;35(5):1082–1092.

29. Mokuno Y, Berthiaume F, Tompkins RG, et al. Technique for expanding the donor liver pool: heat shock preconditioning in a rat fatty liver model. Liver Transpl 2004;10(2):264–272.

30. Matsumoto K, Honda K, Kobayashi N. Protective effect of heat preconditioning of rat liver graft resulting in improved transplant survival. Transplantation 2001;71(7):862–868.

31. Kato Y, Shimazu M, Kondo M, et al. Bilirubin rinse: a simple protectant against the rat liver graft injury mimicking heme oxygenase-1 preconditioning. Hepatology 2003;38(2):364–373.

32. Ploeg RJ, D'Alessandro AM, Knechtle SJ, et al. Risk factors for primary dysfunction after liver transplantation – a multivariate analysis. Transplantation 1993;55(4): 807–813.

33. Selzner N, Selzner M, Jochum W, et al. Ischemic preconditioning protects the steatotic mouse liver against reperfusion injury: an ATP dependent mechanism. J Hepatol 2003;39(1):55–61.

34. Fernandez L, Carrasco-Chaumel E, Serafin A, et al. Is ischemic preconditioning a useful strategy in steatotic liver transplantation? Am J Transplant 2004;4(6):888–899.

35. Serafin A, Rosello-Catafau J, Prats N, et al. Ischemic preconditioning increases the tolerance of fatty liver to hepatic ischemia–reperfusion injury in the rat. Am J Pathol 2002;161(2):587–601.

36. Gao W, Connor HD, Lemasters JJ, et al. Primary nonfunction of fatty livers produced by alcohol is associated with a new, antioxidant-insensitive free radical species. Transplantation 1995;59(5):674–679.

37. Seglen PO. Preparation of isolated rat liver cells. Methods Cell Biol 1976;13:29–83.

38. Fox IJ, Chowdhury JR. Hepatocyte transplantation. Am J Transplant 2004;4(suppl): 7–13.

39. Lee Sung W, Wang X, Chowdhury JR, et al. Hepatocyte transplantation: state of the art and strategies for overcoming existing hurdles. Ann Hepatol 2004;3: 48–53.

40. Matas AJ, Sutherland DE, Steffes MW, et al. Hepatocellular transplantation for metabolic deficiencies: decrease of plasma bilirubin in Gunn rats. Science 1976;192: 892–894.

41. Sutherland DE, Numata M, Matas AJ, et al. Hepatocellular transplantation in acute liver failure. Surgery 1977;82:124–132.

42. Kusano M, Mito M. Observation on the fine structure of long-survived isolated hepatocytes inoculated into rat spleen. Gastroenterology 1982;81:616–628.

43. Andreoletti M, Loux N, Vons C, et al. Engraftment of autologous retrovirally transduced hepatocytes after intraportal transplantation into nonhuman primates: implication for ex vivo gene therapy. Hum Gene Ther 2001;12:169–179.

44. Vons C, Loux N, Simon L, et al. Transplantation of hepatocytes in nonhuman primates: a preclinical model for the treatment of hepatic metabolic diseases. Transplantation 2001;72:811–818.

45. Gupta S, Chowdhury RJ. Hepatocyte transplantation: back to the future. Hepatology 1992;15:156–162.

46. Arkadopoulos N, Chen SC, Khalili TM. Transplantation of hepatocytes for prevention of intracranial hypertension in pigs with ischemic liver failure. Cell Transplant 1998;7:357–363.

47. Rugstad HE, Robinson SH, Yannoni C, et al. Transfer of bilirubin uridine diphosphate–diglucuronyltransferase to enzyme-deficient rats. Science 1970;170:553–555.

48. Fabrega AJ, Bommineni V, Blanchard J, et al. Amelioration of analbuminemia by transplantation of allogenic hepatocytes in tolerized rats. Transplantation 1995;59:1362–1364.

49. Yoshida Y, Tokusashi Y, Lee G, et al. Intrasplenic transplantation of normal hepatocytes prevents Wilson's disease in Long-Evans cinnamon rats. Gastroenterology 1996;111:1654–1660.

50. Widerkehr JC, Kondos GT, Pollak R. Hepatocyte transplantation for the low-density lipoprotein receptor-deficient state. A study in the Watanabe rabbit. Transplantation 1990;50:446–471.

51. Strom SC, Fisher RA, Thompson MR, et al. Hepatocyte transplantation as a bridge to orthotopic liver transplantation in terminal liver failure. Transplantation 1997;63:559–569.

52. Bilir BM, Guinette D, Karrer F, et al. Hepatocyte transplantation in acute liver failure. Liver Transpl 2000;6:32–40.

53. Mito M, Kusano M. Hepatocyte transplantation in man. Cell Transplant 1993;2:65–74.

54. Reyes J, Rubenstein WS, Mieles L, et al. The use of cultured hepatocyte infusion via the portal vein for the treatment of ornithine transcarbamoylase deficiency by transplantation of enzymatically competent ABO/Rh-matched cells. Hepatology 1996;24:308A.

55. Muraca M, Gerunda G, Neri D, et al. Hepatocyte transplantation as a treatment for glycogen storage disease type 1a. Lancet 2002;359:317–318.

56. Fox IJ, Roy Chowdhury JR, Kaufmann SS, et al. Treatment of Crigler–Najjar syndrome type 1 with hepatocyte transplantation. N Engl J Med 1998;338:1422–1426.

57. Schuurman H, Cheng J, Lam T. Pathology of xenograft rejection: a commentary. Xenotransplantation 2003;10:293–299.

58. Robson S, Schulte-am-Esch J, Bach F. Factor in xenograft rejection. Ann N Y Acad Sci 1999;875:261–276.

59. Cramer D. Natural antibodies and the host immune responses to xenografts. Xenotransplantation 2000;7:83–92.

60. Soin B, Vial C, Frind P. Xenotransplantation. Br J Surg 2000;87(2):138–148.

61. Galili U, Clark M, Shohet S, et al. Evolutionary relationship between the natural anti-Gal antibody and the Gal alpha 1-3Gal epitope in primates. Proc Natl Acad Sci USA 1987;84:1369–1373.

62. Mollnes T, Fiane A. Perspectives on complement in xenotransplantation. Mol Immunol 2003;40:135–143.

63. Chen G, Sun Q, Wang X, et al. Improved suppression of circulating complement does not block acute vascular rejection of pig-to-rhesus monkey cardiac transplant. Xenotransplantation 2004;11:123–132.

64. Phelps CJ, Koike C, Vaught TD, et al. Production of alpha 1,3-galactosyltransferase-deficient pigs. Science 2003;299:411–414.

65. Kuwaki K, Tseng YL, Dor FJ, et al. Heart transplantation in baboons using alpha1,3-galactosyltransferase gene-knockout pigs as donors: initial experience. Nat Med 2005;11:29–31.

66. Calne RY, White HJO, Hebertson BM, et al. Pig to baboon liver xenografts. Lancet 1968;1:1176–1178.

67. Powelson J, Cosimi AB, Austen W, et al. Porcine to primate orthotopic liver transplantation. Transplant Proc 1994;26:1353–1354.

68. Ramirez P, Chavez R, Jajado M, et al. Life-supporting human complement regulator decay accelerating factor transgenic pig liver xenograft maintains the metabolic function and coagulation in the nonhuman primate for up to 8 days. Transplantation 2000;70:989–998.

69. Makowka L, Wu GD, Hoffman A, et al. Immunohistopathologic lesions associated with the rejection of a pig to human liver xenograft. Transplant Proc 1998;26:1074–1075.

70. Nagata H, Ito M, Cai J, et al. Treatment of cirrhosis and liver failure in rats by hepatocyte xenotransplantation. Gastroenterology 2003;124:422–431.

71. Ferrari G, Cusella-De Angelis G, Coletta M, et al. Muscle regeneration by bone marrow-derived myogenic progenitors. Science 1998;279:1528–1530.

72. Pittenger MF, Mackay AM, Beck SC, et al. Multilineage potential of adult human mesenchymal stem cells. Science 1999;284:143–147.

73. Mezey E, Chandross KJ, Harta G, et al. Turning blood into brain: cells bearing neuronals antigens generated in vivo from bone marrow. Science 2000;290:1672–1674.

74. Lagasse E, Connors H, Al-Dhalimy M, et al. Purified hematopoietic stem cells can differentiate into hepatocytes in vivo. Nat Med 2000;6:1229–1234.

75. Körbling M, Katz RL, Khanna A, et al. Hepatocytes and epithelial cells of donor origin in recipients of peripheral-blood stem cells. N Engl J Med 2002;346:738–746.

76. Jiang Y, Jahagirdar BN, Reinhardt RL, et al. Pluripotency of mesenchymal stem cells derived from adult marrow. Nature 2002;418:41–49.

77. Schwartz RE, Reyes M, Koodie L, et al. Multipotent adult progenitor cells from bone marrow differentiate into functional hepatocyte-like cells. J Clin Invest 2002;109:1291–1302.

78. Lee KD, Kuo TKC, Whang-Peng J, et al. In vitro hepatic differentiation of human mesenchymal stem cells. Hepatology 2004;40:1275–1284.

Index

Pages numbered in *italics* represents figures, those in **bold** represent tables.